Publisher
Digital Educational Publishing, Inc.
PO Box 43515
Cincinnati, Ohio 45243

Executive Producer
Timothy J. Mullican

NUTRITION OF THE PRETERM INFANT

ISBN 1-58352-100-3

Forward

Pre-term births are common in developing and industrialized countries. Some of the underlying factors include low socio-economic class, inadequate antenatal care, lack of access of mothers to clinical advice and services, and maternal ill-health, infections and undernutrition before and during pregnancy. In many instances no cause can be identified.

The numerous, serious complications that can affect preterm infants can compromise their prospects for survival and their prognosis for subsequent growth and cognitive development. The high rates of disability, disease and deaths associated with preterm births have a very high cost in terms of health, education and community social services, mainly through governments, and on families and communities. The health costs relate to immediate, clinical care of the affected infant and to his or her long-term management of a range of possible complications. Some of these involve severely affected infants who require long-term institutional accommodation and care. The personal and financial burdens on families can be very substantial.

Prevention of preterm births is obviously of great importance. But treatment of affected infants is crucial in order to enhance their chances of survival, to lessen the possibility of complications, including disabilities, and to increase their prospects of leading high-quality lives. Treatment strategies include skilled transfer to appropriate treatment centers, resuscitation, treatment of infections and management of metabolic complications.

Nutritional treatment is a cornerstone in the management of preterm infants. Recent advances in this important field have helped greatly in achieving better outcomes for these patients. This book brings together many eminent international workers in this field to present their latest findings, review the relevant literature and to discuss these issues in an open forum. The topics are very wide-ranging; they include recommendations for nutrients and energy, the role of specific nutrients such as proteins, carbohydrates, lipids, water and electrolytes, and vitamins and minerals.

There are also chapters on the roles of breast milk, enteral and parenteral nutrition, and, very importantly, a chapter on feeding the infant after hospital discharge and about subsequent growth, development and long-term effects.

There can be a temptation to consider that skilled hospital care and nutritional management of preterm infants closes that chapter in their very young lives. But this is just the beginning of a much longer process that should give these patients the opportunity to lead healthy lives. For some, unfortunately, the outcomes may not be so encouraging and different long-term treatments and strategies will be needed. Pediatricians must play a role in all of these aspects of the care of these patients.

This book presents these highly important issues in a refreshing way by which international authorities on the nutrition of pre-term infants contribute their views and discuss the latest developments in this field.

It should be of great interest to all pediatricians.

Michael Gracey, MD, PhD, FRACP, FAAP (Hon)
President, International Pediatric Association

Preface

This book was written as a sequel to "Vitamin and Mineral Requirements in Preterm Infants" (1984), and "Nutrient Requirements in Preterm Infants" (1993). In all three instances, an education grant from Mead Johnson Bristol-Myers Squibb was essential to bring the authors together for a full two days of interaction and mutual review. This integrated team approach has been a critical reason we believe why this book series has stood the test of time and value. The authors gathered in Chicago this time at O'Hare Airport. We wasted little time, but quickly engaged in lively constructive discussions, honing in on how each nutrient requirement was derived, and the advances of the last decade. Much has transpired in the last two decades in terms of understanding nutrient importance for optimal survival, especially in the increasingly smaller preterm infants we now take care of in the nursery. A great deal of attention was focused on practical issues of nutrient delivery, and the special circumstances of specific groups of preterm infants.

Many manuscripts were mailed ahead of time by authors for preview, except for a few who were still editing their manuscripts on site on their laptop computers. Indeed many discussions prompted instant revision of the laptop-based manuscripts; such is the nature of modern manuscript writing. After thorough review and vetting, all papers were again sent to a web-based repository of manuscripts for access and change, on the web, by selected "internal" (ie, other book authors) and "external" (non-authors) reviewers. All joined in the fray with good vigor (and humor in some instances). The process has been long and arduous, with many complications (illness, lost mail, changes in jobs, etc.), but finally we are here!

The present editorial team is a seasoned team. Ricardo Uauy and Stan Zlotkin were former co-editors, and Bert Koletzko was a thoroughly involved author of the previous edition. We instantly "bonded" again and moved to perfect this book, which many have told us is the "bible" for nutrient requirements for preterm infants. The enthusiasm and patience of the team have been inspirational.

Throughout all of this, our publisher, who had been similarly involved in previous books with the Editors (especially Nutrition in Infancy), has been thoroughly engaged. A veterinarian by profession (now a fish doctor he tells me), and publisher/biomedical communications entrepreneur by "hobby", it has been a good and fruitful partnership with Tim Mullican, DVM.

One touch omitted from this edition is any royal endorsements! Anne, HRH the Princess Royal of the British Isles, wrote in the last edition "the whole process ... was conducted with good grace and remarkably little acrimony, – a commendable (and surprising?) achievement for medical experts. I would expect this book to be most influential and warmly received and to set a high and hopefully consistent, international standard of nutritional care for premature infants." We certainly hope the present edition lives up to its previous reputation and HRH Princess Anne's expectations, to bring us to another level of excellence.

Reginald Tsang
Editor-in-Chief

Contributors

Stephen Abrams, M.D.
Department of Pediatrics
Baylor College of Medicine
Baylor University
Houston, Texas

Stephanie A. Atkinson, Ph.D.
Department of Pediatrics
McMaster University
Hamilton, Ontario
Canada

Stephen Baumgart, M.D.
Department of Neonatology
Children's National Medical Center
Washington, D.C.

Edward F. Bell, M.D.
Department of Pediatrics
University of Iowa
Iowa City, Iowa

Hans Boehles, M.D.
Klinik für Kinderheilkunde I
Johann Wolfgang Goethe-Universität
Frankfurt, Germany

Hans Buller, M.D.
University of Amsterdam
Amsterdam, Netherlands

Jane D. Carver, Ph.D., M.P.H.
Department of Pediatrics, Division of Neonatology
University of South Florida College of Medicine
Tampa, Florida

David A. Clark, M.D.
Department of Pediatrics
Children's Hospital at Albany Medical Center
Albany, New York

Richard Cooke, M.D.
Newborn Center
University of Tennessee
Center for Health Sciences
Memphis, Tennessee

Scott C. Denne, M.D.
James Whitcomb Riley Hospital
Indiana University School of Medicine
Indianapolis, Indiana

James K. Friel, Ph.D.
Department of Pediatrics
Memorial University
St. Johns, Newfoundland
Canada

Christoph Fusch, M.D.
Neonatologie
Zentrum fur Kinder-und Jugendmedizin
Greifswald, Germany

Michael Georgieff, M.D.
Department of Pediatrics
University of Minnesota School of Medicine
Minneapolis, Minnesota

Harry L. Greene, M.D.
Slim Fast Foods Company
West Palm Beach, Florida

Frank Greer, M.D.
University of Wisconsin
Madison, Wisconsin

Margit Hamosh, Ph.D.
Professor Emeritus, Pediatrics
Georgetown University Medical Center
Bethesda, Maryland

William W. Hay, Jr., M.D.
Perinatal Research Center
University of Colorado Health Sciences Center
Aurora, Colorado

William C. Heird, M.D.
Department of Pediatrics
USDA/ARS Children's Nutrition Research Center
Baylor University College of Medicine
Houston, Texas

Sheila M. Innis, Ph.D.
Department of Pediatrics
University of British Columbia
Vancouver, British Columbia
Canada

F. Jochum, M.D.
Intensivmedizin
Zentrum für Kinderheilkunde
Universität Greifswald
Greifswald, Germany

Satish C. Kalhan, M.D.
Center for Metabolism & Nutrition
MetroHealth Medical Center
Cleveland, Ohio

Sudha Kashyap, M.D.
Babies & Children's Hospital of New York
Columbia Presbyterian Medical Center
New York, New York

Berthold Koletzko, M.D.
Kinderklinik und Kinderpoliklinik
Dr. von Haunersches Kinderspital
University of Munich
Munich, Germany

Harry N. Lafeber, M.D.
Department of Pediatrics/Division of Neonatology
Free University Hospital
Amsterdam, Netherlands

Catherine A. Leitch, Ph.D.
Department of Pediatrics
Indiana University School of Medicine
Indianapolis, Indiana

Carlos H. Lifschitz, M.D.
USDA/ARS Children's Nutrition Research Center
Baylor University College of Medicine
Houston, Texas

Jean-Leopold Micheli, M.D.
Department of Pediatrics
CHUV University Hospital
Lausanne, Switzerland

Manuel Moya, M.D.
Hospital San Juan
San Juan, Alicante
Spain

Josef Neu, M.D.
Department of Pediatrics/Neonatology
University of Florida
Gainesville, Florida

Buford L. Nichols, M.D.
Department of Pediatrics
Children's Nutrition Research Center
Baylor University College of Medicine
Houston, Texas

Frank Pohlandt, M.D.
Department of Pediatrics
University of Ulm
Ulm, Germany

Prabu Parimi, M.D.
Center for Metabolism & Nutrition
MetroHealth Medical Center
Cleveland, Ohio

Contributors *(cont.)*

Hildegard Przyrembel, M.D., Ph.D.
Federal Institute for Risk Assessment
Berlin, Germany

Raghavendra Rao, M.D.
Department of Pediatrics
University of Minnesota School of Medicine
Minneapolis, Minnesota

Jacque Rigo, M.D., Ph.D.
Department of Pediatrics
University of Liege
Liege, Belgium

Reg Sauve, M.D.
Department of Pediatrics
University of Calgary
Calgary, Alberta
Canada

P.J.J. Sauer, M.D.
Department of Pediatrics
University Hospital
Groningen, Netherlands

Richard J. Schanler, M.D.
Albert Einstein College of Medicine
Schneider Children's Hospital at North Shore
Manhasset, New York

Karen Simmer, M.M.B.S., Ph.D.
King Edward Memorial Hospital for Women
and Princess Margaret Hospital for Children
Subiaco, Western Australia
Australia

Hiroshi Tamai, M.D.
Department of Pediatrics
Osaka Medical College
Takatsuki, Osaka
Japan

Patti J. Thureen, M.D.
Department of Pediatrics/Section of Neonatology
University of Colorado Health Sciences Center
Denver, Colorado

Reginald Tsang, M.D.
Department of Pediatrics
Cincinnati Children's Hospital Medical Center
Cincinnati, Ohio

Ricardo Uauy, M.D., Ph.D.
INTA University of Chile
Santiago, Chile

John E. Van Aerde, M.D.
Children's Health Centre
Department of Pediatrics
University of Alberta
Edmonton, Canada

Victor Y.H. Yu, M.D.
Department of Neonatal Intensive Care
Monash Medical Center
Monash University
Victoria, Australia

Stanley H. Zlotkin, M.D., Ph.D.
Division of Gastroenterology and Nutrition
The Hospital for Sick Children
Toronto, Ontario
Canada

Contents

Concepts, Definitions and Approaches to Define the Nutritional Needs of LBW Infants

Ricardo Uauy, M.D., Ph.D., Reginald Tsang, M.B.B.S.,
Berthold Koletzko, M.D., Ph.D., and Stanley Zlotkin, M.D., Ph.D.

Reviewed by Buford L. Nichols, M.D.

Concepts and Definitions to Describe Nutritional Needs of Individuals and Populations

The following concepts and definitions are intended to characterize nutrient intakes from enteral and parenteral sources required to promote growth and development, and to prevent health risks associated with nutritional deficiency or excess in low birth weight (LBW) neonates.

Requirement: is defined as the intake level that will meet specified criteria of nutritional adequacy, preventing risk of deficit or excess. These criteria encompass a gradient of biological effects related to specific nutrient intakes. Dose response to nutrients will be assumed in this discussion to have a gaussian distribution if it has not been characterized. Thus a risk function for deficiency and excess can be derived (see Figure 1a). The relevance of biological effects starts with the most extreme case, i.e., the prevention of death. For nutrients where sufficient data on mortality are not available, preventing clinical disease or subclinical pathological conditions identified by biochemical or functional assays is used. The next set of markers that can be used to define requirements includes measures of nutrient stores, critical tissue pools or functional effects on relevant organ systems. Intakes to assure replete body stores are particularly important when deficiency conditions are highly prevalent. Presently, approaches to define requirements of most nutrients use several criteria in combination, and functional assays of sub-clinical conditions are considered the most relevant. These biomarkers ideally should be sensitive to changes in nutritional state and specific in terms of identifying sub-clinical deficiency

conditions. The criteria used to define requirements become important, since nutrient intake to meet requirements will vary depending on what serves to define adequacy.[1-3] The information base to scientifically support the definition of nutritional needs of neonates, especially VLBW neonates, are extremely limited for most nutrients. Where relevant, requirement estimates should include allowance for variations in bioavailability and utilization by the enteral and or parenteral route.

Estimated average requirement (EAR): is the average requirement value obtained from a group of individuals based on given criteria. These are usually nutrient-specific, and vary depending on the specified nutrient. The estimation of requirements starts by defining the criteria that will be used to define adequacy and establishing the necessary corrections for physiological and dietary factors. Once a mean value is obtained from a group of subjects, the value is adjusted for interindividual variability. If distribution of values is not known, a gaussian distribution is assumed, that is, a mean plus/minus 2 SD is expected to cover 97.5% of the population. If the SD is not known, a value of 10% of the mean is assumed. Recommended daily allowance (RDA) or recommended nutrient intake (RNI) as used in Europe corresponds to the EAR plus 2 SDs. In this chapter we will use RDA as used in the US National Academy of Science/Food and Nutrition Board (NAS/FNB) Dietary Recommended Intakes (DRI) process.[1,2]

Recommended daily allowance (RDA): the daily intake that meets the nutrient requirements of almost all (97.5 %) apparently "healthy" individuals; in our case "medically stable" for a specific gestational age

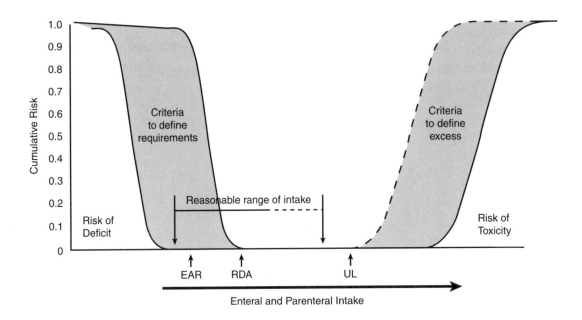

Figure 1a: LBW infants are at risk for deficit and excess. There is cumulative risk associated with deficit or excess according to level of intake by enteral or parenteral route. As intake decreases so does the risk of deficit; after the Upper Tolerance Level, UL, is exceeded, risk of toxicity rises. EAR is the estimated average requirement value obtained from a group of individuals based on a specified criteria. RDA is the recommended nutrient intake to meet the needs of most individuals in the population (EAR + 2SD). UL defines the tolerable upper intake level at which no evidence of toxicity is demonstrable. The shaded range corresponds to different approaches used to define criteria for requirements and excess. The reasonable range of intake (RRI) used in the current book corresponds to intakes associated with minimal risk of deficit or excess. This model can be used to examine the risk of inadequacy for a specific level of intake.

and/or birth weight specific population group is more appropriate. Daily intake corresponds to an average over a given period; it does not need to be fulfilled every day. However, since stores are limited and needs are high, LBW infants should receive their recommended intakes within days of birth. However, older and more mature infants that have reserves of some nutrients (i.e. energy) should receive adequate intakes for their need at least within a week of birth.

Upper tolerable nutrient intake level (UL): for some nutrients, a UL is defined if adverse effects have been identified. This is the maximum intake that is unlikely to pose risk of adverse health effects in almost all (97.5%) medically stable individuals in a specific population group. ULs should be based on long term exposure to the nutrient from all sources, combining the enteral and parenteral route. In the special situation of ELBW and VLBW infants, where parenteral vitamins and minerals may be added to the enteral macronutrient intake and lead to potential excess, the problem should be addressed by carefully monitoring intake of critical nutrients, avoiding exceeding the UL.

Most nutrient requirement estimates assume they are intended for apparently "healthy" individuals; healthy is defined by absence of disease based on clinical signs and symptoms, and functional normalcy assessed by routine laboratory methods and physical evaluation. Unfortunately, many VLBW and most ELBW infants are sick and thus the definition of their nutritional requirements cannot be simply extrapolated from the needs of healthy infants. Moreover, the science base to adjust nutrient needs for the effects of disease in many cases is just not available.[1-3]

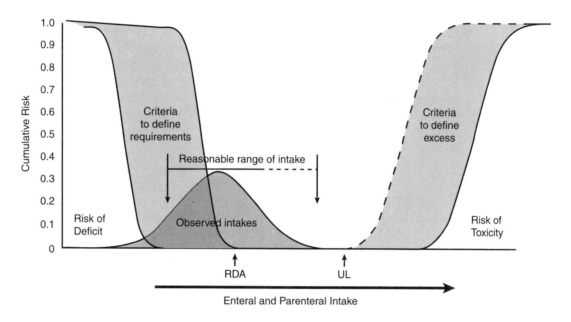

Figure 1b: (model as described under 1a): LBW infants are at risk for deficit and excess. The model now includes a darkly shaded area under the bell shaped curve representing the distribution of observed intakes within the RRI. Cumulative risk associated with deficit or excess as shown.

Reasonable range of intakes (RRI): based on the above limitations the authors of the text suggest the use of the term reasonable range of intake (RRI) for LBW infants defined as the range of average intakes derived from observations or evaluated under controlled conditions that appear to sustain adequate nutrition, based on absence of abnormal clinical signs and symptoms, or biochemical/functional normalcy. The lower value of the RRI will be the EAR, if one has been established for the given birthweight-specific group. The upper value will generally be lower than the UL if one has been established for the specific population group, or if no UL can be derived, the upper value of the range will be defined based on an intake that is considered safe from available data on observed dietary intake of "medically stable" neonates. The RRI for many nutrients should be considered as the best "guesstimate" from expert opinion, plus careful analysis of the limited database available. Figures 1a, b and c illustrate the RRI for LBW and ELBW infants demonstrating the narrowing in this range for more immature infants, since they have higher needs but

also a lower UL. The distribution of observed intakes as seen in Figure 1b is usually within the RRI and does not exceed the UL; under some conditions such as parenteral nutrition, sub-groups of infants receive substantially less or substantially more than their need, as may be the case for calcium and riboflavin respectively. The RRI applies to a range of intake for individuals within a group that is homogenous in terms of age, birth weight and other characteristics believed to affect nutrient requirement. Moreover, since postnatal adaptations are critical in defining nutrient needs, we have provided RRI for the initial feeding, the transitional phase and the goals that should be reached for optimal growth and development of ELBW and VLBW infants as summarized in Appendix I.

Recommendations presented in this book are presented, wherever possible, as a range of intakes for a given category rather than the exact intake for an individual. However ELBW, VLBW and LBW infants can hardly if ever be considered homogenous because of concurrent medical conditions and variability in

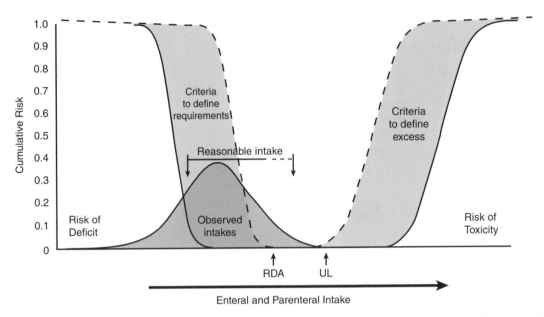

Figure 1c: ELBW infants are at greater risk for deficit and excess. This figure depicts the model applied to extremely LBW infants illustrating a narrower range for adequacy; these infants have higher needs and also are more susceptible to excess, and thus are at increased risk of deficit as well as excess.

physiological development. Thus, health professionals caring for these special groups should, where possible, individualize nutritional care based on individual tolerance to feedings, and adjust nutrient delivery according to restrictions imposed by disease conditions and needs related to developmental stage.[3,4]

Approaches Used in Estimating Nutrient Intakes for Optimal Health (Prevent Deficit and Avoid Excess)

Different approaches to assess nutritional needs of LBW infants have been developed over the past decades. Nutrition for this vulnerable group should consider not only health risks associated with deficits of all essential and conditionally essential nutrients, but also the potential risks from toxicity associated with excess.[4,5]

The traditional criteria to define essentiality of nutrients for human health require a) the presence of disease, or functional or structural abnormalities, if the nutrient is absent or deficient in the diet; and b) that the abnormalities are related to, or a consequence

of, specific biochemical or functional changes that can be reversed by the presence of the essential dietary component. Endpoints considered in recent investigations of essentiality of nutrients in experimental animals and humans include: reductions in ponderal or linear growth rates, altered body composition, compromised host defense systems, impairment of gastrointestinal or immune function, abnormal cognitive performance, increased susceptibility to disease, increased morbidity and changes in biochemical measures of nutrient status. To establish such criteria for particular nutrients requires an understanding of their biological effects, as well as sensitive instrumentation to measure the effects and the amounts of nutrients supplied by enteral and/or parenteral diets.

More recently the concept of conditional essential nutrient has been advanced, based on the fact that some nutrients can be formed by the body but not in sufficient quantities to meet the requirement for normal growth and development, or for optimal function. In some situations, providing the pre-formed product of endogenous synthesis has a measurable effect on a specific organ function; this is the case for taurine and retinal function; glutamine enhancement of immune function; and the provision of long chain PUFAs and visual acuity maturation.[6] For other nutrients, providing the pre-formed product spares the body from the energy and/or protein cost of having to synthesize them *de novo*; this may be the case for preformed nucleotides specially needed by rapidly dividing cells such as the gut or the immune system.[7,8]

A starting point in defining nutritional requirements is the use of factorial estimates of nutritional need. The "factorial model" is based on the minimum requirement of the nutrient: a) for replacement of losses from excretion and utilization at low intakes, and in some cases no intake; b) that does not reduce body stores; and c) which is usually sufficient for prevention of clinical deficiency. Factorial methods are used only as a first approximation for the assessment of individual requirements, or when functional clinical or biochemical criteria of adequacy have not been established.

Nutrient balance calculations include input and output, and requirement is established at the point of equilibrium plus considering the additional needs for growth or tissue deposition. In most cases, balance based on input-output measurements is greatly influenced by prior level of intake; that is, subjects adjust to high intakes by increasing output; conversely they lower output when intake is low. Thus, if sufficient time is provided to accommodate a given level of intake, balance can be achieved. The exclusive use of nutrient balance to define requirements should be avoided whenever possible.[9,10] However, in the absence of other data it may be used. If balance can be attained at multiple levels of intake, it does not serve to estimate requirements. The same can be said of nutrient blood concentrations or even tissue content: they usually will reflect level of intake and absorption rather than functional state. Unless balance data, and data on plasma or tissue concentrations, are related to abnormal function or disease conditions, they are inadequate as the sole criteria to support the definition of requirements.

Functional responses. Present efforts in defining nutrient needs for optimal function include assessment of:

1) Neurodevelopment maturation: using electro-physiologic responses to defined sensory stimuli, sleep-wake cycle organization, and neurobehavioral tests.[11]

2) Bone health: bone mineral density, markers of collagen synthesis and turnover and hormonal responses associated with bone anabolism and catabolism.[12,13]

3) Biochemical normalcy: measuring plasma and tissue concentrations of substrates or nutrient responsive enzymes, hormones or other indices of anabolic (synthesis) and catabolic (oxidative) activity, plasma concentrations and tissue retention in response to a fixed nutrient load, substrate oxidation rates, and non-oxidative disappearance as an index of synthetic rates.[14,15]

4) Immune function: humoral and cellular response to antigens and mitogens *in vitro* or *in vivo*, antibody response to weak antigens such as immunizations; T-cell populations, cytokine responses, and mediators of inflammation related to tissue protection and damage.[8,16]

5) Body composition and tissue metabolic status: stable isotope assessment of body compartments (body water, lean and fat mass), radiation-determined body compartments, including bone density measured by dual energy X-ray absorptiometry (DEXA) and computerized tomography (CT), electrical impedance and conductivity to determine (body water, lean and fat mass) body compartments, and magnetic resonance imaging and spectroscopy-determined body compartments and organ compartments (liver glycogen, brain ATP, muscle high energy phosphate).[17-19]

6) Energy expenditure: energy needs are presently defined based on measured expenditure using oxygen consumption or doubly labeled water. Macronutrient needs can be assessed by evaluation of oxidative rates and metabolism using stable isotope (13C, 2H, 15N) labeled substrates.[20,21]

7) Gene expression: rapid developments in the area

of micro array technology presently permit the use of multiple specific human cDNAs (corresponding to 5-10 thousand genes at a time), fluorescent probes and laser detection. These tools provide a powerful method to assess the amount of nutrient required to trigger a specific mRNA response in a given tissue. This is already being used to define selenium needs without having to measure the respective selenium-dependent GSH peroxidase, and is based on the mRNA response to selenium supply rather than measuring the protein product or the corresponding enzyme. Micro array systems tailored to evaluate nutrient-modulated gene expression may become a new way to assess human nutritional requirements.[22]

These biomarkers and multiple other markers are presently being used to assess organ specific functions. If no other method is available, the customary intake based on human milk composition and volume of intake is a reasonable default position. As a matter of fact, nutrient needs for the term infant are based on the paradigm that human milk is the optimal food for growth and development. Thus, all other criteria are subservient to that estimate obtained from assessment of the range of documented intake observed in the full term breast-fed infant.

Risk Assessment of Nutrient Deficit or Excess

The aim is to develop guidelines for the specific nutrient that apply to a population group; thus the estimate should include a measure of variability in order to define the distribution of requirements and toxicity for the specific population. This review attempts to include the spectrum of biological effects starting with the most extreme such as death; and completing the list of effects with those that may be very sensitive in their response to deficit or excess but are less specific, and result in a high proportion of false positives. It is common to start by selecting the best data from human studies, but if none exists, to select relevant animal studies. It is necessary to review experimental studies in which several intake/exposure levels have been evaluated, in order to estimate requirements and/or toxic effects.

Death and disease related to acute or chronic exposure/intake of essential elements occurs and should be critically assessed; unfortunately, few of these accidental or unintended occurrences are reported in the literature. It is even more difficult to determine cause and effect, since the cause of death may be apparently unrelated to the nutrient exposure. An example of this situation was the increased occurrence of necrotizing enterocolitis (NEC)/sepsis and corresponding death after exposure to high tocopherol intake; it became apparent only because investigators in the study were observant and knowledgeable of the effect of excess tocopherol on leukocyte bactericidal capacity.[23] In many cases death resulting from nutrient deficit or excess may be associated with intervening factors, such as disease conditions. The trial of early intravenous lipid associated with increased mortality from respiratory insufficiency was again noticeable mainly because of close monitoring of the study outcome. In this case the increased mortality was only observed in the 1000-1200 gram birthweight category, and was not significant for the whole group.[24] In these cases, it is particularly difficult to establish a causal relationship, unless the situation is observed under conditions of controlled randomized studies. The controlled clinical trial is the closest proof of causality; eliminating the element (in the case of toxic effects) or incorporating the agent (in the case of deficit) in a group of subjects randomized to control or experimental conditions is necessary to test the hypothesis of a causal relationship. There are very few nutrients where this type of data is available from humans subjected to chronic exposure or acute toxic doses. In the case of animals, LD_{50} and LD_5 and LD_{95} have been defined for some elements, but are not available for most elements. The limitation of human data on lethality from deficit or toxicity is that they are not population-based, since they are usually linked to single case reports or at best a cluster of cases due to unusual circumstances.

For most essential nutrients, disease conditions associated with deficit have been well described (Vitamin A, E, Fe, Cu, Zn); yet few of these data correspond to observations in VLBW infants. Much less is known of pathologic conditions linked to excess, and few of these have been well characterized. In both cases, deficit and excess, disease has sometimes been linked to genetic conditions which favor the occurrence of deficiency or toxicity by modifying requirements, decreasing or increasing intestinal absorption, or altering excretion. In many pathologic conditions specific data on chronic levels of intake/exposure leading to disease from excess or deficit may be lacking, but information on the levels required to cure the condition may be indicative of level of exposure/intake which can be considered safe. For example we know the level of zinc intake required to prevent growth failure in infants[25] or the level of iron excess, which may induce hemolysis in susceptible individuals.[26] However, in many cases the pathologic effect of these metals may occur only in the presence of another concurrent factor: concurrent viral infection in the case of myocardial degenerative effects induced by selenium deficiency (Keshan disease),[27] or copper toxicity in patients on total parenteral nutrition (TPN) with impaired biliary excretion associated with the lack of enteral feedings.[5] The data from intake/exposure levels to prevent disease states, if available, represent the best option to define RRI, since there is no question that preventing disease and protecting health is the essence of a reasonable range of intake.

The next level of evidence in evaluating data to estimate RRI is the assessment of studies that evaluate biologically significant effects at various exposure/intake levels. The difficulty here is establishing what will be considered biologically significant and what will be considered a non-significant effect. A suitable definition for biological significance in this context is the capacity of the biologic indicator to be modified by intake/exposure and predict the occurrence of deficiency or toxicity disease associated with the corresponding element. For example, elevated serum ferritin may serve to predict liver damage induced by elevated iron exposure in susceptible individuals.[28] A functional assay, such as red cell resistance to peroxide stress may also predict the risk of hemolysis from tocopherol deficit. However, the elevation of superoxide dismutase in this same condition may   represent an adaptive response to

oxidant stress without pathologic implication.[29] Unfortunately most biochemical or functional biomarkers have not been validated in terms of their ability to anticipate the occurrence of disease due to excess or deficit. In this context, the most valid indicators are those that relate to the limits of RRI; for example, levels of intake that are associated with excessive or deficient retention of the specific element. For example, negative Zn balance over time will lead to a disease state; markedly positive copper balance may serve to indicate excessive level of intake, which over time may lead to toxicity. For the purpose of quantifying RRI, a key biomarker may be the change in bioavailability of other nutrients induced by high or low intake, since this may be the most sensitive indicator of excess or deficit. For example, high zinc intake is associated with decreased copper bioavailability, as measured by labeled copper studies using stable isotopes, which permit the separation of exogenous from endogenous excreted copper.[30] Following these concepts, one could develop quantitative estimates of RRI on the basis of a lethal effect, prevention of disease or assuring normal range of biomarkers with biological significance. The most stringent criteria will undoubtedly be the former; but in terms of practicality, prevention of disease and normalcy of biomarkers are most likely to be used. Yet, very few specific relevant data are available from VLBW and ELBW infants to provide the scientific basis to define RRI.

A key consideration in defining RRI is the biologic handling of the nutrient that may affect the biologic impact in terms of deficit or excess. This includes absorption, transport, metabolism, excretion and storage of the element and the possible interaction with other elements or factors, which modify these processes. Consideration of these factors in adjusting the level of RRI up or down in a given context is important since these elements or other factors may modify the biological effect significantly. Factors that affect biokinetics differ for each element, but basically include interaction of elements amongst themselves, interactions with other dietary factors and the effect of environmental agents that may affect biokinetics. For example, low protein and/or low zinc intakes will interfere with Vitamin A metabolism and mobilization; thus retinol needs may be falsely elevated in infants who are subjected to low protein or zinc diets. Ascorbic acid will enhance the absorption of iron;[31] thus the lower limit for iron intake may be smaller if cow milk formulas are supplemented with ascorbic acid; on the contrary, if zinc and copper intake is high, iron absorption may be less.[31] Many essential elements are oxidized or excreted in relation to intake; in these cases measurement of oxidative rates or urinary excretion may serve to signal excess intake. In the case of metals or other nutrients that are not metabolized, they will accumulate if not adequately excreted, and once storage capacity is saturated, excess may lead to toxicity. In these cases high retention may be indicative of possible toxic effects. There is no efficient way to excrete iron except by blood loss[32], while copper is mainly excreted by the biliary route. Thus, in biliary atresia, or decreased bile flow during TPN, copper storage in the liver may lead to toxic manifestations.[5]

Another key point in the definition of an RRI is the assessment of the critical effects of deficiency and toxicity relevant to human health. The most sensitive indices of excess or deficiency may be biomarkers without clear functional or health significance. At the other extreme, death associated with organ damage, induced by excess or deficit, is clearly of health significance but is not relevant as a sensitive indicator of health risk. Clinical effects such as bone fractures in the case of calcium deficit leading to osteopenia, or liver dysfunction due to fibrosis in the case of copper excess, are clearly significant in terms of health risk[33], but are difficult to assess in controlled studies since ethical principles in human investigation may preclude a precise quantitative definition of these endpoints. Death from bacterial infection associated with tocopherol excess or increased intracranial pressure associated with excess retinol are clearly not applicable endpoints to define ranges of RRI, although they are of unquestionable significance. Biochemical changes, such as red cell superoxide dismutase (SOD) activity as an index of copper deficit[34] or changes in plasma albumin as an index of protein deficit, are sensitive but non-specific indicators of health risks.[35]

In general the RRI range should be defined by the intake level that prevents the appearance of sub clinical adverse effects either from deficit or excess. One should select effects of similar health significance to define upper and lower ranges of RRI. For example, in the case of phosphorus, the low intake associated with diaphragmatic muscle failure is much lower than the lower limit of the RRI; the corresponding high intake associated with a rise in serum parathyroid hormone as an index of excess phosphorus is closer to the upper limit of the RRI. Thus, since these two measures are markedly dissimilar, we could more likely choose the phosphorus need to support adequate calcium retention or bone density rather than diaphragmatic failure or changes in parathyroid hormone concentrations. This is an example of the principle of selection of comparable effects to define excess and deficit.

Another approach to estimate RRI in quantitative terms is based on examining the range of intake of healthy infant populations. This assumes that if the population is in good health the exposure must be "safe." This is particularly helpful if experimental human information available is limited. A starting point in the definition of RRI can be the customary intake/exposure observed in "healthy" populations: in our case, the healthy full term infant fed human milk provided by a well-nourished omnivorous woman.[36] For example, if we were to select how much taurine or linoleic acid was needed to feed a low birthweight infant, we could start by estimating the range of intakes per unit body weight observed in the fully breast fed infant. We would need to know the range in breast milk content, the range in volume of intake and the corresponding infant weight.

A key issue in health risk assessment is the need to evaluate exposure/intake from all possible sources. For example, the sodium intake needs to consider not only that supplied by enteral and parenteral nutrition sources but also the sodium included as salt in medications to increase solubility of the corresponding drug. Some antibiotics are now provided as arginine salts, which in a single dose provide a rather large arginine load and may in fact accumulate with repeated dosing.[37] The provision of cysteine HCL, added to the parenteral nutrition solution, provides not only the required cysteine but a large acid load, which may induce a metabolic acidosis.[38] Excess aluminum is presently virtually unavoidable because of contaminants present in most enteral and parenteral calcium compounds used; toxicity is potentially severe in patients with prolonged parenteral nutrition.[39]

Another guiding principle in defining RRI is that the acceptable oral intake/exposure range should be safe for the group, but should not be expected to meet the requirements or prevent excess for special situations. For example, the zinc needs of patients with short gut syndrome or malabsorption may fall outside the RRI. In these cases, intakes that are of potential risk for the "common" population may be required to meet the special needs of these patients. Safe zinc intake/exposure levels for these special needs patients may be excessive for most LBW infants. RRI are clearly not intended to meet the special needs of subgroups with genetic alterations of nutrient metabolism; for example, achrodermatitis enteropatica (AE), a disease of zinc metabolism in which intestinal absorption is extremely low.[40] In fact, because of an intestinal transport defect, AE patients need 2-3 times the usual zinc intake; this level of intake may interfere with copper absorption, increasing the risk of copper deficit in normal subjects. In another example, patients with Menkes syndrome will not benefit from raising copper levels in formula, but instead need copper delivered to their central nervous system (CNS), possibly using parenteral copper-hystidine to help traverse the blood-brain barrier.

Levels of Evidence to Establish Nutritional and Feeding Practices

The strength of evidence that supports the recommended reasonable range of intake for birth-weight specific groups includes:

- Anecdotal case studies of deficiency and or toxicity: this is sometimes the first indication of health consequences of nutrient deficit or excess. Unfortunately, case studies do not permit a precise definition of dose, nor do they provide

adequate documentation of causality.

- Presence in human milk within established ranges: the concept that human milk is the optimal food for human infants may be tenable in the case of the full-term healthy infant, but cannot be taken as a dogma for ELBW, VLBW or LBW infants. However, as will be documented for several nutrients in the corresponding chapters, human milk provides a first indication of RRI.

- Dose response of nutrient intake required to achieve given outcomes: prevention of clinical disease, indices of growth (weight, length, other), nutrient balance, biochemical response, plasma responses, tissue content, short-term functional outcome, and long-term functional effect. Most of the nutritional studies in the pediatric literature provide evidence for biological effects and in some cases efficacy in disease prevention or amelioration, by providing the right amount of a given nutrient. This should be the ideal approach to define quantitative estimates of nutrient-based recommendations. Unfortunately, very few nutrients have been systematically evaluated using this approach in VLBW or ELBW infants. Moreover, as pointed out previously, these infants are not homogenous but highly variable in their responses. In addition, disease acts as a powerful uncontrolled confounder in clinical studies, so that research observations are usually conducted in relatively "healthy" infants rather than on a truly representative sample of patients who populate NICUs.

- Randomized clinical trial of controlled intake with clinically relevant outcome (disease prevention, relevant morbidity, infection, immune response, growth, body composition, neurodevelopment and cognition): if we examine the Cochrane and other data bases for systematic randomized clinical trials (RCT) of nutrient intakes, we are disappointed to find out that very few nutrient recommendations have been subjected to formal RCT. For some nutrients,

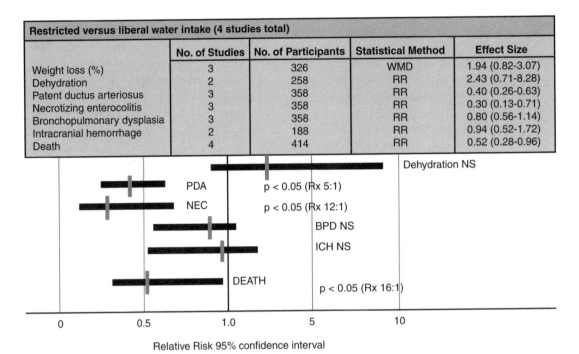

Restricted versus liberal water intake (4 studies total)				
	No. of Studies	**No. of Participants**	**Statistical Method**	**Effect Size**
Weight loss (%)	3	326	WMD	1.94 (0.82-3.07)
Dehydration	2	258	RR	2.43 (0.71-8.28)
Patent ductus arteriosus	3	358	RR	0.40 (0.26-0.63)
Necrotizing enterocolitis	3	358	RR	0.30 (0.13-0.71)
Bronchopulmonary dysplasia	3	358	RR	0.80 (0.56-1.14)
Intracranial hemorrhage	2	188	RR	0.94 (0.52-1.72)
Death	4	414	RR	0.52 (0.28-0.96)

Dehydration NS

PDA $p < 0.05$ (Rx 5:1)

NEC $p < 0.05$ (Rx 12:1)

BPD NS

ICH NS

DEATH

$p < 0.05$ (Rx 16:1)

0   0.5   1.0   5   10

Relative Risk 95% confidence interval

Figure 2: Comparison of restricted versus liberal water supply in LBW infants[42]. The table in the top panel is the result of the meta-analysis combining data drawn from four studies; number of subjects is included. Weighted mean difference (WMD) is presented for % weight loss; other variables presented as relative risks (RR) and 95% confidence intervals. The figure in the bottom panel shows treatment effects; RRs that lie to the left of the no effect vertical line (RR= 1) correspond to results which favor the experimental group. For example the relative risk of a patent ductus is 0.4 meaning that in comparison to liberal water supply, those restricted have a 60 % decrease in the risk of developing the condition. The bracketed numbers represent the number of patients that need to be treated (Rx) to prevent one case of the specific condition, for example to prevent one case of PDA, one needs to restrict water supply in five LBW infants.

efficacy studies have been conducted but very few safety assessments with sufficient power have been reported. *(www.nichd.nih.gov/cochrane/cochrane.htm)*
•Large scale randomized controlled clinical trial exploring the health effects associated with deficit and excess of given nutrients, and meta-analysis of several separate RCTs supporting clinical benefits from recommended range of intake, are the ideal way to scientifically base nutrient intake recommendations. The advantages of clinical practice based on systematic studies and review using rigorous predefined methods are many. Combining different studies in meta-analysis improves the extrinsic validity

of the results; that is, they have greater generalizability, since they are derived from different populations and under different environments. The larger number provides greater power to assess safety as well as efficacy in close to real-life conditions; rare adverse effects are usually undetected in small or medium size trials. It is possible to address specific subgroup analyses in terms of safety and efficacy and provide recommendations for further research addressing special groups of patients.[41]
Meta-analysis requires that we combine different measures of treatment effect. For categorical dichotomous data, both relative estimators (odds ratio,

relative risk) and absolute estimators (risk difference) are used. For data measured on a continuous scale, the effect of treatment is expressed as the mean difference. For each outcome, standard statistical methods are used to calculate the treatment effect for each trial and in the set of included trials as a whole (point estimate and 95% confidence interval) as shown in Figure 2.[42] In this latter estimate, the "typical effect" is a weighted average, the weights being the inverse of the variance of the estimate provided by each participating trial. Thus, large trials have more effect on the typical effect than do small trials. These methods are based on either fixed effect or random effects models. The Cochrane neonatal reviews generally use a fixed effect model.

The statistical significance of a treatment effect is demonstrated when the confidence interval around the point estimate of treatment effect excludes "no difference." This would occur when the confidence interval of the estimate for odds ratio or relative risk does not include one, or when the confidence interval for absolute risk reduction or mean difference does not include zero. By convention, the proportion of adverse events, rather than favorable outcomes, is used as the treatment effect. As an illustration, a study of water intake examined the treatment effect of development of patent ductus arteriosus in LBW infants. As shown in Figure 2, treatment effects that lie to the left of the no effect vertical line or to the left of an odds ratio (OR) of 1 indicate a result that favors the experimental group. For example, in Figure 2 the relative risk of a patent ductus arteriosus is 0.4, meaning that in comparison with liberal water supply, those restricted have a 60% decrease in the risk of developing the condition. In addition, one may derive the number of patients that need to be treated to prevent one case of PDA; in this case, 5 need to be treated. In this same study, using % weight loss to illustrate a continuous variable, the weighted mean difference is 1.94 %, based on combining studies and adjusting for sample size. This means that if one fluid restricts, one can expect on average around a 2% difference in weight loss, relative to providing a liberal water supply. From these results the authors proposed implications for practice and for future research:

"Based on this analysis, the most prudent prescription for water intake to premature infants would seem to be careful restriction of water intake so that physiological needs are met without allowing significant dehydration. This practice could be expected to decrease the risks of patent ductus arteriosus and necrotizing enterocolitis, and perhaps the overall risk of death, without significantly increased risk of adverse consequences. Implications for future research in this area might be directed toward refining the critical period during which water intake must be controlled in order to achieve the desired reduction in complications of prematurity. It would also be valuable to develop models to predict optimal water intakes that take into account the most important determinants of water requirement, such as birthweight, gestational age, postnatal age, and ambient humidity. Finally, future studies should target the most vulnerable group: ELBW infants."[42]

Adaptations to Extrauterine Life and Consequences for Nutrient Delivery

Most neonatal morbidity and nutritional problems can be explained by untimely delivery that affects adaptation to life *ex utero* and progressively compromises specific organ function. The occurrence of hyaline membrane disease in babies born prior to 34 weeks gestation, i.e., before surfactant production is adequate, is a good example of developmental pathology; the high prevalence of hypoglycemia in low birthweight infants represents abnormalities in both storage and/or mobilization of glycogen associated with immaturity. Cardiovascular adaptations required by neonates include a drastic reduction in pulmonary vascular resistance leading to increased lung blood flow and reduced right to left shunt through the ductus arteriosus. Subsequently, closure of the ductus arteriosus establishes separate right and left cardiac pump function. Pulmonary adaptations include continuous rhythmic ventilatory movements to assure oxygenation; the maturation of lung alveolar structure and a capillary network sufficient for gas exchange; and the biochemical development of the surfactant system including production, release and recycling of disaturated phosphatydyl choline and phosphatydyl glycerol. Given the wide shifts in oxygenation, cellular metabolism must be able to alternate between aerobic and anaerobic conditions for energy-yielding processes[43].

Metabolic maturational events include the regulation of substrate flux and metabolism necessary for maintenance and growth needs and the excretion of waste products including acid, nitrogen, various electrolytes and other minerals. As part of this successful adaptation to extrauterine life, the newborn must generate heat and maintain thermal balance independently. Heat production in the neonate is dependent on metabolic thermogenesis rather than muscular activity (shivering which appears several months after birth). Successful metabolic adaptation requires that the neonate be able to mobilize energy reserves (from glycogen and adipose tissue); generate glucose from amino acids; and lactate and regulate fuel supply to key organs by the interaction of various hormones including insulin, glucagon, cortisol and catecholamines. With the interruption of the continuous nutrient supply through the placenta, the neonate must adapt to intermittent flow of nutrients that may require alternate metabolic processing before entry into the systemic circulation. The intestine during fetal life will recycle water and absorb some protein contained in amniotic fluid. *Ex utero*, it digests and absorbs intact proteins as well as amino acids and peptides; it emulsifies, hydrolyses and re-esterifies fat and converts lactose to glucose and galactose before absorption. Many of these maturational events have now been characterized structurally and biochemically; their cellular and molecular basis is now better known.

Several systemic and gut hormones, as well as growth factors, regulate the genes responsible for the development of gut function. Overall, these adaptive responses are integrated and mediated by the neuroendocrine system, which acts as a focal point to assure successful adaptation. Gastrointestinal and metabolic maturation is dependent on adequate nutritional substrates and the action of a variety of hormones including insulin, thyroid and steroidal hormones, as well as the mediation of an array of

growth factors such as IGF-I, IGF-II and epidermal growth factor. During fetal development there are important interactions among nutritional status, hormonal responses and growth factors. Insulin, as one of the principal hormones influencing fetal somatic growth, regulates fetal lipogenic activity and has a permissive role in hepatic glycogen deposition and protein synthesis. Fetuses with insulin deficiency secondary to pancreatic agenesis or with a defective insulin receptor as in "leprechaun" syndrome have marked intrauterine growth retardation (IUGR) with decreased adipose tissue and little weight gain during the last trimester of pregnancy. Conversely, fetal hyperinsulinism results in increased adiposity in human infants of diabetic mothers. Protein feeding as well as several essential and non-essential amino acids stimulate insulin secretion in the fetus and neonate. Protein intake induces plasma insulin and urinary C-peptide, whereas increased arginine plasma concentrations increase serum insulin levels in newborn infants. The significant correlation of urinary C-peptide excretion with weight gain suggests that insulin may be a growth promoting factor for infants. The clinical implications of this are just beginning to be unraveled; evidence from a single controlled clinical study in extremely small preterm infants has shown increased tolerance to glucose and higher weight gain in infants infused with insulin during their initial postnatal days.[44]

Epidermal growth factor (EGF), present in human milk and TGF-a, influences growth and differentiation of epithelial cells, including lung and gut. Receptors for EGF are present throughout development and are increased in number in placenta and lung in fetuses with growth restriction induced by uterine artery ligation, suggesting a role for EGF in fetal growth retardation. Additional evidence for an effect of EGF on somatic growth is the observation that exogenous EGF administered to rats less than 2 weeks of age suppresses plasma IGF-1 and decreases fetal growth. Other "classic" hormones including thyroxin, corticosteroids and sex hormones have important influences on specific organ development and on functional and metabolic adaptation but have little influence on somatic growth during fetal life. For example, thyroid hormone is important for CNS and skeletal maturation, steroids modulate lung maturation and androgens are critical for sex differentiation. The isolation of placental leptin and the higher levels of leptin in newborn infants support a role in intrauterine and neonatal adipose tissue development .

The changes in blood flow that characterize the hemodynamic response to fetal nutrient restriction are also partly modulated by endocrine mechanisms. Fetal nutrient-restricted fetuses have increased circulating levels of arginine vasopressin, which may contribute to decreased splanchnic blood flow and increased blood flow to the brain that is associated with "brain sparing" during growth retardation. Vasoactive prostaglandins are likely of importance in modulating blood flow to the fetus and the hemodynamic changes resulting in brain sparing. The fetus exposed to placental malfunction has decreased responsiveness of peripheral adipose tissue and muscle to insulin; this insulin resistance secures substrates for brain and visceral organ development, but may have adverse long-term consequences.[45]

Glucose is the major energy substrate for the fetus and the newborn, although the fetus is also capable of utilizing lactate, free fatty acids or ketone bodies under special conditions. During the last trimester of pregnancy, it is estimated that 12-15 mg of glucose per kilogram of body weight per minute are transferred across the placenta. The liver, heart and brain of the fetus receive a greater proportion of cardiac output relative to their weight. This distribution provides these organs with greater substrate availability and serves to cover their high-energy needs. These organs have the highest energy expenditure per unit of weight and are able to utilize glucose aerobically or anaerobically. The complete oxidation of one mole of glucose by the anaerobic pathway generates only two moles of ATP and lactate; in contrast, 38 moles of ATP are produced by its complete oxidation in the mitochondria via the Krebs cycle. Glucose, by a pathway, can enter the pentose shunt and form ribose. Ribose and deoxyribose constitute important

precursors for the synthesis of nucleic acids necessary for cell replication and growth. Glycogen synthesis in liver and muscle utilizes glucose and 3 carbon precursors such as lactate or pyruvate. This process is initiated late in the second trimester of gestation and progressively increases until term. It is completed during the third trimester before delivery. Liver glycogen deposits represent stored glucose, which is rapidly available for export to satisfy the needs of other organs, especially the brain. Cerebral hexokinase has the highest affinity for glucose, giving that organ preferential access to the use of this fuel relative to liver, muscle and kidney. Fetal liver progressively increases its glycogen concentration throughout gestation, reaching a maximum of 10% of organ weight at the time of birth. However, because glycogen within liver cells is in a hydrated state at a ratio of 1:4, and not as a starch powder, the total energy stored is quite limited. In the very low birthweight newborn, liver glycogen stores account roughly for a total of 20-30 kilocalories, which is barely sufficient to cover energy needs longer than a couple of hours. These infants with diminished liver glycogen stores and immature glycogen phosphorylase are therefore, susceptible to hypoglycemia. Some organs such as the liver, skeletal muscle or heart are able to directly oxidize free fatty acids derived from lipolysis of triglycerides stored in adipose tissue. Adipose tissue represents the main energy reserve, not only because the oxidation of 1 gram of fat generates 9 kcal per gram but also because triglycerides are stored within adipose tissue in a water-free environment giving adipose tissue an energy density of around 8 kcal per gram, as opposed to 1 kcal per gram of wet liver. Due to very small amounts of peripheral adipose tissue, a 1000 g VLBW infant will use up this reserve within a couple of days, and if sick, even sooner.[46]

Protein synthesis in the fetus and in early postnatal life has been estimated to be 15-20 grams per kilogram body weight per day. This is 5-8 times greater than that observed in the adult. Based on amino acid transfer data from experimental studies and the fetal accretion of protein, it can be estimated that, during late gestation, placental transport of amino acid is on the order of 2.0-2.5 grams per kilogram per day. The rapid

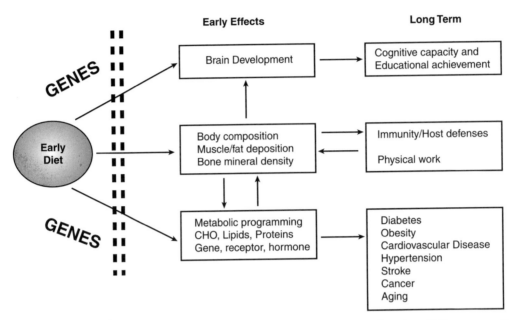

Figure 3: Interaction between early diet and genes in defining relevant health and quality of life outcomes. Early nutrition affects not only brain development, and growth and body composition, but also metabolic programming that has possible long-term effects on adult burden of disease. Nutrition impacts prevalence of diet-related adult chronic disease, immunity, capacity for physical work, and cognitive and educational performance.

anabolic rate of the fetus plus the presence of placental nitrogen exchange precludes the need for significant elimination of nitrogen waste by the fetus. The enzymes necessary for ammonia production and urea formation are all low in fetal life and exhibit significant rises in postnatal life as the protein load from both endogenous catabolism and dietary sources increases. Liver and kidney metabolism of nitrogen by-products is greatly increased postnatally. This increase is coupled to urea formation by the liver and ammonia genesis by the kidney that serves to excrete both nitrogenous waste products and acid equivalents.

Perinatal gastrointestinal development consists of a series of sequential steps leading ultimately to successful digestion, absorption and metabolism of nutrients necessary for maintenance and growth. Early enteral feeding triggers the release of gastrin and other enteric hormones that enhance intestinal maturation. Gut hormones play an important role in determining mucosal growth, smooth muscle contractions and enzymatic maturation. Motilin and bombesin levels

are also elevated after enteral feeds; the former modulates gut contractions and the latter enhances gastrin release. Enteral feeding increases other gut hormones such as enteroglucagon, neurotensin, cholecystokinin, neuropeptide Y, and gastric inhibitory peptide. Even minimal human milk or formula enteral feedings, 5-15 Kcal per kg per day, is sufficient to maintain gut hormonal responses. Feeding tolerance and progression to full enteral feeding appear to be enhanced if minimal enteral feeding is established soon after birth.[47] However, nutrients supplied in excess of what can be tolerated at a given stage of functional development may increase the risk of acquiring necrotizing enterocolitis (NEC).[48] Corticosteroids administered prenatally to mothers may enhance the biochemical, structural and functional maturation of the gut and may help decrease the risk of NEC.[49] Gastrointestinal motility measured manometrically in the duodenum becomes established by 28-30 weeks gestation, even in the absence of enteral feedings. The onset and strength of duodenal contractions is enhanced by maternal betamethasone administration. Prenatal steroids also enhance the rise in beta glycosidases; lactase activity is particularly responsive to corticosteroids. Thus, steroid administration to the mother not only contributes to lung maturation but may also enhance gut maturation, explaining a lower risk of NEC.

Consequences of Malnutrition During Early Life

Nutrition plays a key role in the development of multiple organ systems. Figure 3 illustrates the early and late effects of neonatal malnutrition. Multiple studies over the past 4 decades demonstrate the important effects of early human malnutrition on central nervous system (CNS) development in experimental animals and man.[50,51] From the results of these studies, one can conclude that a reduction in energy and or essential nutrient supply during the first stages of life can have profound effects on somatic growth and organ structural and functional development, especially for the brain. Malnutrition impairs brain development, reducing cell replication cycles and dendritic connections. Different regions of the brain are affected in specific ways; cell number as measured by DNA content is specially affected by intrauterine malnutrition and early postnatal malnutrition; synaptic connectivity is particularly affected if malnutrition occurs after birth but before the third year of life. After 18 months of age, when the "brain's growth spurt" is complete, alterations in dietary precursors may determine in part neurotransmitter availability. Serotonin, norepinephrine, dopamine, acetylcholine are all synthesized from dietary precursors. These effects may differ in specific brain regions; essential fatty acids and non-essential lipid supply may affect the structural composition of the brain and of myelin sheaths. Functional correlates are also significantly modified by malnutrition: waking electroencephalographic (EEG) activity; auditory evoked potentials; and sleep-wake organization as well as neurovegetative activities during sleep are disturbed by early human malnutrition.

The linkage between retarded somatic growth and altered brain development is strong if the nutritional deprivation model is one of early protein energy malnutrition (PEM). This principle has guided many experimental studies and epidemiological evaluations of nutrition versus mental development relationships. Yet, there are multiple instances where somatic growth may proceed unabated while brain structure and function are significantly altered. The effect of early anemia on brain function does not affect somatic growth; the impact of taurine deficiency on retinal and brain development in non-human primates and in human infants is not dependent on structural proteins, since this sulfonic amino acid is not incorporated in protein synthesis. The role of n-3 fatty acids as structural components of the brain is not associated with effects on growth, but rather on modifying membrane function and electrical responses. Examples in the opposite direction, namely of normal mental development and poor growth, are more difficult to find, suggesting that normal somatic growth is a necessary but insufficient condition to attain normal mental development. Early malnutrition from pyloric stenosis or cystic fibrosis illustrate the capacity of the brain to recover from malnutrition, but are not by themselves sufficient to negate the effect of sustained nutritional deprivation on the developing CNS. An important contribution to understanding the relationship between nutritional deficiencies and brain development has been the concept that effects of PEM on child development should not be viewed in a simplistic way, since PEM coexists with other nutritional deficiencies that can also disrupt child development. The influence of specific nutrients on brain development in infants and children has been insufficiently studied. Fetal growth retardation and PEM are not models of isolated nutritional deprivation, but rather a combination of many restrictions: oxygen, blood supply, many nutrients and various growth factors and hormones.[52]

Undernutrition is the most common cause of secondary immunodeficiency in the world. Severe nutritional deficiency markedly affects host defense mechanisms. The most consistent changes in immunocompetence are observed in cell-mediated

Cardiovascular
1. Reduction of pulmonary vasculature resistance
2. Increase lung blood flow
3. Closure of ductus arteriosus
4. Separate right and left cardiac pumps

Pulmonary
1. Maturation of alveoli and capillary network
2. Development of the surfactant system
3. Rhythmic respiration
4. Maturation of antioxidant enzyme systems.

Metabolic-Endocrine
1. Neuroendocrine responsiveness to changes in nutrients and temperature
2. Thermogenesis and temperature regulation
3. Glucose homeostasis (glycogenolysis, gluconeogenesis)
4. Enzymatic maturation for nutrient metabolism and detoxification of excess.

Nutritional/Gastrointestinal
1. Intermittent rather than continuous feeds
2. Digestion and absorption of nutrients
3. Metabolism, storage and mobilization of energy substrates
4. Metabolism and excretion of protein and other nitrogenous compounds
5. Maintenance of nutrient supply for growth and development

Renal/water/electrolyte homeostasis
1. Regulation of renal blood flow and glomerular filtration.
2. Hormonal control of intravascular volume and urinary output
3. Control of electrolyte balance and excretion
4. Excretion of excess electrolytes, nitrogen and acid load
5. Maturation of dermal barrier to prevent water loss

Neurodevelopmental
1. Integrated responses to environmental stimuli
2. Maintenance of autonomic regulation under new conditions
3. Activation of sensory input and processing necessary for learning
4. Operation of reflexes and behaviors needed for survival

Table 1: Neonatal adaptations necessary for extrauterine life.

immunity, bactericidal function of neutrophils, complement system and secretory IgA response. The effects of protein-energy malnutrition on the immune response are difficult to distinguish from those related to deficits of specific nutrients that may occur in conjunction with undernutrition. It is virtually impossible to fully isolate the effect of one specific nutrient from other dietary factors that may also be in deficit. In addition, the immune response is greatly affected by concurrent factors that are difficult to control, such as infection. Animal models allow for a better control of these confounding factors; however, the extrapolation of animal data to humans is always questionable. Malnutrition during the immediate postnatal period may aggravate an already immature immune system and further compromise host resistance to infection. Undernutrition in the critical early months of development will have a greater impact and may have long-lasting effects on immunity as compared to nutritional deficiency acquired in later life. The available evidence indicates that small-for-gestational age low birthweight infants have impaired cell-mediated immune responses and that their neutrophils have reduced bactericidal capacity. Depressed T-cell number and function may persist for several months or even years after birth. Infants with intrauterine growth retardation have diminished chemotaxis following stimulation with chemo attractant derived from E coli; abnormal nitroblue tretazolium oxidative reduction; and deficient microbicidal activity. Maternal nutritional status has also been shown to affect the immune response of the infant. Low birthweight infants born from malnourished mothers have decreased thymic weight and spleen, and their cell-mediated immune response is impaired. T-lymphocyte number and function are defective, and maternal-fetal transfer of IgG is reduced.[8,16]

Specific essential nutrients such as vitamins or trace mineral deficiencies can also have modulating effects on the immune response. Vitamin A (retinol) and its derivative retinoic acid are necessary for cell differentiation and regulation of gene expression of key glycoproteins. Thus, retinoids are important for normal epithelial integrity, cell repair processes, T-cell proliferative response and cell growth in general.[53] Low plasma retinol concentrations are a common finding in the LBW population, especially in those receiving parenteral nutrition. Trace minerals such as iron, zinc and copper are also important for both T-cell function as well as phagocytic and bactericidal capacity of polymorphonuclear leukocytes (PMN). Deficits in these trace elements are common in both parenterally and enterally-fed infants, especially in those with intestinal injury, fistula or resections. The premature infant appears to be more susceptible to severe acute zinc deficiency states compared with the term infant, yet evidence for mild deficiency states is surprisingly limited. Zinc deficiency causes atrophy of lymphoid tissue, impaired delayed cutaneous hypersensitivity reaction, decreased lymphocyte response to mitogens and antigens, and impaired chemotaxis of monocytes and PMN leukocytes.[10] Interactions between zinc and vitamin A have attracted a great deal of attention and may be of clinical significance. Low serum vitamin A concentrations occur in zinc-deficient animals and in humans with low plasma zinc concentrations. Conversely, excess zinc may depress phagocytic and bactericidal activity of leukocytes. Iron deficiency with or without anemia may also be observed in LBW infants. It produces increased susceptibility to infection, by impairing cell-mediated immune response, intracellular killing of bacteria, and secretory IgA antibody response.[8]

Economic Consequences of Malnutrition in Early Life

Several approaches can be used to estimate the costs of neonatal malnutrition to society. A common way of assessing the costs is to define the number of preventable deaths and estimate the lost economic productivity based on remaining years (life expectancy), mean salary, percent unemployment, and discount rate to bring future economic benefit to present terms. The assumptions of this model are that the value of a life lost can be measured in economic terms. Similarly, we can estimate the cost of disability, as in the case of nutritional deficits that affect mental development. For example, mild iodine deficiency in early life affects later IQ by 5-7 points even if treated

later on; this can be translated in economic terms by decreased educational achievement and lower productivity that in turn affects income. In some cases, such as in overall malnutrition, we may need to add the impact related to disability to that of death. In either situation we should include not only the direct costs linked to lost productivity but also the analysis of economic loss of the resources wasted in early stimulation, special education, and health programs, since malnutrition will affect the impact of these programs. This approach has been generically called "investment in human capital", considering that society has not only physical capital in terms of infrastructure and monetary resources, but also human capital which includes physical as well as mental capital. Both components of human capital can be linked to nutrition during early life.[51]

More recently economists have used the concept of disability adjusted life years (DALYs), to estimate the burden of disease to society; no effort is made to separate different health outcomes or establish differences based on potential monetary worth of a life. It considers all health outcomes the same; no difference is made on a healthy life year gained by a poor or rich person, black or white, old or young. Only age and gender are considered, since they affect the number of remaining healthy years independent of all other conditions. The concept of adjusting for disability serves to define the impact of non-fatal outcomes. Life years lost due to premature death, discounting future health, adjusted by age is incorporated in DALYs. The basic concept behind DALYs is that the best measure of lost health is the loss in duration of healthy life itself and not monetary units or arbitrary measures of productivity. Time lost due to premature death is a function of death rate from a specific condition and the expected duration of life lost to death at a given early age.[54]

This concept makes a strong case for investment in newborn care, since the potential healthy life years saved are much greater than those spared in treating an adult with a stroke or coronary disease. Since disability may not be permanent or may not occur in all cases, the incidence and expected duration of disability based

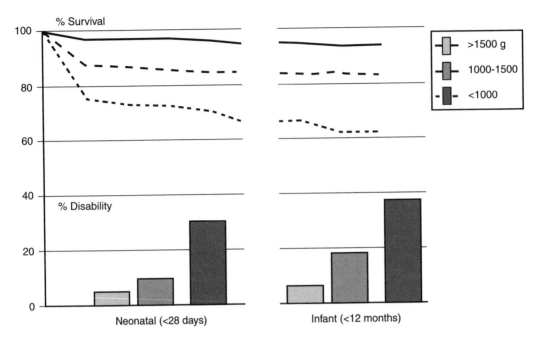

Figure 4: Top panel depicts improvement in neonatal (< 28 days) and infant (< 1 year of age) birthweight specific % survival of very low birthweight infants. Better obstetric and neonatal medical care; understanding of thermal/ energy homeostasis, lung and brain maturation, novel treatments for respiratory distress and better nutrition have led to the survival of progressively smaller neonates. Improved follow-up care throughout the first year of life has contributed to improved infant survival and lower prevalence of mental and physical disability. Bars in lower panel represent birthweight-specific prevalence of physical and mental disability rates expressed as %; current data compiled from various sources.[56,57]

on case fatality and remission rates needs to be incorporated in the calculation. The advantage of DALYs is that it widens the scope of the interventions that can be evaluated beyond those with a direct biomedical focus. For example, the education of socially disadvantaged adolescent girls to prevent undesired pregnancy and premature birth may prove to be more cost effective, measured in terms of DALYs lost due to neonatal mortality and disability, than death and disability related to neonatal bleeding due to vitamin K deficiency. The assumptions placed on these analyses are that we consider all death and disability equally undesirable, and that society will benefit as a whole from providing health and education for all. On a global scales the World Bank estimates that the total costs associated with the prevention of micronutrient deficiency (iodine, vitamin A and iron) in early life is

less than US $50 per DALY gained. A DALY gained does not have an absolute monetary value, but for most societies, yearly per capita income greatly exceeds this amount. In real terms this means that most individuals in the world would be willing and able to pay US $50 for an extra year of healthy life. The benefit-to-cost ratio of this intervention has been estimated to be at least 17 to 1.[55]

Conclusions

We have reviewed the science base to define requirements and this approach will be used as much as possible in establishing recommendations throughout the rest of the book. We expect this knowledge will serve to better understand and provide a framework for what will be presented in the following chapters of this book. Yet we have not fully addressed the ultimate goal of our effort; understanding why we need estimates of nutritional requirements, and utilizing this knowledge to affect the health and well being of infants. The aim of nutrition for the LBW, VLBW and ELBW infant, as we see it, is not only to improve survival as depicted in the top sections of Figure 4, but also to decrease physical and mental disability as shown in the bottom panels. Perhaps we should start emulating the development bankers of this world, and not focus solely on preventing death but also on preserving quality of life and physical and mental function for the rest of life. Neonatal care is indeed an excellent investment, to be measured not by the large number of dollars spent, but measured by the few dollars spent for the number of DALYs produced. What we do, or fail to do, with an infant's nutrition will impact his/her parents' life, and affect our patient's quality of life for years to come.

References

1. Young VR. 2001 W.O. Atwater Memorial Lecture and the 2001 ASNS President's Lecture: Human nutrient requirements: the challenge of the post-genome era. *J Nutr* 2002. Apr;132(4):621-9.

2. Uauy-Dagach R, Hertrampf E. Food-based Dietary Recommendations: Possibilities and Limitations. *Present Knowledge in Nutrition.* 8th edition eds B. Bowman and R. Russell pp 636-649. ILSI Press Washington DC 2001.

3. Aggett PJ, Bresson J, Haschke F, Hernell O, Koletzko B, Lafeber HN, Michaelsen KF, Micheli J, Ormisson A, Rey J, Salazar de Sousa J, Weaver L. Recommended Dietary Allowances (RDAs), Recommended Dietary Intakes (RDIs), Recommended Nutrient Intakes (RNIs), and Population Reference Intakes (PRIs) are not "recommended intakes." *J Pediatr Gastroenterol Nutr* 1997. Aug;25(2):236-41.

4. Hay WW Jr, Lucas A, Heird WC, Ziegler E, Levin E, Grave GD, Catz CS, Yaffe SJ. Workshop summary: nutrition of the extremely low birthweight infant. *Pediatrics* 1999. Dec;104(6):1360-8.

5. Olivares M, Araya M, Uauy R. Copper homeostasis in infant nutrition: deficit and excess. *J Pediatr Gastroenterol Nutr* 2000. Aug;31(2):102-11.

6. Uauy R, Hoffman DR, Peirano P, Birch DG, Birch EE. Essential fatty acids in visual and brain development. *Lipids* 2001. Sep;36(9):885-95.

7. Koletzko B, Aggett PJ, Bindels JG, Bung P, Ferre P, Gil A, Lentze MJ, Roberfroid M, Strobel S. Growth, development and differentiation: a functional food science approach. *Br J Nutr* 1998. Aug;80 Suppl 1:S5-45.

8. Schlesinger L, Uauy R. Nutrition and neonatal immune function. *Semin Perinatol* 1991. Dec;15(6):469-77.

9. Mize CE, Uauy R, Waidelich D, Neylan MJ, Jacobs J. Effect of phosphorus supply on mineral balance at high calcium intakes in very low birthweight infants. *Am J Clin Nutr* 1995. Aug;62(2):385-91.

10. Loui A, Raab A, Obladen M, Bratter P Nutritional zinc balance in extremely low-birth-weight infants. *J Pediatr Gastroenterol Nutr* 2001. Apr;32(4):438-42.

11. Carlson SE, Neuringer M. Polyunsaturated fatty acid status and neurodevelopment: a summary and critical analysis of the literature. *Lipids* 1999. Feb;34(2):171-8.

12. Rigo J, De Curtis M, Pieltain C, Picaud JC, Salle BL, Senterre J Bone mineral metabolism in the micropremie. *Clin Perinatol* 2000. Mar;27(1):147-70.

13. Atkinson SA.Human milk feeding of the micropremie. *Clin Perinatol* 2000. Mar;27(1):235-47.

14. Kashyap S, Schulze KF, Ramakrishnan R, Dell RB, Heird WC. Evaluation of a mathematical model for predicting the relationship between protein and energy intakes of low-birth-weight infants and the rate and composition of weight gain. *Pediatr Res* 1994. Jun;35(6):704-12.

15. Castillo L, DeRojas-Walker T, Yu YM, Sanchez M, Chapman TE, Shannon D,Tannenbaum S, Burke JF, Young VR.Whole body arginine metabolism and nitric oxide synthesis in newborns with persistent pulmonary hypertension. *Pediatr Res* 1995. Jul;38(1):17-24.

16. Hanson LA, Hahn-Zoric M, Wiedermann U, Lundin S, Dahlman-Hoglund A, Saalman R, Erling V, Dahlgren U, Telemo E. Early dietary influence on later immunocompetence. *Nutr Rev* 1996. Feb;54 (2 Pt 2):S23-30.

17. Pieltain C, De Curtis M, Gerard P, Rigo J. Weight gain composition in preterm infants with dual energy X-ray absorptiometry. *Pediatr Res* 2001. Jan;49(1):120-4.

18. Mayfield, S.R., Uauy R, Waidelich D. Body composition of low-birth-weight infants determined by using bioelectrical resistance and reactance. *Am J Clin Nut* 1991. 54:296-303.

19. Bertocci LA, Mize CE, Uauy R. Muscle phosphorus energy state in very-low-birth-weight infants: Effect of exercise. *Am J Physiol* 1992. Mar;262(3 Pt 1):E289-94.

20. Leitch CA, Ahlrichs J, Karn C, Denne SC Energy expenditure and energy intake during dexamethasone therapy for chronic lung disease. *Pediatr Res* 1999. Jul;46(1):109-13.

21. Denne SC, Karn CA, Wang J, Liechty EA. Effect of intravenous glucose and lipid on proteolysis and glucose production in normal newborns. *Am J Physiol* 1995. Aug;269(2 Pt 1):E361-7.

22. Weiss Sachdev S, Sunde RA.Selenium regulation of transcript abundance and translational efficiency of glutathione peroxidase-1 and -4 in rat liver. *Biochem J* 2001. Aug 1;357(Pt 3):851-8.

23. Finer NN, Peters KL, Hayek Z, Merkel CL. Vitamin E and necrotizing enterocolitis. *Pediatrics* 1984. Mar;73(3):387-93.

24. Sosenko IR, Rodriguez-Pierce M, Bancalari E.Effect of early initiation of intravenous lipid administration on the incidence and severity of chronic lung disease in premature infants. *J Pediatr* 1993. Dec;123(6):975-82.

25. Wauben I, Gibson R, Atkinson S. Premature infants fed mothers' milk to 6 months corrected age demonstrate adequate growth and zinc status in the first year. *Early Hum Dev* 1999. Mar;54(2):181-94.

26. Williams ML, Shoot RJ, O'Neal PL, Oski FA. Role of dietary iron and fat on vitamin E deficiency anemia of infancy. *N Engl J Med* 1975. Apr 24;292(17):887-90.

27. Levander OA, Beck MA.Selenium and viral virulence. *Br Med Bull* 1999. 55(3):528-33.

28. Niederau C, Strohmeyer G. Strategies for early diagnosis of haemochromatosis. *Eur J Gastroenterol Hepatol* 2002. Mar;14(3):217-21

29. Huertas JR, Palomino N, Ochoa JJ, Quiles JL, Ramirez-Tortosa MC, Battino M, Robles R, Mataix J. Lipid peroxidation and antioxidants in erythrocyte membranes of full-term and preterm newborns. *Biofactors* 1998. 8(1-2):133-7.

30. Lonnerdal B. Bioavailability of copper. *Am J Clin Nutr* 1996. May;63(5):821S-9S.

31. Cook JD, Reddy MB. Effect of ascorbic acid intake on nonheme-iron absorption from a complete diet. *Am J Clin Nutr* 2001. Jan;73(1):93-8.

32. Albonico M, Stoltzfus RJ, Savioli L, Tielsch JM, Chwaya HM, Ercole E, Cancrini G. Epidemiological evidence for a differential effect of hookworm species, Ancylostoma duodenale or Necator americanus, on iron status of children. *Int J Epidemiol* 1998. Jun;27(3):530-7.

33. Loudianos G, Gitlin JD. Wilson's disease. *Semin Liver Dis* 2000. 20(3):353-64.

34. Prohaska JR, Brokate B.Lower copper, zinc-superoxide dismutase protein but not mRNA in organs of copper-deficient rats. *Arch Biochem Biophys* 2001. Sep 1;393(1):170-6.

35. Briassoulis G, Zavras N, Hatzis T Malnutrition, nutritional indices, and early enteral feeding in critically ill children. *Nutrition* 2001. Jul-Aug;17(7-8):548-57.

36. Koletzko B, Thiel I, Abiodun PO The fatty acid composition of human milk in Europe and Africa. *J Pediatr* 1992. Apr;120(4 Pt 2):S62-70.

37. Uauy R, Mize C, Argyle C, McCracken G Jr. Metabolic tolerance to arginine: implications for the safe use of arginine salt-aztreonam combination in the neonatal period. *J Pediatr* 1991. Jun;118(6):965-70.

38. Manz F L-cysteine in metabolic acidosis of low-birth-weight infants. *Am J Clin Nutr* 1991. Sep;54(3):565-7.

39. Klein GL Metabolic bone disease of total parenteral nutrition. *Nutrition* 1998. Jan;14(1):149-52.

40. Sandstrom B, Cederblad A, Lindblad BS, Lonnerdal B. Acrodermatitis enteropathica, zinc metabolism, copper status, and immune function. *Arch Pediatr Adolesc Med* 1994. Sep;148(9):980-5.

41. Pearman J, Rey J. eds Clinical Trials in Infant Nutrition. Nestlé Nutrition Workshop. 20 Raven Press, New York USA. 1998.

42. Bell EF, Acarregui M. Restricted versus liberal water intake for the prevention of morbidity and mortality in preterm infants (Cochrane Review). *The Cochrane Library*, Issue 4, 1998. Oxford: Update Software.

43. Uauy, R., Mena P, S., Warshaw JB. Growth and Metabolic Adaptation of the Fetus and Newborn. *Principles and Practice of Pediatrics*. Oski FA, DeAngelis C, Feigin RD and Warshaw JB (eds). Lippincott Philadelphia. p.261-268, 1998.

44. Collins JW Jr, Hoppe M, Brown K, Edidin DV, Padbury J, Ogata ES. A controlled trial of insulin infusion and parenteral nutrition in extremely low birthweight infants with glucose intolerance. *J Pediatr* 1991 Jun;118(6):921-7

45. Vaessen N, Janssen JA, Heutink P, Hofman A, Lamberts SW, Oostra BA, Pols HA, van Duijn CM Association between genetic variation in the gene for insulin-like growth factor-I and low birthweight. *Lancet* 2002. Mar 23;359(9311):1036-7.

46. Mena P, Llanos A, Uauy R. Insulin homeostasis in the extremely low birthweight infant. *Semin Perinatol* 2001. Dec;25(6):436-46.

47. Berseth CL.Assessment in intestinal motility as a guide in the feeding management of the newborn. *Clin Perinatol* 1999. Dec;26(4):1007-15.

48. Uauy RD, Fanaroff AA, Korones SB, Phillips EA, Phillips JB, Wright LL. Necrotizing enterocolitis in very low birthweight infants: biodemographic and clinical correlates. National Institute of Child Health and Human Development Neonatal Research Network. *J Pediatr* 1991. Oct;119(4):630-8.

49. Halac E, Halac J, Begue EF, Casanas JM, Indiveri DR, Petit JF, Figueroa MJ,Olmas JM, Rodriguez LA, Obregon RJ, et al. Prenatal and postnatal corticosteroid therapy to prevent neonatal necrotizing enterocolitis: A controlled trial. *J Pediatr* 1990. Jul;117(1 Pt 1):132-8.

50. Winick M Fetal malnutrition and brain development. *J Pediatr Gastroenterol Nutr* 1983. 2 Suppl 1:S68-72.

51. Fenstrom J, Uauy R, Arroyo P. Eds. Nutrition and Brain. Karger Basel Switzerland. 2001.

52. Prada JA, Tsang RC. Biological mechanisms of environmentally induced causes of IUGR. *Eur J Clin Nutr* 1998. Jan;52 Suppl 1:S21-7.

53. Shenai JP, Chytil F, Parker RA, Stahlman MT. Vitamin A status and airway infection in mechanically ventilated very-low-birth-weight neonates. *Pediatr Pulmonol* 1995. May;19(5):256-61.

54. Murray CJ, Lopez AD Global mortality, disability, and the contribution of risk factors: Global Burden of Disease Study. *Lancet* 1997. May 17;349(9063):1436-42.

55. Javitt JC. Health economic analysis of micronutrient supplementation: the World Bank perspective. *Public Health Rev* 2000. 28(1-4):159-62.

56. Lemons JA, Bauer CR, Oh W, Korones SB, Papile LA, Stoll BJ, Verter J, Temprosa M, Wright LL, Ehrenkranz RA, Fanaroff AA, Stark A, Carlo W, Tyson JE, Donovan EF, Shankaran S, Stevenson DK. Very low birthweight outcomes of the National Institute of Child health and human development neonatal research network, January 1995 through December 1996. NICHD Neonatal Research Network. *Pediatrics* 2001. Jan;107(1):E1

57. Hagberg B, Hagberg G, Beckung E, Uvebrant P. Changing panorama of cerebral palsy in Sweden. VIII. Prevalence and origin in the birth year period 1991-94. *Acta Paediatr* 2001. Mar;90(3):27

Energy
Catherine A. Leitch, Ph.D. and Scott C. Denne, M.D.

Reviewed by Harry Lafeber, M.D., and William Heird, M.D.

We gratefully acknowledge the significant contributions by Guy Putet, M.D.,
the previous author of this chapter.

Determining nutritional requirements in preterm infants requires an agreed-upon reference standard. The most commonly applied and accepted standard is that of intrauterine growth.[1-3] However, the premature newborn and fetus differ markedly in physiology and metabolism, so the standard of intrauterine growth may not entirely be appropriate.[1] It is also apparent that this standard is rarely achieved in clinical practice, either in terms of growth rate or body composition.[3, 4] Nevertheless, intrauterine growth remains a reasonable ideal goal, and it is from this perspective that this chapter is written.

Using the rate of fetal energy accretion as the standard, careful nutritional balance measurements are necessary in order to assess whether these goals are achieved in premature infants. This requires determining energy intakes, absorption, and perhaps most importantly, losses. Accurate determinations of energy expenditure are necessary, preferably over relatively long periods. Although a significant amount of this information exists for healthy growing premature infants, substantially less information is available for sick premature infants, including neonates with respiratory disease requiring mechanical ventilation, necrotizing enterocolitis, sepsis, and extremely low birth weight.

Fetal Energy Accretion

Ziegler et al, in a classic article, describe the body composition of the reference fetus using carefully selected literature reports of whole body chemical analysis of fetuses born prematurely.[5] It is important to note that because of the small size of the fetuses included in this report, fetal accretion rates may be somewhat underestimated. Nevertheless, this report remains the most widely accepted representation of human fetal nutrient accretion.

The rate of fetal nutrient accretion and weight gain changes throughout gestation, as is shown in Figure 1. Fetal energy accretion is ~ 24kcal/kg/d between 24 and 28 weeks, and increases slightly to ~ 28kcal/kg/d for the rest of gestation. Thus, an energy balance (energy intake minus energy expenditure) of ~ 25-30kcal/kg/d represents a reasonable goal for premature infants. It is important to note, however, that this energy balance is specific to a particular rate of protein and fat accretion. Protein accretion at the beginning of the third trimester is ~ 2g/kg/d and declines slightly as gestation progresses. In contrast, fat accretion increases gradually throughout the third trimester. Therefore, early gestation is characterized by accumulation of predominantly lean tissue; by late gestation, considerably more fat and less lean tissue is accreted. Because fat tissue is calorie dense (~ 9 kcal/g) compared to lean tissue (~ 1 kcal/g), the rate of weight gain diminishes from 18g/kg/d at 24-28 wks to 16g/kg/d at 32-36 wks.

Energy and Energy Expenditure Measurements
Energy

The chemical energy produced during oxidation of nutrients is the only available source of energy for man and animals. Energy liberated during these reactions cannot be used directly and must be converted into an appropriate chemical form, mostly adenosine-5-triphosphate (ATP). Later, when hydrolyzed to adenosine-5-diphosphate (ADP), ATP will provide

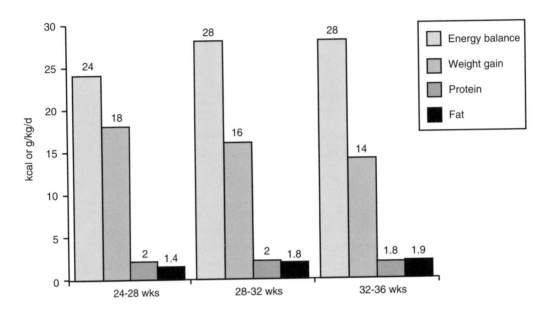

Figure 1: Fetal energy balance, weight gain, protein and fat accretion from 24-36 wks gestation (adapted from Ziegler et al).[5]

the energy necessary for activities such as muscular contraction and synthesis of new molecules.

To understand the methods used to estimate energy expenditure measurement,[6-8] it is important to consider the classic relationship between the liberation of energy during nutrient oxidation and during oxygen consumption. For instance, glucose oxidation will consume oxygen and produce carbon dioxide, water, and energy:

$$C_6H_{12}O_6 + 6O_2 \rightarrow 6CO_2 + 6H_2O - 673 \text{ kcal}$$

Heat liberated by the oxidation of one molecule of glucose is – 673 kcal (the minus sign indicates that heat is liberated). The respiratory quotient (RQ), which is the ratio between the volume of CO_2 produced and the volume of O_2 consumed (VCO_2:VO_2) and which varies according to the type of nutrient oxidized, equals 1 with glucose and other carbohydrates. The heat produced by 1 g of glucose is 673÷180 (with 180 indicating the molecular weight of glucose), or 3.74 kcal/g, and the heat liberated by 1 L of oxygen consumed during this reaction is 673÷

(6 x 22.4), or 5.01 kcal/L of oxygen (22.4 = conversion factor of 1 mol of gas to 22.4 liters under standard conditions of pressure, temperature, and humidity).

Table 1 summarizes these classic parameters for glucose, palmitate (representing fat), and protein. These parameters may vary according to the type of carbohydrate, fat, and protein oxidized.

Energy Expenditure Measurements

Energy expenditure can be determined either directly, by measuring the total heat loss from the body, or indirectly, by measuring O_2 consumption and CO_2 production. Direct calorimetry requires the use of an enclosed chamber in which radiant and convective heat losses are measured, but the heat transferred to the walls of the chamber and evaporative heat loss is measured by the water content of the air entering and exiting the chamber.[9,10] Although this technique provides accurate determinations of energy expenditure and has been used with neonates[9,11], it is difficult and often impractical to implement, requiring the use of complex equipment over long periods while restricting access to the patient. Due to

	Glucose (180)[†]	Palmitate (256.4)[†]	Protein (88)[†]
(a) Heat liberated			
per mol oxidized	673	2398	475
per gram oxidized	3.74	9.3	5.4
(b) O_2 consumed			
(mol)	66	23	5.1
(liters)	134	515	114
(c) CO_2 produced			
(mol)	66	16	4.1
(liters)	134	358	92
(d) Number of ATP[‡] produced[§]			
(mol)	36	129	23
ATP cost:			
Energy kcal/mol of ATP (a/d)**	18.7	18.3	20.7
O_2 L/mol (b/d)	3.72	3.99	4.96
CO_2 L/mol (b/d)	3.72	2.77	4.00
Respiratory quotient (c/b)	1	0.7	0.81
Energy equivalent of (or produced by) one liter of oxygen oxidized (kcal/L)	5.02	4.66	4.17

* Adapted from Ferrannini[8]

[†] Molecular weight. Molecular weight and caloric values may vary according to the type of carbohydrate, fat, and protein oxidized.

[‡] ATP = adenosine-5-triphosphate

[§] Biologically available

** Ratio of (a):(d)

Table 1: Energy balance data for the three main types of nutrients*.

these limitations, energy expenditure studies involving neonates are generally performed using indirect calorimetry.

Open circuit indirect respiratory calorimetry is performed with a patient under a plastic hood, and air is constantly pulled through the hood by a suction pump. From the measured flow rate and changes in the O_2 and CO_2 concentrations, O_2 consumption and CO_2 production can be determined. This method is noninvasive and can be utilized over long periods while allowing access to the patient for routine care. However, the method requires precise measurements of constant O_2 concentrations and may be inaccurate in patients receiving supplemental O_2.[12-14] In addition to measuring energy expenditure, this method also measures the respiratory quotient (RQ=VCO_2/VO_2),

which provides information about the metabolic fuels used for oxidation.

More recently, the doubly labeled water method has been used for measuring energy expenditure. This is a non-invasive technique for determining total daily energy expenditure over a long period. The technique uses water labeled with trace amounts of the stable isotopes deuterium (^2H) and ^{18}O. These tracers distribute throughout the body water pool within a short time period (approximately 4-12 hours). Over time (3-10 days in neonates, 1-3 weeks in adults), both labels are lost from the body. However, the elimination rates of the two isotopes are not equal. As shown in Figure 2, the ^2H label is eliminated solely as ^2H_2O (from urinary and evaporative losses). The ^{18}O label is also lost as $H_2^{18}O$; in addition, some of the ^{18}O

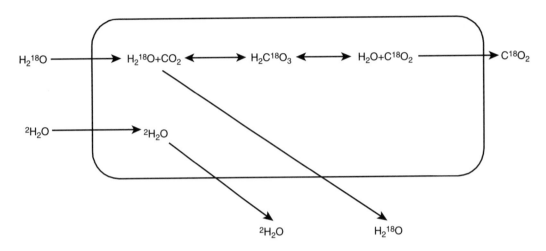

Figure 2: Schematic of the doubly labeled water method for measurement of total energy expenditure. Water labeled with ^2H and ^{18}O is administered and the labels equilibrate in the body water pool (represented by the rectangle). Both labels are eliminated over time. The ^2H label is eliminated solely as labeled ^2H_2O. The ^{18}O label is eliminated as labeled $H_2^{18}O$ and $C^{18}O_2$.

equilibrates with the bicarbonate pool and is eliminated as $C^{18}O_2$. The difference between the two elimination rates (Figure 3) reflects the rate of CO_2 production. From the measured CO_2 production rate and an assumed or measured RQ, energy expenditure can be calculated. The significant advantage to this method is that total energy expenditure can be determined non-invasively in free-living individuals over fairly long periods.

The assumptions of the method, and the studies testing these assumptions, are discussed in detail by Schoeller.[15] The doubly labeled water method has been validated in preterm[16-18] and term[19,20] infants, as well as infants recovering from surgery.[21,22] This method is potentially more sensitive to errors in extremely premature infants due to their higher body water pool sizes and relatively rapid rates of H_2O turnover compared to the rate of CO_2 production.

Energy Requirements in Growing Very Low-Birthweight Infants

Estimation of the energy requirements of the growing preterm infant requires knowledge of the outcome of the energy given. This is shown in the classic energy (E) balance equation:

E *intake* = E *excreted* + E *stored* + E *expended*

Energy intake or gross energy is the energy provided by food. Energy excreted occurs mainly in the feces and to a small extent in the urine. The difference between E intake and E excreted is the metabolizable energy. (Metabolizable energy is often confused with absorbed energy, which is the difference between energy intake and energy excreted in the stools, and does not take into account energy which may be lost in urine. In practice, both values are similar.) Energy stored is the energy laid down in newly formed tissue (mainly as fat and protein); energy expended comprises the energy used for resting metabolism, thermoregulation, and the activity and synthesis of new tissue.

Each term of this equation can be estimated in the preterm infant using methods such as indirect calorimetry and nutrient balance measurements. From such measurements and accurate anthropometry data, weight gain composition can be estimated, as explained in Figure 4.

Complete energy balances, including nutrient balances and concomitant energy expenditure measurements, have been performed in VLBW infants, most of them healthy, growing infants.

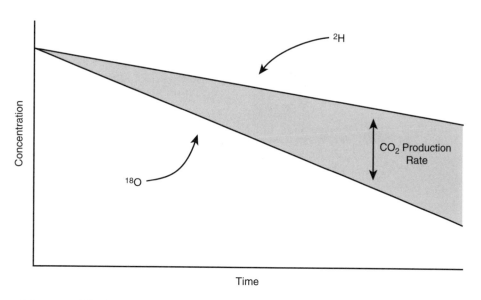

Figure 3: Schematic of the doubly labeled water method for measurement of total energy expenditure. The ^2H and ^{18}O elimination rates are not equal. Since both labels are lost as labeled H_2O, the difference between the elimination rates reflects the rate of CO_2 production. Energy expenditure can be calculated from the rate of CO_2 production and the assumed or measured RQ.

Figure 2.5 presents most of the studies[23-32] in which both techniques were performed. Few nutrient balances have been performed during the first 2 weeks[33] or in sick infants. These published data allow reasonable estimation of the level of each term of the energy balance equation in preterm infants.

Energy Excretion

Energy excretion is mainly due to fat and protein losses via the feces (and to a small extent due to urinary urea excretion), the major factor being the long-chain saturated fatty acid malabsorption of the VLBW infant. From published data,[23-32, 34,35] an average retention of 90% (standard deviation 3%) of the energy intake may be expected by 2 to 3 weeks of age (Figure 5); few data are available for infants weighing <1,000 g or during the first and second weeks of life. However, according to the data of Atkinson et al., an energy absorption of around 80% may be expected during this early postnatal period.[33]

Energy Expenditure

Energy expenditure includes energy for resting metabolism, activity, thermoregulation, and synthesis of new tissue. Most of the information available on energy expenditure has been derived from indirect calorimetry measurements performed in a thermoneutral environment over several hours, knowing that measurements performed over 8 to 12 hours may be representative of total energy expenditure over 24 hours.[36-38]

Components of Energy Expenditure: The usual comparative measurement in the neonate is resting energy expenditure, or resting metabolic rate (RMR), since measurement of the so-called basal metabolic rate (BMR), which requires at least a 12-hour fast, cannot ethically be performed in the preterm infants. Resting metabolic rate differs from BMR in that it includes BMR together with a part of energy used for growth (see following). On average, RMR estimations vary from 45 to 60 kcal/kg/day: lower values have been reported,[39] though, especially during the first week of life. Resting metabolic rate rises during the first week of life[40-42] due partly to an increase in energy intake, and is higher in small-for-gestational-age (SGA) infants.[42,43]

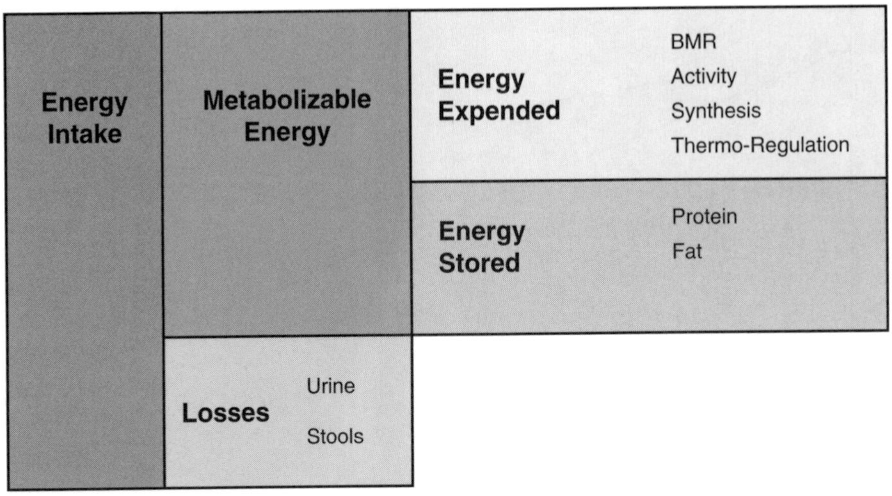

Figure 4: The classic energy balance equation is energy intake = energy expended + energy stored + energy excreted. Metabolizable energy (energy intake minus energy losses) is the energy available for use and can be either expended or stored. Metabolizable energy can be determined through nutritional balance studies. Energy expenditure can be determined through respiratory calorimetry over short periods (hours), or by the doubly labeled water method over longer periods (days). The amount of energy stored is equal to the difference between metabolizable energy and energy expended. In the growing preterm infant, energy is stored mainly as protein and fat. If weight gain is known, the composition of newly accreted tissue can be estimated.

Activity has been shown to increase energy expenditure two– to threefold over short periods. Estimations over 24 hours are more difficult to achieve. Activity cost has been estimated at 3.6 kcal/kg/day by Freymond,[32] 4.3 kcal/kg/day by Reichman,[41] and 7.4 kcal/kg/day by Sauer.[11] Recently, Thureen et al directly measured an energy of activity of 2.4 kcal/kg/day in premature infants using a force plate system, confirming these earlier estimates. [44]

It is likely that during clinical studies, handling of the infants is decreased in comparison with normal nursing conditions. Yeh[45] has estimated nursing procedures to amount to approximately 2% to 12% of the total daily energy expenditure. A total activity cost of 5 to 10 kcal/kg/day is a reasonable estimate.

In VLBW infants, energy lost in thermoregulation should be minimized by careful adherence to standard methods for maintaining a thermoneutral environment.[46] However, temperature instability is frequent during nursing procedures[47]; very modest thermal stresses may increase energy expenditure by 7 to 8 kcal/kg/day.[48] Thermal losses may be further increased when a sick preterm infant is handled frequently, or when a stable growing infant is bathed or nursed. Great importance must be given to thermal losses because they, more than any of the other components of energy expenditure, can be controlled by adequate nursing.

The energy cost of growth includes energy utilized for the synthesis of new tissues and the energy stored in these new tissues. The estimation of energy utilized for synthesis in preterm infants is controversial, and published values demonstrate great variability: 0.26,[11] 0.55,[39] 0.67,[41] and 1.2[24] kcal/g of weight gain (4.8, 6.2, 11.3, and 18 kcal/kg/day, respectively). Hommes,[49] using Atkinson's metabolic price system, estimated the energy needs for synthesis at 0.3 kcal/g of weight gain in term infants. These discrepancies relate in part to the fact that the composition of weight gain is not similar in all studies (the cost of deposition of 1 g of protein is not equal to the cost of deposition of 1 g of fat). It is difficult to provide a more precise

N	Birthweight g	Gestational Age wk	Weight at Study g	Age at Study d	Weight gain g/kg/d	Energy Intake kcal/kg/d	Total Energy Expenditure kcal/kg/d	Method	Ref
9	1260	30.6	1510	20	-	101	59.8	RC	(36)
12	1228	29.6	1465	32	-	120-150	60.6	RC	(38)
9	1740	33	-	21	16.6	110	68	RC	(32)
8	1274	32	1515	22	20.3	120	59.9	RC	(116)
8	1274	32	1515	22	20.3	120	57.5	DLW	(116)
12	1335	30.3	1674	31	15.4	118	68.6	RC	(18)
12	1335	30.3	1674	31	15.4	118	68.3	DLW	(18)
4	1592	30.5	1695	23	13.9	-	56.1	RC	(37)
4	1592	30.5	1695	23	13.9	-	56.3	DLW	(16)
8	1550	32	1700	17	25	131	59	DLW	(50)

Table 2: 24-hr energy expenditure measurements in healthy, growing premature infants.

estimation of energy required for synthesis, and an average of 10 kcal/kg/day for growth is acceptable in view of these data and of total energy expenditure measurements obtained in these infants.

Total Energy Expenditure Estimation: Table 2 summarizes the available data for 24-hour energy expenditure measurements in healthy, growing VLBW infants. Three sets of data[32,36,38] were obtained using respiratory calorimetry over a 24 hour period; one[50] was obtained by the doubly labeled water method; and three[16-18,37] used both techniques in the same infants. Agreement among the different studies is very good and the results indicate that a growing preterm infant born at around 31 weeks gestation has a total daily energy expenditure of approximately 60 to 65 kcal/kg/d at around 24 days of postnatal life.

Energy Stored

Estimates of fat, protein, and energy accretion during fetal growth are shown in Figure 1. For a mean weight gain of 15 g/kg/day, a value of 25 to 30 kcal/kg may be estimated to be stored every day during the last trimester.

During postnatal growth, energy and protein metabolism are tightly linked with respect to growth

and quality of growth. Studies carried out by Kashyap et al demonstrated that protein accretion is related directly to protein intake (to a protein intake of 3.6 g/kg/day), and fat accretion is related primarily to energy intake.[23,51,52] Thus, as energy and protein intake are varied in studies of premature infants, absolute rates of weight gain and composition of weight gain can markedly differ. For example, at similar energy intakes (120 kcal/kg/day) but different protein intakes (2.8 versus 3.8 g/kg/day), similar energy balances are achieved, but the rate of weight gain is significantly greater in the high protein group (19 vs 16 g/kg/day).[51] This is due to increased protein accretion (as lean tissue) and decreased fat accumulation in the high protein group. This clearly demonstrates that the composition of weight gain is an important determinant of growth rate. These concepts are further illustrated by Figure 6. Small increases in energy and protein intake lead to increases in energy and fat accretion with minimal changes in the rate of weight gain; further increases in energy intake without a change in protein intake result in a higher rate of weight gain, all accounted for by increased fat accretion.

Most complete nutrient balance studies have

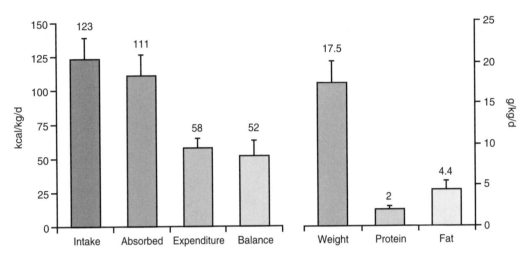

Figure 5: Summary of nutrient balance studies conducted in 223 healthy growing premature infants.[3,23,25-29, 31,32,51,119] Energy intake, energy absorbed, energy expenditure and energy balance shown in the panel on the left, and weight gain, protein and fat accretion is shown on the panel on the right.

demonstrated a much higher rate of fat accretion in enterally-fed premature infants compared to that observed *in utero* (Figure 1, Figure 5). However, it must be noted that these fat accretion rates are calculated from energy balance and not directly measured. Therefore, these fat accretion rates are highly sensitive to underestimations of energy expenditure. In a recent study by Fairey et al, measured energy expenditure was higher than that obtained by previous investigations (76 kcal/kg/day), leading to a fat accretion rate similar to that obtained *in utero*[53] from these data it is possible that previous fat accretion rates for healthy, growing premature infants may have been overestimated to some degree. Nevertheless, the bulk of the evidence continues to suggest relatively high fat accretion rates. The long-term consequences of increased fat accretion in premature infants remain unknown.

A number of studies in infancy provide some reassurance. DeGamarra et al have shown that preterm infants, subject to rapid growth during the neonatal period with 20% of weight gain as fat, experience "normalization" of adiposity within the first two years of life.[54] Cooper et al, comparing three

types of feedings (human milk, standard formula, and preterm formula) that produced wide differences in skin fold thickness during the neonatal period, did not find differences in growth parameters at three years of age.[55] On the other hand, Agras et al have found that greater adiposity at birth was a predictive factor of greater fatness at six years of age.[56] At this point, it is unclear what the impact of a higher rate of fat accretion in premature infants will be in later childhood and adult life.

Energy Intake Recommendations for Enteral Feeding in Growing VLBW Infants

From the available data discussed above, recommended energy intakes of 110 to 130 kcal/kg/day for healthy, growing, premature infants can be made; this recommendation is summarized in Table 3. This energy intake assumes a weight gain of 16 to 20 g/kg/day, a protein retention of 2 g/kg/day, and an energy absorption rate of 90%. It must be noted that this leads to an energy balance higher than that achieved *in utero*, and consequently more fat accretion. This may in part compensate for early postnatal energy deficits. This recommendation is consistent with those of the American Academy of

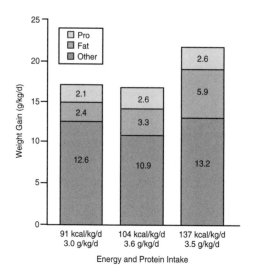

Figure 6: Composition of weight gain in VLBW infants receiving three levels of protein and metabolizable energy intake. Metabolizable energy intakes above 104 kcal/kg/d do not result in additional protein accretion, but rather lead to increased fat accretion. Data from[23, 28].

Pediatrics and Canadian Pediatric Society (120 to 130 kcal/kg/day), as well as the European Society for Gastroenterology and Nutrition (130 kcal/kg/day).[57-61]

Small-for-Gestational-Age Infants

Current nutritional recommendations[57-59, 62] do not differentiate between the needs of SGA and AGA VLBW infants. There are no reported studies specifically examining the energy expenditures of ELBW (Extremely Low Birth Weight) SGA infants compared to AGA infants. However, as summarized in Leitch et al.[63], several studies of energy expenditure in ELBW infants included one or more SGA infants.[17,44,64-66] No significant differences were found in energy expenditure, intake or growth rate between the SGA and AGA ELBW infants. Several investigators compared the energy expenditures of SGA and AGA infants with gestational ages around 33 weeks and birth weights <1500 gm at approximately 1 month of post-natal age. Some reported somewhat higher (~10%) rates of resting energy expenditure in growing SGA infants compared to AGA infants[67-69],

although others have shown slightly lower rates of resting energy expenditure in SGA infants.[70] Davies et al[71] examined total energy expenditure and body composition in term SGA and AGA infants at 5 weeks of life and found significant differences in body composition between groups with the SGA infants having a significantly lower % body fat. Total energy expenditure was increased in SGA infants relative to AGA infants (84 kcal/kg/d vs. 69 kcal/kg/d); the difference in total energy expenditure between the groups was statistically significant when normalized to lean body mass (LBM) (96 kcal/kgLBM/d vs. 82 kcal/kgLBM/d). Although the data would seem to indicate a trend of increasing differences in energy expenditure between SGA and AGA infants with longer gestation, the trend may merely reflect increasing differences in fat mass between the groups.

The majority of reports indicate that weight gain is not statistically different between SGA and AGA infants receiving similar energy intakes.[67,68,71,72] However, Bohler et al[69] showed a significantly greater rate of weight gain in SGA infants compared to AGA infants receiving similar caloric intakes, despite a higher energy expenditure in the SGA group. Term SGA infants given high-energy formulas showed slightly better weight gain and head growth than those receiving standard formula.[73] Although the available data are not completely definitive, energy requirements in SGA infants appear to be similar or only slightly higher than their AGA counterparts.

Early Postnatal Life

The initial goal for premature infants in early postnatal life is to provide sufficient energy intake to at least match rates of energy expenditure in order to preserve body energy stores. In this regard, two factors must be taken into consideration. First, weight changes in early postnatal life are due to both fluid losses and catabolism[74,75]; Bower et al demonstrated that the weight loss in 26 to 30 week premature infants in the first week of life was primarily related to changes in interstitial volume.[75] Therefore, weight changes in early postnatal life are not a good indication of energy balance. Second, energy expenditure may be mini-

	All values in kcal/kg/d
Resting Metabolic Rate	50
Energy of Activity	5
Thermoregulation	10
Total Energy Expenditure	65
Energy Excreted	15
Energy Stored	30-50
Recommended Energy Intake	110-130

Table 3: Energy requirement estimates for growing premature infants.

mized in early postnatal life by low energy intakes; there is a clear relationship between energy intake and energy expenditure.[11,76,77] Therefore, as energy intake is advanced, some increase in overall energy expenditure must be anticipated.

Multiple measures of energy expenditure have been made in non-ventilated 30 to 34 week premature infants in the first week of life over the past two decades. Remarkably consistent results have been obtained, with energy expenditure ranging from 40 to 50 kcal/kg/day.[11,76,78-81] It is important to recognize that all these determinations were made using indirect respiratory calorimetry, usually over fairly short periods of time. Therefore, these measures best represent resting rather than total energy expenditure. Total energy expenditure for these infants is likely to be somewhat higher.

Energy expenditure increases in the second week of life, as would be expected with increased energy intake. Energy expenditures have been measured at 55 to 65 kcal/kg/day during this time[11,76], again using respiratory calorimetry, suggesting that total energy expenditures may be slightly higher.

Given the available information, 60 to 70 kcal/kg/day of energy intake (which includes protein intake) is a reasonable clinical goal to achieve a neutral or slightly positive energy balance in 30 to 34 week premature infants who do not require mechanical ventilation in the first week of life. In the second week of life, 70 to 80 kcal/kg/day may be required to produce the same effect. Further increases in energy intake should be done as quickly as possible to achieve adequate growth. These recommendations are for relatively mature and minimally to moderately sick premature infants; other clinical conditions which may alter energy expenditure (respiratory distress, extremely low birthweight, bronchopulmonary dysplasia, necrotizing entercolitis) are discussed below.

Respiratory Distress Requiring Mechanical Ventilation

Over the last ten years, a number of investigators have measured energy expenditure in very low birthweight infants requiring mechanical ventilation in the first week of life.[77,78,82-86] Although technical concerns remain about this technique because of endotrachial tube leaks and the difficulty of accurate measurements in a supplemental oxygen environment[87], these studies have provided an initial estimate of energy requirements for premature infants with respiratory disease. Remarkably, a majority of these studies have measured energy expenditures of 38 to 45 kcal/kg/day in infants requiring mechanical ventilation, similar to measurements in non-ventilated infants.[77,78,85,86] Moreover, Forsythe and Crighton determined energy expenditure in both ventilated and non-ventilated infants and showed no differences between these groups.[78] Hazon et al observed no change in energy expenditure after surfactant administration, despite significant respiratory improvement.[83] Thus, respiratory disease requiring mechanical ventilation may not substantially alter energy expenditure.

However, three studies in ventilated premature infants measured somewhat higher energy expenditures of 58 to 74 kcal/kg/day in the first week of life.[82-84] Wahlig et al also observed a correlation between energy expenditure and degree of respiratory illness[85], although a study by DeMarie et al, which included a larger number of infants, did not confirm this relationship.[77]

No. of Infants	Population	GA wk	BW g	Study wt g	Age d	EE kcal/kg/d	EI kcal/kg/d	Growth g/kg/d	End Note
5	-	-	-	702	2	49	30	-	(85)
2	-	28.1	780	1542	54	70	120	17.8	(18)
3	BPD	27.3	853	2563	129	78	129	-	(90)
4	-	30.8	790	1244	38	68	114	17.8	(117)
14	SGA	30.5	939	1892	54	67	-	16.1	(66)
1	-	29.0	990	-	17	74	138	14.6	(118)
4	SGA	28.8	850	1534	45	76	130	-	(44)
1	SGA	31.0	900	1750	42	70	96	20.5	(64)
1	-	28.0	950	1310	26	55	115	15.7	(24)
24	-	28.0	1010	-	3	55	37	-	(82)
15	SGA	30.5	939	1276	35	61	123	15.8	(65)
1	SGA	35.0	955	1139	17	66	120	20.2	(17)
	Mean	29.7	905.1	1495.1	38.4	66.6	104.7	17.3	
	SD	2.2	77.2	442.9	331	4.8	28.6	2.2	

Table 4: Energy expenditure determinations by respiratory calorimetry in ELBW infants.

In a recent study using the doubly labeled water technique, total energy expenditure in near-term infants with severe respiratory disease requiring high frequency ventilation was not different than the normal controls.[88]

The precise energy effect of respiratory disease requiring mechanical ventilation in premature infants remains incompletely defined, but any increase in energy expenditure appears to be rather modest. From a clinical perspective, an energy intake of 70 kcal/kg/day (including protein intake) is likely to maintain body energy stores in premature infants requiring mechanical ventilation in the first week of life.

Extremely Low Birthweight Infants

Relatively little data exists on the energy expenditures of extremely low birthweight infants, and the majority of the existing data are from studies on older infants. Very little information exists on the energy needs of these infants immediately after birth or of sick ELBW infants. The existing literature data obtained by respiratory calorimetry is summarized in Table 4. The results of 12 studies involving 75 infants are shown. It must be noted that it was not the primary purpose of most of these studies to determine energy expenditure in extremely premature or extremely low birth weight infants. Most of the determinations in appropriate for gestational age (AGA) infants were made in ventilated, oxygen-dependent patients. Five studies (35 infants) investigated small for gestational age (SGA) infants. The SGA infants had a statistically greater gestational age compared to AGA infants (31.2 + 2.3 weeks vs. 28.5 + 1.2 weeks, p<0.05), but were not significantly different in birthweight, weight or age at study, energy expenditure or intake, and growth rate.

Figure 7 shows energy expenditure as a function of age at time of study for these infants. There is a significant (p < 0.001) positive correlation between energy expenditure and age. As discussed previously, there are several co-existing reasons for the observed increase of energy expenditure with post-natal age.

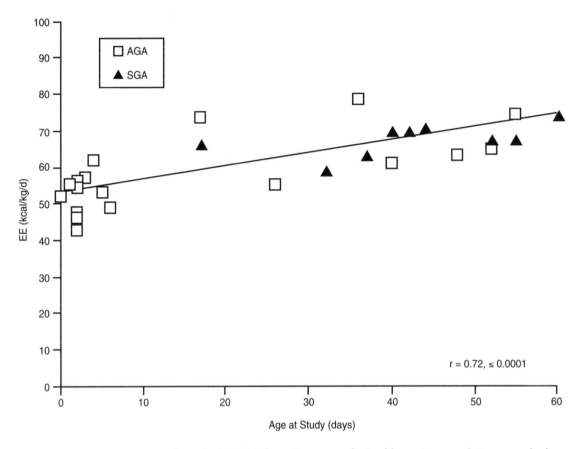

Figure 7: Age versus energy expenditure for ELBW infants. Data were obtained by respiratory calorimetry and taken from[17, 18, 24, 44, 64-66, 82, 85, 90, 117, 118].

In the early neonatal period, infants receive parenteral nutrition. Caloric intakes of infants receiving total parenteral nutrition are lower than those of enterally-fed infants; hence, energy expenditure would be expected to be lower, reflecting lower energy intake. Physical activity, although a small component of energy expenditure in this population, will increase with age.

It is clear that the available data describing energy expenditure in extremely premature infants suffer from severe limitations. The quantity of observations is small, important variables influencing energy expenditure have not been controlled, and the respiratory calorimetry methods employed in this population may be of questionable validity. It is interesting to note, however, that the average energy

expenditure in ELBW infants in these studies is 67 kcal/kg/day, substantially higher than the 52 kcal/kg/day determined in more mature premature infants (all measurements by respiratory calorimetry).

The doubly labeled water technique has been recently used to measure total energy expenditure in extremely low birth weight infants in early postnatal life.[88] Measurements were made in ELBW infants with minimal respiratory disease requiring low ventilator support over a 7 day period ending on day-of-life ten; total energy expenditure was also measured in critically ill near-term infants requiring high frequency oscillator ventilation and in normal healthy controls over the same period. Total energy expenditure in these minimally sick ELBW infants was ~ 80 kcal/kg/day, significantly higher than their more critically ill near

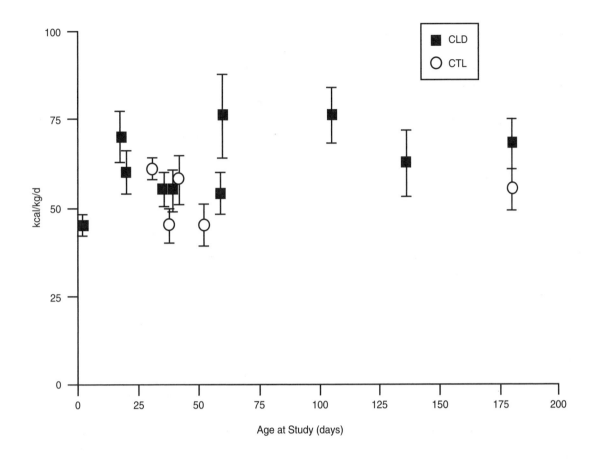

Figure 8: Energy expenditure measured by respiratory calorimetry in preterm infants with chronic lung disease (CLD) and controls (CTL). Data are shown as mean + sd from 9 studies.[13,14,85,90-95]

term counterparts (~ 50 kcal/kg/day). Additional information obtained from the doubly labeled water technique is available in extremely low birth weight infants who have continued to require ventilator support at 3 and 5 weeks postnatal age.[89] Total energy expenditure was measured at 86 to 94 kcal/kg/day in twelve 26-week gestation 900 g birth weight infants; these rates of total energy expenditure at 3 to 5 weeks are consistent with measures of energy expenditure in early postnatal life.

Although limited and incomplete, the available evidence is consistent with elevated energy expenditure in ELBW infants; these high rates of energy expenditure are consistent with the poor growth outcomes currently experienced by this population of infants.[4] At this point, only tentative recommendations can be made for this population. In very early postnatal life, energy intakes may be somewhat limited by glucose and lipid tolerance. However, achieving a parenteral energy intake (including protein) of 80 kcal/kg/day as early as possible appears to be necessary to simply maintain body energy stores. To achieve acceptable rates of growth on parenteral nutrition, 105 to 115 kcal/kg/day (including 3.5 g/kg/day of protein) is likely to be required. For enteral nutrition, assuming an energy absorption of 90%, at least 130 kcal/kg/day of enteral energy intake seems necessary to achieve an energy balance of 25 to 30 kcal/kg/day in ELBW infants. Up to 150 kcal/kg/day may be required in order to achieve an energy balance closer to that of healthy, growing, more mature premature infants. It must be noted that at least a proportional increase in protein intake is likely to be required to accompany the higher energy intakes.

Chronic Lung Disease

A number of studies over the last 20 years have investigated the question of whether premature infants with chronic lung disease have elevated rates of energy expenditure. The results of most of the studies measuring energy expenditure with respiratory calorimetry in infants with chronic lung disease are shown in Figure 8[13,14,85,90-95]; from these data , it is difficult to come to a definitive conclusion about energy expenditure in these infants. In addition, these studies have significant limitations in design (missing or poorly matched control groups) and methodology (inaccuracy of respiratory calorimetry in an oxygen-supplemented environment).[12]

The doubly labeled water technique is now beginning to be applied to important questions regarding neonatal energy expenditure. Preliminary information is emerging regarding energy expenditure in extremely premature infants with early chronic lung disease; from these data, total energy expenditure is approximately 25% greater (91 vs. 73 kcal/kg/day) in ventilated extremely premature infants than in their non-ventilated counterparts.[96]

The doubly labeled water method has also been used to examine the effect of dexamethasone therapy on energy expenditure and balance in extremely premature infants. Dexamethasone therapy substantially reduces growth rates in premature infants[97,98] and steroids have been shown to increase energy expenditure in adults[99]; therefore, increased energy expenditure in premature infants in response to dexamethasone therapy would seem to be a plausible explanation for altered rates of weight gain. Using a cross over, double-blind, placebo controlled study design, Leitch et al[89] determined total energy expenditure and balance in twelve 26-week gestation premature infants during treatment with dexamethasone and placebo. Although the rate of weight gain was reduced 70% during dexamethasone

treatment, total energy expenditure was unchanged (Figure 9). Furthermore, energy balance during dexamethasone treatment and placebo treatment was virtually identical. This result of similar energy balance and substantially altered weight gain strongly suggests that dexamethasone alters the composition of newly accreted tissue toward fat and away from protein; studies in preterm infants, human adults, and animals support this probability.[99-101] Based on the findings from this study, it seems unlikely that a strategy directed simply at increasing caloric intakes in infants receiving dexamethasone will be successful in achieving normal growth.

The doubly labeled water technique has also been used to evaluate energy expenditure in non-ventilated premature infants with chronic lung disease at two months of age. De Meer and colleagues[102] reported higher rates of energy expenditure in two month old 29-week gestation infants with chronic lung disease (73 kcal/kg/d) compared to one-month-old control infants (63 kcal/kg/d). The fact that the control and chronic lung disease groups were not well matched for postnatal age is a limitation; nevertheless, from total energy expenditure determinations in both early and established chronic lung disease, it appears energy needs in this population are increased 15-25% over controls, although further work is clearly necessary.

It is an attractive hypothesis to attribute the increase in energy expenditure in infants with chronic lung disease to increased work of breathing. In fact, a number of studies have observed a correlation between energy expenditure and some measure of respiratory status.[85,91,102] However, Kao et al[92] examined the relationship between work of breathing and energy expenditure more rigorously. The energy cost of breathing was calculated at approximately 1-2 kcal/kg/d, unlikely to contribute significantly to increased energy expenditure in infants with chronic lung disease. Alternative explanations for increased energy expenditure, such as inflammation, appear more likely.

Further information about energy metabolism in patients with chronic lung disease is clearly necessary, especially additional determinations of total energy

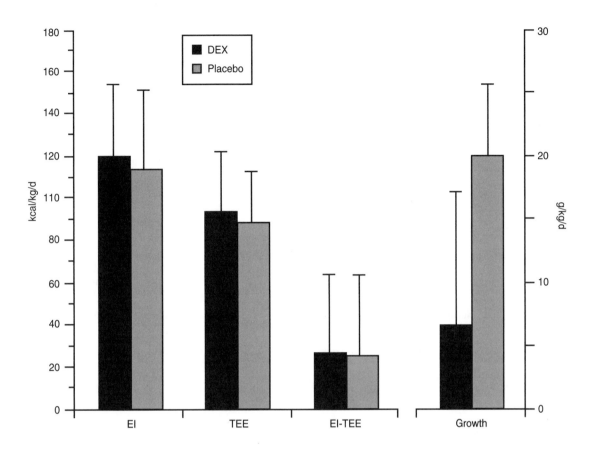

Figure 9: Energy intake (EI), total energy expenditure (TEE), energy balance (EI-TEE), and growth of infants receiving dexamethasone (DEX) or placebo treatment. Growth rates are significantly decreased during DEX treatment despite no differences in energy balance between the treatment phases. Data are taken from Leitch et al.[89]

expenditure and body composition. Acknowledging the limitations of the available data, energy expenditure in premature infants with chronic lung disease may be increased by 10 to 15 kcal/kg/day. Therefore, energy intakes of 120 to 140 kcal/kg/day, with a proportional increase in protein intake, may be reasonable.

Energy Intake During Total Parenteral Nutrition

As with enteral nutrition, the primary determinant of energy requirements during parenteral nutrition is energy expenditure. The route of energy intake (parenteral or enteral) does not seem to substantially alter overall energy expenditure. In a crossover study of premature infants in the first week of life, isocaloric intakes of parenteral or enteral nutrition resulted in virtually identical rates of energy expenditure.[79] Similar results have been obtained in a study that measured energy expenditure in premature infants receiving either enteral or parenteral nutrition in early postnatal life.[78]

Unlike enteral nutrition, energy absorption during parenteral nutrition is essentially complete; the small energy losses during parenteral nutrition (i.e. urine, skin, small stools) can be practically ignored. Therefore, parenteral energy intake is provided to match the underlying rate of energy expenditure to conserve body energy stores. It is crucial that protein must be included in this parenteral intake (approximately 1.5 to 2 g/kg/day) in order to preserve body protein stores.[103-105] A parenteral energy intake of approximately 60 kcal/kg/day (including protein) should effectively preserve energy stores in a 30 to 34 week non-ventilated premature infant in the first week of life. However, extremely low birth weight infants during the same period are likely to require 80 to 85 kcal/kg/day (including protein). To achieve normal growth, positive energy balance of 25 to 30 kcal/kg/day must be achieved. Therefore, for non-ventilated premature infants in the first week of life, a reasonable parenteral energy intake would be 85 to 95 kcal/kg/day (including a protein intake of approximately 3 g/kg/day; for an extremely low birth weight infant parenteral energy intake of ~ 105 to 115 kcal/kg/day including a protein intake of 3 to 3.5 g/kg/day may be necessary.[88] A classic study by Zlotkin et al in 29-week gestation premature infants at ~ 3 weeks of age supports these estimates.[106] Parenteral protein and energy intakes were varied in four groups of infants; parenteral energy intakes of 96 kcal/kg/day (including a protein intake of 3 g/kg/day) produce reasonable weight gains of approximately 16 g/kg/day in this group.

Nonprotein energy can be provided in parenteral nutrition as glucose alone or as a combination of glucose and intravenous fat. Van Aerde et al demonstrated significantly higher energy expenditure in neonates who received glucose alone as the nonprotein energy source compared with a combination of glucose and intravenous fat.[107] Similar results have been obtained in studies of infants and older children.[108,109] Most of the available data support a combined glucose and lipid nonprotein energy supply to maximize nutrient accretion. These results are not surprising given that lipogenesis from glucose is an energy expensive process. In addition to maximizing energy efficiency, some authors have also suggested that a balanced glucose/lipid nonprotein energy source may improve protein accretion.[108, 110]

Necrotizing Enterocolitis and Sepsis

There is very limited information regarding the effect of necrotizing enterocolitis and sepsis on energy

expenditure in premature infants. In a pilot study of 6 infants with necrotizing enterocolitis, energy expenditure was measured using indirect calorimetry during the acute stage of their disease and again when their clinical condition had stabilized (approximately 4 days later).[111] Somewhat surprisingly, energy expenditure did not appear to be elevated in either the acute phase (43 kcal/kg/day) or the recovery phase (51 kcal/kg/day). Although unexpected, this result is consistent with studies in critically ill infants and neonates following trauma or major surgery which also have been unable to document an increase in energy expenditure.[112,113] These findings may represent a diversion of energy from growth toward tissue repair, although clearly further work is necessary.

Mrozek et al evaluated the effect of sepsis on energy expenditure in septic and non-septic near-term infants using respiratory calorimetry.[114] Energy expenditure was similar in the septic and non-septic infants (approximately 50 kcal/kg/day in each group). Energy expenditure in septic infants after recovery was not significantly different than during the septic period. In contrast, preliminary data in extremely low birth weight infants using the doubly labeled water method to measure total energy expenditure show a substantially higher rate of energy expenditure during sepsis (95 kcal/kg/day) than during the post septic period (53 kcal/kg/day).[115] Discrepancies between these two studies may be due to the differences in patient population and/or measurement techniques, but substantially more work must be performed in order to document the effects of sepsis on energy expenditure requirements in premature infants.

Future Areas of Research Include:

1) Longitudinal studies measuring total energy expenditure in ELBW infants from birth to discharge.

2) Nutrient tolerance during the first days of life in ELBW infants.

3) Further delineation of energy expenditure and balance during specific clinical conditions (necrotizing enterocolitis, sepsis, severe respiratory distress, bronchopulmonary dysplasia).

4) Follow-up studies of energy requirements in

ELBW infants after NICU discharge and beyond.

5) Long-term longitudinal follow-up studies of body composition of preterm infants fed various protein/energy ratio formulas in order to detect potential consequences (insulin resistance and cardiovascular disease) of different rates of growth and fat accretion.

Case History

A 750 g female infant was born at 25 weeks gestation to a 26-year-old primiparous mother with an uncomplicated pregnancy. The infant required immediate intubation and the Apgar score at 5 minutes was 7. She received surfactant administration, and the ventilator and supplemental oxygen were weaned quickly to minimal settings (Peak Inspiratory Pressure 14, Positive End Expiratory Pressure 4, Rate 25, 21% oxygen). She was begun on intravenous fluids of 10% dextrose at 120 ml/kg/day (41 kcal/kg/day). On day 4, 0.5 g/kg/day of lipid and 0.5 g/kg of amino acids were added to her intravenous fluids (48 kcal/kg/day). Intravenous amino acids and lipids were slowly advanced at 0.5 g/kg/day to a maximum of 2.5 g/kg/day of amino acids and 2.0 g/kg/day of lipid; total fluids were advanced to 150 ml/kg/day cc/kg including D10W (total calories 81 kcal/kg/day by day 8). At day 10, the infant weighed 650 g.

Commentary

This extremely low birthweight infant with minimal respiratory disease has experienced significant energy deficits in the first 8 days of postnatal life. Based on recent evidence, total energy expenditure in these infants is approximately 80 kcal/kg/day; this level of energy intake was achieved in this infant only after 8 days. Some of the weight loss at 10 days of age represents fluid shifts, but at least some proportion of the weight at 8 days of life also represents loss of body energy stores. Although tolerance to lipid and glucose intake may be limiting in ELBW infants in early post natal life, initiation of both protein (1.5 to 2 g/kg/day) and lipid (0.5 to 1.5 g/kg/day) on day 1 can help minimize energy and deficits. Amino acids and lipids can be gradually advanced (by 0.5 to 1 g/kg/day) to

achieve an intake of 3.5 g/kg/day of each; glucose intake can also be gradually increased to provide intakes of 16 to 17.5 g/kg/day, for a total caloric intake of 105 to 110 kcal/kg/day which should support a reasonable rate of growth. Low volume enteral feeding (preferably 20 cc/kg/day, with human milk) should also be considered beginning on day 1 in order to facilitate the transition to full enteral feedings. Using such an aggressive nutritional approach, Wilson et al minimized early energy (and protein) deficits and improved growth outcomes in sick, very low birth weight infants.[116]

References

1. Swyer PR. New perspectives in neonatal nutrition. *Biology of the Neonate* 1987;52:4-16.

2. American Academy of Pediatrics. Nutritional needs of preterm infants. In: Kleinman RE, ed. *Pediatric Nutrition Handbook.* 4th ed. Elk Grove Village: American Academy of Pediatrics, 1998:55-87.

3. Putet G. Energy. In: Tsang RC, Lucas A, Uauy R, Zlotkin S, eds. Nutritional needs of the preterm infants. Scientific basis and practical guidelines. Pawling: Caduceus Medical Publishers, Inc., 1993:15-28.

4. Lemons JA, Bauer CR, Oh W, et al. Very low birth weight outcomes of the National Institute of Child Health and Human Development Neonatal Research Network, January 1995 through December 1996. *Pediatrics* 2001;107.

5. Ziegler EE, O'Donnell AM, Nelson SE, Fomon SJ. Body composition of the reference fetus. *Growth* 1976;40:329-341.

6. Frayn KN. Calculation of substrate oxidation rates in vivo from gaseous exchange. *J Appl Physiol* 1983;55:628-34.

7. Jequier E, Acheson K, Schutz Y. Assessment of energy expenditure and fuel utilization in man. *Annu Rev Nutr* 1987;7:187-208.

8. Ferrannini E. The theoretical bases of indirect calorimetry: a review. *Metabolism* 1988;37:287-301.

9. Sulyok E, Jequier E, Prod'hom L. Thermal balance of the newborn infant in a heat-gaining environment. *Pediatr Res* 1973;7:888-900.

10. Jequier E, Felber J-P. Indirect calorimetry. *Baillere's Clinical Endocrinology and Metabolism* 1987;1: 911-935.

11. Sauer P, Dane H, Visser H. Longitudinal studies on metabolic rate, heat loss, and energy cost of growth in low birth weight infants. *Pediatr Res* 1984;18:254-259.

12. Denne S, Kalhan S. Glucose carbon recycling oxidation in human newborns. *Am J Physiol* 1986;251:E71-E77.

13. Yeh T, McClenan D, Ajayi O, Pildes R. Metabolic rate and energy balance in infants with bronchopulmonary dysplasia. *J Pediatr* 1989;114:448-451.

14. Yunis K, Oh W. Effects of intravenous glucose loading on oxygen consumption, carbon dioxide production, and resting energy expenditure in infants with bronchopulmonary dysplasia. *J Pediatr* 1989;115: 127-132.

15. Schoeller D. Measurement of energy expenditure in free-living humans by using doubly labeled water. *J Nutr* 1988;118:1278-1289.

16. Roberts S, Coward W, Schlingenseipen K-H, Nohria V, Lucas A. Comparison of the doubly labeled water (2H218O) method with indirect calorimetry and a nutrient-balance study for simultaneous determination of energy expenditure, water intake, and metabolizable energy intake in preterm infants. *American Journal of Clinical Nutrition* 1986;44:315-322.

17. Westerterp K, Lafeber H, Sulkers E, Sauer P. Comparison of short term indirect calorimetry and doubly labeled water method for the assessment of energy expenditure in preterm infants. *Biol Neonate* 1991;60:75-82.

18. Jensen CL, Butte NF, Wong WW, Moon JK. Determining energy expenditure in preterm infants: Comparison of 2H218O method and indirect calorimetry. *Am J Physiol* 1992;263:R685-R692.

19. Roberts S, Coward W, Ewing G, Savage J, Cole T, Lucas A. Effect of weaning on accuracy of doubly labeled water method in infants. *Am J Physiol* 1988;254:R622-R627.

20. Bronstein M, Davies P, Hambidge K, Accurso F. Normal energy expenditure in the infant with presymptomatic cystic fibrosis. *J Pediatr* 1995;126: 28-33.

21. Jones PJH, Winthrop AL, Schoeller DA, et al. Validation of doubly labeled water for assessing energy expenditure in infants. *Pediatric Research* 1987;21: 242-246.

22. Jones P, Winthrop A, Schoeller D, et al. Evaluation of doubly labeled water for measuring energy expenditure during changing nutrition. *Am J Clin Nutr* 1988;47:799-804.

23. Schulze KF, Stefanski M, Masterson J, et al. Energy expenditure, energy balance, and composition of weight gain in low birth weight infants fed diets of different protein and energy content. *Journal of Pediatrics* 1987;110:753-759.

24. Catzeflis C, Schutz Y, Micheli J-L, Welsch C, Arnaud M, Jequier E. Whole body protein synthesis and energy expenditure in very low birth weight infants. *Pediatr Res* 1985;19:679-687.

25. Whyte RK, Haslam R, Vlainic C, et al. Energy balance and nitrogen balance in growing low birthweight infants fed human milk or formula. *Pediatric Research* 1983;17:891-898.

26. Reichman B, Chessex P, Verellen G, et al. Dietary composition and macronutrient storage in preterm infants. *Pediatrics* 1983;72:322-328.

27. Putet G, Senterre J, Rigo J, Salle B. Nutrient balance, energy utilization, and composition of weight gain in very-low-birth-weight infants fed pooled human milk or a preterm formula. *Journal of Pediatrics* 1984;105: 79-85.

28. Putet G, Rigo J, Salle B, Senterre J. Supplementation of pooled human milk with casein hydrolysate: energy and nitrogen balance and weight gain composition very low-birthweight infants. *Pediatric Research* 1987;21:458-461.

29. Whyte RK, Campbell D, Stanhope R, Bayley HS, Sinclair JC. Energy balance in low birth weight infants fed formula of high or low medium-chain triglyceride content. *Journal of Pediatrics* 1986;108:964-971.

30. Kashyap S, Schulze KF, Forsyth M, Dell RB, Ramakrishnan R, Heird WC. Growth, nutrient retention, and metabolic response of low-birth-weight infants fed supplemented and unsupplemented preterm human milk. *Am J Clin Nutr* 1990;52:254-62.

31. Roberts SB, Lucas A. Energetic efficiency and nutrient accretion in preterm infants fed extremes of dietary intake. *Human Nutrition: Clinical Nutrition* 1987;41C:105-113.

32. Freymond D, Schutz Y, Decombaz J, Micheli J-L, Jequier E. Energy balance, physical activity, and thermogenic effect of feeding in premature infants. *Pediatric Research* 1986;20:638-645.

33. Atkinson SA, Bryan MH, Anderson GH. Human milk feeding in premature infants: protein, fat, and carbohydrate balances in the first two weeks of life. *J Pediatr* 1981;99:617-24.

34. Schanler RJ, Garza C, Nichols BL. Fortified mothers' milk for very low birth weight infants: results of growth and nutrient balance studies. *J Pediatr* 1985;107:437-45.

35. De Curtis M, Brooke O. Energy and nitrogen balances in very low birthweight infants. *Archives of Disease in Childhood* 1987;62:830-832.

36. Bell E, Rios G, Wilmoth P. Estimation of 24-hour energy expenditure from shorter measurement periods in premature infants. *Pediatr Res* 1986;20:646-649.

37. Roberts S, Murgatroyd P, Crisp J, Nohria V, Schlingenseipen K-H, Lucas A. Long-term variation in oxygen consumption rate in preterm infants. *Biol Neonate* 1987;52:1-8.

38. Schulze K, Stefanski M, Masterson J, et al. An analysis of the variability in estimates of bioenergetic variables in preterm infants. *Pediatr Res* 1986;20:422-7.

39. Gudinchet F, Schutz Y, Micheli JL, Stettler E, Jequier E. Metabolic cost of growth in very low-birth-weight infants. *Pediatr Res* 1982;16:1025-30.

40. Sinclair JC. Energy balance of the newborn. In: Sinclair JC, ed. Temperature regulation and energy metabolism in the newborn. New York: Grune Stratton, 1978: 187-204.

41. Reichman B, Chessex P, Putet G, et al. Partition of energy metabolism and energy cost of growth in the very-low-birth-weight infant. *Pediatrics* 1982;69: 446-451.

42. Hill J, Robinson D. Oxygen consumption in normally grown, small-for-dates and large-for-dates new-born infants. *J Physiol* 1968;199:685-703.

43. Bhakoo O, Scopes J. Minimal rates of oxygen consumption in small-for-dates babies during the first week of life. *Arch Dis Child* 1974;49:583-585.

44. Thureen P, Phillips R, Baron K, DeMarie M, Hay WJ. Direct measurement of the energy expenditure of physical activity in preterm infants. *J Appl Physiol* 1998;85:223-230.

45. Yeh TF, Lilien LD, Leu ST, Pildes RS. Increased O$_2$ consumption and energy loss in premature infants following medical care procedures. *Biol Neonate* 1984;46:157-62.

46. Hey E. Thermal neutrality. *Br Med Bull* 1975;31: 69-74.

47. Mok Q, Bass CA, Ducker DA, McIntosh N. Temperature instability during nursing procedures in preterm neonates. *Arch Dis Child* 1991;66:783-6.

48. Glass L, Silverman WA, Sinclair JC. Effect of the thermal environment on cold resistance and growth of small infants after the first week of life. *Pediatrics* 1968;41:1033-46.

49. Hommes FA. The energy requirement for growth-a re-evaluation. *Nutr Metab* 1980;24:110-113.

50. Fjeld CR, Cole FS, Bier DM. Energy expenditure, lipolysis, and glucose production in preterm infants treated with theophylline. *Pediatr Res* 1992;32: 693-698.

51. Kashyap S, Schulze KF, Forsyth M, et al. Growth, nutrient retention, and metabolic response in low birth weight infants fed varying intakes of protein and energy. *Journal of Pediatrics* 1988;113:713-721.

52. Kashyap S, Forsyth M, Zucker C, Ramakrishnan R, Dell R, Heird W. Effects of varying protein and energy intakes on growth and metabolic response in low birth weight infants. *J Pediatr* 1986;108:955-963.

53. Fairey A, Butte N, Mehta N, Thotathuchery M, Schanler R, Heird W. Nutrient Accretion in Preterm Infants Fed Formula with Different Protein: Energy Ratios. *JPGN* 1997;25:37-45.

54. de Gamarra M, Schutz Y, Catzeflis C, et al. Composition of weight gain during the neonatal period and longitudinal growth follow-up in premature babies. *Biol Neonate* 1987;52:181-187.

55. Cooper PA, Rothberg AD, Davies VA, Horn J, Vogelman L. Three-year growth and developmental follow-up of very low birth weight infants fed own mother's milk, a premature infant formula, or one of two standard formulas. *J Pediatr Gastroenterol Nutr* 1989;8:348-54.

56. Agras WS, Kraemer HC, Berkowitz RI, Hammer LD.

Influence of early feeding style on adiposity at 6 years of age. *J Pediatr* 1990;116:805-9.

57. ESPGAN. Guidelines on infant nutrition. *Acta Paediatr Scan Suppl* 1987;262:1.

58. ESPGAN. Nutrition and feeding of preterm infants. *Acta Paediatr* 1987;336:1-14.

59. ESPGAN. Committee report: comment on the content and composition of lipids in infant formulas. *Acta Paediatr Scand* 1991;80:887.

60. Pediatrics AAo. Pediatric Nutrition Handbook. Elk Grove Village: American Academy of Pediatrics, 1998.

61. Nutrition Committee CPS. Nutrient needs and feeding of premature infants. *Can Med Assoc J* 1995;152: 1765-1785.

62. Nutrition Co. Pediatric Nutrition Handbook. 4th Edition ed. Elk Grove Village, Illinois: American *Academy of Pediatrics* 1998.

63. Leitch C, Denne S. Energy expenditure in the extremely low-birth weight infant. *Clinics in Perinatology* 2000;27:181-195.

64. Brooke O. Energy requirements and utilization of the low birthweight infant. *Acta Paediatr Scand* 1982;296:67-70.

65. van Toledo-Eppinga L, Houdijk MC, Delemarre-van de Waal HA, Jakobs C, Lafeber HN. Leucine and glucose kinetics during growth hormone treatment in intrauterine growth-retarded preterm infants. *Am J Physiol* 1996;270 (*Endocrinol Metab* 33):E451-E455.

66. van Toledo-Eppinga L, Houdijk E, Cranendonk A, Delemarre-Van de Waal H, Lageber H. Effects of recombinant human growth hormone treatment in intrauterine growth-retarded preterm newborn infants on growth, body composition and energy expenditure. *Acta Paediatr* 1996;85:476-81.

67. Cauderay M, Schutz Y, Micheli JL, Calame A, Jequier E. Energy-nitrogen balances and protein turnover in small and appropriate for gestational age low birthweight infants. *Eur J Clin Nutr* 1988;42: 125-36.

68. Chessex P, Reichman B, Verellen G, et al. Metabolic consequences of intrauterine growth retardation in very low birthweight infants. *Pediatr Res* 1984;18:709-713.

69. Bohler T, Kramer T, Janecke A, Hoffmann G, Linderkamp O. Increased energy expenditure and fecal fat excretion do not impair weight gain in small-for-gestational-age preterm infants. *Early Human Development* 1999;54:223-234.

70. Picaud J-C, Putet G, Rigo J, Salle B, Senterre J. Metabolic and energy balance in small- and appropriate-for-gestational-age, very low-birth-weight infants. *Acta Paediatr Suppl* 1994;405:54-59.

71. Davies PSW, Clough H, Bishop NJ, Lucas A, Cole JJ, Cole TJ. Total energy expenditure in small for gestational age infants. *Arch Dis Child* 1996;74:F208-F210.

72. Pencharz PB, Masson M, Desgranges F, Papageorgiou A. Total-body protein turnover in human premature neonates: effects of birth weight, intra-uterine nutritional status and diet. *Clin Sci (Colch)* 1981;61:207-15.

73. Brooke OG, Kinsey JM. High energy feeding in small for gestation infants. *Archives of Disease in Childhood* 1985;60:42-6.

74. Georgieff M, Amarnath U, Mills M. Determinants of arm muscle and fat accretion during the first postnatal month in preterm newborn infants. *J Pediatr Gastroenterol Nutr* 1989;9:219-224.

75. Bauer K, Bovermann G, Roithmaier A, Gotz M, Prolss A, Versmold H. Body composition, nutrition, and fluid balance during the first two weeks of life in preterm neonates weighing less than 1500 grams. *J Pediatr* 1991;118:615-20.

76. Chessex P, Reichman B, Verellen G, et al. Influence of postnatal age, energy intake, and weight gain on energy metabolism in the very low-birth-weight infant. *J Pediatr* 1981;99:761-766.

77. DeMarie MP, Hoffenberg A, Biggerstaff SLB, Jeffers BW, Hay WW, Thureen PJ. Determinants of Energy Expenditure in Ventilated Preterm Infants. *J Perinat Med* 1999;27:465-472.

78. Forsyth JS, Crighton A. Low birthweight infants and total parenteral nutrition immediately after birth. I. Energy expenditure and respiratory quotient of ventilated and non-ventilated infants. *Arch Dis Child Fetal Neonatal Ed* 1995;73:F4-7.

79. Denne S, Karn C, Liu Y, Leitch C, Liechty E. Effect of enteralversus parenteral feeding on leucine kinetics and fuel utilization in premature newborns. *Pediatr Res* 1994;36:429-435.

80. Fok TF, Gu JS, Lim CN, Ng PC, Wong HL, So KW. Oxygen Consumption and Resting Energy Expediture During Phototherapy in Full Term and Preterm Newborn Infants. *Arch Dis Child Fetal Neonatal Ed* 2001;85:F49-F52.

81. Carnielli VP, Verlato G, Benini F, et al. Metabolic and Respiratory Effects od Theophylline in the Preterm Infant. *Arch Dis Child Fetal Neonatal Ed* 2000;83: F39-F43.

82. Samiec TD, Radmacher P, Hill T, Adamkin DH. Measured energy expenditure in mechanically ventilated very low birth weight infants. *Am J Med Sci* 1994;307:182-4.

83. Hazan J, Chessex P, Piedboeuf B, Bourgeois M, Bard H, Long W. Energy expenditure during synthetic surfactant replacement therapy for neonatal respiratory distress syndrome. *J Pediatr* 1992;120:S29-S33.

84. Mayfield SR. Technical and clinical testing of a computerized indirect calorimeter for use in mechanically ventilated neonates. *Am J Clin Nutr* 1991;54:30-34.

85. Wahlig T, Gatto C, Boros S, Mammel M, Mills M, Georgieff M. Metabolic response of preterm infants to variable degrees of respiratory illness. *J Pediatr* 1994;124:283-8.

86. Forsyth JS, Crighton A. An indirect calorimetry system for ventilator dependent very low birthweight infants. *Arch Dis Child* 1992;67:315-9.

87. Kalhan SC, Denne SC. Energy consumption in infants with bronchopulmonary dysplasia. *Journal of Pediatrics* 1990;116:662-664.

88. Carr BJ, Denne SC, Leitch CA. Total energy expenditure in extremely premature and term infants in early postnatal life. *Pediatric Research* 2000;47:284A.

89. Leitch CA, Ahlrichs JA, Karn CA, Denne SC. Energy expenditure and energy intake during dexamethasone therapy for chronic lung disease. *Pediatric Research* 1999;46:109-113.

90. de Gamarra E. Energy expenditure in premature newborns with bronchopulmonary dysplasia. *Biol Neonate* 1992;61:337-344.

91. Billeaud C, Piedboeuf B, Chessex P. Energy expenditure and severity of respiratory disease in very low birth weight infants receiving long-term ventilatory support. *J Pediatr* 1992;120:461-4.

92. Kao L, Durand D, Nickerson B. Improving pulmonary function does not decrease oxygen consumption in infants with bronchopulmonary dysplasia. *J Pediatr* 1988;112:616-621.

93. Weinstein M, Oh W. Oxygen consumption in infants with bronchopulmonary dysplasia. *J Pediatr* 1981;99:958-961.

94. Chessex P, Belanger S, Piedboeuf B, Pineault M. Influence of energy substrates on respiratory gas exchange during conventional mechanical ventilation of preterm infants. *J Pediatr* 1995;126:619-24.

95. Merth I, de Winter J, Zonderland H, Borsboom G, Quanjer P. Pulmonary function in infants with neonatal chronic lung disease with or without hyaline membrane disease at birth. *Eur Respir J* 1997;10:1606-1613.

96. Leitch C, Denne S. Increased energy expenditure in premature infants with chronic lung disease. *Pediatr Res* 2000;47:291A.

97. Yeh T, Torre J, Rastogi A, Anyebuno M, Pildes R. Early postnatal dexamethasone therapy in premature infants with severe respiratory distress syndrome: a double-blind, controlled study. *J Pediatr* 1990;117:273-282.

98. Papile L, Tyson J, Stoll B, et al. Multi-center trial of two dexamethasone therapy ragimes in ventilator-dependent premature infants. *N Engl J Med* 1998;338:1112-1118.

99. Tataranni PA, Larson DE, Snitker S, Young JB, Flatt JP, Ravussin E. Effects of glucocorticoids on energy metabolism and food intake in humans. *Am J Physiol Endocrinol Metab* 1996;271:E317-E325.

100. Van Goudoever J, Wattimena J, Carnielli V, Sulkers E, Degenhart H, Sauer P. Effect of dexamethasone on protein metabolism in infants with bronchopulmonary dysplasia. *J Pediatr* 1994;124:112-118.

101. Weiler HA, WAng Z, Atkinson SA. Whole body lean mass is altered by dexamethasone treatment through reductions in protein and energy utilization in piglets. *Biol Neonate* 1997;71:53-59.

102. de Meer K, Westerterp K, Houwen R, Brouwers H, Berger R, Okken A. Total energy expenditure in infants with bronchopulmonary dysplasia is associated with respiratory status. *Eur J Pediatr* 1997;156: 299-304.

103. Rivera A, Bell EF, Bier DM. Effect of intravenous amino acids on protein metabolism of preterm infants during the first three days of life. *Pediatric Research* 1993;33:106-111.

104. Van Lingen RA, Van Goudoever JB, Luijendijk IHT, Wattimena JLD, Sauder PJJ. Effects of early amino acid administration during total parenteral nutrition on protein metabolism in pre-term infants. *Clinical Science* 1992;82:199-203.

105. Van Goudoever JB, Colen T, Wattimena JLD, Huijmans JGM, Carnielli VP, Sauer PJJ. Immediate commencement of amino acid supplementation in preterm infants: Effect on serum amino acid concentrations and protein klinetics on the first day of life. *Journal of Pediatrics* 1995;127:458-465.

106. Zlotkin SH, Bryan MH, Anderson GH. Intravenous nitrogen and energy intakes required to duplicate in utero nitrogen accretion in prematurely born human infants. *Journal of Pediatrics* 1981;99:115-120.

107. Van Aerde J, Sauer P, Pencharz P, Smith J, Swyer P. Effect of replacing glucose with lipid on the energy metabolism of newborn infants. *Clinical Science* 1989;76:581-588.

108. Nose O, Tipton J, Ament M, Yabuuchi H. Effect of the energy source on changes in energy expenditure, respiratory quotient, and nitrogen balance during total parenteral nutrition in children. *Pediatric Research* 1987;21:538-541.

109. Bresson J, Narcy P, Putet G, Ricour C, Sachs C, Rey J. Energy substrate utilization in infants receiving total parenteral nutrition with different glucose to fat ratios. *Pediatric Research* 1989;25:645-648.

110. Bresson JL, Bader B, Rocchiccioli F, et al. Protein-metabolism kinetics and energy-substrate utilization in infants fed parenteral solutions with different glucose-fat ratios. *Am J Clin Nutr* 1991;54:370-376.

111. Powis MR, Smith K, Rennie M, Halliday D, Pierro A. Characteristics of protein and energy metabolism in neonates with necrotizing enterocolitis--a pilot study. *J Pediatr Surg* 1999;34:5-10; discussion 10-2.

112. Powis MR, Smith K, Rennie M, Halliday D, Pierro A. Effect of major abdominal operations on energy and protein metabolism in infants and children. *Journal of Pediatric Surgery* 1998;33:49-53.

113. Letton R, Chwals W, Jamie A, Charles B. Early postoperative alterations in infant energy use increase the risk of overfeeding. *J Pediatr Surg* 1995;30:988-993.

114. Mrozek JD, Georgieff MK, Blazar BR, Mammel MC, Schwarzenberg SJ. Effect of sepsis syndrome on neonatal protein and energy metabolism. *Journal of Perinatology* 2000;2:96-100.

115. Torine IJ, Wright-Coltart SI, Denne SC, Leitch CA. Energy expenditure in extremely premature infants with sepsis. *Pediatr Res* 2001;49:261A.

116. Wilson DC, Cairns P, Halliday HL, Reid M, McClure G, Dodge JA. Randomised controlled trial of an aggressive nutritional regimen in sick very low birth-weight infants. *Archives of Disease in Childhood Fetal & Neonatal Edition* 1997;77:4F-11F.

Protein, Amino Acid and Other Nitrogen Compounds
J. Rigo, M.D., Ph.D.

Reviewed by Hildegard Przyrembel, M.D., Ph.D., Pieter Sauer, M.D., and JL Micheli, M.D.

We gratefully acknowledge the important contributions of J.L. Micheli and
Y. Schutz the authors of this chaper in the previous edition.

Introduction

Nutritional problems of preterm babies have become particularly relevant in the last decade because of the increased survival of very-low-birthweight (<1500 g) and gestational-age (<32 weeks) infants, and the numerous studies underlining the importance of early feeding on short- and long-term development. The recommended nutrient intakes of preterm infants are still a matter of debate in spite of extensive experimental and clinical studies. Such a difficulty is probably mainly the result of the sum of metabolic challenges arising during the transition of intrauterine to extrauterine life and the lack of consensus on short- and long-term objectives for early nutrition.

Current nutritional recommendations from various international committees[1-5] are based on healthy preterm infant studies and designed to provide nutrients to approximate the rate of growth and composition of weight gain of that of a normal fetus of the same corrected age. In practice, the shorter the gestation of a neonate the more challenging are the limiting influences of immaturity and accompanying morbidity on nutritional provision during the early weeks of life.[6-8] **As a result, cumulative nutritional deficits resulting from the initial adaptative period may be high, and recommended intakes do not compensate for this early nutritional gap.**[7,9]

Superimposed on this, the use after birth of the gastrointestinal tract instead of placental transfer does not allow quantitative or qualitative provision of all the various nutrients necessary to optimize growth approximating the normal fetus of similar corrected age.[10-12] Additional nutritional deprivations arise from

neonatal illnesses such as bronchopulmonary dysplasia, necrotizing enterocolitis, or infectious diseases[7,13] when recommended nutrient supplies are frequently interrupted and when endogenous repositories of nutrient are compromised by mobilization of stores and tissue catabolism.

As a result of this cumulative nutritional deficit during early life, most growth parameters remain subnormal by the time the preterm infant reaches a corrected age of 40 weeks,[9,14,15] and this phenomenon worsens in the case of VLBW and ELBW infants[15,16] suggesting that the current nutritional recommendations need to be re-evaluated in order to reduce the initial gap during the first days of life and to promote a compensatory catch-up growth before the corrected term.

The Basis of Re-Evaluating Protein Requirements for Preterm Infants
Actual Recommendations for Protein Requirements in Preterm Infants

Actual nutritional and protein recommendations for preterm infants (Table 1) were developed between 1985 and 1995 on the basis of the fetal accretion rate during gestation by the Committee of Nutrition of the AAP in 1985[1] and the Committee of Nutrition of the ESPGHAN in 1987.[2] Those data have been re-evaluated in 1993 by Micheli and Schutz,[3,17] taking into account the factorial approach and data on the metabolic and neurodevelopmental implications of protein metabolism, as well as in 1995 by the Committee of Nutrition of the CPS[4] and more recently by an expert panel in a LSRO/ASNS report.[5]

In practice those recommendations have been

Advisable protein intake (g/kg*d)		
AAP 1985	26-28 wks GA 800-1200 g *4.0 g/kg*d*	28-31 wks GA 1200-1800 g *3.5 g/kg*d*
ESPGHAN 1987	28-32 wks GA 1000-1800 g *2.9-3.6 g/kg*d*	
International guidelines Micheli, JL and Schutz, Y 1993	≤27 wks GA ≤1000 g *3.6-3.8 g/kg*d*	29-31 wks GA 1200-1800 g *3.0-3.6 g/kg*d*
CPS 1995	<1000 g *3.5-4.0 g/kg*d*	≥1000 g *3.0-3.6 g/kg*d*
Expert panel LSRO/ASNS 2001	Minimum *3.4 g/kg*d* *2.5-2.8 g/100 kcal*	Maximum *4.3-4.9 g/kg*d* *3.6 g/100 kcal*

Table 1: Recommended protein intake by various international committees.[1-5,17]

summarized by Micheli[18] who has developed a chart to obtain a practical nutritional survey by comparing the actual daily intake of an individual infant in comparison to recommended intakes (Figure 1).

The Postnatal Cumulative Nutritional Deficit in Preterm Infants

Recent nutritional studies focused on the daily parenteral and oral nutrient supplies in preterm infants in comparison to current recommended intakes of energy and protein to evaluate the contribution of poor nutrition as rate limiting on growth status at the time of discharge. [7,9,16] According to those data, establishment of an adequate intake is difficult during the early weeks of life especially in extremely immature and sick infants. The protein and energy deficits are maximal during the transition period (Figure 1) inducing an important reduction in growth rate as illustrated by rapid losses in body weight and body length Z score.[7,9]

These studies also show that during the second period, from full enteral feeding up to discharge,

recommended nutritional intakes are rarely maintained due to various clinical conditions. In addition (Table 2), the use of human milk fortifiers (HMF) and conventional preterm formulas (PTF) with a mean protein content of 2.5 and 2.8 per 100 kcal, respectively, does not allow growth and weight gain composition similar to fetal growth but contributes to an additional postnatal growth retardation.[9,19] Reduced gain was more marked in infants fed HMF than in those fed PTF, suggesting that poorer growth reflected an inadequate protein intake. However, in their study, Embleton et al 2001,[7] suggested that the cumulative nutritional deficit explained only close to 50% of the reduction in growth Z scores before discharge. Additional non-nutritional factors must also play a role in the postnatal growth deficit of preterm infants.

Protein Gain and Changes in Whole Body Composition During Fetal Life

Measurements of body composition are of major importance and represent the basis for estimating the protein needs in preterm infants.[17,20-24] At present we have no better model for the growing preterm infant than the growing fetus of the same gestational age. During fetal life, the growth velocity is particularly high approximating 1.6%/day for body weight and 1.0%/day for body length,[5,25-28] whereas body composition changes dramatically. Whole body composition of fetuses of various gestational ages has been collected from chemical carcass analysis of approximately 169 deceased fetuses and stillborn newborn infants[22] since the first report by H Fehling in 1877.[29] Although, as noted by Ziegler et al, 1976,[30] the published data fall considerably short of the ideal for numerous reasons, such as accuracy of gestational estimation, method of chemical analysis, and completeness of medical information on gestation, those data remain of considerable interest. From the data obtained in a limited number of those infants, the body composition of the "reference fetus" according to gestational age was characterized and is referred to in numerous studies. More recently, additional information obtained by other techniques, such as

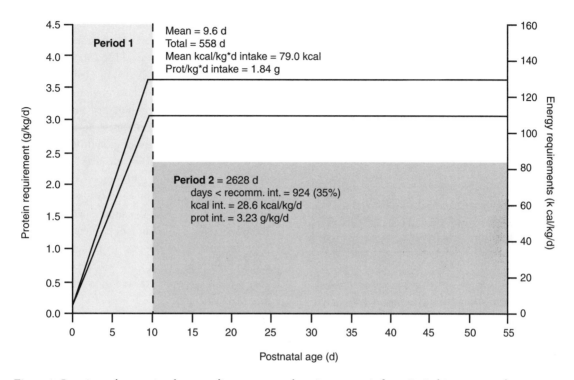

Figure 1: Protein and energy intakes according to postnatal age in preterm infants. Period 1 represents the transitory period when protein and energy supplies are progressively increased up to the recommended values. The black lines represent the minimal and maximal recommendations at once for protein and energy supplies for stable growing preterm infants.[18] Data for periods 1 and 2 were obtained in 58 VLBW infants (BW<1500 g).[9]

neutron activation[31] and DEXA[32,33] performed at birth, confirmed the reference values. At 22 weeks of gestational age, the fetus is composed almost exclusively of lean body mass (LBM). The protein content accounts for ±9% of body weight (BW) or LBM. At term, lean body mass represents about 87% of BW with a protein content of 12% of BW or 14% of the LBM. From those data, optimal weight gain, lean body mass gain and protein accretion can be estimated for preterm infants of similar gestational age (Figure 2). Considering that fat mass deposition is always significantly higher postnatally, lean body mass gain is preferable to weight gain in the evaluation of postnatal growth in preterm infants. Similarly, the contribution of protein gain to lean body mass gain appears as a more suitable reference. As shown in Figure 3, that value increases from 12 to 18% during the last trimester of gestation.

Factors Affecting Protein Metabolism in Preterm Infants

Protein turnover: A large body of literature has been published over the years using isotopic tracer kinetics for evaluating protein and nitrogen metabolism in neonates.[23,34-60] The use of isotopic tracer technique is based on the assumption that the tracer is representative of the unlabeled amino acids and can therefore be used as an indicator of the protein turnover. However, each amino acid is only representative of its own turnover inside of the protein pool. [39,41,54-56] In spite of methodological variations in the use of different tracers and models for the calculation of whole body protein parameters in preterm infants, the protein turnover (synthesis and breakdown) in growing preterm neonates has consistently been found high compared to term infants and older children. It has been suggested that the more immature the infant,

Per kg/d	HMF (n=48)	PTF (n=86)	p
Weight gain (g)	15.7±2.3	19.6±3.1	<0.001
Length gain (cm/wk)	0.95±0.34	1.07±0.35	=0.06
HC gain (cm/wk)	0.97±0.25	1.05±0.30	=0.010
LBM (g)	12.4±2.3	14.7±3.0	<0.001
Fat mass (g)	3.2±1.6	4.7±1.8	<0.001
BMC (mg)	215±86	263±83	=0.002
BA (cm²)	1.18±0.41	1.51±0.39	<0.001
Vol intake (ml)	164±12	152±12	<0.001
Energy (kcal)	118±10	119±12	=0.57
Protein (g)	2.9±0.3	3.3±0.4	<0.001

Table 2: Growth, weight gain composition and nutritional intake in preterm infants fed fortified human milk (HMF) and preterm formulas (PTF) (mean±SD). [19 and Rigo unpublished data]

the higher the rate of protein turnover.[17,18,40] Thus an inverse relationship was observed between post-conceptional age and the protein synthesis to gain ratio.

Whether or not preterm infants respond to nutrient administration predominantly by increasing protein synthesis or by suppression of protein breakdown is still a matter of debate.[23] First of all, it appears that energy supplied as glucose or fat has no significant effect on protein turnover and proteolysis.[47-49] When both energy and protein were provided, normal healthy neonates respond to enteral application by increasing protein synthesis instead of suppression of protein breakdown,[50] and to parenteral application by an increased rate of protein synthesis plus a significant reduction of proteolysis.[51] In preterm infants, several reports consistently showed that in response to protein and energy supply, both orally and parenterally, there is a corresponding increase in whole body protein turnover with a smaller decrease in protein breakdown from endogenous sources.[23,47,48,51-56] In response to nutrient administration, VLBW infants continue to have a higher rate of proteolysis than larger infants[51] but respond to exogenous infusion of amino acids by a reduction of endogenous protein

breakdown.[57,58] The variable degree of suppression of proteolysis observed in the various studies in response to nutrient administration could partly be the result of confounding factors, such as associated illness or the clinical support required in those preterm infants.[23]

Similar observations were obtained in SGA infants where catch-up growth increases protein turnover rate, but where a faster rate of growth was promoted by a lower value of protein turnover and a better protein synthesis to gain ratio compared to preterm infants with similar birth weight.[17,37,59,60] From data evaluating the dynamic aspects of protein metabolism using stable isotopes in preterm infants, it can be suggested that the cost of protein deposition could be slightly higher in ELBW infants as a result of higher protein turnover rates and a less efficient protein synthesis to gain ratio.[17,23]

Protein absorption and retention: Many factors are known to affect the various parameters of protein absorption and utilization in preterm infants.[17] The stomach does not contribute significantly to overall protein digestion. The breakdown of most large molecular weight proteins into smaller peptides and amino acids is the result of intestinal luminal hydrolysis and subsequent peptidase activities located at the level of microvillus membrane or within the enterocyte.[61] This activity may be affected by immaturity, the quality of the protein supply, and the technical process used for feeding design.[62-66] In addition, protein utilization is known to be affected by protein and nitrogen intakes, the biological value of ingested proteins, the energy: protein ratio, nutritional status, catch-up growth, hormonal environment and clinical status. Therefore, all thr protein or nitrogen supplies are not equivalent in terms of net protein utilization.

One of the most extensively used methods to evaluate protein metabolism in newborn infants is the relatively simple evaluation of protein intake and protein excretion, which allows the quantitative estimation of protein absorption (intake – fecal), protein retention (absorbed – urinary), retention rate (retention/absorption) or protein utilization (retention/intake). For more than twenty years, we

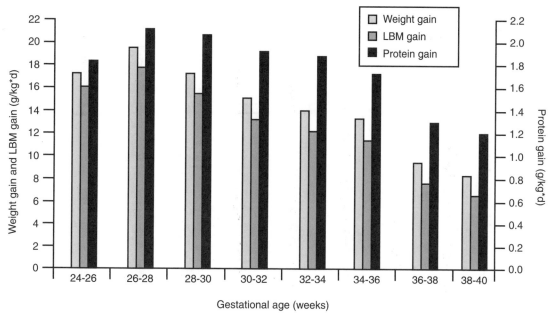

Figure 2: Weight gain, lean body mass (LBM) gain and protein accretion during the last trimester of gestation. Adapted from Widdowson 1981 [20], Ziegler 1986[21], Sparks 1984[22], Micheli 1993[17], and Kalhan 2000[23]

have performed metabolic balances studies in preterm infants fed human milk, supplemented or not with various human milk fortifiers or fed formulas.[66-76] In all, up to 358 balances with 30 different regimens were evaluated.[66]

Nitrogen Absorption: Fecal nitrogen excretion represents the sum of endogenous fecal nitrogen derived from the gastrointestinal tract (desquamation, secretion) and the non-absorbed fraction of nitrogen intake. The nitrogen absorption rate (absorbed/intake) differs significantly according to feeding regimen (Figure 4). It was higher with powder preterm formulas (90.7 ± 3.3 %) than with human milk ± Human Milk Fortifier (82.7 ± 4.8 %), protein hydrolyzed formulas (84.3 ± 4.0 %) or ready-to-use liquid preterm formulas (86.0 ± 5.0%) (Figure 4). These differences result from the variable nature of the protein. In human milk, non-nutritional proteins (eg, lactoferrin, IgA) or non-protein nitrogen (eg, oligosaccharides) are less well absorbed than the nutritional proteins (whey proteins, caseins)

and contribute to the fecal nitrogen excretion. An interesting observation is the relatively lower absorption rate of ready-to-use liquid preterm formulas or protein hydrolyzed preterm formulas. The technical process seems to impair nitrogen absorption by eg, heat treatment which induces some Maillard reaction, or by preliminary hydrolysis which alters the physiological absorption process in the lumen or at the border of the gastrointestinal tract.[62-64,77,78]

Computing the results of numerous metabolic balance studies reported by various groups, Micheli and Schutz, 1993,[17] suggested that nitrogen absorption could be directly related to gestational age and that immaturity of ELBW infants could significantly reduce absorbed nitrogen. The multivariate analysis of our data does not confirm this hypothesis but suggests that nitrogen absorption was independent of weight or gestational age at the time of the balance study (Figure 5). Whether the data observed in VLBW infants can be extrapolated to ELBW infants is still to be evaluated.

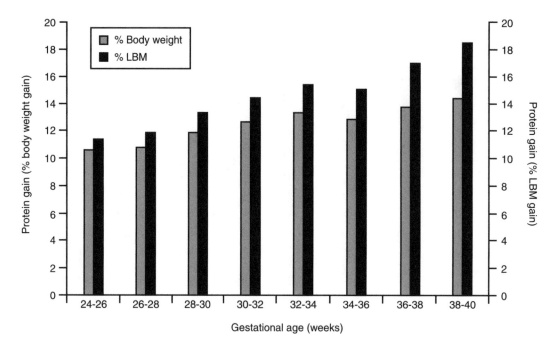

Figure 3: Contribution of protein gain to body weight (BW) gain and to lean body mass (LBM) gain during the last trimester of gestation. Adapted from Widdowson 1981[20], Ziegler 1986[21], Sparks 1984[22], Micheli 1993[17] and Kalhan 2000[23]

Nitrogen utilization: The efficiency of protein gain (or the biological value of the protein source) can be estimated by the ratio between retained and metabolizable nitrogen (absorbed) as well as by the slope of the regression line calculated between nitrogen retention and nitrogen absorbed (Figure 6). The efficiency of protein gain differs according to the feeding regimen (Table 2) the highest values were obtained in preterm infants fed powder and ready-to-use preterm formulas ($77.6 \pm 5.4\%$). It was significantly reduced in those fed protein hydrolyzed preterm fourmula (Prot Hydr PTF) ($74.0 \pm 6.9\%$) and HMF ($72.1 \pm 7.6\%$). The lower value obtained with HMF may be related to the non-protein nitrogen (NPN) fraction of human milk, which represents 20 to 25% of the total nitrogen content of human milk, and still 13.5 to 17% of total nitrogen content of HMF fortified human milk.[79-81] As demonstrated for urea nitrogen, the contribution of this metabolizable NPN fraction to protein gain (urea availability) is lower than that of the alpha-lactalbumin or the casein of human milk. By contrast, the

significantly lower protein gain value obtained with Prot Hydr PTF suggests that the process of hydrolysis by itself reduces the biological value of hydrolysed protein.[67,78]

Therefore, with regard to net protein utilization (N retained/N intake), preterm formulas appear to be more efficient than human milk with or without protein supplementation. However, in formulas the net protein utilization can be altered by various technical processes such as heat treatment or hydrolysis.

Computing numerous metabolic balance studies in preterm infants, Micheli and Schutz, 1993,[17] showed that the efficiency of protein gain, ie, the ratio between nitrogen retained and metabolizable nitrogen (nitrogen absorbed), seems to be independent from gestational age. By contrast, in preterm infants fed HMF or preterm formulas, in powder and liquid form, the efficiency of protein gain (retained/metabolizable ratio) was inversely related to body weight suggesting a higher efficiency of protein deposition in ELBW infants (Figure 7).

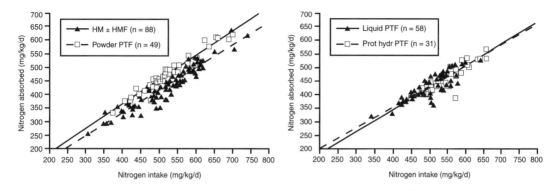

Figure 4: Nitrogen absorption according to nitrogen intakes in preterm infants fed human milk with and without human milk fortifier (n=88), powder (n=49), liquid (n=58) or protein hydrolysed (n=31) preterm formulas (PTF).[66]

Plasma Amino Acid Concentrations

Several amino acid metabolic pathways are immature in preterm infants. These infants are, therefore, at risk of semi-essential amino acid deficiency or essential amino acid overload. The optimal value for plasma amino acid concentrations in preterm infants is a matter of discussion. At least three different "gold standards" have been proposed for the premature infant:[17,79-85] first, the amino acid concentrations in umbilical cord plasma obtained by fetal cord puncture or after birth; second, that of rapidly growing preterm infants receiving their own mother's milk or human milk supplemented with human milk proteins; third, that of healthy breast-fed term infants. For LBW infants, levels obtained during the last trimester of gestation or in well-growing preterm infants fed optimal intakes of human milk protein appear to be safe. However, considering that large differences are observed for some amino acids (THR, VAL, TYR PHE, LYS and HIS) between fetal and postnatal values, a combined reference has been proposed (Figure 8) taking into account the mean ± 1SD of the values obtained in cord blood and in preterm infants fed human milk supplemented with human milk protein.[86-88]

> **The basis of re-evaluating protein requirements for preterm infants:**
> • Previous recommendations
> • Needs for the compensation of the initial protein gap and the early catch up growth.

> • Fetal reference related to lean body mass and protein gain instead of weight gain.
> • All protein supplies are not equivalent in term of net protein utilizaiton affected by immaturity, protein quality and technological processes.
> • AA requirements instead of protein requirement need additional evaluations in enteral and parenteral nutrition (optimal AA composition).
> • Protein energy ratio affect protein deposition and relative lean body mass gain.

It is still a matter of debate whether the plasma amino acid disturbances frequently observed in preterm infants on oral or parenteral nutrition are harmful for development. Nevertheless, when one essential amino acid is administered both in excessive as well as deficient amounts in relation to other amino acids for protein synthesis, the metabolic fate of the excessive amino acids will be, besides imbalances, oxidation rather than protein synthesis. Therefore, efforts have been made to maintain the plasma amino acid concentrations in an acceptable level whatever the protein diet and the route of administration.

Human milk protein quality is considered the golden standard, even if its nitrogen content is not adapted to the high protein requirement of preterm infants. Considering that bovine whey and casein have a different amino acid composition compared to human milk, and that human milk contains a large proportion of non-protein nitrogen which is partially available for protein synthesis, it is virtually

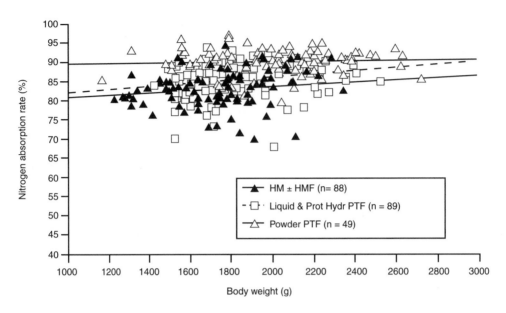

Figure 5: Absence of relationship between nitrogen absorption rate and body weight in preterm infants fed human milk with and without human milk fortifier (n=88), powder (n=49), liquid (n=58), or protein hydrolysed (n=31) preterm formulas (PTF).[66]

impossible to obtain cow milk based formulas with a nitrogen content and amino acid pattern identical to human milk.

Preterm infants fed human milk fortified with cow milk whole protein or casein hydrolysate have plasma amino acid concentrations approximating the normal range. By contrast, the use of whey hydrolysate as fortifier induces significant increases in plasma threonine and a relative reduction in phenylalanine.[74,86]

Numerous studies have evaluated indices of protein metabolism and plasma amino acid concentrations in preterm infants fed formula with various whey:casein ratios.[77,89-91] From more recent data,[77] it is suggested that the type of protein has no effect on metabolic stress, acidosis, uremia or hyperammonemia, contrary to data reported in preterm infants receiving older preterm formulas.[92-94] Present day formulas for preterm infants differ from formulas used in the 1970s, not only by their higher metabolizable nitrogen content, but also by considerably higher sodium and phosphorus contents. Considering the intrauterine relationship between sodium and phosphorus accretion and the accretion of nitrogen, it is conceivable that an inadequate intake of those nutrients required for protein synthesis of new tissue will inhibit the use of nitrogen for production of lean body mass.

However, the whey:casein ratio significantly influences the individual amino acid supply and the plasma amino acid concentrations. Thus, plasma threonine is increased and histidine relatively decreased in infants fed whey predominant formula, whereas methionine and aromatic amino acids are increased in those fed casein predominant formula.[77] The high plasma threonine concentration observed in preterm infants fed whey predominant formulas is related to the glycomacropeptide obtained from casein by enzymatic casein precipitation of cow milk proteins. Acidic precipitation, by contrast, removes the glycomacropeptide rich in threonine from the soluble phase.[95-97] Therefore, it is presently possible to design whey predominant formulas (WPF) with a lower threonine content.[97-100] Fourteen preterm infants receiving either an enzymatic or an acidic whey predominant formula showed a sharp reduction in plasma threonine concentration while fed the acidic WPF (27.9 ± 8.5 µmol/dl), compared to those

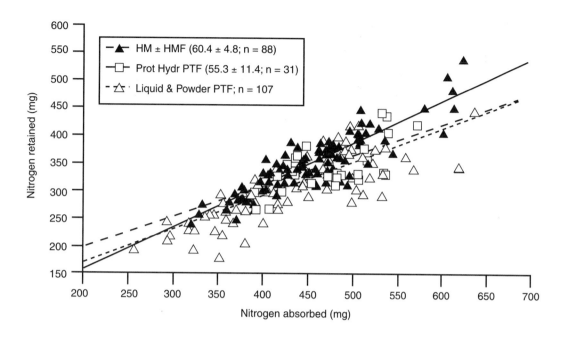

Figure 6: Relationship between nitrogen retained and nitrogen absorbed in preterm infants fed human milk with or without human milk fortifier (n=88), powder (n=49), liquid (n=58), or protein hydrolysed (n=31) preterm formulas (PTF).[62]

receiving the conventional WPF (37.5 ± 8.4 µmol/dl). All other plasma amino acid concentrations were similar with the exception of valine (reduced in the acidic WPF fed infants).[97]

The mixture of proteins in human milk is particularly rich in tryptophan and cystein and low in methionine, a pattern difficult to achieve with commercially available proteins due to the low alpha-lactalbumin content of cow milk proteins. Considering that tryptophan is essential to brain maturation and development and that tryptophan could be a limiting amino acid in highly growing preterm infants, enrichment of preterm formula with bovine alpha-lactalbumin could be of interest.[65,101]

Formulas based on hydrolyzed proteins have been recently proposed for the feeding of preterm infants to reduce gastrointestinal disturbances[67,73,102] such as delayed gastric emptying, abdominal distention, hard stools and feeding intolerance. The technological processes necessary to perform hydrolysis and reduce protein antigenicity may, however, modify amino acid content and/or amino acid bioavailability.[78] The use of a higher percentage of whey in the protein hydrolyzed formulas worsens the plasma amino acid distortions previously observed with the use of whey predominant formulas, increasing threonine and decreasing aromatic amino acid concentrations.[67] Moreover, sharp decreases in plasma histidine and tryptophan concentrations were also observed which could be due to a relative reduction in amino acid bioavailability. Thus, additional histidine and tryptophan supplementation and more appropriate technology have been developed for these formulas.[98,103-105]

Nevertheless, considering that the nutritional strategy for preterm infants is to provide indispensable amino acids at a level sufficient to meet the demands for protein synthesis while avoiding an excessive supply, further studies are requested to re-evaluate the individual amino acid requirements in ELBW infants. For this purpose, the use of the amino acid oxidation methodology to evaluate the individual amino acid requirements appears as a promising technique.[41,106]

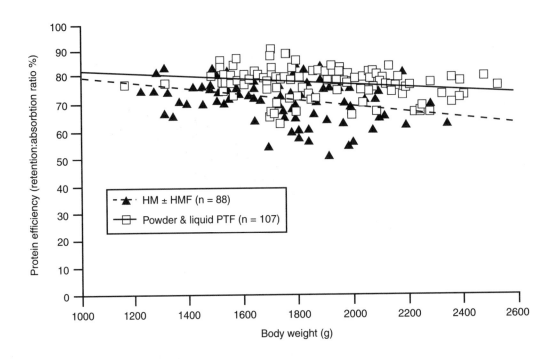

Figure 7: Relationship between protein efficiency and body weight in preterm infants fed human milk with and without human milk fortifier (n=88), powder (n=49) or liquid (n=58) preterm formulas (PTF).[66]

Protein Energy Interaction

In addition to the relationships between whole body rate of protein synthesis and protein gain as well as nitrogen intake and nitrogen retention, there is a relationship between energy expenditure and protein gain.[17] It has been suggested that the energy cost for the deposition of 1g of protein is between 5.5 and 10 kcal in preterm infants.[18,107] These data, which exceed by far the theoretical energy necessary for the biochemical synthesis of 1g of protein from isolated amino acids (±1 kcal/g), illustrate the dynamic aspect of protein turnover where protein gain results from the difference between protein synthesis and breakdown so that each gram of protein deposition requests five to six times more protein to be synthesized. Therefore, protein gain is not only related to protein intake but also to energy intake, and rapid growth is a situation where protein-energy interrelationships are of special relevance. Protein and energy are supplied concurrently, and it is reasonable to assume that there is an optimal range of protein-energy intake for each

newborn. In fasting adults, the provision of carbohydrate equivalent to about 20% of energy requirement can reduce the irreversible protein-nitrogen loss to a minimum. In preterm infants, the nitrogen loss in the prolonged fasting state has not been evaluated for ethical reasons. Nevertheless, several studies, mainly in parenteral nutrition,[108,109] have shown that preterm infants, who are not receiving exogenous nitrogen, use endogenous protein as an energy source with urinary nitrogen losses representing around 150 mg/kg*d (±1 g of protein). When metabolizable energy intake is lower than maintenance requirements, dietary nitrogen is not retained efficiently. An intake of 50 kcal/kg/d induces some nitrogen saving, whereas a provision of >300 mg/kg*d of nitrogen allows positive nitrogen balance. When energy intake is sub-optimal (metabolizable energy between 50 and 90 kcal/kg*d), the newborn infant is in a very sensitive range of protein-energy interaction. An increase in either the energy or protein intake will result in an increase in nitrogen retention. By contrast,

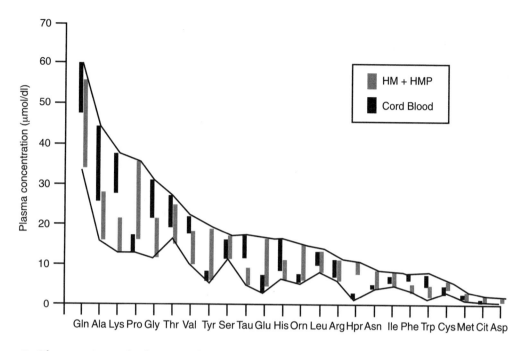

Figure 8: Plasma amino acid reference combining the mean ± 1SD of the values obtain in cord blood and preterm infants fed human milk supplemented with human milk protein.[86,88]

when metabolizable non-protein calories exceed 70-80 kcal/kg*d, the level of nitrogen intake is the primary determinant of nitrogen retention. Thus, it is probably important to separate protein saving from proteolysis. Protein saving is a decrease in irreversible nitrogen loss due to protein oxidation and is responsive to the availability of energy. Proteolysis is protein breakdown and release of amino acid as an important component of tissue remodelling and protein accretion, but it is less responsive to energy administration.[23]

With an intermediate intake of energy (100 kcal/kg*d) and protein (2.5 g/kg*d), the major effect of increasing the energy intake is the promotion of weight gain by fat mass deposition, whereas, the major effect of increasing the protein supply is weight gain through promotion of lean body mass accretion with a concomitant relative reduction in fat mass deposition.[24] It is still a matter of discussion if this effect persists at higher levels of energy and protein supply, and if it is useful to increase the protein:energy ratio over 3.3 g/100 kcal.[24]

This matter has been investigated by Kashyap et al 1994[110] evaluating a mathematical model for predicting the rate and composition of weight gain in relation to the protein and energy intakes in low-birth-weight (LBW) infants. However, infants fed a 3.6 g/100 kcal formula, providing 625 mg of metabolizable nitrogen/kg*d for 111 kcal/kg*d of metabolizable energy, did not show a rate and composition of weight gain comparable to that of a fetus at postconceptional age at discharge. Protein retention was lower than expected, and some indices of protein overload were observed. The provision of additional metabolizable energy up to 150 kcal/kg*d increased weight gain and fat deposition without major changes in nitrogen retention.[107,110-112] In addition, a recent study from the same group[113] suggests that energy supplied as carbohydrate is more effective than energy supplied as fat in sparing protein oxidation. From these studies, it seems that preterm infants require a protein:energy ratio higher than that of current LBW infant formula to obtain significant catch-up growth without fat accretion vastly in excess of the intrauterine rate.[114] Nevertheless, presently, it seems unrealistic and probably not necessary to mimic the quality of fetal tissue

	Group I	Group II	Group III	Group IV
HMF/PTF	6/4	3/5	1/7	0/1
Protein intake (g/kg*d)	2.7	3.6	3.4	4.1
Energy intake (kcal/kg*d)	118	113	143	142
Protein energy ratio (g/100 kcal)	2.27	3.21	2.39	2.88
N infants	107	85	79	15
Birth weight (g)	1353	1369	1379	1325
Gestational age (wks)	31	31	31	31
Weight gain (g/kg*d)	16.4	18.0	20.4	24
Length gain (cm/wks)	1.5	1.13	1.14	1.39
LBM gain (g/kg*d)	12.2	14.7	14.9	18.5
Fat mass gain (g/kg*d)	4.22	3.37	5.55	5.54
Protein gain (g/kg*d)	1.78	2.35	2.37	2.87
Protein gain (% BW gain)	10.9	13.0	11.6	12.0
Protein gain (% LBM gain)	14.7	16.1	16.2	15.6

Table 3: *Weight gain and weight gain composition in preterm infants. Data related to protein intake and protein:energy ratio were obtained after computing the various studies evaluating growth and weight gain composition in preterm infants fed human milk,[46,115-120] human milk fortifiers[115,118,121-126] and preterm formulas.[46,68,70,110,116,119-121,124,125,127,128]*

deposition in LBW infants. The optimal postnatal fat mass deposition is still on debate. Therefore, it seems more appropriate to take into account the lean body and the length gain to appreciate the catch-up growth in those preterm infants.

Compilation of various studies in preterm infants fed human milk,[46,115-120] human milk fortifiers[115,118,121-126] and various preterm formulas[46,68,70,110,116,119-121,124,125,127,128] allows evaluation of the main determinants of weight gain, nitrogen retention and fat mass deposition. These data represent about 286 preterm infants with a mean birth weight of 1354 g and a gestational age of 30.5 weeks; 22 groups were fed human milk with/without human milk fortifiers and 25 received various preterm formulas. Table 3 shows the results available on growth, nitrogen retention and nonprotein energy stored distributed in four groups related to energy and protein supply. From those published data, the major determinants of weight gain, lean body mass

gain, fat accretion and protein retention may be determined using stepwise regression analysis. Protein intake and protein:energy ratio (PER) are the main determinants of weight gain, whereas protein intake is the only determinant of LBM gain. By contrast, fat mass gain is positively related to energy intake and negatively influenced by the protein:energy ratio. Protein gain and lean body mass gain increase significantly with protein supply without any additional significant influence of energy intake and protein:energy ratio. As suggested by Figures 9 and 10, protein intake and protein:energy ratio are the main determinants of growth and body composition in preterm infants.

Route of Administration

The amino acid profile and concentration in parenteral nutrition solution generally reflect those in oral diets. However, there is some evidence that

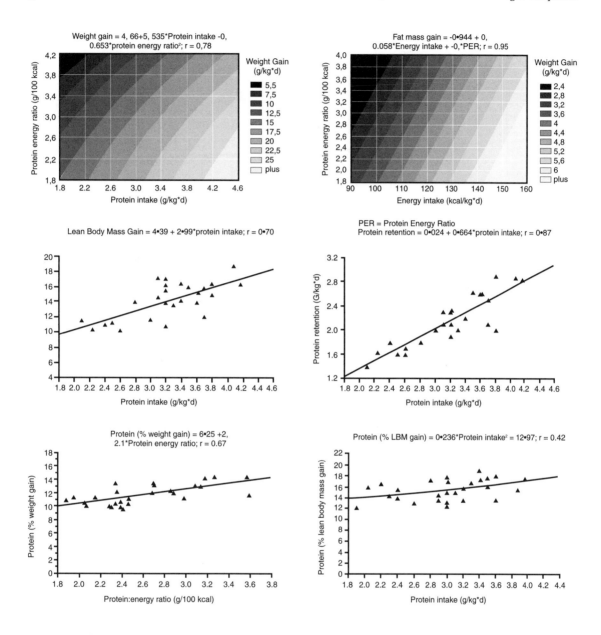

Figure 9: Influence of nutrient supplies on weight gain and weight gain composition in stable growing preterm infants fed human milk,[46,115-120] human milk fortifiers[115,118,121-126] and preterm formulas.[46,68,70,110,116,119-121, 124,125,127,128]

parenteral amino acid requirements could be affected from by-passing nutrient absorption and first-pass metabolism by splanchnic tissues. By contrast, the nitrogen content of parenteral amino acid solution represents the sum of the nitrogen content of the individual amino acids. Thus, nitrogen content of 1g of amino acid is related to its amino acid composition and is frequently lower than that of 1g of protein.[86] A more important difference between parenteral and enteral nutrition could be the individual amino acid

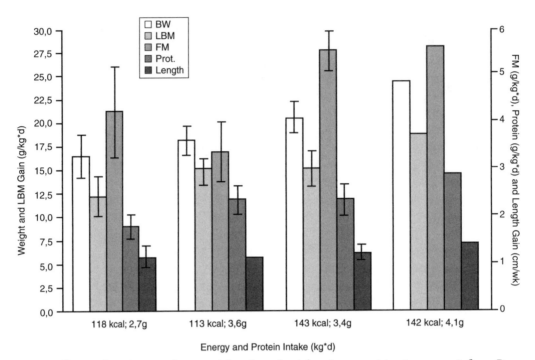

Figure 10: Influence of nutrient supplies on weight gain and weight gain composition in preterm infants. Data were obtained after computing the various studies evaluating growth and weight gain composition in preterm infants fed human milk[46,115-120], human milk fortifiers[115,118,121-126] and preterm formulas.[46,68,70,110,116,119-121,124,125,127,128]

requirements. Indeed, gut and liver metabolism could differently affect the individual indispensable amino acid metabolism. Recent data suggest that specific studies need to re-evaluate the individual amino acid profile of parenteral amino acid solution for preterm infants.[41,129]

Revised Recommendation for Protein Intake in Preterm Infants

The quality of clinical care offered to extremely premature infants has improved since the publication of the previous recommendations for feeding premature infants. Several reports stress the point that severe postnatal growth restriction, which frequently occurs in those infants, has the potential of long-term deleterious effects on growth, neurodevelopmental outcome and adult health. Most of the actual nutritional recommendations were designed with the aim to provide postnatal protein retention during the "stable-growing" period equivalent to the intrauterine protein

gain of a normal fetus and without considering the relatively long transitional period necessary to reach the recommended energy and protein supplies, which induces the cumulative nutritional deficit and requires an early catch-up growth. It is, therefore, appropriate to revise the recommendations concerning nutrition for preterm infants.

The recommendations for "stable-growing" preterm infants are based on recent data, which suggest that preterm infants fed human milk fortifier or various preterm formulas providing nutritional supplies in the range of the previous recommendations develop a significant growth deficit until the time of discharge and of corrected term. In order to better approach the protein requirement for optimal intrauterine reference growth, the development of LBM gain instead of weight gain is taken into account, while keeping in mind the dramatic change in fat mass deposition that occurs postnatally during the stable growing period in newborn infants. In consideration of the decreasing

Revised advisable protein recommendation for growing preterm infants		
	Without need of catch-up growth	With need of catch-up growth
26-30 wks PCA: 16-18 g/kg*d LBM 14% prot retention	3.8-4.2 g/kg*d PER: ~3.3	4.4 g/kg*d PER: ~3.4
30-36 wks PCA: 14-15 g/kg*d LBM 15% prot retention	3.4-3.6 g/kg*d PER: ~2.8	3.8-4.2 g/kg*d PER: ~3.3
36-40 wks PCA: 13 g/kg*d LBM 17% prot retention	2.8-3.2 g/kg*d PER: 2.4-2.6	3.0-3.4 g/kg*d PER: 2.6-2.8

Table 4: Revised recommended protein intake and protein:energy ratio (PER) for preterm infants according to postconceptional age and the need of catch-up growth.

LBM gain and protein retention with increasing gestational age, and in agreement with studies on protein metabolism in preterm infants of various gestational age, the revised values were adapted for the postconceptional age instead of gestational age or birth weight to integrate the dynamic aspect of growth and protein metabolism in the recommendation. In addition, the data available on growth and weight gain composition in preterm infants were re-analyzed with respect to nutrient intake. Because the results suggest that protein intake and protein to energy ratio are the main determinants of growth and body composition during the stable growing period, these two aspects of protein supply were integrated in the recommendations. Nutritional deprivations arise in the early adaptative period as well as from several neonatal events and illness; therefore, additional recommendations are suggested to promote early catch-up growth before discharge. Despite differences in several aspects, the updated recommendations (Table 4) are in line with previous guidelines from other Committees as summarized in Table 1.

Large randomized controlled trials are unfortunately unavailable, but most of the available cohort studies were considered and combined in the analysis. There is much more information on low-birth-weight (greater than 1000 g) infants than on those with extremely low birth weights (less than 750 g). Thus, estimates of the intake required by infants with extremely low birth weights were mainly extrapolated from data involving larger premature infants. Therefore, recommendations for these infants are more tentative than those for larger infants.

In a recent evaluation which combined various growth and body composition parameters to design a mathematical model for predicting the relationship between protein and energy intakes and the rate and composition of weight gain, Kashyap et al, 1994,[110] underline that the rate and composition of weight gain can be manipulated by intake. In their validation study, they observed that values correlated closely with the predicted outcomes even if the individual outcomes were less satisfactory. This could be the result of multiple poorly identified biological independent variables influencing variations in growth. In the study of Embleton, 2001,[7] about 45% of the variation of growth was not explained by the recorded nutritional parameters. Therefore, these studies underline the need to control as closely as possible for additional parameters that can potentially affect growth and interfere with the accurate evaluation of revised recommendations in a randomized controlled multi-center study on short- and long-term outcomes. Nutritional factors include Ca, P, Na, trace elements, vitamins, etc. Non-nutritional factors include diseases, drugs and hormonal environment. For this study, the use of DEXA to evaluate the three compartments of weight gain composition could be

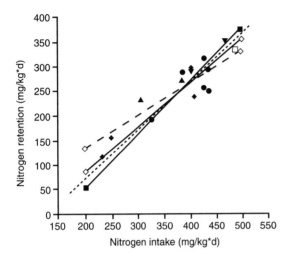

Figure 11: Relationship between nitrogen retention and nitrogen intake in parenterally fed preterm infants. Mean data (individual figures) and retention to intake regression lines were obtained from various studies.[36,139-148]

helpful to avoid more invasive processes such as metabolic balance and indirect calorimetry.

Particular Aspects of Recommendations
Parenteral Nutrition

The current issues have been the object of excellent reviews.[130-136]

Nitrogen utilization: Considerable improvements in parenteral amino acid (AA) solutions have been achieved since the late 1960s, when casein hydrolysate was the source of intravenous protein. The use of crystalline amino acid mixtures in the early 1980s improved nitrogen utilization, and specific pediatric amino acid solutions have been designed in the early 1990s with high essential:non-essential AA ratios and conditionally essential amino acid content adapted for use in LBW infants. Mixtures were designed to mimic the human milk amino acid content[137] to achieve plasma amino acid concentrations of healthy 30 day-old breast-fed term infants 2 hours post-prandial[138,139] or to obtain a plasma amino acid profile in the range of the cord blood values.[140] In spite of the diversity in composition, parenteral amino acid solutions used in pediatric care do not change

significantly nitrogen utilization.[86,88] However, the amino acid nitrogen content is related to the amino acid composition and varies from 134 to 158 mg/g of AA.[86] It is, therefore, preferable to consider nitrogen intake rather than amino acid intake. Results of nitrogen balances in preterm infants[36,139-148] show that a nitrogen retention of 380 mg/kg*d can be obtained with a nitrogen intake of 530 mg/kg*d, which corresponds to a nitrogen efficiency of 70%. This is a slightly higher value than that recorded in oral nutrition (Figure 11).[86,88] From these data it can be concluded that the amino acid requirement in parenteral nutrition is close to that of protein requirement for enteral nutrition.

Amino acid composition: Optimal supply of amino acids is also crucial in parenteral nutrition. If the pattern of amino acid is not well balanced, the first limiting amino acid will compromise protein synthesis. Alternatively, parenterally fed preterm infants are at risk of amino acid toxicity from excessive intake, immaturity of degradative pathways, immaturity of kidney function for nitrogen excretion, lack of small intestinal metabolism, or absence of "first hepatic pass." The optimal amino acid pattern of parenteral amino acid solutions for preterm infants still needs to be determined.[135] It should be guided by the following principles:[134]

- The requirement of essential amino acids is larger than in full-term neonates or larger infants.[149]
- The activities of tyrosine aminotransferase and 4-hydroxyphenylpyruvate dioxygenase are considered to be immature during the neonatal period.[150]
- The activity of cystathionase in the neonate is low and cysteine synthesis from methionine is reduced.[150,151]
- Attention is required for the nutritional supply of taurine during the neonatal period. Although cysteine sulphinic acid decarboxylase activity has been demonstrated in preterm infants, taurine is probably a conditionally essential amino acid in the neonate.[152]
- In addition to cysteine and tyrosine, histidine, glycine and arginine are categorized as semi-essential in neonates.[153]

- Organ dysfunction tends to occur with excess or default of individual amino acids: liver disease with methionine excess,[130,154] pulmonary hypertension and necrotizing enterocolitis with low plasma glutamine and arginine concentrations.[155,156]

Phenylalanine and tyrosine supply: Hyperphenyl-alaninemia has been observed in some TPN fed preterm infants receiving a high phenylalanine supply of 7.9% of total amino acids.[157-159] Relative hypertyrosinemia has been observed in the more immature infants in spite of the limited tyrosine supply due to its poor solubility.[88,142,159] In addition, a negative effect of leucine intake on plasma aromatic AA was also observed.[86,160] Because of the low solubility of tyrosine, N-acetyl tyrosine has been used as a soluble compound. Unfortunately, the newborn infant has a low capacity of deacetylation, and most of the acetylated AA appears unchanged in the plasma and was excreted in the urine.[161] Recently, using the soluble dipeptide glycyl-L-tyrosine, Roberts et al, 1998,[162] evaluated the PHE and TYR requirement in parenteral nutrition. They suggest that the safe aromatic AA intake that meets the needs of the term neonate is approximately 7.9% of the AA supply with a PHE:TYR ratio of 56:44. Whether those requirements are identical for ELBW infants needs to be evaluated.

Methionine and cystine supply: Cysteine is a conditionally essential amino acid in newborn infants due to the low activity of the rate limiting enzyme cystathionase in premature infants.[143,151] Cysteine is unstable in solution and easily oxidized to the insoluble form cystine. Therefore, most of the commercial solutions contain very low (or no) cysteine and variable amounts of methionine (1.8 to 5.5%) to meet the total sulphur requirement.

There are continuing controversies over cysteine supplementation as cysteine hydrochloride or acetyl-cysteine in premature human infants. Indeed, although plasma cystine concentration appears to be highly predictive of protein synthesis on the fourth day of life[163] and despite some evidence that plasma cystine concentrations increase with cystein supplementation, clinical condition or nitrogen retention does not

appear to be improved, whereas there is a risk of worsening metabolic acidosis with supplemented parenteral nutrition.[161,164] In preterm infants the activity of cystathionase increases with gestational age.[86,88] In the absence of cysteine supply the cysteine requirement must be covered by the methionine supply. Such a relative high methionine supply leads to an increase in plasma methionine concentration and has been implicated in the parenteral nutrition induced cholestasis.[165,166] Therefore, the effect of replacing a portion of methionine with cysteine in intravenous solutions for human neonates should be carefully evaluated. This is necessary in view of animal studies, which showed that the methionine intake required to maximize protein synthesis in newborn piglets fed intravenously was only 69% of the intragastric requirement.[129,135] In addition, there are not much lot of data showing that taurine is also considered a conditionally essential amino acid due to the reduction of liver cysteine sulphinic acid decarboxylase activity in newborn infants. When fed taurine deficient diets a significant reduction in plasma and urinary taurine concentrations occurred.[152] While we still await more evidence for taurine essentiality, taurine supplementation at a level close to human milk content has become widespread both in parenteral solutions and formula for preterm and term infants.[167,168]

Amino Acids for Special Purpose in Oral or Parenteral Nutrition

Arginine: Arginine is a precursor of nitric oxide. An inadequate availability has been implicated in various neonatal diseases, such as persistent pulmonary hypertension[155] and necrotizing enterocolitis.[169] Recent evidence suggests that de novo arginine synthesis in the neonate depends upon small intestinal metabolism, and dietary arginine requirements could be higher in parentally fed infants.[129,135] Presently, arginine content varies widely in pediatric parenteral solutions, illustrating that the dietary requirement in parenteral and oral nutrition needs to be elucidated.

Glutamine: Glutamine is the most abundant amino acid in the human body and the predominant amino acid supplied to the fetus through the placenta.[170] Glutamine is an important fuel for rapidly dividing cells such as enterocytes and lymphocytes.[171] It is a regulator of acid-base balance via ammonium and an important precursor of nucleic acids, nucleotides, amino-sugars and protein.[172] There is, however, little information on the role of glutamine in children and infants, or whether glutamine supplementation is beneficial in preterm babies. In ELBW infants and during critical illness, glutamine could be a conditionally essential amino acid.[172] Glutamine supplementation in preterm infants might enhance gut mucosal integrity, thus improving enteral feed tolerance and reduce time spent on parenteral nutrition, thereby improving weight gain and ultimately shortening the hospital stay.[173] Improving gut barrier function and lymphocyte production might reduce the rate of sepsis.[174] Although parenteral glutamine failed to enhance rates of protein synthesis, glutamine may have an acute protein-sparing effect, as it suppressed leucine oxidation and protein breakdown in parenterally fed very-low-birth-weight infants.[175] Up to now, there is no clear evidence of a beneficial effect of supplementing glutamine to the oral and parenteral nutrition of preterm infants.[176-178] This may be a promising field for research, and we need to await the results of large randomized controlled trials presently under evaluation.

Additional Nitrogen Compounds

Carnitine: Carnitine, a quaternary amino acid, plays an important role in the oxidation of long-chain fatty acids. Both breast milk and infant formulas contain carnitine. It is not routinely provided in parenteral nutrition solutions. Non-supplemented parenterally fed infants have reduced carnitine levels. The clinical significance of this is uncertain. Carnitine deficiency may be an etiological factor in the limited ability of premature babies to utilize parenteral lipids. Among infants supplemented with carnitine, there was no evidence of effect on weight gain, lipid utilization or ketogenesis. Up to now, there is no evidence to support the routine supplementation of parenterally fed neonates with carnitine.[179]

Nucleotides: Nucleotides are ubiquitous intracellular compounds of crucial importance for cellular function and metabolism.[180] Because nucleotides are components of the non-protein nitrogen fraction of human milk,[181-183] nucleotide supplementation of preterm formulas has been introduced in various countries. Dietary nucleotides have been shown to have important effects on several components of the immune system.[184] They appear to facilitate phagocytosis and increase natural killer cell activity. Production of interleukin-2 by stimulated mononuclear cells was higher in infants fed supplemented formula.[185] Nucleotides promote iron absorption, and this action might partly explain the higher iron absorption rate from human milk.[186] Nucleotides affect lipoprotein and long-chain polyunsaturated fatty acid metabolism.[187] Dietary nucleotides play a role in hepatic and enterocyte lipoprotein synthesis leading to HDL and VLDL lipoprotein profiles similar to human-milk-fed infants.[188] In addition, they promote the plasma and phospholipid membrane content in ω-6 PUFA.[189-190] The latter effect could be the result of effects on the fecal flora, because the bifidobacterial flora possesses the necessary enzymes for elongation and desaturation of fatty acids, or of a direct modulation of chain elongation and desaturation in the enterocyte or in the liver.[180] In the intestine, nucleotide supplementation seems to enhance maturation and growth.[191] This trophic effect on the intestine might explain the beneficial effect reported on growth in IUGR infants.[192] Therefore, the European Union has recognized nucleotides as semi-essential components of initial formula and has drafted norms to regulate nucleotide-supplemented formula.[193] However, up to now, there is no general consensus on the necessity for nucleotide supplementation, and further work is necessary to identify the beneficial role of nucleotides in preterm infants.

Practical Aspects of Clinical Nutrition in the Preterm Infant

In preterm infants, practical aspects of clinical nutrition can be described for two successive periods; the early adaptive or "transition" period from birth to

	Eoprotin (Milupa) powder	FM-85 (Nestl) powder	BMF (Nutricia) sachet 1.5 g	EHMF1 (M-J)* sachet 0.9 g	SHMF (Abbott) sachet 0.9 g	WHMF (Whyeth) sachet 2 g	EHMF2 (M-J)* sachet 0.8 g	EHMF3 (M-J) sachet 0.7 g
Protein (g)	1	1	1	1	1	1	1	1
Monoglyceride (g/g prot)	0	0	0	0	0.36	0	0.58	0.91
CH (g/g prot)	3.8	4.3	2.86	3.9*	1.8	2.0*	1.0*	0.2
Na (mg/g prot)	12.4	32.3	8.7	10.3	15.0	15.0	1.0	15.0
K (mg/g prot)	9.7	13.8	5.7	23.0	62.9	20.0	18.2	26.0
Ca (mg/g prot)	81	61	87	136	117	80	82	82
Mg (mg/g prot)	7.5	2.4	8.6	1.5	7.0	2.0	0.9	0.9
P (mg/g prot)	56	40.7	58.4	66.8	67.2	40.0	41.0	45.0
Cl (mg/g prot)	8.7	22.2	10.1	26.0	37.9	14.0	8.2	12.0
Energy (kcal/g prot)	19	21.4	14.3	20.7	14.0	13.0	12.7	12.7
Osmol/g/g prot	96	96	85	177	90	136	59	40

*Including glycerophosphate content

Table 5: Composition of various human milk fortifiers (HMF) per gram of protein content.

the second week of life, and the "stable-growing" period up to discharge from the neonatal unit, which is generally close to term post-conceptional age (35-37 wks PCA). Depending on birth weight and gestational age, the transition period may be severely extended, particularly in ELBW infants with major clinical disorders.

The Transition Period

During the early transition period, infants (particularly those with a birth weight below 1000 g) are likely to lose weight and be clinically and metabolically unstable, primarily as a result of shifts in water balance and relative starvation. The minimum achievable goal during this period is the provision of sufficient nutrients, parenterally or enterally, to prevent nutrient deficiencies and substrate catabolism, and to initiate positive nitrogen retention. If the infant is quite stable, increasing intakes can be provided to reach the optimal requirements and to reduce the transition period.

During the early transition period, protein (amino-acids) should be given to prevent breakdown of endogenous tissue. Numerous studies[36,55,194-199] underline the importance of an early introduction of protein/

amino acid supply in ELBW infants even on the first day of life to improve protein metabolism. The minimum protein requirement to achieve a zero nitrogen balance in healthy growing preterm infants receiving full enteral feeding providing 110 kcal/kg*d (460 kj/kg*d) corresponds to about 0.75 g/kg*d.[106] By contrast, during the first days of life, when only a "maintenance" energy intake of 50 to 60 kcal/kg (209 to 250 kJ/kg) per day is provided, approximately 1.0-1.5 g of amino acid/kg*d is required parenterally.[194] An early higher protein/amino acid supply of 1.5-2.0 g/kg/d could also be beneficial in preterm infants with increased protein breakdown, such as induced by prenatal maternal or postnatal corticosteroid therapy and by catabolic stress due to diseases or early neonatal surgery.[199-205] When positive nitrogen balance is expected, a more aggressive nutritional strategy is necessary. Increasing the amino acid supply from 1 g to 3 g/kg*d with a "maintenance" energy intake of 50 to 60 kcal/kg (209 to 250 kJ/kg) per day allows early positive nitrogen balance without inducing negative side effects. No differences were observed in blood pH, ammonia, and urea concentrations with this approach.[206]

> **Protein intake during the transition period:**
> - To achieve a zero nitrogen balance:
>   - 0.75 g/kg/d in healthy growing preterm infants
>   - 1.0-1.5 g/kg*d during the first days of life when energy supply is limited
>   - 1.5-2.0 g/kg/d during the first days of life if concomitant catabolic conditions are present
> - To achieve a positive nitrogen balance:
>   - 2.5-3.0 g/kg/d during the first days of life when energy supply is limited
> - Progressive increase in energy and protein supplies up to recommended values for conceptional age

The general practice in the NICU to increase both the energy and protein supply in parallel during the first few days of life, is one of the major clinical factors limiting the practical protein supply during the transition period in ELBW infants due to the relative glucose intolerance frequently observed after the first day of life. Hyperglycemia is not only the result of the glucose intake but the result of an impaired neonatal glucose homeostasis. The endogenous glucose production rate is high in VLBW infants and is not suppressed by a modest glucose infusion rate. In addition, relative peripheral insulin resistance is associated with a reduction of the insulin sensitivity of the hepatocyte.[206] Both lipid and amino acid infusions, separately or together, augment the glycemic effect of the glucose supply.

Several studies have suggest the potential benefit of continuous insulin administration to improve glucose tolerance and permit increases of the early parenteral nutrition intakes in VLBW infants.[199,206-211] Weight gain was also increased; however, the effect on whole body composition and protein metabolism is still not clear. Insulin is an important anabolic hormone in adults and an important growth hormone during fetal life. In early postnatal life, insulin secretion depends on glucose concentrations as well as those of amino acids such as leucine and arginine. The use of early high amino acid supply (±3 g/kg*d) doubled approximately the insulin concentration compared to early low amino acid supply (1 g/kg*d).[206] An additional advantage of such a strategy could be to reduce the limited glucose

tolerance and to increase the progression of energy supply by stimulating endogenous insulin secretion as well as to stimulate growth by enhancing the secretion of insulin and insulin-like growth factors.[207] Indeed, from both fetal and postnatal animal results, during a euglycemic, euaminoacidemic, hyperinsulinemic clamp, a sharp increase in the net uptake rate of nitrogen derived from amino acids was observed.[212,213] Up to now, very limited studies evaluated the benefit of these early and aggressive parenteral nutritional policies during the transition period, particularly of the use of continuous insulin perfusion, on longitudinal growth in preterm infants. Nevertheless, the first studies are promising.[209-210, 214]

In addition to parenteral nutrition, early oral nutrition is indicated in preterm infants for promoting feeding tolerance, decreasing time to reach full feedings, and preventing morbidity in parenterally fed infants. Different concepts have been proposed: trophic feeding, minimal enteral feeding and early enteral feeding. Although the border between these different denominations is not clear from several studies, it is suggested that "early" enteral feeding stimulates surges in secretion of intestinal polypeptide hormone,[215,216] an important determinant of postnatal intestinal adaptation, which increases intestinal motility,[217-219] improves host defense at the mucosal level, and may play an important role in development of the mucosal barrier and microflora with a reduction in bacterial translocation.[220-222] The main reported effects are reduction in days to full enteral feeding, improvement in energy intake and weight gain,[218,223,224] and an increase in mother's milk supply. These results were obtained without increasing NEC incidence and other apparent adverse effects.[225] Duration of minimal enteral feeding and safety of early advancing feeding volumes during the transition period is still controversial. In a recent study, Berseth et al 2003 suggest that early advancing feeding volumes from the second day of life in preterm infants below 32 weeks of gestational age increase the risk of necrotizing enterocolitis without providing benefits for motor function or feeding tolerance.[227] Although this study needs confirmation in a larger multicenter trial, it suggests that enteral feeding needs to be cautiously increased during the transition period.

The Stable-Growing Period

The stable-growing period begins when the infant can tolerate the recommended energy and protein supplies and ends when the infant is discharged from the neonatal unit. During this period, the primary nutritional goal is to obtain full enteral feeding with growth and nutrient-retention rates at least similar to those that would have been achieved in utero, taking into account that fat mass deposition is significantly lower prenatally than postnatally. Therefore, it is preferable to focus on length gain and lean body mass gain instead of weight gain. An additional objective of this period, when necessary, is to obtain catch-up growth to reduce growth deficit occurring during the transition period. With the exception of preterm infants with serious clinical or surgical gastrointestinal diseases, enteral nutrition will be the exclusive route of nutrition during this period. Fortified preterm mother's milk or alternatively, formula designed for preterm infants, is the feeding of choice for premature infants. Even though the energy needs are relatively stable during that period, the protein supplies need to be adapted according to postconceptional age and slowly decrease up to discharge, when the infant is able to nurse effectively. The benefits of fortified preterm mother's milk and the need for a preterm infant formula become less apparent as the infant approaches the weight and gestational age of a term infant. However, an exact weight or gestational-age cut-off cannot be defined. It is probably dependent on the residual postnatal growth retardation.

Preterm Mother's Milk

The use of human milk as a sole source of nutrients for preterm infants has been the subject of controversy and debate during recent years (see Chapter 12). Early preterm mother's milk (from the first production of colostrum to 4 weeks after birth) is more dense in some nutrients than milk from mothers delivered at term and thus comes closer to providing the nutrient requirements of preterm infants. This observation supports the position that such milk should be considered the optimal primary nutrition for preterm infants.[226,228-229] In addition to the nutritional properties of human milk, breast-feeding has psychological benefits for the mother and anti-infective and functional benefits for the infant.[226,228] Moreover, the use of preterm mother's milk may be associated with long-term neuro-developmental advantages.[230, 231] The only restrictive aspect for the use of preterm human milk is the fact that human immunodeficiency virus, human T-lymphotropic virus type 1, cytomegalovirus and other viruses are excreted in breast milk.[232] Therefore, the use of human milk from milk banks requires greater safeguards, and there is consensus to promote the exclusive use of the own preterm mother's fresh milk in LBW infants.

Own Preterm Mother's Milk and Human Milk Fortifiers

The protein density of preterm mother's milk is generally higher than that of term mother's milk during the early postnatal weeks.[228] However, it decreases rapidly during lactation, and the precise difference in nutritional protein content between preterm and term milk is still a matter of discussion. Nevertheless, it has been shown that preterm infants fed preterm mother's milk show better growth than those fed human milk.[233-235] However, preterm mother's milk does not provide adequate amounts of protein and other nutrients to support the optimal growth of the stable-growing period in preterm infants.[235, 236] One reason is the large variation in the macronutrient composition of the expressed own preterm mother's milk used in feeding LBW and ELBW infants. The variations concern not only the protein content but also other essential nutrients for growth, such as fat, minerals and sodium.[228,237] Therefore, it is not surprising that inadequacies of calcium, phosphorus, protein, sodium and energy are observed in the premature infant fed unfortified preterm mother's milk. Various human milk fortifiers have been developed to increase the protein, energy, minerals, electrolytes, trace elements and vitamins supplies (Table 5) and have been studied to evaluate growth, metabolic balance and weight gain composition.[1,19,66,68,69,71,73,74,83,91,115,117,118,122] [123,124-128,226,228,230,233-247] As shown in Table 2, growth and the various parameters of weight gain composition were significantly lower than those observed in infants fed preterm formula. These differences could be related to the lower protein content but also to the reduction in metabolizable protein and energy available for new tissue synthesis.[237]

The properties of human milk may be changed by nutrient fortification. The addition of human milk fortifier induces a rapid and clinically significant increase in osmolality, frequently above 400 mosm/kg H_2O, a value 40% higher than that of human milk (280 mosm/kg H_2O).[248] This is the result of the osmotic content of the fortifier but also of the rapid and continuous activity of human milk amylase on the dextrin content of HMF. Such an increase in osmolality may at least partly explain some minimal clinical disturbances, such as abdominal discomfort and delayed gastric emptying frequently observed in clinical practice. It could also explain the two fold increase of the incidence of necrotizing enterocolitis in preterm infants 2.2% compared to 5.8%; p=0.12 found in a study of 275 preterm infants fed human milk and fortified human milk.[249] Although this difference was not significant, the authors suggest that a larger study would be required to detect a two- to three-fold increase in incidence at the 5% significance level. Both nutrient fortification and storage alter some of the defense properties of human milk.[250] The total bacterial colony count was slightly but significantly higher, whereas the IgA concentration remained stable. In another study, lysozyme activity was reduced by the addition of HMF (-19%) although to a lesser extent than by the addition of formula.[251-253] All cow-milk-based formulas, but not HMF, decreased the inhibition of bacterial growth of human milk. The effect of HMF on the microflora colonization of the newborn intestine needs still to be evaluated as an additional causal factor of the occurrence of NEC in preterm infants.[254] More recently, new HMF have been designed providing energy supply as fat instead of carbohydrate to reduce the osmotic load and to allow

higher nutrients fortification.[125,243] Although the use of the more recent HMF improves growth, it has not resulted in optimal nutrient intakes and growth in preterm infants.

Preterm Formulas

In spite of the important nutritional and non nutritional benefits of human milk, the feeding of preterm infants with preterm mother's milk leads to a sub-optimal growth of preterm infants and does not compensate for the cumulative nitrogen deficit frequently observed in VLBW and ELBW infants.[9,19,226] In addition, there are numerous circumstances in which feeding an infant preterm mother's milk is impossible or extremely limited, and cow-milk-based formulas for preterm infants must be used. Assuming a protein requirement of 3.85 g/kg/d to obtain nitrogen retention and LBM gain similar to in utero, the estimated cumulative protein deficit at three to four postnatal weeks amounts to 30 to 40 g/kg in an ELBW infants.[7,9] Thus, the additional protein supply necessary to replace the cumulative deficit over a period of 40 days is 1 to 1.4 g/kg*d, assuming a net protein utilization of approximately 70%. Such an intake is higher than that provided by most of the preterm formulas in Europe and North America, which provide 80 kcal/100 ml with a protein:energy ratio of 2.5 to 3 g/100kcal. Therefore, new formulas with higher protein:energy ratios up to 3.3-3.5 g/ 100 kcal need to be developed.[114] The potential risk of such an aggressive nutritional strategy is to induce metabolic stress resulting from protein overload or unbalanced amino acid supply. Therefore, the most recent technologies will be necessary to improve nitrogen bioavailability, reduce Maillard reactions, and provide the most balanced amino acid composition.[98,255] Further studies are also needed to identify more sensitive markers for protein toxicity to determine the safety and efficacy of such a high protein supply and to evaluate the beneficial impact on short- and long-term growth and development. Formulas do not contain any of the biologically active immune substances, nor the enzymes, hormones or growth factors found in human milk. The long-term significance of the lack of these components has not been determined. Several studies have been performed to evaluate the functional properties of non-nutritional compounds, such as nucleotides,[180] polyamines,[256] growth factors or prebiotics,[257] which could potentially be implemented in the new formulas. In general, large multicenter, randomized studies need to evaluate the improvement in growth and body composition, as well as the reduction in incidence of postnatal growth restriction expected from an aggressive nutritional policy in preterm infants.

Clinical Conditions Affecting Protein Requirements

The clinical status of LBW and ELBW infants is frequently unstable during several days in NICU due to suppress illnesses which induce metabolic stress. To what extent these pathological conditions affect protein metabolism is incompletely understood.

Small for Gestational Age

The incidence of growth retardation at birth is high and concerns up to 35% of the VLBW infants. Two distinct groups of infants are growth retarded at birth: SGA infants with frequently asymmetric growth retardation, and capacity for normal growth, and the IUGR infants who are more symmetric and have a decreased capacity for normal growth. The decreased fetal growth rate associated with IUGR is an adaptation to an unfavorable intrauterine environment and may result in permanent alterations in metabolism, growth and development. Relatively limited and conflicting data have been obtained on protein metabolism in infants with growth retardation at birth and clear distinctions between the two groups are lacking. SGA infants are particularly deficient in muscle mass. Protein gain and composition of weight gain is very similar in SGA and AGA infants.[73] The rate of protein synthesis was lower in SGA as compared to AGA, which suggests a more efficient protein gain:protein synthesis ratio in SGA, because they show a slower protein turnover for the same weight and protein gains.[17,37] The authors emphasize that postconceptional age seems to be an important factor in the regulation of protein turnover. However, others studies disagree with the results suggesting a similar or a higher turnover rate in SGA versus AGA infants.[258] On nutritional intervention, SGA infants, being more mature, tend to have a better transition period with less weight loss and a shorter time to regain birth weight. Nutritional intervention studies have not been performed during the stable-growing period to investigate the potential catch-up growth of SGA infants on higher protein supply. Nevertheless, it seems reasonable to assume that, contrary to IUGR infants, SGA infants have similar metabolic requirements as postnatally growth-retarded preterm infants of similar postconceptional age.

Conclusions

From the review of the recent data on protein metabolism in preterm infants it is suggested that the actual recommendations should be updated to reduce postnatal growth retardation and to prevent long-term deleterious effects. Recent studies suggest to use early more aggressive nutrition strategy promoting high protein supply from the first days of life resulting in positive nitrogen balance and reducing early postnatal cumulative nitrogen deficit in VLBW infants. There is also a general consensus to increase not only the protein supply but also the protein to energy ratio during the stable growing period in order to better promote protein accretion, lean body mass deposition and length growth. Consequently, protein requirements have been reviewed to optimize the lean body mass and longitudinal growth but also to promote an early catch up growth. However, other nutritional and non-nutritional parameters interfere with growth and need to be considered. Following delivery, the major change for the fetus is not only the interruption of the continuous parenteral nutrition from the mother but also the separation from an hormonal and metabolic environment promoting the growth velocity rate of the fetus. Further clinical research is necessary to provide data on the efficacy and safety of the proposed higher protein supply at short-term, around discharge, but also on neurodevelopmental outcome and later health. A better understanding of the beneficial effects of the fetal hormonal environment on growth as well as of the potential improvements of protein metabolism in disease and various clinical situations is expected to further its potential application in ELBW infants.

Case Study

A 850 g male infant was delivered at 27.5 gestational weeks. The mother, a 25-year-od primipara, had been hospitalized since the 25th postmenstrual week for premature labor, tocolysis and lung maturation. Unfortunately, premature rupture of the membrane (PROM) occurred after 15 days. Fetal monitoring remained within the normal range up to vaginal delivery, occurring within 18 hours after inset of PROM. In all, the mother received two complete courses of betamethasone. Resuscitating the infant was minimal, requiring quiet mask and bag ventilation followed by nasal CPAP with and FiO$_2$ of 0.25. Venous umbilical catheter was inserted with the distal tip into the inferior vena cava and lung X-Ray suggested a minimal wet lung syndrome. At 2 hours of life, he appeard to be clinically stable without respiratory distress with a blood pressure and blood gases within normal ranges.

Question: *How and what should this infant be fed during the early transitional period?*

Answer: *At 2 hours post-natal age, the inravenous (IV) maintenance (dextrose 10%) was replaced by a total parenteral (TPN) solution containing 3.0 g amino acids, 14.4 g glucose, 2.4 g lipid, plus minerals and electrolytes for 100 ml. Over the first 24 hours, parenteral fluids accounted for 60 ml/kg*d, 50 ml of the TPN solution, with addition of 1 g of AA (10 ml), providing in all 2.5 g AA and 48 kcal/kg*d. At 24 and 48 hours of age, parenteral fluids were increased to 70 ml/kg*d (60 TPN + 10 AA) and 85 ml/kg*d (80 TPN + 5 AA) providing 2.8, 2.9 g AA and 56 and 72 kcal/kg*d respectively. Thereafter, nasal CPAP was removed and from day 4 to 7, the TPN solution alone was progressively increased up to 125 ml/kg*d, reaching 3.8 g AA and 11o kcal/kg*d, whereas minimal enteral nasogastric tube feeding was intitated with 12 x 1-2 ml/24 hours with own mother's milk or preterm formula. At that time, his respiratory condition had improved, and his body weight was close to birth weight at 840 g.*

Question: *What is the result of this early nutritional policy in terms of cumulative nutritional supplies?*

Answer: *Estimated from the daily nutritional supply during the early transitional period, mean parenteral AA and energy intakes were 3.1 g AA and 82 kcal/kg*d; and minimal enteral feeding accounted for 0.22 g protein and 12 kcal/kg*d on average, respectively. On this basis the cumulative protein and energy deficit at the end of the first week of life represented about 4.2 g of protein and 180 kcal.*

Question: *How should enteral feeding be resumed?*

Answer: *Over the next 14 days, enteral feeding of preterm formula was gradually increased from 12 x 2 ml/24 hour to .8 x 20 ml/24 hour by continuous gastric feeding with fortified human milk or preterm formula; concomitantly, the parenteral solution of amino acid was tapered off. Own human milk was supplemented with 1.3 g of protein/100 ml to obtain a protein energy ratio close to 3.3 g/100 kcal. The fortifier was selected to minimize the increase in osmolality of the mixture. When own human milk was not available, preterm formula, 3.3 g/100 kcal was provided to maintain the protein and energy intakes of 4.2 g and 125-130 kcal/kg*d respectively. Full enteral feeding with 160 ml/kg was obtained and well-tolerated during the third week of life. Weight gain increased progressively during the second and the third weeks of life to reach 20-25 g/kg*d. At 33 weeks post-conceptional age a preterm formula 3.0 g/100 kcal was substituted for the previous one to reduce the protein supply. From the second week to discharge at 36 weeks gestational age crown-heel length increased at 1.2 cm/wk from 36.5 cm to 46 cm. At discharge, whoe body composition was determined by DEXA; body weight was 2340 g with a fat mass of 280 g or 12% BW. At that time, the boy was appropriate for post-conceptional age and a formula 2.7 g of protein/100 kcal was recommended up to corrected term age.*

References

1. American Academy of Pediatrics Committee on Nutrition. Nutritional needs of low-birth-weight infants *Pediatrics* 1985;75:976-986.

2. European Society of Pediatric Gastroenterology and Nutrition, Committee on Nutrition of the Preterm

Infant. Nutrition and feeding of preterm infants. Oxford, UK: Blackwell Scientific Publications; *Acta Paediatr Scand Suppl.* 1987;336:1-14.

3. Nutritional Needs of the Preterm Infant: Scientific Basis and Practical Guidelines. Tsang RC, Lucas A, Uauy R and Zlotkin S, eds. Williams and Wilkins, Baltimore, MD. 1993:pp.301.

4. Canadian Pediatrics Society & Nutrition Committee. Nutrient needs and feeding of premature infants. *Can Med Assoc J* 1995;152:1765-1785.

5. Klein CJ. Nutrient requirements for preterm infant formulas. *J Nutr* 2002;132:1395S-577S.

6. Georgieff MK. Chapter 23. Nutrition; In: Avery GB, Fletcher MA and MacDonald MG, eds. Neonatology: Pathophysiology and Management of the Newborn. 5th ed. Lippincott, Williams and Wilkins, Philadephia, PA,1999:pp 363-394.

7. Embleton NE, Pang N, Cooke RJ. Postnatal malnutrition and growth retardation: an inevitable consequence of current recommendations in preterm infants? *Pediatrics* 2001;107: 270-273.

8. Thorp JW, Tucker R, Chen J, Chng YM, Vohr BR. Ability to provide adequate nutrition to very-low-birth-weight (VLBW) infants in a neonatal intensive unit. *Pediatr Res* 47:298A (abs. 1758).

9. Rigo J, De Curtis M, Pieltain C. Nutritional assessment in preterm infants with special reference to body composition. Seminars in Neonatology, 2002,6 (in press).

10. De Curtis M, Pieltain C, Rigo J. Nutrition of preterm infants on discharge from hospital. In: Raïha NCR, Rubaltelli FF eds. Infant formula: closer to the reference. Nestle Nutrition Workshop Series, Nestec Ltd, Vevey/lippincott Williams & Wilkins, Philadelphia, 2002;47:149-163.

11. Rigo J, De Curtis M, Pieltain C, Picaud JC, Salle BL, Senterre J. Metabolism and nutrition of the micropremie, bone mineral metabolism. *Clinics in Perinatology* 2000, 27:147-170.

12. Rigo J, Boboli H, Franckart G, Pieltain C, De Curtis M. Surveillance de l'ancien prématuré: croissance et nutrition. *Arch Pédiatrie* 1998;5:449-453.

13. Premer DM and Georgieff MK. Nutrition for Ill Neonates. *Pediatrics in Review* 1999 20: 56-62.

14. Wright K., Dawson J.P., Fallis D., Vogt E., Lorch V. New postnatal growth grids for very-low-birth-weight infants. *Pediatrics* 1993;91: 922-926.

15. Lucas A. Nutrition, growth, and development of postdischarge preterm infants. In: Posthospital nutrition in the preterm infant. Report of the 106th Ross Conference on Pediatric Research, 1996:81-89.

16. Carlson SJ, Ziegler EE. Nutrient intake and growth of very-low-birth-weight infants. *J Perinatol* 1998;18:252-258.

17. Micheli JL, Schutz Y. Protein. In : Tsang RC, Lucas A, Aauy R, Zlotkin S (eds). Nutritional Needs of the Preterm Infant. Pawkings: Williams and Wilkins 1993;29-46.

18. Micheli JL, Fawer CL, Schutz Y. Protein requirement of the Extremely Low-Birth-weight Preterm Infant. In: Ziegler EE, Lucas A, Moro GE,eds. Nutrition of the Very-Low-Birth-weight Infant. Nestle Nutrition Workshop Series, Nestec Ltd, Vevey/Lippincott Williams & Wilkins, Philadelphia, 1999;43:155-178.

19. Pieltain C, De Curtis M, Gerard P, Rigo J. Weight gain composition in preterm infants fed fortified human milk or preterm formula. *Pediatr Res* 49, 2001:120-124.

20. Widdowson EM. Changes in body composition during growth. In:Davis JA, Dobbing J; Scientific Foundation of Pediatrics, 2nd ed. Heinemann Medical Books Ltd; London, 1981.

21. Ziegler EE. Protein requirements of preterm infants. In: Energy and Protein Needs During Infancy. Fomon SJ and Heird WC, eds. Academic Press, Inc., New York, NY.,1986: 69-85.

22. Sparks JW. Human intrauterine growth and nutrient accretion. *Semin Perinatol* 1984;8:74-93.

23. Kalhan SC, Iben S. Protein metabolism in the extremely low-birth-weight infant. *Clin Perinatol* 2000;27:23-56.

24. Putet G. Protein. In : Tsang RC, Lucas A, Uauy R, Zlotkin S, eds. Nutritional Needs of the Preterm Infant. Scientific Basis and Practical Guidelines. Williams and Wilkins, New-York, 1993 :15-28.

25. Lubchenco LO, Hansman C, Boyd E. Intrauterine growth in length and head circumference as estimated from live births at gestational ages from 26 to 42 weeks. *Pediatr* 1966;47:403-408.

26. Usher R, Mc Lean F. Intrauterine growth of liveborn

Caucasian infants at sea level: standard obtained from measurements in 7 dimensions of infants born between 25 and 44 weeks of gestation. *J Pediatr* 1969; 74:901-910.

27. Thomas P, Peabody J, Turnier V, Clark RH. A new look at intrauterine growth and the impact of race, altitude and gender. *Pediatr* 2000;106:e21.

28. Alexander GR, Mor JM, Kogan MD, Leland NL, Kieffer E. Pregnancy outcomes of US-born and foreign-born Japanese Americans. *Am J Public Health* 1996; 86:820-824.

29. Fehling H. Beitrage. Zur Physiologie des placentaren Stoffverkkehrs. *Arch Gynakol* 1877;11:523.

30. Ziegler EE, OíDonnell AM, Nelson SE, Fomon SJ. Body composition of the reference fetus. *Growth* 1976;40:329-341.

31. Ellis KJ, Shypailo RJ, Schanler RJ, Langston C. Body elemental composition of the neonate: new reference data. *Am J Hum Biol* 1993;5:323-330.

32. Rigo J, Nyamugabo K, Picaud JC, Gerard P, Pieltain C, De Curtis M. Reference values of body composition by dual energy x-ray absorptiometry in preterm and term infants. *J Pediatr Gastrol Nutr* 1998;27:184-190.

33. Koo WWK, Walters J, Bush AJ, Chesney RW, Carlson SE. Dual-energy-x-ray absorptiometry studies of bone mineral status in newborn infants. *J Bone Min Res* 1996;11:997-1002.

34. Yudkoff M, Nissim I. Methods for determining the protein requirement of infants. *Clin Perinatol* 1986;13:123-132.

35. Catzeflis C, Schutz Y, Micheli JL, Welsch C, Amaud MJ, Jéquier E. Whole body protein synthesis and energy expenditure in very-low-birth-weight infants. *Pediatr Res* 1985;19:679-687.

36. Duffy B, Gunn T, Collinge J, Pencharz P. The effect of varying protein quality and energy intake on the nitrogen metabolism of parenterally fed very-low-birth-weight (<600g) infants. *Pediatr Res* 1981;15: 1040-1044.

37. Cauderay M, Schutz Y, Micheli JL, Calame A, Jéquier E. Energy-nitrogen balances and protein turnover in small and appropriate for gestational age low-birth-weight infant. *Eur J Clin Nutr* 1988;42: 125-136.

38. De Benoist B, Abdulrazzak Y, Brooke OG, Hallyday D, Millward D. The measurement of whole body protein turnover in the preterm infant with intragastric infusion of L-[1-13C] leucine and sampling of the urinary leucine pool. *Clin Sci* 1984;66:155-164.

39. Jackson AA, Shaw JCL, Barber A, Golden MHN. Nitrogen metabolism in preterm infants fed human donor breast milk: the possible essentiality of glycine. *Pediatr Res* 1981;15:1454-1461.

40. Nissim I, Yudkoff M, Pereira G, Segal S. Effects of conceptual age and dietary intake on protein metabolism in premature infants. *J Pediatr Gastroent Nutr* 1983;2:507-516.

41. Pencharz PB. The 1987 Borden Award Lecture: protein metabolism in premature human infants. *Can J Physiol Pharmacol* 1988;66:1247-1252.

42. Pencharz PB, Beesley J, Sauer P et al. Total-body protein turnover in parenterally fed neonates: effects of energy source studied by using [15N] glycine and [1-13C] leucine 1-3. *Am J Clin Nutr* 1989;50: 1395-1400.

43. Pencharz PB, Clarke R, Papageorgiou A, Farri L. A reappraisal of protein turnover values in neonates fed human milk or formula. *Can J Physiol Pharmacol* 1989;67:282-286.

44. Plath C, Heine Willi, Wutzke KD, Uhlemann M. 15N-tracer studies in formula-fed preterm infants: the role of glycine supply in protein turnover. *J Pediatr Gastroenterol Nutr* 1996;23:287-297.

45. Denne SC, Karn CA, Liu YM, Leitch CA, Liechty EA. Effect of enteral versus parenteral feeding on leucine kinetics and fuel utilization in premature newborns. *Pediatr Res* 1994;36:29-35.

46. Pencharz PB, Farri L, Papageorgiou A. The effect of human milk and low-protein formulae on the rates of total body protein turnover and urinary 3-methylhistidine excretion of preterm infants. *Clin Sci (Colch)* 1983;64:611-616.

47. Hertz DE, Karn CA, Liu YM, Liechty EA, Denne SC. Intravenous glucose suppresses glucose production but not proteolysis in extremely premature newborn. *J Clin Invest* 1993;92:1752-1758.

48. Denne SC, Karn CA, Liechty EA. Leucine kinetics after a brief fast and in response to feeding in premature

infants. *Am J Clin Nutr* 1992;56:899-904.

49. Denne SC, Karn CA, Wang J, Liechty EA. Effect of intravenous glucose and lipid on porteolysis and glucose production in normal newborns. *Am J Physiol* 1995;269:E361-E367.

50. Denne SC, Rossi EM, Kalhan SC. Leucine kinetics during feeding in normal newborns. *Pediatr Res* 1991;30:23-27.

51. Denne SC, Karn CA, Ahlrichs JA, Dorotheo AR, Wang J, Liechty EA. Proteolysis and phenylalanine hydroxylation in response to parenteral nutrition in extremely premature and normal newborns. *J Clin Invest* 1996; 97:746-754.

52. Battista MA, Price PT, Kalhan SC. Efffect of parenteral amino acids on leucine and urea kinetics in preterm infants. *J Pediatr* 1996;128:130-134.

53. Beaufrere B, Putet G, Pachiaudi C, Salle B. Whole body protein turnover measured with 13C leucine and energy expenditure in preterm infants. *Pediatr Res* 1990;28:147-152.

54. Mitton SG, Garlick PJ. Changes in protein turnover after the introduction of parenteral nutrition in premature infants: comparison of breast milk and egg protein-based amino acid solutions. *Pediatr Res* 1992;32:447-454.

55. Van Toledo-Eppinga L, Kalhan SC, Kulik W, Jakobs C, Lafeber HN. Relative kinetics of phenylalanine and leucine in low-birth-weight infants during nutrient administration. *Pediatr Res* 1996;40:41-46.

56. Wykes LJ, Ball RO, Menendez CE, Ginther DM, Pencharz PB. Glycine, leucine and phenylalanine flux in low-birth-weight infants during parenteral and enteral feeding. *Am J Clin Nutr* 1992;55:971-975.

57. Clark SE, Karn CA, Ahlrichs JA, Wang J, Leitch CA, Leichty EA, Denne SC. Acute changes in leucine and phenylalanine kinetics produced by parenteral nutrition in premature infants. *Pediatr Res* 1997;41:568-574.

58. Kilani RA, Cole FS, Bier DM. Phenylalanine hydroxylase activity in preterm infants: is tyrosine a conditionally essential amino acid? *Am J Clin Nutr* 1995;61:1218-1223.

59. Penchartz PB, Parsons H, Motil K, Duffy B. Total body protein turnover and growth in children: is it a futile cycle? *Med Hypoth* 1981;7:155-160.

60. Pencharz PB, Mason M, Desgranges F, Papageorgiou A. The effects of postnatal age on the whole body protein metabolism and the urinary 3-methyl histidine excretion of premature infants. *Nut Res* 1984;4:9-19.

61. Hamosh M. Digestion in the newborn. *Clin Perinatol* 1996;23:191-209.

62. Rudloff S, Lonnerdal B. Solubility and digestibility of milk proteins in infant formulas exposed to different heat treatments. *J Pediatr Gastroenterol Nutr* 1992;15:25-33.

63. Sarwar G, Botting HG. Liquid concentrates are lower in bioavailable tryptophan than powdered infant formulas, and tryptophan supplementation of formulas increases brain tryptophan and serotonin in rats. *J Nutr* 1999;129:1692-7.

64. Donovan SM, Lönnerdal B. Non-protein nitrogen and true protein in infants formulas. *Acta Paediatr Scand* 1989:78:497-504.

65. Sarwar G. Amino acid ratings of different forms of infant formulas based on varying degrees of processing. *Adv Exp Med Biol* 1991;289:389-402.

66. Rigo J, Putet G, Picaud JC, Pieltain C, De Curtis M, Salle BL, Senterre J. Nitrogen balance and plasma amino acids in the evaluation of protein sources for extremely low-birth-weight infants. In: Ziegler EE, Lucas A, Moro GE, eds. Nutrition of the very-low-birth-weight infant. Nestle Nutrition Workshop Series, Nestec Ltd, Vevey/lippincott Williams and Wilkins. Philadelphia, Pennsylvania, 1999;43:139-153.

67. Rigo J, Salle BL, Picaud J-C, Putet G, Senterre J. Nutritional evaluation of protein hydrolysate formulas. *Eur J Clin Nutr* 1995;49:S26-S38.

68. Putet G, Senterre J, Rigo G, Salle B. Nutrient balance, energy utilization and composition of weight gain in very-low-birth-weight infants fed pooled human milk or preterm formula. *J Pediatr* 1984;105:79-85.

69. Putet G, Rigo J, Salle B, Senterre J. Supplementation of pooled human milk with casein hydrolysate: energy and nitrogen balance and weight gain composition in very-low-birth-weight-infants. *Pediatr Res* 1987;21:458-461.

70. De Curtis M, Brooke OG. Energy and nitrogen balances in very-low-birth-weight infants. *Arch Dis Child* 1987;62:830-832.

71. Senterre J, Voyer M, Putet G, Rigo J. Nitrogen, fat and

mineral balance studies in preterm infants fed bank human milk, a human milk formula, or a low-birth-weight infant formula. In: Baum, ed. Human milk processing, fractionation, and the nutrition of the low-birth-weight baby, Nestle nutrition worshop series.New York: Raven Press,1983;3:102-111.

72. Senterre J, Rigo J. Nutritional requirements of low-birth-weight infants. In: Gracey M, Falkner F, eds.Nutritional needs and assessment of normal growth. Nestle nutrition worshop series, New York: Raven Press, 1985;7:45-49.

73. Picaud JC, Putet G, Rigo J, Salle BL, Senterre J. Metabolic and energy balance in small-and-appropriate for gestational age in very-low-birth-weight infants. *Acta Paediatr* 1994; Suppl 405:54-59.

74. Rigo J, Senterre J, Putet G, Salle B . Various human milk fortifiers in low-birth-weight infants fed pooled human milk: plasma and urinary amino acid concentrations. In: Koletzko B, Okken A, Rey J, Salle B, Van Biervliet JP, eds. Recent advances in infant feeding, Georg ThiemVerlag Stuttgart,New-York,1992 :164-170.

75. Rigo J, Senterre J. Metabolic balance studies and plasma amino acid concentrations in preterm infants fed experimental protein hydrolysate preterm formulas. *Acta Paediatr* 1994;Suppl 405:98-104.

76. Picaud JC, Rigo J, Lapillonne A, Salle B, Senterre J. Metabolic balance and plasma amino acid concentrations in VLBW infants fed a new acidic whey hydrolysate preterm formula. *J Pediatr Gastrol and Nutr* 1997;24:A459.

77. Cooke R, Watson D, Werkman S, Conner C. Effects of type of dietary protein on acid-base status, protein nutritional status, plasma levels of amino acids, and nutrient balance in the very-low-birth-weight infant. *J Pediatr* 1992;121: 444-451.

78. Lee YH. Food-processing approaches to altering allergenic potential of milk-based formula. *J Pediatr*1992;121:S47-50.

79. Kalhan SC. Urea and its bioavailability in newborns. *Arch Dis Child* 1994;71:F233.

80. Jackson AA. Urea as a nutrient: bioavailability and role in nitrogen economy. *Arch Dis Child* 1994;70:3-4.

81. Donovan SM, Lonnerdal B, Atkinson SA. Bioavailability of urea nitrogen for the low-birth-weight infant. *Acta Paediatr Scand* 1990;79:899-905.

82. Hanning RM, Zlotkin SH. Amino acid and protein needs of the neonate: effects of excess and deficiency. *Semin Perinatol* 1989;13:131-141.

83. Polberger S, Axelsson I, Räihä N. Amino acid concentrations in plasma and urine in very-low-birth-weigth infants fed non proteinenriched or human milk protein enriched human milk. *Pediatrics* 1990;86: 909-915.

84. McIntosh N, Rodeck CH, Heath R. Plasma amino acids of the mid trimester human fetus. *Biol Neonate* 1984;45:218-224.

85. Atkinson SA, Hanning RM. Amino acid metabolism and requirements of the premature infant: does human milk feeding represent the "gold standard"? In: Atkinson SA, Lonnerdal B, eds. Protein and nonprotein nitrogen in human milk. Boca Raton, FL:CRC Press;1989.

86. Rigo J. Azote et acides aminés. In: Ricour C, Ghisolfi J, Putet G, Goulet O, eds. *Traité de Nutrition Pédiatrique*, Paris, Maloine:1993:852-866.

87. Rigo J, Senterre J. Significance of plasma amino acid pattern in preterm infants. *Biol Neonate* 1987;52: 41-49.

88. Rigo J. Les besoins en acides aminés des prématurés alimentés par voie orale ou parentérale. Thèse, Université de Liège. Derouaux-Ordina eds, Liège, 1991; 1-181.

89. Janas LM, Picciano MF, Hatch TF. Indices of protein metabolism in term infants fed either human milk or formulas with reduced protein concentration and various whey/casein ratios. *J Pediatr* 1987;110:838-848.

90. Kashyap S, Okamoto E, Kanaya S, Zucker C, Abildskov K, Dell RB, Heird WC. Protein quality in feeding low-birth-weight infants: a comparison of whey-predominant versus casein-predominant formulas. *Pediatrics* 1987;79:748-755.

91. Priolisi A, Didato M, Gioeli R, Fazzolari-Nesci A, Raiha NC. Milk protein quality in low-birth-weight infants: effects of proteinfortified human milk and formulas with three different whey-to-casein ratios on growth and plasma amino acid profiles. *J Pediatr Gastroenterol Nutr* 1992;14:450-455.

92. Tikanoja T, Simell O, Jarvenpaa AL, Raiha NC. Plasma

amino acids in preterm infants after a feed of human milk or formula. *J Pediatr* 1982;101:248-52.

93. Rassin DK, Gaull GE, Heinonen K, Raih NC. Milk protein quantity and quality in low-birth-weight infants: II. Effects on selected aliphatic amino acids in plasma and urine. *Pediatrics* 1977;59:407-422.

94. Rassin DK, Gaull GE, Raiha NC, Heinonen K. Milk protein quantity and quality in low-birth-weight infants. IV. Effects on tyrosine and phenylalanine in plasma and urine. *J Pediatr* 1977;90:356-360.

95. Rigo J, Senterre J. Optimal threonine intake for preterm infants fed on oral or parenteral nutrition. *JPEN* 1980;4:15-17.

96. Boehm G, Cervantes H, Georgi G, Jelinek J, Sawatzki G, Wermuth B, Colombo JP. Effect of increasing dietary threonine intakes on amino acid metabolism of central nervous system and peripheral tissues in growing rats. *Pediatr Res* 1998;44:900-906.

97. Rigo J, Boehm G, Georgi G, Jelinek J, Nyamugabo K, Sawatski G, Studzinski F. An infants formula free of glycomacropeptide prevents hyperthreoninemia in formula-fed preterm infants. *J Pediatr Gastroenterol Nutr* 2001;32:127-130.

98. Picaud JC, Rigo J, Normand S, Lapillonne A, Reygrobellet B, Claris O, Salle BL. Nutritional efficacy of preterm formula with a partially hydrolyzed protein source: a randomized pilot study. *J Pediatr Gastroenterol Nutr* 2001; 32,5:555-561.

99. Raïhïa NCR, Nesci AF, Cajozzo C, Puccio G, Minoli I, Moro GE, Monestier A, Haschke-Becher E, CarriÈ AL, Haschke F. Protein quantity and quality in infant formula: closer to the reference. In: Raïhï NCR, Rubaltelli FF, eds. *Infant Formula: Closer to the Reference*. Nestle Nutrition Workshop Series. Philadelphia: Nestec Ltd, Vevey/Lippincott Williams and Wilkins: 2002; 47:53-69.

100. Bachmann C, Haschke-Becher E. Plasma amino acid concentrations in breast-fed and formula-fed infants and reference intervals. In: Raïhï NCR, Rubaltelli FF, eds. *Infant Formula: Closer to the Reference*. Nestle Nutrition Workshop Series. Philadelphia: Nestec Ltd, Vevey/Lippincott Williams and Wilkins: 2002;47: 121-137.

101. Heine WE, Klein PD, Reeds PJ. The importance of alphalactalbumin in infant nutrition. *J Nutr* 1991;121:277-83.

102. Mihatsh WA, Hogel J, Pohlandt F. Hydrolysed protein accellerates the gastrointestinal transport of formula in preterm infants. *Acta Paediatr* 2001;90:196-198.

103. Lajoie N, Gauthier SF, Pouliot Y. Improved storage stability of model infant formula by whey peptides fractions. J Agric Food Chem 2001;49:1999-2007.

104. Mihatsh WA, Pohlandt F. Protein hydrolysate formula maintains homeostasis of plasma amino acids in preterm infatns. *J Pediatr Gastroenterol Nutr* 1999;29(4):406-410.

105. Szajewska H. Probiotics in the treatment and prevention of acute infectious diarrhea in infants and children: a systematic review of published randomized. *J Pediatr Gastroenterol Nutr* 2001;33,(2):S17-25.

106. Zello GA, Menendez CE, Rafii M, Clarke R, Wykes LJ, Ball RO, Pencharz PB. Minimum protein intake for the preterm neonate determined by protein and amino acid kinetics. *Pediatr Res* 2003;53:338-44.

107. Towers HM, Schulze KF, Ramakrishnan R, Kashyap S. Energy expended by low-birth-weight infants in the deposition of protein and fat. *Pediatr Res* 1997;41: 584-589.

108. Pencharz PB, Steffee WP, Cochran W, Scrimshaw NS, Rand WM, Young VR. Protein metabolism in human neonates: nitrogenbalance studies, estimated obligatory losses of nitrogen and wholebody turnover of nitrogen. *Clin Sci (Colch)* 1977;52: 485-498.

109. Saini J, MacMahon P, Morgan JB, Kovar IZ. Early parenteral feeding of amino acids. *Arch Dis Child* 1989;64:1362-1366.

110. Kashyap S, Schuylze KF, Ramakrishan R, Dell R, Heird WC. Evaluation of a mathematical model for predicting the relationship between protein and energy intakes of low-birth-weight infants and the rate and composition of weight gain. *Pediatr Res* 1994;35: 704-712.

111. Kashyap S, Schulze KF, Sorsyth M, Zucher C,Dell RB, Ramakrishnan R, Heird WC. Growth, nutrient retention, and metabolic response in low-birth-weight infants fed varying intakes of protein and energy. *J Pediatr* 1988; 113: 713-721.

112. Kashyap S, Ohira-Kist K, Abildskov K, Towers HM,

Sahni R, Ramakrishnana, Schulze K. Effect of quality of energy intake on growth and metabolic response of enterally fed low-birth-weight infants. *Pediatric Res* 2001; 50:390-397.

113. Kashyap S, Towers HM, Sahni R, Ohira-Kist K, Abildskov K, Schulze KF. Effects of quality of energy on substrate oxidation in enterally fed, low-birth-weight infants. *Am J Clin Nutr* 2001;74:374-380.

114. Cooke RJ, Rigo J, Embleton ND, Ziegler EE. Nutrient balance and metabolic status in preterm infants fed two levels of dietary protein. *Pediatr Res* 2002;4:318A.

115. Putet G, Picaud JC, Salle BL, Rigo J, Senterre J. Utilization and storage of energy. In: Salle BL, Swyer PR, eds. Nutrition of the Low-Birth-weight Infant. Nestle Nutrition Workshop Series. Nestec Ltd., Vevey/Raven Press, Ltd., New York:1993;32:61-69.

116. Whyte RK, Haslam R, Vlainic C, Shannon SR, Samulski K, Campbell D, Bayley HS, Sinclair JC. Energy balance and nitrogen balance in growing low-birth-weight infants fed human milk or formula. *Pediatr Res* 1983;17: 891-898.

117. Kashyap S, Forsyth M, Zucker C, Ramakrishnan R, Dell RB, Heird WC. Effect of varying protein and energy intakes on growth and metabolic response in low-birth-weight infants. *J Pediatr* 1986;108:955-963.

118. Kashyap S, Schulze KF, Forsyth M, Dell RB, Ramakrishnan R, Heird WC. Growth, nutrient retention and metabolic response of low-birth-weight infants fed supplemented and unsupplemented preterm human milk. *Am J Clin Nutr* 1990;52: 254-262.

119. Roberts SB, Lucas A. Energetic efficiency and nutrient accretion in preterm infants fed extremes of dietary intake. *Clin Nutr* 1987;416:105-113.

120. Schultze KF, Stefanski M, Masterson J, Spinnazola R, Ramakrishnan R, Dell RB, Heird WC. Energy expenditure, energy balance and composition of weight gain in low-birth-weight infants fed diets of different protein and energy content. *J Pediatr* 1987;110: 753-759.

121. Reichman B, Chessex P, Verellen G, Putet G, Smith JM, Heim T, Swyer PR. Dietary composition and macronutrient storiage in preterm infants.

Pediatrics 1983; 72: 322-328.

122. Boehm G, Muller DM, Senger H, Borte M, Moro G. Nitrogen and fat balances in very-low-birth-weight infants fed formula fortifier with human milk or bovine milk protein. *Eur J Pediatr* 1993;152: 236-239.

123. Schanler RJ, Abrams SA. Postnatal attainment of intrauterine macromineral accretion rate birth weight infants fed fortified human milk. *J Pediatr* 1995;126(3):441-447.

124. Polberger S, Raihä, P Juvonen, Moro GE, Minoli I, Warm A. Individualised protein fortification of human milk for preterm infants: comparison of ultrafiltrated human milk protein and a bovine whey fortifier. *J Pediatr Gastroenterol Nutr* 1999;29: 332-338.

125. Reis BB, Hall RT, Schanler RJ, Berseth CL, Chan G, Ernst JA, Lemons J, Adamkin D, Baggs G, O'Connor D. Enhanced growth of preterm infants fed a new powdered human milk fortifier: A randomized, controlled trial. *Pediatrics* 2000;106: 581-588.

126. Porcelli P, Schanler R, Greer F, Chan G, Gross S, Mehta N, Spear M, Kerner J, Euler AR. Growth in human milk-fed very-low-birth-weight infants receiving a new human milk fortifier. *Ann Nutr Metab* 2000;44:2-10.

127. Freymond D, Schutz Y, Decombaz J, Micheli JL, Jéquier E. Energy balance, physical activity and thermogenic effect of feeding in premature infants. *Pediatr Res* 1986;20:638-645.

128. Putet G, Senterre J, Rigo J, Salle B. Energy balance and composition of body weight. *Biol Neonate* 1987;52 suppl.1:17-24.

129. Bertolo RF, Pencharz PB, Ball RO. Organ and plasma amino acid concentrations are profoundly different in piglets fed identical diets via gastric, central venous or portal venous routes. *J Nutr* 2000;130:1261-6.

130. Heird WC, Kashyap S, Gomze MR. Parenteral alimentation of the neonate. *Seminars in Perinatology* 1991;15:493-502.

131. Denne SC, Clark SE, Poindexter BB, Leictch CA, Ernst JA, Lemons PK, Lemons JA, Hertz DE, Liechty EA. Nutrition and Metabolism in the high-risk

neonate. In: Fanaroff AA, Martin RJ eds. *Diseases of the Fetus and Infant.* Neonatal-Perinatal Medicine. Mosby-Year Book. St. Louis:1997:586-588.

132. Collier S, Lo C. Advances in parenteral nutrition. *Curr Opin Pediatr* 1996;8,5:476-482.

133. Heird WC. Amino acids in pediatric and neonatal nutrition. *Curr Opin Clin Nutr Metab Care* 1998; 1:73-78.

134. Imura K, Okada A. Amino acid metabolism in pediatric patients. *Nutrition* 1998; 14:143-148.

135. Brunton JA, Ball RO, Pencharz PB. Current total parenteral nutrition solutions for the neonate are inadequate. *Curr Opin Clin Nutr Metab Care* 2000;3:299-304.

136. Thureen, PJ, and Hay, Jr., WW. Intravenous nutrition and postnatal growth of the micropremie. *Clin Perinatol* 2000;27:197-219.

137. Puntis JW, Ball PA, Preece MA, Green A, Brown GA, Booth IW. Egg and breast milk based nitrogen sources compared. *Arch Dis Child* 1989;64:1472-1475.

138. Heird WC, Dell RB, Helms RA, Greene HL, Ament Me, Karna P, Storm MC. Amino acid mixture designed to maintain normal plasma amino acid patterns in infants and children requiring parenteral nutrition. *Pediatrics* 1987;80:401-408.

139. Heird WC, Hay W, Helms RA, Storm MC, Kashyap S, Dell RB. Pediatric parenteral amino acid mixture in low-birth-weight infants. *Pediatrics* 1988;81:41-50.

140. Rigo J, Senterre J, Putet G, Salle B. A new amino acid solution specially adapted to preterm infants. *Clin Nutr* 1987;6:105-109.

141. Bell EF, Filer LJ Jr, Pon Wong A, Steging LD. Effects of a parenteral nutrition regimen containing dicarboxylic amino acids on plasma, erythrocyte, and urinary amino acid concentrations of young infants. *Am J Clin Nutr* 1983;37:99-107.

142. Rigo J, Senterre J. Parenteral nutrition in the very low-birth-weight infant. In: Kretchmer N, Minkowski A, eds. *Nutritional Adaptation of the Gastrointestinal Tract of the Newborn.* New York: Raven Press 1983:191-207.

143. Zlotkin SH, Brayn MH, Anderson GH. Cysteine supplementation to cysteine free intravenous feeding

regimens in newborn infants. *Am J Clin Nutr* 1981;34:914.

144. Malloy MH, Rassin DK, Richardson JC. Total parenteral nutrition in sick preterm infants: effects of cysteine supplementation with nitrogen intakes of 240 and 400 mg/kg/day. *J Pediatr Gastroenterol Nutr* 1984;3:239-244.

145. Chessex P, Zebiche H, Pineault M, Lepage D, Dallaire L. Effect of amino acid composition of parenteral solutions on nitrogen retention and metabolic response in very-low-birth-weight infants. *J Pediatr* 1985;106:111-117.

146. Pineault M, Chessex P, Bisaillon S, Brisson G. Total parenteral nutrition in the newborn: impact of the quality of infused energy on nitrogen metabolism. *Am J Clin Nutr* 1988;47:298-304.

147. Kovar IZ, Saini J, Morgan JB. The sick very-low-birth-weight infant fed by parenteral nutrition: studies of nitrogen and energy. *Eur J Clin Nutr* 1989;43: 339-346.

148. Coran AG, Drongowski RA. Studies on the toxicity and efficacity of a new amino acid solution in pediatric parenteral nutrition. *J Parenter Enter Nutr* 1987; 11:368-377.

149. Munro HN. Amino acid requirements and metabolism and their relevance to parenteral nutrition. In: Wilkinson AW, ed. *Parenteral Nutrition.* London: Churchill Livingstone 1972;34.

150. Raiha NCR. Biochemical basis for nutritional management of preterm infants. *Pediatrics* 1974;53: 147-156.

151. Gaull G, Sturman JA, RaÔha NCR. Developement of mammalian sulfur metabolism: absence of cystathionase in human fetal tissues. *Pediatr Res* 1972;6:538-547.

152. Rigo J, Senterre J. Is taurine essential for the neonate? *Biol Neonate* 1977;32:73-76.

153. Holt LE, Snyderman SE. The amino acid requirement of infants. *JAMA* 1961;174:100.

154. Olney JW, Ho OI, Rhee V. Brain-damaging potential of protein hydrolysates. *N Engl J Med* 1973;289: 391-395.

155. Pearson DL, Dawling S, Walsh WF, Haines JL, Christman BW, Bazyk A, Scott N, Summar ML.

Neonatal pulmonary hypertension—urea-cycle intermediates, nitric oxide production, and carbamoylphosphate synthetase function. *N Engl J Med* 2001;14,344:1832-1838.

156. Becker RM, Wu G, Galanko JA, Chen W, Maynor AR, Bose CL, Rhoads JM. Reduced serum amino acid concentrations in infants with necrotizing enterocolitis. *J Pediatr* 2000;137:785-793

157. Puntis JW, Edwards MA, Green A, Morgan I, Booth IW, Ball PA. Hyperphenylalaninaemia in parenterally fed newborn babies. *Lancet* 1986; 29,2:1105-1106.

158. Walker V, Hall MA, Bulusu S, Allan A. Hyperphenylalaninaemia in parenterally fed newborn babies. *Lancet* 1986;29,2:1284.

159. McIntosh N, Mitchell V. A clinical trial of two parenteral nutrition solutions in neonates. *Arch Dis Child* 1990;65: 692-699.

160. Rigo J, Senterre J. Aromatic amino acid in LBW infants. The role of branched chain amino acids. *Clin Nutr* 1985; 4 suppl:71 A.

161. Van Goudoever JB, Sulkers EJ, Timmermans M, Huijmans JG, Langer K, Carnielli VP, Sauer PJ. Amino acid solutions for premature infants during the first week of life: The role of N-acetyl-L-cysteine and N-acetyl-L-tyrosine. *Parenter Enteral Nutr* 1994;18:404-408.

162. Roberts, SA, Ball RO, Filler RM, Moore AM, Pencharz PB. Phenylalanine and tyrosine metabolism in neonates receiving parenteral nutrition differing in pattern of amino acids. *Pediatr Res* 1998;44:907-914.

163. Van Goudoever JB, Colen T, Wattimena JL, Huijmans JG, Carnielli VP, Sauer PJ. Immediate commencement of amino acid supplementation in preterm infants: effect on serum amino acid concentrations and protein kinetics on the first day of life. *J Pediatr* 1995;127:458-465.

164. Stabler SP, Morton RL, Winski SL, Allen RH, White CW. Effects of parenteral cystein and glutathione feeding in a baboon model of severe prematurity. *Am J Clin Nutr* 2000;72:1548-1557.

165. Preisig R, Rennert O. Biliary transport and cholestatic effects of amino acids. *Gastroenterology* 1977;73:1232.

166. Moss RL, Haynes AL, Pastuszyn A, Glew RH.

Methionine infusion reproduces liver injury of parenteral nutrition cholestasis. *Pediatr Res* 1999;45:664-668.

167. Sturman JA, Chesney RW. Taurine in pediatric nutrition. *Pediatr Clin North Am* 1995;42:879-897.

168. Chesney RW, Helms RA, Christensen M, Budreau AM, Han X, Sturman JA. An updated view of the value of taurine in infant nutrition. *Adv Pediatr* 1998a;45:179-200.

169. Zamora SA, Amin HJ, McMillan DD, Kubes P, Fick GH, Butzner JD, Scott RB. Plasma L-arginine concentrations in premature infants with neonatal enterocolitis. *J Pediatr* 1997;131:226-232.

170. Vaughn PR, Lobo C, Battaglia FC, Fennessey PV, Wilkening RB, Meschia G. Glutamine-glutamate exchange between placenta and fetal liver. *Am J Physiol* 1995; 268: E705-E711.

171. Ziegler TR, Szeszycki EE, Estivariz CF, Puckett AB, Leader LM. Glutamine from basic science to clinical applications. *Nutrition* 1996;12:S68-S70.

172. Lacey JM, Wilmore DW. Is glutamine a conditionally essential amino acid? *Nutr Rev* 1990;48:297-309.

173. Lacey JM, Crouch JB, Benfell K, Ringer SA, Wilmore CK, Maguire D, Wilmore DW. The effects of glutamine supplemented parenteral nutrition in premature infants. *J Parenter Enteral Nutr* 1996;20:74-80.

174. Neu J. Glutamine in the fetus and critically ill low-birth-weight neonate: metabolism and mechanism of action. *J Nutr* 2001;131:2585S-2589S.

175. des Robert C, Le Bacquer O, Piloquet H, Roze JC, Darmaun D. Acute effects of intravenous glutamine supplementation on protein metabolism in very-low birth-weight infants: a stable isotope study. *Pediatr Res* 2002;51:87-93.

176. Tubman TR, Thompson SW. Glutamine supplementation for preventing morbidity in preterm. *Cochrane Database Syst Rev* 2000;2:CD001457.

177. Neu, J. Glutamine: Role in the Fetus and Low-birth-weight Infant. *NeoReviews* 2000; 1:e215-e221.

178. Buchman AL. Glutamine: commercially essential or conditionally essential? A critical appraisal of the human data. *Am J Clin Nutr* 2001;74:25-32.

179. Cairns PA, Stalker DJ. Carnitine supplementation of

parenterally fed neonates. The Cochrane Libary 2000: CDOO950.

180. Cosgrove M. Nucleotide. *Nutrition* 1998; 14:748-751.

181. Garofalo RP, Goldman AS. Expression of functional immunomodulatory and anti-inflammatory factors in human milk. *Clinics in Perinatology* 1999;26:361-77.

182. Hamosh M. Bioactive factors in human milk. *Pediatr Clin North Am* 2001;48:69-86.

183. Thorell L, Sjoberg LB, Hernell O. Nucleotides in human milk: sources and metabolism by the newborn infant. *Pediatr Res* 1996;40:845-852.

184. Maldonado J, Navarro J, Narbona E, Gil A. The influence of dietary nucleotides on humoral and cell immunity in the neonate and lactating infant. *Earl Hum Develop* 2001; 65 Suppl: S69-S74.

185. Carver JD, Pimental B, Cox WI, Barness LA. Dietary nucleotide effects upon immune function in infants. *Pediatrics* 1991;88:359-363.

186. McMillan JA, Oski FA, Lourie G, Tomarelli RM, Landaw SA. Iron absorption from human milk, simulated human milk, and proprietary formulas. *Pediatrics* 1977; 60:896-900.

187. Sanchez-Pozo A, Morillas J, Molto L, Robles R, Gil A. Dietary nucleotides influence lipoprotein metabolism in newborn infants. *Pediatr Res* 1994;35:112-116.

188. Van Buren CT, Rudolph F. Dietary nucleotides: a conditional requirement. Nutrition 1997;13:470-472.

189. Gil A, Pita ML, Martinez A, Molina JA, Sanchez-Medina F. Effect of dietary nucleotides on the plasma fatty acids in at-term neonates. *Hum Nut Clin Nutr* 1986;40C:185-195.

190. DeLucchi C, Pita ML, Faus MJ, Molina JA, Uauy R, Gil A. Effects of dietary nucleotides on the fatty acid composition of erythrocyte membrane lipids in term infants. *J Pediatr Gastroenterol Nutr* 1987;6:568-574.

191. Uauy R, Quan R, Gil A. Nucleotides in infants nutrition. In: Gil A, Uauy R, eds. Nutritional and Biological Significance of Dietary Nucleotides and Nucleic Acids. Granada: Abbott Laboratories; 1996:169-180.

192. Cosgrove M, Davies DP, Jenkins HR. Nucleotide supplementation and the growth of term small for gestational age infants. *Arch Dis Child* 1996;74: F122-125.

193. Commission Directive 96/4/CE 1996 amending directive 91/321/EEC on infant formula. *Official Journal L* 049,28/02/96:12-16.

194. Thureen PJ, Hay WW Jr. Intravenous nutrition and postnatal growth of the micropremie. *Clin Perinatol* 2000;27:197-219.

195. Saini J, MacMahon P, Morgan JB, Kovar IZ. Early parenteral feeding of amino acids. *Arch Dis Child* 1989;64:1362-1366.

196. Rivera A Jr, Bell EF, Bier DM Effect of intravenous amino acids on protein metabolism of preterm infants during the first three days of life. *Pediatr Res* 1993;33:106-111.

197. Thureen PJ, Hay WW Jr. Early aggressive nutrition in pretem infants. *Semin Neonatol* 2001;6:403-415

198. van Lingen RA, van Goudoever JB, Luijendijk IHT, Wattimena JLD, Sauer PJJ. Effects of early amino acid administration during total parenteral nutrition on protein metabolism in preterm infants. *Clinical Science* 1992;82:199-203.

199. Thureen PJ, Anderson AH, Baron KA, Melara DL, Hay WW, Fennessey PV. Protein balance in the first week of life in ventilated neonates receiving parenteral nutrition. *Am J Clin Nutr* 1998;68:1128-1135.

200. Tsai FJ, Tsai CH, Wu SF, Liu YH, Yeh TF. Catabolic effect in premature infants with early dexamethasone treatment. *Acta Paediatr* 1996;85:1487-1490.

201. van Goudoever, JB, Sulkers EJ, Timmerman M, Huijmans JGM, Langer K, Carnielli VP, Sauer PJJ. Amino acid solutions for premature infants during the first week of life: The role of N-acetyl-Lcysteine and N-acetyl-L-tyrosine. *J Parent Ent Nutr* 1994;18: 404-408.

202. Premer DM, Georgieff MK. Nutrition for III neonates. *NeoReviews* 1999:e56-e62.

203. Anderson MS, Thureen PJ, Bacon KA, Bass KD, Melara DL, Hay WW Jr. Achieving positive protein balance in the immediate postoperative period in neonates with amino acid administration plus narcotic analgesia. *Pediatr Research* 1999;45:276 A.

204. Shew SB, Keshen TH, Glass NL, Jahoor F, Jaksic T. Ligation of a patent ductus arteriosus under fentanyl anesthesia impoves protein metabolism in premature neonates. 2000;35:1277-1281.

205. Mrozek JD, Georgieff MK, Blazar BR, Mammel MC, Schwarzenberg SJ.Effect of sepsis syndrome on neonatal protein and energy metabolism. *J Perinatol* 2000;20:96-100.

206. Thureen PJ, Melara D, Fennessey PV, Hay WW Jr. Effect of low versus high intravenous amino acid intake on very-low-birth-weight infants in the early neonatal period. *Pediatr Res* 2003;53:24-32.

207. Ziegler EE, Thureen PJ, Carlson SJ. Aggressive nutrition of the very-low-birth-weight infant. *Clin Perinatol* 2002 Jun;29(2):225-44.

208. Binder ND, Raschko PK, Benda GI, Reynolds JW. Insulin infusion with parenteral nutrition in extremely-low-birth-weight infants with hyperglycemia. *J Pediatr* 1989;114:273-280.

209. Collins JW Jr, Hoppe M, Brown K et al. A controlled trial of insulin infusion and parenteral nutrition in extremely-low-birth-weight infants with glucose intolerance. *J Pediatr* 1991;118:921-927.

210. Wilson DC, Cairns P, Halliday HL, Reid M, McClure G, Dodge JA. Randomised controlled trial of an aggressive nutritional regimen in sick very-low-birth-weight infants. *Arch Dis Child Fetal Neonatal Ed* 1997;77:F4-11.

211. Meetze W, Bowsher R, Compton J, Mooredhead H. Hyperglycemia in extremely-low-birth-weight infants. *Biol Neonate* 1998;74:214-221.

212. Thureen PJ, Scheer B, Anderson SM, Tooze JA, Young DA, Hay WW. Effect of hyperinsulinemia on amino acid utilization in the ovine fetus. *Am J Physiol* 2000; 279: E1294-E1304.

213. Wray-Cahen D, Beckett PR, Nguyen HV, Davis TA. Insulinstimulated amino acid utilization during glucose and amino acid clamps decreases with development. *Am J Physiol* 1997;273:E305-14.

214. Paisley JE, Thureen PJ, Baron KA, Hay WW. Safety and efficacy of low versus high parenteral amino acid intakes in extremely-low-birth-weight (ELBW) neonates immediately after birth. *Ped Research* 2000;47: 293A .

215. Lucas A, Bloom SR, Aynsley-Green A. Gut hormones and 'minimal enteral feeding'. *Acta Paediatr Scand* 1986;75:719-723.

216. Meetze WH, Valentine C, McGuigan JE, Conlon M, Sacks N, Neu J. Gastrointestinal priming prior to full enteral nutrition in very-low-birth-weight. *J Pediatr Gastroenterol Nutr* 1992;15:163-170.

217. Berseth CL. Effect of early feeding on maturation of the preterm infant's small intestine. *J Pediatr* 1992;120:947-953.

218. Berseth CL, Nordyke C. Enteral nutrients promote postnatal maturation of intestinal motor activity in preterm infants. *Am J Physiol* 1993;264:G1046-1051.

219. Berseth CL. Minimal enteral feedings. *Clin Perinatol* 1995;22:195-205.

220. Walker WA, Dai D. Protective nutrients for the immature gut. In: Ziegler EE, Lucas A, Moro GE, eds. *Nutrition of the Very-Low-Birth-Weight Infant.* Nestle Nutrition Workshop Series. Nestec Ltd, Vevey/Lippincott Williams and Wilkins. Philadelphia, Pennsylvania:1999; 43:179-197.

221. Lipman TO. Bacterial translocation and enteral nutrition in humans: an outsider looks in. *J Parenter Enteral Nutr* 1995;19:156-165.

222. McClure RJ, Newell SJ. Randomised controlled trial of trophic feeding and gut motility. *Arch Dis Child* 1999;80:F54-F58.

223. Dunn L, Hulman S, Weiner J, Kliegman R. Beneficial effects of early hypocaloric enteral feedingon neonatal gastrointestinal function: preliminary report of a randomized trial. *J Pediatr* 1988;112:622-629.

224. Stagle TA, Gross SJ. Effect of early low-volume enteral substrate on subsequent feeding tolerance in very-low-birth-weight infants. *J Pediatr* 1988; 113:526-531.

225. Kennedy KA, Tyson JE, Chamnanvanikij S. Early versus delayed initiation of progressive enteral feedings for parenterally fed low-birth-weight or preterm infants. *Cochrane Review* 2000:CD01970.

226. Schanler RJ, Shulman RJ, Lau C. Feeding strategies for premature infants: beneficial outcomes of feeding fortified human milk versus preterm formula. *Pediatrics* 1999;103:1150-1157.

227. Berseth CL, Bisquera JA, Paje VU.Prolonging small feeding volumes early in life decreases the incidence of necrotizing enterocolitis in very-low-birth-weight infants. *Pediatrics* 2003 ;111:529-34.

228. Atkinson SA. Human milk feeding of the micropremie. *Clinics in Perinatology* 2000;27:235-247.

229. Lawrence RA. Breastfeeding support benefits very-low-birth-weight infants. *Arch Pediatr Adolesc Med* 2001;155:543-544.

230. Lucas A, Morley R, Cole TJ, Lister G, Leeson-Payne C. Breast milk and subsequent intelligence quotient in children born preterm. *Lancet* 1992 1;339:261-264.

231. Morley R. Nutrition and cognitve development. *Nutrition* 1998;14:752-754.

232. Michie CA, Gilmour J. Breast feeding and the risks of viral transmission. *Arch Dis Child* 2001;84:381-382.

233. Stein H, Cohen D, Herman AA, Rissik J, Ellis U, Bolton K, Pettifor J, MacDougall L. Pooled pasteurized breast milk and untreated own mother's milk in the feeding of very low birth weight babies: a randomized controlled trial. *J Pediatr Gastroenterol Nutr* 1986;5:242-247.

234. Polberger SK, Axelsson IA, Raiha NC. Growth of very low-birth-weight infants on varying amounts of human milk protein. *Pediatr Res* 1989;25:414-419.

235. Greer FR, McCormick A. Improved bone mineralization and growth in premature infants fed fortified own mother's milk. *J Pediatr* 1988; 112:961-969.

236. Voyer M, Senterre J, Rigo J, Charlas J, Satge P. Human milk lacto-engineering. Growth nitrogen metabolism, and energy balance in preterm infants. *Acta Paediatr Scand* 1984;73:302-306.

237. Schanler RJ, Hurst NM, Lau C. The use of human milk and breastfeeding in premature infants. *Clin Perinatol* 1999;26:379-398.

238. Moody GJ, Schanler RJ, Lau C, Shulman RJ. Feeding tolerance in premature infants fed fortified human milk. *J Pediatr Gastroenterol Nutr* 2000;30:408-412.

239. Moro GE, Minoli I, Ostrom M, Jacobs JR, Picone TA, Raiha NC, Ziegler. Fortification of human milk: evaluation of a novel fortification of a new fortifier. *J Pediatr Gastroenterol Nutr* 1995;20:162-172.

240. Moyeur-Mileur L, Chan GM, Gill G. Evaluation of liquid or powdered fortification of human milk on bone mineralization status ofpreterm infants. *J Pediatr Gastroenterol Nutr* 1992;15:370-374.

241. Nicholl RM, Gamsu HR. Changes in growth and metabolism in very-low-birth-weight infants fed with fortified breast milk. *Acta Paediatr* 1999;88:1056-1061.

242. Polberger S, Raïihä, P Juvonen, Moro GE, Minoli I, Warm A. Individualized protein fortification of human milk for preterm infants: comparison of ultrafiltrated human milk protein and a bovine whey fortifier. *J Pediatr Gastroenterol Nutr* 1999;29:332-8.

243. Porcelli P, Schanler R, Greer F, Chan G, Gross S, Mehta N, Spear M, Kerner J, Euler AR. Growth in human milk-fed very-low-birth-weight infants receiving a new human milk fortifier. *Ann Nutr Metab* 2000;44:2-10.

244. Furman L, Schluchter M, Taylor GH, Minich N, Hack M. Feeding fortified maternal milk results in lesser weight gain for very-low-birth-weight (VLBW, <1.5 kg) infants. *Neonatology*:260A.

245. Guerrini P. Human milk fortifiers. *Acta Paediatr Suppl* 1994 ;402 :37-39.

246. Kuschel CA, Harding JE. Protein supplementation of human milk for promoting growth in preterm infants. *Cochrane Review* 2000;2:CD000433.

247. Kushel CA, Harding JE. Multicomponent fortified human milk for promoting growth in preterm infants. Cochrane Review 2000;2:CD000343.

248. De Curtis M, Candusso M, Pieltain C, Rigo J. Effect of fortification on the osmolality of human milk. *Arch Dis Child Fetal Neonatal Ed* 1999;81:F141-143.

249. Lucas A, Fewtrell MS, Morley R, Lucas PJ, Baker BA, Lister G, Bishop. Randomized outcome trial of human milk fortification and development outcome in preterm infants. *Am J Clin Nutr* 1996;64,2:142-151.

250. Jocson MAL, Mason EO, and Schanler RJ. The effects of nutrient fortification and varying storage conditions on host defense properties of human milk. *Pediatrics* 1997;100:240-243.

251. Schanler RJ, Shulman RJ, Lau C. Feeding strategies for premature infants: beneficial outcomes of feeding fortified human milk versus preterm formula. *Pediatrics* 1999;103:1150-1157.

252. Lessaris KJ, Forsythe DW, Wagner CL. Effect of human milk fortifier on the immunodetection and molecular mass profile of transforming growth factor-alpha. *Biol Neonate* 2000;77:156-161.

253. Quan R, Yang C, Rubinstein S, Lewiston NJ, Stevenson DK, Kerner JA. The effect of nutritional

additives on anti-infective factors in human milk. *Clinical Pediatrics* 1994:325-328.

254. Claud EC, Walker WA. Hypothesis: inappropriate colonization of the premature intestine can cause neonatal necrotizing enterocolitis. *FASEB J* 2001; 15:1398-1403.

255. Räihä NCR, Fazzolari A, Cayozzo C, Puccio G, Minoli I, Moro G, Monestier A, Haschke-Becher E, Carrié A, Hashke F. Protein nutrition during infancy: effects on growth and metabolism. *J Pediatr Gastroenterol Nutr* 2002;35:275-281.

256. Loser C. Polyamines in human and animal milk. *Br J Nutr* 2000;84:S55-S58.

257. Collins MD, Gibson GR. Probiotics, prebiotics, and synbiotics: approaches for modulating the microbial ecology of the gut. *Am J Clin Nutr* 1999;69: 1052S-1057S

258. Thureen PJ, Anderson MS, Hay WW Jr. The small-for-gestational age infant. *NeoReviews* 2001: e139-e149.

Carbohydrates Including Oligosaccharides and Inositol

Prabhu Parimi, M.D. and Satish C. Kalhan, M.D.

Reviewed by Hans Buller, M.D. and Carlos Lifschitz, M.D.

Introduction

The macro and micronutrient requirements for the preterm infant remain controversial and unresolved, mostly because of: (a) lack of a consensus regarding the anticipated rate of growth; and (b) the heterogeneity of the premature population, particularly in terms of gestational age. Although several expert committees have recommended that postnatal growth should approach the rate of growth that would have occurred "in utero" for a normal fetus, assuming it to be the best measure or model for subsequent growth and development, it still remains to be demonstrated that such a goal can be achieved in contemporary clinical practice. The discrepancy between extrauterine growth curves and intrauterine rate of growth becomes largest, the more premature the neonate, so that the extrauterine growth curve of the very low birth weight or extremely premature infants (less than 27-weeks gestation) depart the farthest from the intrauterine growth curves.[1] Even though the above discrepancy has often been attributed to limitation in energy intake or adminis-tration, data supporting such an inference are not easily available. In addition, there is no conclusive evidence to justify uncritical acceptance of the recommendation that the extrauterine growth curve should mimic the intrauterine rate of growth of a normal fetus.[2]

The heterogeneity of the preterm population is an additional consideration because of the marked improvement in survival of the extremely low birth weight infants. While the nutrient requirements and growth of less premature infants (32- to 36-weeks gestation) may resemble those of near term infants, it may not necessarily be true for those born at less than 32-weeks gestational age. Recent data cited above[1] show that most low birth weight infants (24- to 29-weeks gestation), at the time of discharge from the hospital, do not achieve the median birth weight of the reference fetus at the same postmenstrual age.

Glucose Utilization and Range of Carbohydrate Intake

Glucose is the major source of energy for humans, including infants and children, and is the primary circulating carbohydrate in the body. It is a major source of energy for the brain, and is an important carbon source for de novo synthesis of fatty acids and a number of non-essential amino acids. The majority of the exogenously administered carbohydrates are metabolized following their conversion to glucose. Exogenously administered carbohydrates, during low energy intakes or during starvation, have been shown to have nitrogen sparing effects in adult humans.[3] However, any relation between carbohydrate intake and nitrogen loss in children has not been evaluated systematically. Kashyap and colleagues[4] report that preterm infants receiving a high carbohydrate (65% of energy intake) formula tend to have lower nitrogen losses and positive nitrogen balance. However, these data should be interpreted with caution, since the high carbohydrate intake resulted in a higher intake of metabolizable energy when compared with a lower carbohydrate, high fat formula group.

The acceptable range of upper and lower limit of carbohydrate intake in infants and children has been reviewed recently.[5,6] Although very few studies have examined whole body metabolism of glucose in the

	Preterm	Term	Child
Glucose Ra			
mg/kg.min	8-9	5.0	4.0
g/kg.d	11.5-12.9	7.2	5.8
Glucose oxidation			
(% of Ra)	-	65	-
g/kg.d	-	4.7	-

Ra = rate of production
kg = kg body weight
Data are averages from several studies. Oxidation was calculated from
respiratory gas exchange.

Table 1: Basal rates of glucose production and oxidation in the newborn infant.

human preterm infant, a few inferences can be drawn from published data.[7] These conclusions can be inferred from measured rates of production and oxidation of glucose, rate of energy expenditure, quantitative contribution of glucose to energy expenditure, impact of exogenous glucose administration, and estimated rate of utilization of glucose by the brain.

The rates of endogenous production of glucose in preterm and term infants are presented in Table 1. Based upon a number of studies and approximated from published reports, it can be inferred that a preterm infant has a higher rate of basal glucose production when compared with the full-term infant (8-9 vs. 5 mg.kg body wt.$^{-1}$min^{-1}).[8-11,15-19] Of this, approximately 30% is contributed by gluconeogenesis from pyruvate[16] and an additional 20% by glycerol.[11-15] In addition, as inferred from the respiratory exchange data, 65-70% of the glucose produced is oxidized to carbon dioxide in full-term infants.[8] Such a rate of oxidation will meet only ~50% of the total energy needs and perhaps account for most of the energy requirement of the brain. No corresponding data are available for preterm infants, in part because they cannot be studied in the basal state due to clinical and ethical considerations.

In response to glucose/carbohydrate administration, the preterm infant has the capacity to oxidize increasing amounts of glucose in order to meet energy demands, so that at high rates of glucose infusion, almost all energy expenditure is met by glucose or carbohydrate oxidation. The data of Sauer et al[21] are displayed in Figure 1. As shown, with increasing glucose intake, range 10-25 g.kg^{-1}.d^{-1}, there was a linear increase in both total glucose utilization as measured by respiratory calorimetry and glucose oxidation as measured by ^{13}C labeled glucose tracer.

Glucose utilization by the brain: The rate of glucose consumption by the brain has been calculated from the published data on oxygen consumption by the brain. The average rate of oxygen consumption by the brain in children is 235 µmol.min^{-1}.100 g brain weight^{-1}, corresponding to 39 µmole of glucose. min^{-1}.100 g brain weight^{-1}. For a full-term newborn with a brain weight of 399 gm, the rate of glucose consumption by the brain will correspond to 37 gm.day^{-1} or 11.5 gm.kg body wt^{-1}.day^{-1}. Thus in order to meet the glucose requirement of the brain, the full-term infant should be given at least 11.5 gm of carbohydrate(glucose).kg body wt^{-1}.day^{-1}.[5] Corresponding data for the preterm infant are not available. However, based on recent studies using positron emission tomography (PET), it appears that there is a lower rate of uptake of glucose by the brain in the neonate, particularly in the immediate period after birth. In addition, regional differences in the local cerebral metabolic rate of glucose were also observed.[22-24] The reasons for the difference in PET data and the arterio-venous gradient data are not easily discerned.

Upper and lower limit of carbohydrate intake: Based upon the above data, acceptable upper and lower limits of carbohydrate intake can be described. It should be underscored that these limits are entirely theoretical, since the impact of carbohydrate intake at such limits on whole body metabolism, growth, nitrogen sparing, etc., has not been evaluated in infants and children, neither in the basal state nor under defined experimental conditions.[5,6]

The upper limit of carbohydrate intake should be described in relation to the minimal need for other macronutrients, ie, protein and fat. Although the entire energy needs of an infant or an adult can be

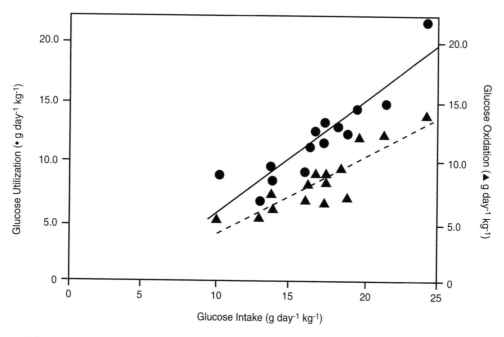

Figure 1: Relation between glucose intake (•) and oxidation (▲) of glucose in preterm infants. The rate of glucose utilization was measured by indirect respiratory calorimetry while oxidation was calculated from the rate of appearance of ^{13}C in expired CO_2 following a continuous infusion of U-[$^{13}C_6$]glucose. Reproduced with permission from Sauer et al.[21]

met by carbohydrates, there is an obligatory need for protein and fat in order to provide for growth and essential nutrients. Thus the upper limits of carbohydrate intake can be calculated as the glucose equivalent of the total energy expenditure. The total energy expenditure of the neonate is estimated to be 70 kcal/kg.d, which corresponds to a carbohydrate equivalent of 17 gm.kg body wt[-1].d[-1]. High carbohydrate intake could, however, potentially cause increased lipogenesis and predisposition to obesity. It should be underscored that high carbohydrate administration in the neonatal period may not only result in obesity in the immediate newborn period, but also may predispose to obesity and insulin resistance in adult life. Data in animal studies provide compelling evidence that a high carbohydrate diet during the suckling period results in permanent obesity in the adult, as well as in the future progeny.[25,26]

In contrast to the upper limit, the lower boundary of carbohydrate intake can be defined based upon: (a) that which meets the energy needs of the brain and other glucose-dependent organs; (b) that which can minimize the irreversible loss of protein and nitrogen and minimize gluconeogenesis; and (c) that which prevents ketosis. For the premature infant, such estimates can only be made based upon their endogenous rate of glucose production, ie, 11.5 g.kg[-1].d[-1] (Table 1), since data regarding prevention of ketosis are not available. It should be emphasized that these estimates assume the premature infants to be a uniform homogeneous group and do not separate the very premature (VLBW) from the less mature infants.

Glucose Uptake by the Gut

Glucose is the major biological carbohydrate, representing the final pathway for the metabolism and oxidation of all carbohydrates in the body. It is not present in significant quantities in milk, from human and animal sources, nor is it present in other nutrient sources.

Glucose is absorbed by the gut via a specific Na+/glucose co-transporter that handles all hexoses. D-glucose and D-galactose are the natural substrates for these transporters.[23] Although the Na+/glucose co-transporter has been identified as a 73-KD integral membrane protein and the gene has been cloned and sequenced, not much is known about its ontogeny in the human fetus.

The kinetics of absorption of glucose by the gut in premature infants were examined by Shulman in 16 infants, birth weight 1120 ± 89 g and gestational age 27.7 ± 0.5 weeks (mean ± SEM).[28] The infants were studied at 32 ± 0.6 days (28-38 d) after birth, when the orogastric intake of formula/human milk was fully established. There was a positive correlation between V_{max}, K_m and postnatal age of the infants at the time of study (K_m: r = 0.6, p = 0.015; V_{max}: r = 0.64, p = 0.008). K_m was also positively related to the amount of feeding the infant received as preterm infant formula. Although the author also found a correlation between gestational age and log V_{max} for glucose (r = 0.52, p = 0.039), suggesting a development-related effect, the observed change may simply have been related to postnatal age rather than gestation. Since the infants were studied late (32 days) after birth, gestation related development change would have been mitigated by the extrauterine environment. This study also showed that at equal glucose loads (mg.min^{-1}.cm^{-1}), glucose absorption was greater when the infusion was delivered in a higher volume (higher rate, lower concentration) than when delivered in a lower volume (lower rate, higher concentration). The latter effect may be due to difference in osmolarity of the infusate. Finally, intrapartum steroids given to the mother appeared to enhance V_{max} for glucose.

The above data are the only carefully conducted study of glucose absorption in preterm infants in the literature. Because the studies were performed between 28 and 38 days after birth, the postnatal age and the duration of enteral feeding appear to be the predominant determinants of K_m and V_{max}, rather than the gestational age of the infant. Indirect evidence suggest that absorption of glucose by the gut is present in the 12-week-old fetus; however, ontogenic changes, if any, have not been demonstrated.[29,30] Other indirect measurements of glucose absorption have not demonstrated any significant differences between preterm and term infants.[31] The K_m values reported by Shulman are comparable to those obtained from studies in human adults.[32]

Thus, absorption of glucose appears to be well developed in enterally fed preterm infants and changes with age (or duration of enteral feeding), and is influenced by the volume of feeding and by glucocorticoids.

Glucose as the exclusive carbohydrate has not been used in infant formula because of the potential for increase in osmolarity of the formula and for its possible non-enzymatic reaction with protein in the formula when heated, which may cause the Maillard Reaction.[33]

Lactose

In the human fetus, intestinal lactase activity is measurable by 10- to 12-weeks gestation. There is a gradual increase in lactase activity with advancing gestation; however, the activity actually remains low until about 36-weeks gestation when it reaches the levels seen in full-term neonates.[30] Based on the low lactase activity in early gestation and the estimated length of the bowel, it was calculated that a preterm infant weighing 1300-1400 g might be expected to have nearly 50-70% of the lactose ingested to pass unabsorbed into the colon.[35] These estimates are higher than those of Kien et al.[36,37] Using stable isotope tracers of glucose and galactose in 14 preterm infants (gestational age 26-31 weeks) who were 31-37 weeks post-conceptional age at the time of study, these investigators demonstrated that the mean lactose digestion was 79 ± 26% (mean ± SD), and that the percentage of lactose that was not absorbed but was instead fermented in the colon, averaged 35 ± 27%.

Whether premature birth or early exposure to lactose-containing nutrients can induce intestinal lactase is not known. Shulman et al[38] recently examined whether the timing of initiation of feeding affected the development of intestinal lactase activity. In a randomized trial, 135 babies (26- to 30-weeks gestation) were assigned to begin feeds either early (4 days) or to the standard practice of 15 days. The intestinal lactase activity was evaluated by measuring the urinary ratios of lactulose/lactose after the two sugars were administered. From their data it appears that early feeding increases intestinal lactase activity in preterm infants.

Lactose and calcium bioavailability: Data from animal studies, particularly rat, have provided strong evidence that lactose has beneficial effects on intestinal calcium absorption and calcium retention in bone. However, the beneficial effect of lactose may be related to lactose's resistance to enzymatic degradation (in rat), since the presence of other non-absorbable sugars can also promote calcium absorption in the rat small intestine.[39] In lactose tolerant normal healthy adults, lactose had no effect on calcium bioavailability as determined by stable-strontium loading test.[39] In contrast to studies in adults and in animals, the data in human newborns are conflicting. In six white healthy infants (birth weight greater than 2500 g) studied during the first few months of life using careful metabolic balance studies, Ziegler and Fomon[40] observed a significant and sustained promoting effect of lactose on absorption of calcium and other minerals. However, it is important to note that in their study the mean calcium intake was significantly higher and fecal excretion of calcium only "somewhat less" (61 ± 30 vs. 66 ± 25 mg/kg.d, mean ± SD) in the infants fed formula containing lactose as compared with those fed formula containing sucrose and cornstarch hydrolysate. In low birth weight infants (n=14, birth weight 960-2230 g, gestational age 29-36 weeks), using stable isotopic tracer of calcium, Stathos et al[41] observed a higher rate of calcium absorption with glucose polymer when compared with similar amount of lactose. Of interest, calcium absorption correlated positively with water and carbohydrate absorption. It should be underscored that the study of Stathos et al used the triple lumen catheter perfusion method;

hence, the calcium absorption kinetics were measured only in the proximal intestine, and the absorption in the distal gut was not quantified. Wirth and colleagues[42] did not find any effect of reducing lactose content of premature infant formulas (from 100% to 50%) on absorption of calcium in preterm infants. In a recent study, Moya et al[43] observed that feeding full-term infants a lactose-free formula resulted in a higher total retention of calcium, even though there was no significant difference in urinary and fecal excretion or total absorption of calcium when compared with infants fed formula which contained lactose.

From these data in human adults and preterm infants, we infer that in lactose tolerant subjects, lactose does not appear to have any beneficial effect on calcium bioavailability. However, in lactose intolerant subjects (such as preterm infants), the presence of non-hydrolyzed lactose in the distal bowel may increase calcium absorption by enhancing passive transport of calcium via the nonsaturable paracellular route that occurs throughout the length of the intestine.

Galactose

Although most human infants and the newborns of several mammalian species ingest large quantities of galactose, the requirements and benefits of galactose feeding remain unknown.[44] The major source of galactose for the human newborn is lactose, which is the predominant carbohydrate in human milk and infant formula. Hydrolysis of lactose at the intestinal brush border results in the release of glucose and galactose which are readily absorbed. The majority of the enterally-absorbed galactose is taken up by the liver during the first pass,[45,46] so that there is minimal change in plasma galactose concentration. Galactose taken up by the liver is either converted to glucose or deposited as glycogen.

In the isolated perfused liver preparation and in in vivo studies in newborn monkey and dog, galactose has been shown to augment hepatic glycogen synthesis and activate hepatic glycogen synthase.[47-50]

Galactose administered parenterally is also cleared rapidly from the plasma.[44] The rate of clearance of galactose appears similar in premature and term neonates, and in older infants. Although galactose has been used for the treatment and prevention of hypoglycemia and hyperglycemia in the newborn infant, the nutritional requirements of galactose for the premature or full-term infant have not been examined. In this context, it is important to note that a significant rate of endogenous synthesis of galactose has been observed in normal healthy human adults by using stable isotopic tracer dilution methods[41] and therefore an obligatory requirement for exogenous galactose, at least in normal health adult humans, is not certain.

Oligosaccharides

The protective effect of human milk against diarrheal diseases and respiratory and ear infections has been documented from a number of clinical epidemiological studies in developed and developing countries. Although this protective effect has been attributed, for the most part, to the presence of secretory immunoglobulins and related components in breast milk, from recent data it appears that some of these anti-infective properties may also be related to the presence of oligosaccharides. These oligosaccharides could function as protective factors via a non-immunological mechanism, eg, by affecting the growth of intestinal flora, preventing the attachment of microorganisms to epithelial cells, and by acting as receptor analogues for adhesion molecules on mucosal cells.[52]

Quantitatively, other than lactose, oligosaccharides are the largest carbohydrate component in mature human milk[53] and represent the third largest solute load after lactose and fat.[54] The concentration of oligosaccharides in human milk has been observed to change with the duration of lactation, being highest in the colostrum, ~20-23 g/L, ~20 g/L on day 4 and ~13 g/L on day 120 of lactation.[55] No significant difference in concentration of neutral oligosaccharides has been documented between preterm human milk and in milk examined at term gestation;[56] however, other oligosaccharides (for example sialic acid containing) may be higher in preterm milk.[53] Most of the oligosaccharides are formed from the sequential

addition of monosaccharide to the molecule of lactose by specific glucosyl transferase of the mammary gland.[54] A large number of different oligosaccharides (~130) have been identified in human milk. Their presence and quantity are determined possibly by genetic and environmental factors. Erney et al[57] examined a large number of human milk samples from diverse geographical populations. Concentrations of the nine neutral oligosaccharides varied quantitatively and qualitatively with geographical origin of donors. The authors attributed these differences to possible genetically determined traits that are not uniformly distributed. Wide quantitative and qualitative distribution patterns of oligosaccharides have also been observed in animal species. Cow milk and, therefore, cow milk derived infant formula, contain very little oligosaccharides. In contrast, the total oligosaccharide concentration in elephant milk was three times higher than human milk and comprised up to 10% of the carbohydrate content. Furthermore, the ratio of neutral:acidic components in the milk of the two species was also different.[58]

Other than the possible anti-infective properties, the biological role of oligosaccharides in human milk is not known. Gnoth et al[59] examined the digestibility of human milk oligosaccharides in vitro using human salivary amylase, porcine pancreatic amylase and porcine brush border membrane vesicle. From their data it appears that less than 5% of the ingested human milk oligosaccharides would be digested in the intestinal tract. Similarly, Engfer et al[60] demonstrated resistance of human milk oligosaccharides to enzymatic hydrolysis by human pancreatic juice and human brush border membrane vesicle or porcine intestinal tissue samples. Brand Miller and colleagues,[61] by using lactulose hydrogen breath test, have shown that human milk oligosaccharides resist digestion in the small intestine of breast fed infants and undergo fermentation in the colon, and may be the source of breath hydrogen in these babies. Quantitatively very few oligosaccharides are excreted in stools of breast fed babies. In contrast, lactose derived oligosaccharides have been demonstrated in the urine, suggesting at least some absorption of intact molecules.[62] In addition, breast fed infants have higher concentrations of sialic acid in their saliva when compared with formula fed babies.[63] It was hypothesized that the higher sialic acid levels were due to the high concentration of sialyated oligosaccharides in human milk. In the large bowel, oligosaccharides have been suggested to be involved in maintenance of normal gut flora, inhibition of the growth of pathogenic bacteria, interference in the attachment of the bacteria to mucosal cell and their fermentation products, mostly short chain fatty acids, and provision of nutrition and energy for the colonocytes and the whole body.[52,53]

Since sialic acid is a structural and functional component of brain gangliosides and is suggested to play a role in neurotransmission and memory, sialyated oligosaccharides have been suggested to play a role in perinatal brain development.[52,53,58] A similar role for galactose containing oligosaccharides has been suggested.[53]

All of these data provide compelling evidence for the beneficial role of oligosaccharides in the nutritional care of the preterm infant. Since commercial infant feeding formulae, derived from cow milk or other sources, do not contain significant quantities of these compounds, these data further emphasize the need to provide human milk for the nutritional support of the preterm babies.

Glucose Polymers

Glucose polymers are pure carbohydrates prepared by controlled acid/enzyme hydrolysis of cornstarch. They consist of polymers of glucose of varying chain length, although the majority are of medium (6-10 glucose units) chain length with a small amount (usually <2%) of free glucose. The glucose polymers are mainly linear, in which the glucose residue are attached by α-1,4 glucosidic bonds. They have been used as nutritional supplement for adults and infants because of their lower osmolality (as compared with glucose or other hexose solutions) and therefore possibly rapid gastric emptying, and for being less sweet as compared with fructose and sucrose.[64,65]

Glucose polymers are hydrolyzed by salivary,

pancreatic and intestinal amylase and maltases to free glucose which is rapidly absorbed. The absorption and oxidation of glucose polymers of different lengths was examined by Shulman and colleagues[64] in twelve healthy 1-month-old infants. Their data show that long-chain glucose polymers are not absorbed as completely as short-chain glucose polymers by some infants, and that colonic bacterial flora play a major role in salvaging the carbohydrate (energy) not absorbed in the small intestine. However, a wide variation was seen between subjects in the measured colonic fermentation of unabsorbed carbohydrate.[64] Studies by Kien et al[66] in preterm infants had shown efficient absorption of glucose polymers. They calculated absorption from the difference between intake and the carbohydrate energy excreted in the stools. In a later study, Kien et al[67] presented evidence for extensive colonic fermentation of carbohydrates in infants fed combined lactose and glucose polymer (50% each) formula. The absorption of lactose and glucose polymers by premature infants was compared by Shulman et al[68] using the double lumen perfusion catheter placed in the duodenum-jejunum. Twenty-one low birth weight infants (gestational age 33 ± 3 weeks, mean ± SD) who were receiving nasogastric tube feedings were studied at a mean postnatal age of 19.3±9 weeks (range 9 to 39 weeks) using test feeds of lactose, lactose-glucose polymer or glucose polymer alone. Absorption of lactose was significantly less than that of either lactose-glucose polymer combination or the glucose polymers alone (0.18 ± 0.24 mg.min^{-1}.cm^{-1} vs. 0.51 ± 0.45 and 0.57 ± 0.59, respectively; $p<0.005$). In addition, lactose absorption was not related to postnatal age at the time of study or to the total duration of enteral feeding prior to the study. In contrast, absorption of glucose-polymers alone or glucose-lactose combination was significantly correlated with postnatal age and the total duration of enteral feeding prior to the study. However, careful evaluation of the data shows that these two correlations may be weighted by two data points in the older age group.

In summary, glucose polymers appear to be rapidly hydrolyzed and absorbed by the neonate, and carbohydrate energy not absorbed in the small intestine is rapidly salvaged by the colonic bacteria. The efficiency of the absorption has only been examined in preterm babies at relatively older postnatal age and not in very low birth weight infants in the first few weeks after birth.

Carbohydrate Supplementation to Promote Growth

Because of the greater efficiency of absorption and assimilation of carbohydrates, and their possible effect on nitrogen and mineral retention in preterm infants as compared with fat, a number of investigators have examined whether addition of carbohydrates would lead to improved growth and development.

Kuschel and Harding[69] searched several published neonatal and perinatal databases in order to determine if the addition of carbohydrate supplements to human milk leads to improved growth and neurodevelopmental outcome without significant adverse effects in preterm infants. There were no studies which specifically evaluated the addition of carbohydrates alone for the purpose of improving growth or neurodevelopmental outcome. All published trials had used carbohydrate as only one component of a multi-component fortifier. Therefore it is difficult to make any conclusive statement or recommendation.

Inositol

Inositol is a six-carbon sugar present in several tissues as myo-inositol. It is synthesized in liver, kidney, brain, testis and mammary gland from D-glucose which is converted to glucose-6-phosphate. Cyclization of glucose-6-phosphate leads to formation of inositol-1-phosphate. Dephosphorylation of inositol-1-phosphate by inositol-1-phosphatase results in formation of inositol. Circulating inositol is transported into tissues against a concentration gradient and exists in its free form, phosphorylated derivatives and as phosphoinositides. The circulating tissue levels of inositol are determined by synthesis (cyclase activity) and clearance by the kidney (inositol oxygenase activity). Inositol has been shown to participate in transmembrane signaling processes,

eicosanoid synthesis, and in the secretion of lipoprotein in animals.[70]

Effect of intravenous inositol supplementation: Since inositol has been related to surfactant synthesis, and since parenteral nutrient mixture contains very low amounts of inositol, the parenteral effect of supplemental inositol has been examined in preterm infants with respiratory distress syndrome. Preterm infants less than 28-weeks gestation were randomized to receive either placebo (glucose) or inositol.[71,72] All infants were mechanically ventilated and required inspired oxygen concentration greater than 40%. Supplemented infants were given 80 mg.kg^{-1}.day^{-1} (440 mmol.kg^{-1}) of intravenous inositol for 5 days. Once the enteral feeds were started, they were fed either their mothers' breastmilk or pooled breastmilk. Infants who received inositol had higher lecithin:sphingomyelin ratio on the second day, significantly lower mortality and a lower incidence of bronchopulmonary dysplasia. However, it is to be emphasized that supplemental inositol had no beneficial effect among infants who received exogenous surfactant.

The study of Hallman et al shows that supplemental inositol may help babies with respiratory distress syndrome by inducing surfactant synthesis. The easy availability and high efficacy of exogenous surfactant has reduced the need to supplement preterm babies suffering from respiratory distress syndrome with inositol.

Inositol is present in human breastmilk at very high concentrations (~1800 mmol/L). Currently available preterm formulas contain inositol at very low concentrations. Therefore, the effects of inositol supplementation of preterm formulas on plasma inositol levels were examined by Carver et al[73] in a group of 72 clinically stable preterm infants (gestational age 25 - 33 weeks and birth weight 750 - 1500 grams) during the first five months. They received inositol-supplemented premature infant formula (1100 mmol/L) when they tolerated 70 ml/kg of enteral feeds. After discharge they were fed 20 calorie formula containing 178 mmol/L of inositol. At birth preterm infants had significantly higher plasma inositol concentrations when compared with term infants. The plasma inositol levels in preterm infants declined in spite of continued supplementation with inositol. The authors suggest the following: (1) the higher plasma inositol concentrations in preterm infants may be a consequence of enhanced synthesis and decrease in renal inositol oxygenase activity; and (2) lack of elevation of plasma inositol concentration in infants receiving enteral supplementation may be the consequence of accelerated disposal.

Based on the limited data presented above, there is no convincing evidence that inositol supplementation has any significant beneficial effect on growth or neonatal morbidity. Other beneficial effects of supplementing preterm formulas with inositol remain to be determined.

Clinical Problems

Hyperglycemia

Hyperglycemia occurs frequently in very low birth weight premature infants. The frequency of hyperglycemia in premature infants has been reported to be between 50% and 80%.[74,75] Although there is no consensus regarding the definition of hyperglycemia, a plasma glucose concentration >150 mg/dl (8.3 mmol/L) is generally considered to be high in neonates. An increase in plasma glucose concentration leads to higher serum osmolality. However, it is to be emphasized that an increase in plasma glucose concentration from 150 mg/dl to 200 mg/dl, ie, an increase of 50 mg/dl, represents an increase in serum osmolality of only 2.7 mOsm/L. Cellular dehydration, electrolyte shifts and increased risk for intracranial hemorrhage have been correlated with increase in serum osmolality. Perturbations in cellular hydration status can also alter cellular metabolism by changing the expression of certain genes and affecting cellular protein metabolism. Hyperglycemia also leads to osmotic diuresis with accompanied urinary electrolyte loss and systemic fluid and electrolyte derangement. The magnitude of glycosuria depends predominantly on the renal tubular threshold for glucose. Cowett et al observed that even in the presence of significant hyperglycemia, the

urinary loss of glucose in preterm babies was relatively small and demonstrated a lack of correlation between glycosuria and plasma glucose concentration.[76]

An understanding of the pathogenesis of hyperglycemia is essential to formulate the strategies for its management. A fine balance between endogenous glucose production and its utilization maintains plasma glucose concentrations in the euglycemic range. Perturbations in either of the above processes can lead to hyperglycemia. The magnitude of hepatic glucose output is influenced by both glycogenolysis and gluconeogenesis. These, in turn, are regulated by glucoregulatory hormones and amount of substrate availability (amino acids, lactate, etc.). Although the exact mechanism/s of hyperglycemia in the low birth weight infant have not been elucidated, both enhanced rate of hepatic glucose output and peripheral muscle insensitivity to insulin action as a result of increased counterregulatory hormones such as glucagon, cortisol, and catecholamines, have been suggested.[77,78]

The primary goal in the management of hyperglycemia is to decrease plasma glucose and serum osmolality. Since sepsis is a major causative factor, all premature infants with a plasma glucose concentration >150 mg/dl should be evaluated for sepsis and treated. Hyperglycemia often improves with optimal treatment of sepsis. The higher plasma glucose concentration can also be reduced by either decreasing the rate of glucose infusion or administering insulin. It should be underscored that reduction of glucose infusion will compromise energy intake. Several studies have been performed using insulin infusion with parenteral nutrition in extremely low birth eight infants with glucose intolerance.[79-83] Although plasma glucose could be normalized, all of these studies were reported to be extremely labor intensive, requiring close monitoring of infants in order to prevent hypoglycemia and other related metabolic disorders.

Hypoglycemia

The supply of glucose from the mother ceases abruptly at birth with the cutting of the umbilical cord. This is accompanied by a surge in a number of glucoregulatory hormones (glucagon, catecholamines) stimulating glucose production and initiation of gluconeogenesis.[84] Most healthy preterm infants are able to mobilize glycogen, initiate gluconeogenesis and produce glucose in the immediate newborn period. However, maternal, fetal and perinatal stressors can perturb normal smooth transition to extrauterine life, leading to abnormal adaptation to glucose metabolism. In addition, it has been suggested that the extremely low birth weight infant may not be able to produce glucose due to very limited glycogen stores. But there are no actual measurements to support this speculation.

The definition of hypoglycemia in the neonate has remained controversial. Cut-off or threshold values of glucose below which the neonate may be at risk for development of deleterious consequences have been suggested.[85,86] However, several unique features of the neonate, such as lack of clinical correlates between plasma glucose concentration and long term sequelae, make it difficult to define the threshold value for intervention. Based upon the available physiological data on glucose metabolism, the threshold values for preterm infants should not be any different from those recommended for the full-term baby. Hypoglycemia in premature infants during neonatal transition is a rare event in most intensive care units. This is because most preterm infants are placed on intravenous glucose infusion shortly after birth for clinical reasons. Prolonged parenteral nutrition with a mixture of glucose, amino acids and intralipids induce higher plasma insulin concentrations in the neonate. Interruption of glucose supply in such infants can lead to hypoglycemia due to prior induced hyperinsulinism. High plasma insulin suppresses glycogenolysis and lipolysis; and therefore, infants are unable to mobilize alternate fuels for energy metabolism.

Bronchopulmonary Dysplasia

Infants with chronic respiratory insufficiency as a result of bronchopulmonary dysplasia (BPD) present with unique problems in relation to macronutrient administration and assimilation. Clinically these infants exhibit tachypnea, suggesting an increased work of breathing. Because these infants often require supplemental oxygen, measurements of rate of oxygen/energy consumption using indirect calorimetry have resulted in conflicting data.[87,88] More recent studies using both indirect calorimetry and doubly-labeled water methods have provided evidence of higher rates of energy consumption in infants with bronchopulmonary dysplasia, irrespective of the need for supplemental oxygen.[88-90] Thus, in order to achieve optimal growth, these infants require supplemental energy intake of approximately 15-20% higher than those for healthy infants. Whether this additional energy should be provided as carbohydrate or fat remains a subject of continued debate. Oxidation of carbohydrate (respiratory quotient: RQ 1.0) results in a higher rate of CO_2 production for the same amount of O_2 consumed when compared with fat (RQ 0.7). Since infants with BPD already have CO_2 retention and a higher rate of CO_2 production (VCO_2), it has been suggested that they should be given a higher amount of lipid in their nutrient mixture as compared with healthy babies. However, such a nutrient regimen has not been shown to affect blood PCO_2. Replacement of glucose with lipid in parenteral nutrients for otherwise healthy preterm infants did not cause any change in arterial PCO_2, although it did result in a decreased rate of CO_2 production.[91-93] These data in healthy preterm babies show an adequate compensation for the increase in the rate of CO_2 production, by change in ventilation without impacting arterial PCO_2. Such data have not been obtained in infants with BPD. However, since arterial PCO_2 is a complex function of pH, respiratory drive, etc., it is likely that infants with BPD who are in a compensated state will also be able to adjust for the quantitatively small increase in VCO_2 caused by nutrient mixtures with a normal proportion of carbohydrates. It is important to underscore that nitrogen accretion and growth in healthy premature babies are closely related to dietary protein and energy intake, and that nitrogen retention and urinary nitrogen excretion are a continuous function of protein:energy ratio of the dietary intake.[94-97] Kashyap et al[96,97] have also shown that a protein intake of 2.8 g/kg.d with an energy intake of 119 kcal/kg.d results in weight gain and nitrogen at rates slightly in excess of intrauterine rates. In this context, recent data of Brunton et al are of interest.[98] They showed that provision of protein at 2.8 g/kg.d and energy at ~117 kcal/kg.d to infants with bronchopulmonary dysplasia resulted in a greater linear growth, lean body mass and bone mass, compared to infants who received the standard premature formula. Such a nutrient regimen also resulted in improved bone mineral content and zinc retention. From these data taken together, we suggest that the goal of nutrient intervention in infants with BPD should be to provide a higher energy intake (~15-20%) with optimal protein intake. Further manipulation of carbohydrate and fat in the nutritional regimen do not appear to provide any distinct clinical benefits.

Acknowledgment

The cited data from the investigators' laboratory were supported by grants HD11089 and RR00080 from the National Institutes of Health. The secretarial assistance of Mrs. Joyce Nolan is gratefully appreciated.

References

1. Ehrenkranz RA, Younes N, Lemons JA, et al. Longitudinal growth of hospitalized very low birth weight infants. *Pediatrics* 1999;104:280-289.

2. Bayes R, Campoy C, Molina-Font JA. Some current controversies on nutritional requirements of full-term and pre-term newborn infants. *Early Human Devel* 1998;53(suppl):S3-S13.

3. Gamble JL. Physiological information gained from studies on the life raft ration. *Harvey Lectures* 1946;42:247-273.

4. Kashyap S, Ohira-Kist K, Abildskov K, et al. Effects of quality of energy intake on growth and metabolic response of enterally fed low-birth-weight infants. *Pediatr Res* 2001;50:390-397.

5. Kalhan S, Kiliç İ. Carbohydrate as nutrient in the infant and child: range of acceptable intake. *Eur J Clin Nutr* 1999;53:S94-S100.

6. Bier DM, Brosnan JT, Flatt JP, et al. Report of the IDECG Working Group on lower and upper limits of carbohydrate and fat intake. International Dietary

7. Kalhan SC. Metabolism of glucose in very low birth weight infants, In: *Year Book of Neonatal* and *Perinatal Medicine*, ed. Fanaroff AA, Klaus M; Chicago: Mosby Year Book, Inc., 1994; xix-xxx.

8. Denne SC, Kalhan SC. Glucose carbon recycling and oxidation in human newborns. *Am J Physiol* 1986;251:E71-E77.

9. Bier DM, Leake RD, Haymond MW, et al. Measurement of "true" glucose production rates in infancy and childhood with 6,6-dideuteroglucose. *Diabetes* 1977;26:1016-1023.

10. Cowett RM, Susa JB, Giletti B, Oh W, Schwartz R. Glucose kinetics in infants of diabetic mothers. *Am J Obstet Gynecol* 1983;146:781-786.

11. Patel D, Kalhan S. Glycerol metabolism and triglyceride-fatty acid cycling in the human newborn: effect of maternal diabetes and intrauterine growth retardation. *Pediatr Res* 1992;31:52-58.

12. Bougneres PF, Karl IE, Hillman LS, Bier DM. Lipid transport in the human newborn. Palmitate and glycerol turnover and the contribution of glycerol to neonatal hepatic glucose output. *J Clin Invest* 1982;70:262-270.

13. Sunehag A, Gustafsson J, Ewald U. Glycerol carbon contributes to hepatic glucose production during the first eight hours in healthy term infants. *Acta Paediatr* 1996;85:1339-1343.

14. Sunehag A, Ewald U, Gustafsson J. Extremely preterm infants (<28 weeks) are capable of gluconeogenesis from glycerol on their first day of life. *Pediatr Res* 1996;40:553-557.

15. Sunehag AL, Haymond MW, Schanler RJ, Reeds PJ, Bier DM. Gluconeogenesis in very low birth weight infants receiving total parenteral nutrition. *Diabetes* 1999;48:791-800.

16. King KC, Tserng K, Kalhan SC. Regulation of glucose production in newborn infants of diabetic mothers. *Pediatr Res* 1982;16:608-612.

17. Hertz DE, Karn CA, Liu YM, Liechty EA, Denne SC. Intravenous glucose suppresses glucose production but not proteolysis in extremely premature newborns. *J Clin Invest* 1993;92:1752-1758.

Energy Consultative Group. *Eur J Clin Nutr* 1999;53:S177-S178.

18. Sunehag A, Ewald U, Larsson A, Gustafsson J. Glucose production rate in extremely immature neonates (<28 weeks) studied by use of deuterated glucose. *Pediatr Res* 1993;33:97-100.

19. VanGoudoever JB, Sulkers EJ, Chapman TE, et al. Glucose kinetics and glucoregulatory hormone levels in ventilated preterm infants on the first day of life. *Pediatr Res* 1993;33:583-589.

20. Kalhan SC, Parimi P, Van Beek R, et al. Estimation of gluconeogenesis in newborn infants. *Am J Physiol* 2001;281:E991-E997.

21. Sauer PJJ, Van Aerde JEE, Pencharz PB, Smith JM, Swyer PR. Glucose oxidation rates in newborn infants measured with indirect calorimetry and [U-^{13}C] glucose. *Clin Sci* 1986;70:587-593.

22. Chugani HT. Positron emission tomography scanning: applications in newborns. *Clin Perinatol* 1993;20: 395-409.

23. Kinnala A, Suhonen-Polvi H, Aarimaa T, et al. Cerebral metabolic rate for glucose during the first six months of life: an FDG positron emission tomography study. *Arch Dis Child* 1996;74:F153-F157.

24. Suhonen-Polvi H, Kero PN, Korvenranta H, et al. Repeated fluorodeoxyglucose positron emission tomography of the brain in infants with suspected hypoxic-ischaemic brain injury. *Eur J Nucl Med* 1993;20:759-765.

25. Vadlamudi S, Hiremagalur BK, Tao L, et al. Long-term effects on pancreatic function of feeding a high-carbohydrate formula to rat pups during the preweaning period. *Am J Physiol* 1993;265: E565-E571.

26. Vadlamudi S, Kalhan SC, Patel MS. Persistence of metabolic consequences of feeding a high carbohydrate formula in early postnatal life in the next generation. *Am J Physiol* 1995;269:E731-E738.

27. Weight EM. The intestinal Na+/glucose cotransporter. *Annu Rev Physiol* 1993;55:575-589.

28. Shulman RJ. In vivo measurements of glucose absorption in preterm infants. *Biol Neonate* 1999;76:10-18.

29. Jirsova V, Koldovsky O, Heringova A, Hoskova J, Jirasek J, Uher J. The development of the functions of the small intestine of the human fetus. *Biol Neonate*

1965; 66:44-49.

30. Levin RJ, Koldovsky O, Hoskova J, Jirsova V, Uher J. Electrical activity across human foetal small intestine associated with absorption processes. *Gut* 1968;9:206-213.

31. McNeish AS, Ducker DA, Warren LF, Davies DP, Harran MH, Hughes CA. The influence of gestational age and size on the absorption of D-xylose and D-glucose from the small intestine of the human neonate. CIBA Foundation Symposium 1979;20:267-276.

32. Modigliani R, Rambaud JC, Bernier JJ. The method of intraluminal perfusion of the human small intestine: Principle and technique. *Digestion* 1973;9:264-290.

33. LSRO Report: Assessment of Nutrient Requirements of Infant Formulae. VII. Carbohydrate. *J Nutr* 1998;128:2131S-2139S.

34. Auricchio S, Rubino A, Murset G. Intestinal glucosidase activity in the human embryo, fetus and newborn. *Pediatrics* 1965;35:944-954.

35. Watkins JB. Developmental aspects of carbohydrate malabsorption in the premature infant. In: Lifshitz F (ed), *Carbohydrate Intolerance in Infancy*. Marcel Dekker, Inc., NY: 1982: pp 61-73.

36. Kien CL, McClead RE, Cordero L Jr. In vivo lactose digestion in preterm infants. *Am J Clin Nutr* 1996;64:700-705.

37. Kien CL, Liechty EA, Myerberg DZ, Mullett MD. Dietary carbohydrate assimilation in the premature infant: evidence for a nutritionally significant bacterial ecosystem in the colon. *Am J Clin Nutr* 1987;46: 456-460.

38. Shulman RJ, Schanler RJ, Lau C, Heitkemper M, Ou C-N, Smith EO. Early feeding, feeding intolerance, and lactase activity in preterm infants. *J Pediatr* 1998;133:645-659.

39. Zittermann A, Bock P, Drummer C, Scheld K, Heer M, Stehle P. Lactose does not enhance calcium bioavailability in lactose-tolerant, healthy adults. *Am J Clin Nutr* 2000;71:931-936.

40. Ziegler EE, Fomon SJ. Lactose enhances mineral absorption in infancy. *J Pediatr Gastroenterol Nutr* 1983;2:288-294.

41. Stathos TH, Shulman RJ, Schanler RJ, Abrams SA. Effect of carbohydrates on calcium absorption in

premature infants. *Pediatr Res* 1996;39:666-670.

42. Wirth FH Jr, Numerof B, Pleban P, Neylan MJ. Effect of lactose on mineral absorption in preterm infants. *J Pediatr* 1990;117:283-287.

43. Moya M, Lifschitz C, Ameen V, Euler AR. A metabolic balance study in term infants fed lactose-containing or lactose-free formula. *Acta Paediatr* 1999;88:1211-1215.

44. Kliegman RM, Sparks JW. Perinatal galactose metabolism. *J Pediatr* 1985; 107:831-840.

45. Kaempf JW, Li H, Groothuis JR, Battaglia FC, Zerbe GO, Sparks JW. Galactose, glucose, and lactate concentrations in the portal venous and arterial circulations of newborn lambs after nursing. *Pediatr Res* 1988;23:598-602.

46. Goresky CA, Bach GG, Nadeau BE. On the uptake of materials by the intact liver. The transport and net removal of galactose. *J Clin Invest* 1973;52:991-1009.

47. Sparks JW, Lynch A, Glinsmann WH. Regulation of rat liver glycogen synthesis and activities of glycogen cycle enzymes by glucose and galactose. *Metabolism* 1976;25:47-55.

48. Kunst C, Kliegman R, Trindade C. The glucose-galactose paradox in neonatal murine hepatic glycogen synthesis. *Am J Physiol* 1989;257:E697-E703.

49. Sparks JW, Lynch A, Chez RA, Glinsmann WH. Glycogen regulation in isolated perfused near term monkey liver. *Pediatr Res* 1976;10:51-56.

50. Kliegman RM, Miettinen E, Kalhan SC, Adam PAJ. The effect of enteric galactose on neonatal canine carbohydrate metabolism. *Metabolism* 1981;30: 1109-1118.

51. Berry GT, Nissim I, Lin Z, Mazur AT, Gibson JB, Segal S. Endogenous synthesis of galactose in normal men and patients with hereditary galactosaemia. *Lancet* 1995;246:1073-1074.

52. Kunz C, Rudloff S, Baier W, Klein N, Strobel S. Oligosaccharides in human milk: structural, functional, and metabolic aspects. *Annu Rev Nutr* 2000;20: 699-722.

53. Brand Miller J, McVeagh P. Human milk oligosaccharides: 130 reasons to breast-feed. *Br J Nutr* 1999;82:333-335.

54. Coppa GV, Pierani P, Zampini L, Carloni I, Carlucci A, Gabrielli O. Oligosaccharides in human milk during

different phases of lactation. *Acta Paediatr Suppl* 1999;430:89-94.

55. Coppa GV, Gabrielli O, Pierani P, Catassi C, Carlucci A, Giorgi A. Changes in carbohydrate composition in human milk over 4 months of lactation. *Pediatrics* 1993;91:637-641.

56. Nakhla T, Fu D, Zopf D, Brodsky NL, Hurt H. Neutral oligosaccharide content of preterm human milk. *Br J Nutr* 1999;82:361-367.

57. Erney RM, Malone WT, Skelding MB, et al. Variability of human milk neutral oligosaccharides in a diverse population. *J Pediatr Gastroent Nutr* 2000;30:181-192.

58. Kunz C, Rudloff S, Schad W, Braun D. Lactose-derived oligosaccharides in the milk of elephants: comparison with human milk. *Br J Nutr* 1999;82:391-399.

59. Gnoth MJ, Kunz C, Kinne-Saffran E, Rudloff S. Human milk oligosaccharides are minimally digested in vitro. *J Nutr* 2000;130:3014-3020.

60. Engfer MB, Stahl B, Finke B, Sawatzki G, Daniel H. Human milk oligosaccharides are resistant to enzymatic hydrolysis in the upper gastrointestinal tract. *Am J Clin Nutr* 2000;71:1589-1596.

61. Brand Miller JC, McVeagh P, McNeil Y, Messer M. Digestion of human milk oligosaccharides by healthy infants evaluated by the lactulose hydrogen breath test. *J Pediatr* 1998;133:95-98.

62. Rudloff S, Pohlentz G, Diekmann L, Egge H, Kunz C. Urinary excretion of lactose and oligosaccharides in preterm infants fed human milk or infant formula. *Acta Paediatr* 1996;85:598-603.

63. Tram TH, Brand Miller JC, McNeil Y, McVeagh P. Sialic acid content of infant saliva: comparison of breast fed with formula fed infants. *Arch Dis Child* 1997;77:315-318.

64. Shulman RJ, Feste A, Ou C. Absorption of lactose, glucose polymers, or combination in premature infants. *J Pediatr* 1995;127:626-631.

65. Foster C, Costill DL, Fink WJ. Gastric emptying characteristics of glucose and glucose polymer solutions. *Res Q Exercise Sport* 1980;51:299-305.

66. Kien CL, Sumners JE, Stetina JS, Heimler R, Grausz JP. A method for assessing carbohydrate energy absorption and its application to premature infants. *Am J Clin Nutr* 1982;36:910-916.

67. Kien CL, Liechty EA, Myerberg DZ, Mullett MD. Dietary carbohydrate assimilation in the premature infant: evidence for a nutritionally significant bacterial ecosystem in the colon. *Am J Clin Nutr* 1987;46: 456-460.

68. Shulman RJ, Feste A, Ou C. Absorption of lactose, glucose polymers, or combination in premature infants. *J Pediatr* 1995;127:626-631.

69. Kuschel CA, Harding JE. Carbohydrate supplementation of human milk to promote growth in preterm infants. Cochrane Neonatal Reviews 1999.

70. Holub BJ. The nutritional importance of inositol and the phosphoinositides. *N Engl J Med* 1992;326: 1285-1287.

71. Hallman M, Bry K, Hoppu K, Lappi J, Pohjavuori M. Inositol supplementation in premature infants with respiratory distress syndrome. *N Engl J Med* 1992;326:1233-1239.

72. Hallman M, Arjomaa P, Hoppu K. Inositol supplementation in respiratory distress syndrome: Relationship between serum concentration, renal excretion, and lung effluent phospholipids. *J Pediatr* 1987;110:604-610.

73. Carver JD, Stromquist CI, Benford VJ, Minervini G, Benford SA, Barness LA. Postnatal inositol levels in preterm infants. J Perinatol 1997;17:389-392.

74. Lilien LD, Rosenfield RL, Baccaro MM, Pildes RS. Hyperglycemia in stressed small premature neonates. *J Pediatr* 1979;94:454-459.

75. Hertz DE, Karn CA, Liu YM, Liechty EA, Denne SC. Intravenous glucose suppresses glucose production but not proteolysis in extremely premature newborns. *J Clin Invest* 1993;92:1752-1758.

76. Cowett RM, Oh W, Pollak A, Schwartz R, Stonestreet BS. Glucose disposal of low birth weight infants: steady state hyperglycemia produced by constant intravenous glucose infusion. *Pediatrics* 1979;63:389-396.

77. Kalhan SC, Parimi P. Disorders of carbohydrate metabolism. In: Fanaroff AA, Martin RJ eds. *Neonatal-Perinatal Medicine. Diseases of the Fetus and Infant, 7th edition.* St. Louis, MO, Mosby-Year Book; 2001 pp 1351-1376.

78. Kalhan SC, Raghavan CV. Metabolism of glucose and methods of investigation in the fetus and newborn. In: Polin RA, Fox WW eds. *Fetal and Neonatal Physiology,* Second Edition. Philadelphia, PA: WB Saunders & Co.; 1998: 543-558.

79. Collins JW, Hoppe M, Brown K, Edidin DV, Padbury J, Ogata ES. A controlled trial of insulin infusion and parenteral nutrition in extremely low birth weight infants with glucose intolerance. *J Pediatr* 1991;118:921-927.

80. Binder ND, Raschko PK, Benda GI, Reynolds JW. Insulin infusion with parenteral nutrition in extremely low birth weight infants with hyperglycemia. *J Pediatr* 1989;114:273-280.

81. Avent M, Whitfield J. Insulin infusions in extremely low birth weight infants. *Pediatrics* 2000;105:915.

82. Simeon PS, Geffner ME, Levin SR, Lindsey AM. Continuous insulin infusions in neonates: Pharmacologic availability of insulin in intravenous solutions. *J Pediatr* 1994;124:818-820.

83. Poindexter BB, Karn CA, Denne SC. Exogenous insulin reduces proteolysis and protein synthesis in extremely low birth weight infants. *J Pediatr* 1998;132:948-53.

84. Kalhan S, Parimi P. Gluconeogenesis in the fetus and neonate. *Sem Perinatol* 2000;24:94-106.

85. Cornblath M, Hawdon JM, Williams AF, et al. Controversies regarding definition of neonatal hypoglycemia: suggested operational thresholds. *Pediatrics* 2000;105:1141-1145.

86. Kalhan SC, Peter-Wohl S. Hypoglycemia: What is it for the neonate? *Am J Perinatol* 2000;17:11-18.

87. Kalhan SC, Denne SC. Energy consumption in infants with bronchopulmonary dysplasia. *J Pediatr* 1190;116:662-664.

88. Denne SC. Energy expenditure in infants with pulmonary insufficiency: is there evidence for increased energy needs? *J Nutr* 2001;131:935S-937S.

89. de Meer K, Westerterp KR, Houwen RHJ, Brouwers HAA, Berger R, Okken A. Total energy expenditure in infants with bronchopulmonary dysplasia is associated with respiratory status. *Eur J Pediatr* 1997;156: 299-304.

90. de Gamarra E. Energy expenditure in premature newborns with bronchopulmonary dysplasia. *Biol Neonate* 1992;61:337-344.

91. Salas-Salvado J, Molina J, Figueras J, Masso J,

Marti-Henneberg C, Jimenez R. Effect of the quality of infused energy on substrate utilization in the newborn receiving total parenteral nutrition. *Pediatr Res* 1993;33:112-117.

92. Van Aerde JEE, Sauer PJJ, Pencharz PB, Smith JM, Swyer PR. Effect of replacing glucose with lipid on the energy metabolism of newborn infants. *Clin Sci* 1989;76:581-588.

93. Chessex P, Belanger S, Piedboeuf B, Pineault M. Influence of energy substrates on respiratory gas exchange during conventional mechanical ventilation of preterm infants. *J Pediatr* 1995;126:619-624.

94. Kashyap S, Forsyth M, Zucker C, Ramakrishnan R, Dell RB, Heird WC. Effects of varying protein and energy intakes on growth and metabolic response in low birth weight infants. *J Pediatr* 1986;108:955-963.

95. Kashyap S, Ramakrishnan R, Heird WC. Effect of concomitant energy intake on nitrogen retention of low birth weight infants. *Pediatr Res* 1990;29:1773 (abstract).

96. Kashyap S, Schulze KF, Ramakrishnan R, Dell RB, Heird WC. Evaluation of a mathematical model for predicting the relationship between protein and energy intakes of low-birth-weight infants and the rate and composition of weight gain. *Pediatr Res* 1994;35: 704-712.

97. Kashyap S, Schulze KF, Forsyth M, et al. Growth, nutrient retention, and metabolic response in low birth weight infants fed varying intakes of protein and energy. *J Pediatr* 1988;113:713-721.

98. Brunton JA, Saigal S, Atkinson SA. Growth and body composition in infants with bronchopulmonary dysplasia up to 3 months corrected age: A randomized trial of a high-energy nutrient-enriched formula fed after hospital discharge. *J Pediatr* 1998;133:340-345.

Lipids
Berthold V. Koletzko, M.D., Ph.D. and Sheila M. Innis, Ph.D.

Reviewed by John E. Van Aerde, M.D., and Margit Hamosh, Ph.D.

The dietary supply of lipids provides the preterm infant with a large portion of energy needs, essential polyunsaturated fatty acids, and lipid soluble vitamins (discussed in Chapter 6). Dietary lipids may interfere with the absorption of other substrates such as calcium. The amount and composition of dietary lipids can have a direct impact on the efficiency of lipid absorption, metabolism and tissue deposition, and hence, on the quality of growth and body composition. Due to the very limited endogenous lipid stores, which amount to only 20 g total lipids in the body of a 1000 g infant,[1] the quantity and quality of the dietary lipid supply is of particular importance in low-birth-weight (LBW, <2500 g) and very-low-birth-weight (VLBW, <1500 g) infants. Lipids serve as indispensable structural components of cell membranes. The availability and metabolism of membrane components such as long-chain polyunsaturated fatty acids (LC-PUFA) have direct implications for cell membrane functions, including the activity of membrane-bound enzymes, receptors, transport proteins, ion channel activities and signal transduction. Brain grey matter and the retina are particularly rich in LC-PUFAs, and complex neural functions are related to energy supply and the composition of dietary fatty acids in LBW infants. Certain LC-PUFAs also regulate gene expression and serve as substrates for formation of bioactive eicosanoids (prostaglandins, thromboxanes, and leukotrienes). These eicosanoids modulate various tissue functions such as thrombocyte aggregation, postnatal closure of the ductus arteriosus, inflammatory reactions, and postnatal development of immune phenotypes. Thus, the quantity and quality of the lipid supply for low-birth-weight infants deserves careful attention.

Body Fat Deposition

Daily intrauterine body fat deposition from about 25 weeks of gestation onwards is in the range of 1-3 g/kg body weight and contributes some 75% of the energy stored in the growing fetus.[1-4] This is equivalent to an average total weight gain of about 15 g/day, with a daily gain of about 3 g adipose tissue/kg during the last trimester.[1]

Intrauterine growth is often considered as a guide for the desirable quality of postnatal growth and body composition in preterm infants. Adipose tissue growth in the preterm infant depends both on the total energy provided and the proportions of protein and non-protein energy. Growing preterm infants tend to have a somewhat higher extrauterine body fat deposition, as compared to the fetus in utero. Extrauterine fat deposition during the first weeks of life in fully enterally fed preterm infants with a birth weight <1750 g was recently estimated with dual energy X-ray absorptiometry.[5] Preterm infants fed fortified human milk showed a weight gain of 15.9 ± 2.2 g/kg/day with a daily body fat deposition of 3.3 ± 1.3 g/kg/day, whereas infants fed formula gained 19.9 ± 3.2 g/kg/day and 5.1 ± 1.9 g/fat/kg. However, a reasonable fat deposition appears desirable since subcutaneous fat can protect the infant against thermal and mechanical stress and hence replace part of the protection offered by the intrauterine environment. Moreover, body fat offers an energy resource for periods of low intake,

	Percentiles						
	2.5	10	25	50	75	90	97.5
Milk fat content (g/dl)	1.84	2.38	2.94	3.61	4.34	5.46	8.90

Table 1: Percentile distribution of fat content in 2554 human milk samples.[7]

such as transient periods with feeding difficulties or diarrhea. In healthy term infants, body fat deposition increases markedly after birth when lipids contribute about 35% of the weight gain or about 90% of the energy retained in the babies' newly formed tissue during the first 6 postnatal months.[6] However, there is little information on the potential relationship of body fat deposition in LBWI relevant to short- and long-term outcomes.

Total Dietary Lipid Intake

Fat is the major source of energy in human milk. The average fat content of human milk is about 3.8-3.9 g/100 ml, but the variability is large. The analysis of 2554 milk samples from 224 Danish mothers taken over 33 months of lactation shows a range between 2 and 9 g fat/100 ml[7] (Table 1). The variation in the amount of fat in human milk is clearly larger than that for protein, and much larger than that for lactose. Although milk fat content increases with duration of lactation, there appears to be little difference between milk from mothers of term and preterm babies.[8] The proportion of human milk energy provided by fat is in the range of 40-55% in most milk samples.[9]

Long-chain triglycerides contain about 9 kcal metabolizable energy per gram and thus about 2.25 times more energy per gram than protein or carbohydrates. The high fat content of human milk provides a high energy density per unit volume of the feed. As a result, a higher energy intake can be achieved for a given volume of milk than would be possible if the same amount of energy were provided as carbohydrate or protein. Moreover, a high fat intake does not expose the infant to the osmotic and metabolic burdens that would occur with very high carbohydrate or protein intakes.

The proportion of dietary energy derived from fat

rather than carbohydrate influences nutrient substrate flux. The large amount of lipids deposited in growing preterm infants theoretically could be synthesized *de novo* from other precursors such as carbohydrates. However, the capacity for endogenous *de novo* lipacidogenesis is rather limited in man.[10] Moreover, occurring *de novo* lipogenesis would result in the synthesis of only non-essential saturated and monounsaturated fatty acids. Of further importance, synthesis of triglycerides for adipose tissue growth from dietary fat energetically is more efficient than synthesis of fat from carbohydrate. This is explained because about 25% of the energy content of glucose is consumed in the conversion of glucose into fatty acid in the liver. The hydrolysis of circulating plasma triglycerides, uptake of fatty acids, and re-esterification to form triglycerides in adipose tissue on the other hand consumes only about 4% of the potential energy of the initial triglyceride molecule.[11] The extent of energy loss in vivo is difficult to determine, but a higher thermogenic effect of dietary carbohydrates and proteins as compared with long-chain lipids is well known.[12,13] Indeed, in parenterally fed infants, energy expenditure was reduced by providing lipid in place of part of the parenteral glucose.[14] Moreover, the addition of lipids at the same level of energy intake, reduces CO_2 production because fatty acid oxidation has a lower respiratory quotient (RQ = CO_2-production/O_2-consumption; about 0.7) than glucose (RQ = 1.0).[15] This reduction of carbon dioxide production, achieved when part of the energy is provided as fat, may be of clinical importance in the choice of nutritional strategies for LBWI with hypercapnia or during the phase of weaning from artificial ventilation.

There is no firm scientific basis for a strict definition of minimal and maximal dietary fat intakes in preterm infants. To some extent, limits for a reasonable fat intake are determined by the requirements for minimal protein and carbohydrate intake, in addition possibly to practical limits with respect to achieving a desirable energy density at acceptable osmolarity of the feed. However, the data reviewed here allows estimation based on the concept that the dietary intake of metabolizable fat (with long-chain fatty acids) should at least equal body fat deposition of the fetus during growth. Assuming a daily intrauterine fat deposition of 3 g/kg,[1] 15% losses due to fat malabsorption[17] (3.45 g/kg), and a further 5% for metabolic losses during conversion of absorbed triglyceride to deposited triglyceride in adipose tissue,[18] the estimated fat intake would then be 3.62 g/kg/day. An arbitrarily chosen, additional uncertainty factor of 33% could be added to account for individual variability. Based on this approach, a minimal dietary fat intake of about 4.83 g/kg per day is suggested. At an energy intake of 110 kcal/kg, this intake is met by the lower range of total fat contents in LBWI formula of 4.4 g/100 kcal (or 39.6% of energy contents) recommended by the Committee on Nutrition of the European Society for Paediatric Gastroenterology, Hepatology and Nutrition (ESPGHAN)[19] and the expert committee convened by the US Life Science Research Office.[20] The same two expert committees recommended upper limits of 6.0 g fat/100 kcal (54% of energy; E%)[19] and of 5.7 g fat/100 kcal (51 E%),[20] which are similar to the upper end of the range usually observed in human milk samples. In the absence of definitive scientific data to justify a wider or a more narrow range, we consider as a reasonable range of fat intake to be:

Total fat: 4.4 - 6.0 g/100 kcal (40-55 E%)

Quality of Dietary Lipids

The quality of lipid is determined both by the lipid class (for example, triglycerides, phospholipids

> ### Human Hindmilk, Fat Intake and Weight Gain
>
> *Human hindmilk, ie, the last portion of breast milk fed during nursing or expressed from the breast and collected, has a much higher fat content than foremilk (the first milk portion expressed).[9] The preferential use of human hindmilk can improve the weight gain of preterm infants who are not meeting anticipated rates of growth. Valentine and co-workers[16] studied a group of 15 preterm infants with a birthweight of 1087 ± 400 g who were fed more than 150 ml expressed, pooled human milk/kg bodyweight and day but who showed an unsatisfactory daily weight gain of less than 15g/kg. The infants were switched to the feeding of hindmilk, ie, the last 60% of their mother's milk expression. Hindmilk contained more fat than pooled total milk expressions (4.78 ± 0.85 vs. 3.96 ± 0.73 g/L, p<0.0001) and thus more energy (824 ± 77 vs. 740 ± 90 kcal/L, p=0.0001). At the same volume of milk intake (158-159 ml/kg), the use of the lipid rich hindmilk increased the infants' daily weight gain by 7.0 ± 4.4 g/kg.*

and cholesterol), and by the fatty acids incorporated into esterified lipids (eg, triglycerides).

Most of the fat and fatty acids in the body are stored as triglycerides. Phospholipids and unesterified cholesterol are essential components of the lipid bilayer of all cell membranes. Phospholipids and cholesterol are also incorporated into the surface of lipoproteins, which together with apoproteins allow the transport of non-polar (oily) lipids (triglycerides and cholesteryl esters) in the aqueous (watery) plasma. Cholesterol is also required in considerable amounts as the precursor for the synthesis of steroid hormones and bile acids.

The major portion of the fat in human milk is found in the form of triglycerides, which account for about 98% by weight of the total milk fat. Phospholipids contribute about 0.7% and cholesterol 0.5% (wt/wt) of the total milk fat.[9] Freshly expressed human milk contains only small amounts of lipolysis products, free fatty acids and mono- and diacylglycerols,[9] which may increase during storage of milk. Milk triglycerides, cholesteryl esters and retinyl esters are predominantly found in the hydrophobic core of the milk fat globules. The surface of milk fat globules is comprised of amphipathic compounds such as phospholipids, proteins, cholesterol and enzymes in a loose network termed the milk fat globule membrane. This amphipathic surface is required for the dispersion of milk fats in the watery environment of milk and for stability of the "oil in water emulsion" that milk represents. Most of the membrane material is derived from the mammary cell apical plasma and mature

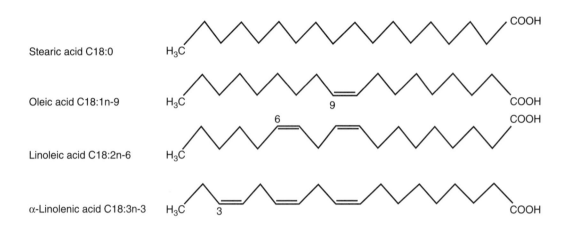

Figure 1: Fatty acids are carboxylic acids that vary in number of carbon atoms and chain length, and number and position of double bonds. Fatty acids can be saturated (contain no double bonds, eg, stearic acid), monounsaturated (contain one double bond, eg, oleic acid) or polyunsaturated (contain more than one double bond, eg, the essential fatty acids linoleic and α-linolenic acids). The usual fatty acid nomenclature indicates the number of carbon atoms found in the fatty acid chain, followed by a colon, then the number of unsaturated bonds in the fatty acid chain. For example, the saturated fatty acid stearic acid with 18 carbon atoms and no double bonds is denoted as C18:0. The notation "n" is used to designate the position of the last double bond counted from the methyl terminus. Thus, the polyunsaturated fatty acid linoleic acid with 18 carbon atoms and 2 double bonds with the last double bond 6 carbon atoms from the methyl terminus, is denoted as C18:2:n-6.

Golgi vesicle membranes, which envelop the globules as they are extruded from the secreting mammary cell. The diameter of the globules ranges from 1 to 10 mm, with most of the globules measuring 1 mm, but those of 4 mm account for most of the weight. The large surface area of the globules (4.5m²/dl) can bind various lipases, and thereby, contribute to effective milk triglyceride digestion.

Considerable amounts of cholesterol are deposited in tissue lipids during growth, and dietary cholesterol contributes to the cholesterol pool in plasma and tissues. However, the major portion of deposited cholesterol appears to be derived from endogenous synthesis primarily in the liver, where the activity of cholesterol synthesis is modulated by dietary factors.[21-24] An inborn defect of endogenous cholesterol synthesis is associated with severe mental retardation in children with the Smith Lemli Opitz-syndrome,[25,26] which points to the importance of cholesterol availability for normal development. Available data, however, suggest that the developing brain synthesizes cholesterol required for membrane growth *de novo*, rather than taking up cholesterol from plasma.[27] Further, there is no evidence that the dietary supply of cholesterol, in individuals with an intact cholesterol synthesis pathway, affects nervous system development. Whether or not the preterm infant would benefit from a dietary supply of preformed cholesterol similar to that provided by human milk is not known, and few data are available to address this.

The supply of dietary phospholipids provides a source of phosphorus and choline and has further biological effects, but again there is little systematic data in LBWI.[28] An impressive effect of dietary phospholipids on disease risk in VLBWI has been reported. In a randomized, double-blind clinical trial, Carlson et al found that preterm infants fed a formula with egg phospholipids which had been added to provide arachidonic acid (20:4n-6) and docosahexaenoic acid (22:6n-3), developed significantly less stage II and III necrotizing enterocolitis (NEC) (2.9 versus 17.6 %, p<0.05) than infants fed a commercial preterm formula containing usual amounts of phospholipid in the formula fat emulsion.[28] Rates of bronchopulmonary dysplasia (23.4 versus 23.5%), septicemia (26 versus 31%), and retinopathy of prematurity (38 versus 40%) were not different between the two groups of infants. Compared with the control formula, the experimental formula provided 7-fold more esterified choline, as well as arachidonic acid (0.4% of total fatty acids) and docosahexaenoic acid (0.13%) which were absent from the control formula. The authors proposed that components of egg phospholipids may have enhanced one or more immature intestinal functions to lower the incidence of NEC. In this respect, they discuss the role of phospholipids as constituents of mucosal membranes and intestinal surfactant, and their components, arachidonic acid and choline, as substrates for intestinal vasodilatory and cytoprotective eicosanoids (arachidonic acid) and the vasodilatory neuro-transmitter, acetylcholine (choline), respectively.

Consistent with a possible beneficial effect of LC-PUFA, Caplan et al found newborn rats stressed with asphyxia had less mortality and death when fed formula with LC-PUFA, and less intestinal inflammation when fed formula with LC-PUFA and nucleotides, as opposed to rats fed unsupplemented formula.[29] These data support the need for a larger randomized trial to test the possible protective effects of formula with phospholipid, and potentially with other sources of LC-PUFA, on NEC.

Lipid Digestion, Absorption and Metabolism

The process of fat digestion and absorption is of great importance in the choice of fats used for the feeding of preterm infants. It can be divided into:

(1.) The luminal phase involving solubilization and hydrolysis of the fat;

(2.) The mucosal phase which includes re-esterification of fatty acids and secretion into the lymphatics in chylomicrons, or release of unesterified fatty acids into the portal venous system; and

(3.) Uptake of the unesterified fatty acid or chylomicron triglyceride into the tissues.

Luminal Phase. Triacylglycerols (triglycerides) comprise about 98% or more of all dietary fats in human milk or formula. Triglycerides are hydrolyzed by colipase-dependent lipase in the upper intestine.[15] This enzyme has a specificity for sn-1,3 ester bonds to give rise to two free fatty acids and one sn-2 monoglyceride (Figure 2). The free fatty acid and sn-2 monoglyceride products become solubilized in the aqueous portion of the intestine by micellar concentrations of bile salts and are absorbed as components of mixed micelles into the intestinal mucosal cells.[15] Newborn infants have a low activity of colipase-dependant pancreatic lipase, a limited bile salt pool, and low intraluminal bile salt concentrations.[30,31] The infant has several alternate mechanisms to overcome the relative deficiency in pancreatic lipase activity and bile salts and to provide for a relatively efficient fat absorption. Triglyceride hydrolysis in infants fed fresh human milk is the result of the combined action of bile salt stimulated lipase produced in the mammary gland and secreted into the milk, and the endogenous gastric lipases and colipase-dependent lipase.[30,31] The major preduodenal enzyme acting in the stomach of infants is gastric lipase.[32,33] The milk fat globule, due to its surface layer of phospholipid, cholesterol and protein, is relatively resistant to colipase-dependent pancreatic lipase or

> ***Fatty Acid Nomenclature***
> *The generally accepted fatty acid nomenclature provides the number of carbon atoms found in the fatty acid chain, then a colon followed by the number of unsaturated bonds in the fatty acid chain. For example, the saturated fatty acid stearic acid with 18 carbon atoms and no double bonds is denoted as C18:0 (Figure 1). The number following the notation "n" is used to designate the position of the first double bond counted from the methyl terminus. Thus, the polyunsaturated fatty acid linoleic acid with 18 carbon atoms and 2 double bonds, with the first double bond 6 carbon atoms from the methyl terminus, is denoted as C18:2:n-6 (Figure 1).*

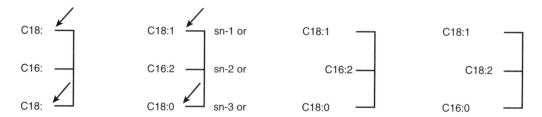

Digestion by pancreatic lipases preferentially in the sn-1 and sn-3 positions.

Figure 2: Triglyceride structure modulates fat absorption. In human milk lipids and structured triglycerides used in some preterm formulas, the saturated fatty acid palmitic acid (16:0) is esterified predominantly in the sn-2 position. Since lipolytic enzymes cleave the fatty acids primarily in sn-1- and sn-3-positions, palmitic acid will appear primarily in the remaining monoglyceride which has a higher water-solubility and is absorbed well. In contrast, if palmitic acid is esterified primarily at the sn-1,3 position of the molecule, as found in vegetable oils, unesterified palmitic acid is released through the action of gastric and colipase-dependent lipase. Unesterified palmitic acid is less well absorbed and tends to form calcium salts, thus reducing the absorption of both fat and calcium.

bile salt-stimulated lipase. The hydrophobic nature of the gastric lipase, however, allows the enzyme to penetrate to the core of the milk fat globule and initiate hydrolysis without disrupting the membrane. Gastric lipase, produced by the chief cells of the gastric mucosa, has functional specificity for the sn-3 ester bond of triglycerides and gives rise to free fatty acids and sn-1,2 diglycerides. Preduodenal lipases have relatively low specific activity, are rapidly inactivated by pancreatic proteases in the presence of bile salts, and are very sensitive to product-inhibition by free fatty acids.[34,35] However, the initial partial hydrolysis may be critically important because the free fatty acids released by gastric lipase induce binding between the colipase-lipase complex and the milk fat globules, thus eliminating the resistance of the globule to hydrolysis.[33] Gastric lipase has been detected in the chief cells of human fetal gastric mucosa as early as 10 weeks of gestation[36] and is present from about 26 weeks of gestation in very-low-birth-weight infants.[37] Thus, it is plausible that gastric lipase activity may improve hydrolysis of human milk fat in premature infants.[38]

In infants fed formulas, gastric lipase and colipase-dependent pancreatic lipase hydrolyze about two-thirds of the triglyceride fatty acids, with the final products being free fatty acids and sn-2 monoglycerides.

Additional hydrolysis of milk fat may occur in infants fed fresh human milk, due to the action of bile salt-stimulated lipase provided with human milk. This enzyme has no positional specificity and can hydrolyze the sn-2 monoglyceride left by pancreatic lipase when mixed with bile salts. This lipase is present in milk from about 26-weeks gestation, has a pH optimum of 7 to 9, and in the presence of bile salts in vitro, hydrolyzes a wide variety of triglycerides to free fatty acids and glycerol.[33,37] Free fatty acids (unesterified fatty acids) are more soluble than monoglycerides in the vesicular phase of the aqueous intraluminal contents, thus possibly improving net fat absorption in infants with low intraluminal bile salt concentrations. However, the sn-2 monoglyceride products of colipase-dependent lipase activity form micelles, and hence, are more readily absorbed than free fatty acids.[34,35]

Little is known about the development of other endogenous enzymes involved in fat hydrolysis in preterm infants. Phospholipase A2 hydrolyzes fatty acids from phospholipids, and it has an absolute requirement for bile salts.[34,35] Pancreatic carboxylic ester hydrolase is functionally and structurally identical to bile salt-stimulated lipase,[40] and has been thought to be important for the hydrolysis of LC-PUFA such as arachidonic acid (20:4n-6), from triglycerides.[31] The assumed low activity of colipase-dependent lipase in the newborn suggests that the activity of other pancreatic enzymes of fat hydrolysis, such as phospholipase A2, cholesterol esterase and carboxylic ester hydrolase, may also be a limiting factor in fat assimilation. Two pancreatic proteins, pancreatic lipase related proteins 1 and 2, with strong nucleotide and amino acid sequence homology to pancreatic triglyceride lipase, have a broad substrate specificity and also hydrolyze phospholipids and galactolipids, two fats that are not substrates for pancreatic triglyceride lipase. Pancreatic lipase-related protein 2 mRNA appears before birth and persists into adulthood. Thus, pancreatic lipase-related protein 2 may play a relevant role in the lipid digestion of premature infants, but little evidence on its effects in low-birth-weight babies in vivo is available.[41]

The coefficient of fat absorption in preterm infants depends on gastrointestinal maturity, the fat composition of the formula fed, and any storage or processing of expressed human milk. Preterm infants <1500 g absorb fat from fresh human milk to about 85% to 95%, which is similar to the fat absorption in term gestation infants.[17,33,42] Total fat absorption may be lower from formulas, depending primarily on the composition of the formula fat used.[38]

The efficacy of infant fat absorption is modulated by the chain length and degree of unsaturation of the fatty acids found in human milk and formula fat. The efficiency of absorption of the monounsaturated oleic acid (18:1) and the polyunsaturated linoleic acid (18:2n-6) from vegetable oil triglycerides is high (>90%).[43] However, the coefficient of absorption of the saturated fatty acids myristic acid (14:0), palmitic acid (16:0), and stearic acid (18:0), is lower and decreases with increasing fatty acid chain length (approximately 89%, 75%, and 62%, respectively).

Approximately 75% of fatty acids absorbed in the sn-2 position as monoglycerides are conserved during reassembly of the triglyceride, whereas fatty acids originating from the sn-1,3 positions are re-esterified at random to the sn-1 and 3 positions during triacylglcyerol formation via the monoacylglycerol pathway. Following reassembly, the triacylglcyerols are

secreted as components of chylomicrons. Indeed, lymphatic transport of medium-chain fatty acids (MCFA) has been shown to be greater for MCFA absorbed as sn-2 monoglycerides than for MCFA located on the sn-1,3 position of the diet fat.[44] This may be expected to occur due to the reassembly of monoacylglycerols absorbed into the enterocyte via the monoacylglycerol path.

Mucosal Phase. The route of transport of absorbed fat is determined by the absorption as free fatty acids or sn-2 monoglycerides, the polarity of the fatty acids, and the specificity of fatty acid-binding proteins involved in mucosal triglyceride transport and reassembly. Intestinal cells have been shown to produce pancreatic triacylglycerol lipase and acid lipase,[45,46] but their role in vivo remains to be determined. Medium-chain triglycerides may be incorporated directly into mucosal cells and hydrolyzed. Liberated medium-chain fatty acids are then transported bound to albumin predominantly via the portal system. The separation of MCFA to be transported as unesterified, albumin-bound fatty acids via the portal venous route, and of fatty acids of carbon chain length 14 and longer to be transported in chylomicron triglycerides via the lymphatics, is not complete. Physiologically significant amounts of saturated and unsaturated fatty acids, including linoleic acid (18:2n-6) and α-linolenic acid (18:3n-3), are transported via the portal pathway,[47] while MCFA are found in chylomicron triglycerides.[48]

Metabolism of Absorbed Lipid. Hydrolysis of triglyceride constituents of intestinal chylomicrons and hepatic very low-density lipoprotein (VLDL) is the result of lipoprotein lipase activity released from adipose tissue, muscle, and possibly other tissues to the capillary endothelium. Compared to the lipoprotein lipase activity in infants born at term, lipoprotein lipase activity seems to be lower in infants <28-weeks gestation but not different in infants >32-weeks gestation.[49] Whether the relative deficiency of lipase activity in very small infants <28-weeks gestation is due to immaturity of lipoprotein lipase enzyme synthesis or to limited adipose tissue (ie, the major site of fat deposition), is not clear. The small adipose mass of infants <1000 g, however, has possible implications for the metabolism of products of triglyceride hydrolysis. A limited capacity for adipose tissue assimilation of free fatty acids could result in uptake by the liver, then resecretion as VLDL triglyceride.[50]

Dietary Factors Affecting Fat Absorption in Preterm Infants

Medium-chain triglycerides (MCT). These are used in LBWI formulas to increase fat absorption. MCT oils are produced by fractionation of coconut oil and contain primarily saturated fatty acids with 8 and 10 carbon atoms (octanoic and decanoic acids). While octanoic and decanoic acids usually contribute less than 2% of all fatty acids in human milk lipids,[8,9] preterm infant formulas in the USA contain up to 50%, and in Europe up to 40% of all fat as MCT. MCT have high water solubility, are rapidly cleaved by lipases, and are readily absorbed even in the presence of low intraluminal bile salts and pancreatic lipases.[51] Arguments for the use of MCT when compared to fats containing longer chain sources of saturated fatty acids in LBWI formulas include an improved fat absorption together with possible advantages related to rapid, portal venous transport of the albumin-bound MCFA to the liver, carnitine-independent transport into the mitochondria, and subsequent oxidation that is more rapid than for longer-chain fatty acids. Indeed, most balance studies show a higher fat absorption in premature infants fed formula if part of the formula fat is contributed by MCT. For example, Sulkers et al[52] studied 28 clinically stable VLBWI at 4 weeks of age and found a higher overall fat absorption of 88% with a formula containing 38% MCT, compared to only 79% fat absorption from a formula with 6% MCT (p<0.05). However, some studies have also reported no difference in fat absorption between preterm infants fed formulas without or with MCT.[53] It needs to be noted though that benefits in improvement of fat absorption are likely only in comparison between long-chain saturated fatty acids (16:0 and 18:0) and medium-chain saturated fatty acids, since the absorption of unsaturated 18:1 and 18:2n-6 is high. Comparison of formulas containing high amounts of

unsaturated fatty acids with formulas with medium-chain triglycerides, or between formulas with relatively small differences in the amount of 16:0 and 18:0 are not likely to yield appreciable differences in fat absorption.

The higher absorption of MCT than of longer-chain saturated triglycerides (LCT) does not necessarily lead to an increased supply of metabolizable energy. Due to the shorter chain length of their fatty acids, the energy content of MCT (per g) is about 15% lower than that of LCT. On the basis of this difference in chemical energy content, one can estimate that the inclusion of 38% MCT in the formula fat used in the study of Sulkers and coworkers[52] would not have led to any appreciable difference in the available energy supply. This may also explain why several clinical studies have not found any advantage in replacing part of the fat in LBWI formulas with MCT based on energy or nitrogen balance, or weight gain of the recipient premature infants.[54-57]

MCT are very rapidly oxidized and have a high thermogenic effect. Medium-chain fatty acids are predominantly transported to the liver directly via the portal vein without prior incorporation into chylomicrons. In the liver, they quickly enter mitochondria for β-oxidation. This occurs in large part without the need for binding to coenzyme A and carnitine regulated transport into the mitochondria, which explains the increase of resting metabolic rate induced by MCT.[51,58,59] Dietary medium-chain fatty acids, however, may affect carnitine metabolism in non-hepatic tissues.[60-62] Providing MCT in infant formula does result in an increased rate of fatty acid oxidation in the liver, which exceeds the ability for usual oxidation of acetyl CoA in the tricarboxylic acid cycle. This results in increased omega (ω)-oxidation of fatty acids, which involves cytochrome P-450 in the endoplasmic reticulum and cytosolic dehydrogenase, and the excretion of their dicarboxylic acid products in the urine.[56,63-67] The excretion of dicarboxylic acids is not signficantly increased in infants fed formulas with 5% MCT in the fat blend, but increases linearly with increasing amounts of MCT in formula. Higher plasma ketones are evident in infants fed formulas with

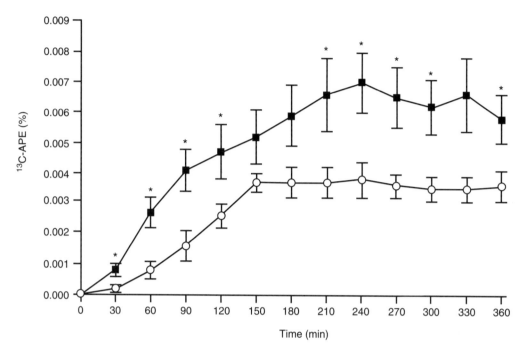

Figure 3: Dietary MCT can spare essential fatty acids from oxidation and thus enhance their availability for tissue incorporation. The oxidation of ¹³C-labeled linoleic acid (¹³C-Atom Percent Excess values, APE, means + SEM, in breath CO₂) measured in preterm infants fed control (■)formula is higher than in infants fed a formula with 40 % of fat provided as MCT (○), *p<0.05. Modified from (78)

20% MCT (about 10% total energy) or more.[64,65,67,68] Small amounts of dicarboxylic acids, primarily of adipic (C6), suberic (C8) and sebacic (C10) acid, are found in the urine of normal breast-fed infants. The increase in dicarboxylic acid excretion in infants fed MCT is largely the result of a marked increase in β-oxidation of decanoic acid (10:0). Concentrations 200-fold above normal have been reported for infants fed formula with 40% fat as MCT oils.[64] The total amount of energy lost to the urine is low, and there is at present no evidence that the significant production of dicarboxylic acid caused by MCT feeding has any deleterious effect on growth or development of infants <1750 g, except in infants with a congenital medium-chain acyl dehydrogenase deficiency (MCAD-deficiency).[69] The concentrations of dicarboxylic acids found in infants fed MCT are also lower than those found to be related to any neurological adverse effects.

The mild degree of ketonemia induced by formulas with MCT is of uncertain benefit. Ketone body synthesis occurs when the rate of formation of acetyl CoA from fat oxidation exceeds the capacity for entry to the tricarboxylic acid cycle. Undoubtedly, ketone bodies can be used by the developing brain for energy and as a substrate for synthesis of myelin cholesterol and fatty acids,[70,71] but adenosine triphosphate is required for the uptake of ketone bodies into the brain. Instead, glucose can be oxidized by the developing brain and should not be limited in the appropriately nourished preterm infant. An argument for including large amounts of MCT in formulas in order to provide ketones for the brain of preterm infants is not convincing at present, although this has not been systematically studied.

Studies of whole body oxidation of dietary MCT using stable isotope methodology have indicated that only 32% to 64% of the medium-chain fatty acid 8:0

is oxidized by preterm infants with a mean birth weight of 1150 g fed a formula with 40% of fat as MCT.[66] Analyses of adipose tissue fatty acids with methods to limit losses during extraction or high-temperature gas-liquid chromatography have also shown that very little of the medium-chain fatty acids with 8 and 10 carbon atoms are deposited in the infants' adipose tissues. Lauric acid (12:0), which is formed by elongation of MCFA, is incorporated in amounts related to the formula content of the shorter chain precursors.[72] Stable isotope studies have confirmed that preterm infants can chain elongate dietary medium-chain fatty acids, an energy consuming pathway.[73] In line with the observations in infants, the feeding of MCT oils, rather than long-chain fatty acids, to young rodents was reported to result in diminished fat deposition and adipose tissue cellularity.[63,74,75] Since MCT hardly contribute to tissue fat deposition, it is uncertain whether the MCT fraction of formula lipids should be included in the definition of minimal total fat supply if the calculation of the desirable minimal dietary fat intake of preterm infants is based on fat deposition rates.

A potentially beneficial effect of MCT supply is related to the rapid oxidation of a large portion of dietary MCT, which can spare other substrates such as glucose from oxidation.[76] As a result, plasma glucose levels in preterm infants can be increased.[77] Similarly, dietary MCT can spare PUFA from oxidation. Using stable isotope methodology, Rodriguez et al studied the effects of MCT in formulas on linoleic acid metabolism in preterm infants.[78] Enterally fed preterm infants were randomly assigned to formula with 40% of fat as MCT, or without MCT but otherwise similar in composition. At study day 5, infants received orally 2 mg/kg body weight of uniformly ^{13}C labelled linoleic acid. Fatty acids in plasma lipid classes and ^{13}C enrichment of phospholipid fatty acids were measured at 24h and 48h thereafter, and tracer oxidation was monitored by breath gas analysis. In comparison to the control group, the MCT group showed lower enrichment of ^{13}C in breath CO_2 (Figure 3) and higher plasma lipid octanoic acid, decanoic acid and several polyunsaturated fatty acids, as well as higher

total triglyceride LC-PUFA (57.1 ± 4.4 µmol/L vs. 37.9 ± 4.8 µmol/L, p <0.01). ^{13}C-concentrations in phospholipid n-6 fatty acids have indicated no difference in the relative conversion of linoleic to arachidonic acid. Thus, oral MCT may effectively reduce polyunsaturated fatty acid oxidation in preterm infants and enhance their availability for tissue incorporation and desaturation.

The use of MCT instead of the long-chain saturated fatty acids 16:0 and 18:0 in preterm infant formulas can also reduce the formation of calcium and magnesium soaps with unabsorbed long-chain saturated fatty acids, which can thereby increase calcium and magnesium absorption.[79] However, similar benefits on calcium and magnesium bioavailability can be achieved by using fats containing long-chain saturated fatty acids at the sn-2 position of the triglyceride or polyunsaturated fatty acids to limit the amount of excreted long-chain saturated fatty acids, rather than saturated vegetable oils with 16:0 esterifed at the triglyceride sn-1,3 positions.

LBWI formulas in the USA currently contain up to 50% of fat as MCT, while in Europe the Committee on Nutrition of the European Society of Paediatric Gastroenterology, Hepatology and Nutrition (ESPGHAN) has recommended a maximum content of MCT in LBWI formulas of 40% of the total fat content. At the present time, there is insufficient evidence to document a net benefit of including 40-50% MCT in preterm formulas. However, MCT as part of the fat source may be preferable to inclusion of high amounts of polyunsaturated or saturated fats.

As inferred above, the triglyceride structure also influences the efficacy of fat absorption. The saturated fatty acids in vegetable oils are largely esterified at the outer sn-1,3 positions of the triglyceride molecule. Unlike this, the major portion (about 60%) of the saturated fatty acid palmitic acid (16:0) and also stearic acid (18:0) in human milk triglycerides is located in the sn-2-position.[80] Since the lipolytic enzymes gastric and colipase-dependent lipase cleave fatty acids preferentially in sn-1- and sn-3-positions, human milk palmitic acid will appear primarily in the remaining monoglyceride which has a higher water-solubility than free palmitic acid (Figure 2). Thereby, absorption is facilitated because palmitic acid present as a monoglyceride is more polar than the nonesterifed palmitic acid. Hence, most of the palmitic acid (16:0) sn-2 monoglyceride is absorbed, and this structure is expected to be partly preserved through and beyond the intestinal wall. This has been shown to be so through studies on the distribution of fatty acids in chylomicon lipids of breast-fed infants.[81] Clinical trials in formula fed preterm infants have confirmed a significantly better absorption of palmitic acid from triglycerides when more of the palmitic acid was esterifed at the sn-2 position (beta-palmitate) compared to the sn-1,3 position.[74,82]

The overall effect on energy balance may be considered modest, but there are additional effects on mineral absorption. In clinical trials, the formula content of palmitic acid (16:0) and stearic acid (18:0) influenced not only the efficiency of fat absorption, but also that of some minerals. This finding is explained by the formation of insoluble soaps of calcium and magnesium with free palmitic acid (16:0) and stearic acid (18:0) as well as myristic acid (14:0) in the stomach or intestine.[43,75] Supplementation with calcium also resulted in a reduction in fat absorption of approximately 10% from frozen human milk or preterm infant formula containing palmitic acid (16:0) and stearic acid (18:0) from oleo oils. The fecal fatty acid analyses showed greater malabsorption of palmitic acid (16:0) and stearic acid (18:0) than of monounsaturated or polyunsaturated n-6 and n-3 fatty acids.[43,75] Other studies suggest that the fat and mineral malabsorption is predominantly the result of fat malabsorption, not the amount of calcium in the formula. The available data show the importance of avoiding large amounts of palmitic and stearic acid in the sn-1,3 positions of the formula fat. In preterm infants, calcium absorption was increased from 42% in infants fed a control formula to 57% in infants fed a formula containing 74% of palmitate esterified in the triglyceride sn-2 position (beta-palmitate).[74] Different options are available to increase the amount of palmitic acid (16:0) and stearic acid (18:0) in the

sn-2 position of formula fats. Fats that contain long-chain saturated fatty acids at the sn-2 position include lard, which is not acceptable to some population groups, and triglycerides specifically synthesized using randomization or co-randomization, or with immobilized enzyme technology. In randomization, the fatty acids in one or more oils are hydrolyzed from the triglyceride then re-esterified at random across the 3 positons of the triglyceride molecule. This results in an equal distribution of saturated fatty acids across all 3 carbon positions of the triglyceride. In processes using enzyme technology, fatty acids are re-esterifed, and triglycerides are selected that are specifcally enriched in palmitic acid at the triglyceride sn-2 position. Although a number of clinical and animal studies have been done, only a few preterm infant formulas contain these triglycerides today. Further, some commercial preterm infant formulas with beta-palmitate available today contain lower proportions of this synthesized triglyceride than previously evaluated in clinical trials. Thus, one would anticipate that any beneficial effect on the absorption of calcium or other divalent cations would be lower than that demonstrated in clinical trials.

Heat treatment of expressed human milk. Heat treatment may alter the absorption of milk lipids. Heat treatment of human milk is frequently applied in hospitals to reduce bacterial contamination and the risk of cytomegaly virus transmission, particularly for feeding human milk to preterm infants.[83,84] Pasteurization and sterilization may induce oxidative losses of unsaturated lipids and vitamins as well as inactivation of enzymes and immunological factors. Milk pasteurization (62.5° C/30 min) leads to inactivation of the milk bile salt-stimulated lipase.[85,86] This inactivation of the milk lipase, as well as possible changes in the milk fat globule structure, may explain the observed reduction in the coefficient of fat absorption to 75% from 90% in preterm infants fed heat-treated milk.[87] Although the total lipid content of human milk does not change during frozen storage, there is a gradual loss of triglyceride and an increase in free fatty acids at temperatures up to -20° C, whereas milk seems to remain rather stable at -80° C.[88] Milk sterilization (120° C/30 min) can reduce the fat content available to the recipient infant by >10% due to fat adherence to the container surface after sterilization.[89] However, neither pasteurization nor sterilization of human milk change the percentage composition of saturated, monounsaturated and polyunsaturated fatty acids both of the n-6 (18:3, 20:2, 20:3, 22:4) and n-3 series (18:3 20:5, 22:5, 22:6).[89]

Use of recombinant bile salt-stimulated lipase. Human bile salt-stimulated lipase has been cloned and shown to be identical to pancreatic cholesterol ester hydrolase.[40,90,91] Based on this information, the recombinant enzyme has been expressed and produced in transgenic mice as well as cultured cells, and has been shown to have catalytic activity.[92-94] Thus, it appears theoretically possible to add this or other lipolytic enzymes to heat treated human milk or to LBWI formulas, in order to improve the recipient infant's fat absorption. Obviously, this very promising novel approach would require a detailed characterization of its safety and efficacy,[95,96] and potential benefits would have to be weighed against the cost of the addition. One important question would be whether the enzyme would cleave saturated fatty acids, palmitic acid and stearic acid from the sn-2 position of the milk triglyceride, and thus lower both saturated fat and mineral absorption.

Fatty Acids

Fatty acids are important components of the phospholipids which make up the structural matrix of all cellular and subcellular membranes. The composition of membrane lipids is known to affect membrane functions such as receptor activities, transmembranous transport and membrane enzyme activities. In addition, the LC-PUFA di-homo-γ-linolenic acid (20:3n-6), arachidonic acid (20:4n-6) and eicosapentaenoic acid (20:5n-3) are precursors for synthesis of highly active oxygenated metabolites, ie, leukotrienes, thromboxanes, prostaglandins and prostacyclins, collectively known as eicosanoids (Figure 3). These eicosanoids, particularly those derived from arachidonic acid (20:4n-6), are important modulators and mediators of a variety of

physiological and developmental processes, such as patency of the ductus arteriosus, platelet-vessel wall interactions, regulation of pulmonary and systemic vascular resustance, immune function and renal function. Recently, the LC-PUFA docosahexaenoic acid (DHA, 22:6n-3) was identified to act in brain tissue as a specific ligand and activator of the retinoid X receptor (RXR), a nuclear receptor that functions as a ligand-activated transcription factor.[97] From these data, it is suggested that DHA may influence gene expression and neural function through activation of an RXR signaling pathway. It has long been known that in animals a deficiency of linoleic acid (18:2n6) or α-linolenic acid (18:3n-3) during early brain development results in long-term problems in learning and visual function, which may be irreversible in later life, even if a fatty acid sufficient diet is provided.[15,98,99] These problems have been related to reduced amounts of arachidonic acid (20:4n-6) and docosahexaenoic acid (22:6n-3) in the brain and retina. The goal of fatty acid nutrition in the premature infant is the support of normal pathways of eicosanoid metabolism and optimum levels of metabolically essential n-6 and n-3 fatty acids in membranes of the central nervous system (CNS), as well as other organs.

Fatty Acid Metabolism

Most fatty acids in the diet are supplied in triglycerides, with small amounts also obtained from phospholipids and cholesterol esters. Of particular importance is the greater solubility in water of caprylic acid (8:0) and capric acid (10:0), known as medium-chain fatty acids (MCFA), compared to fatty acids of carbon chain length 16 or more – for example, palmitic acid (16:0) and oleic acid (18:1) – which results in several important differences in physical and biochemical properties. Lauric acid (12:0) and myristic acid (14:0) have an intermediate position, sharing some of the properties of both MCFA and of long-chain fatty acids.

Saturated fatty acids, and unsaturated fatty acids of the n-9 and n-7 series, can be synthesized *de novo* from acetyl CoA. In contrast, humans cannot introduce double bonds in the n-6 or n-3 positions, therefore,

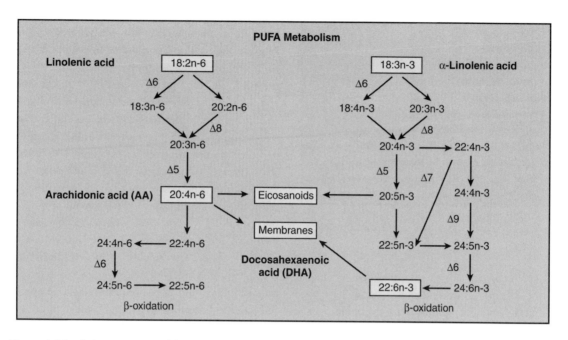

Figure 4: Metabolic conversion of the essential fatty acids linoleic acid (18:2 n-6) and linolenic acid (18:3 n-3) to long-chain polyunsaturated fatty acids (LC-PUFA).

n-6 polyunsaturated fatty acids (n-6 PUFA, linoleic acid and metabolites) and n-3 PUFA (α-linolenic acid and metabolites) are essential nutrients that must be provided with the enteral or parenteral substrate supply. The n-6 and n-3 fatty acids are not interconvertible either in the body or in their essential metabolic functions. Further, metabolism of the dietary precursor essential fatty acids, linoleic acid (18:2n-6) and α-linolenic acid (18:3n-3), occurs by alternating desaturation (insertion of double bonds) and elongation (addition of 2 carbon units) of the carbon chain. The result is a series of more highly unsaturated, long-chain polyunsaturated (LC-PUFA) fatty acids with 20 and 22 carbon atoms and 3 to 6 double bonds (Figure 4). The LC-PUFA arachidonic acid (20:4n-6; AA) and docosahexaenoic acid (22:6n-3; DHA) are of particular metabolic importance in infant growth and development.

Many of the metabolic functions of the n-6 and n-3 fatty acids, particularly those related to CNS function, are not fully understood. Arachidonic acid (20:4n-6) is the precursor of series 2 eicosanoids and series

4 leukotrienes.[15] Docosahexaenoic acid (22:6n-3) is essential for visual function.[15,99] Linoleic acid (18:2n-6) also seems to have independent essential metabolic roles perhaps related to normal triglyceride and cholesterol metabolism and specific water barrier functions of linoleic acid containing ceramides, in addition to providing substrate for synthesis of arachidonic acid (20:4n-6). Possible functions of α-linolenic acid (18:3n-3) that extend beyond its role as a precursor for longer-chain omega-3 fatty acids, eicosapentaenoic acid (EPA, 20:5n-3) and docosahexaenoic acid, (22:6n-3) are less well understood.

The biochemistry and metabolism of essential fatty acids is complex, involving differences in metabolism and competition among various n-6 and n-3 fatty acids. The desaturase enzymes are known to show substrate preference in the order n-3>n-6>n-9, and are inhibited by products of either the n-6 or n-3 fatty acid series.[15,99] Consequently, the rate of desaturation of linoleic acid (18:2n-6) to arachidonic acid (20:4n-6) and of α-linolenic acid (18:3n-3) to docosahexaenoic

- Scaly, hyperkeratotic dermatitis
- Loss of hair
- ↓ Weight gain and growth
- ↓ Energy utilization
- ↓ Nitrogen retention
- ↑ Susceptibility to infection
- Disturbed wound healing
- Fatty liver, hepatomegaly, ↑ ALAT and ASAT
- Thrombopenia, anemia, ↓ platelet aggregation
- ↑ Ratio Mead acid (20:3n-9)/Arachidonic acid (20:4n-6) in plasma and tissue lipids

Table 2: Signs and symptoms of linoleic acid deficiency in infants.

acid (22:6n-3) depends on the quantities of linoleic acid (18:2n-6) and α-linolenic acid (18:3n-3) substrates, and of preformed arachidonic acid (20:4n-6, AA) and/or docosahexaenoic acid (22:6n-3, DHA) in the diet. Eicosapentaenoic acid (20:5n-3, EPA), which is found predominantly in fatty fish and fish oils, inhibits the synthesis of arachidonic acid (20:4n-6), possibly due to inhibition of the desaturation of linoleic acid (18:2n-6) to arachidonic acid (20:4n-6, AA). Eicosapentaenoic acid (20:5n-3, EPA) also replaces arachidonic acid in tissue structural lipids. The infant's ability to maintain tissue arachidonic acid (20:4n-6, AA) levels may be lost if in appropriately high amounts of eicosapentaenoic acid (20:5n-3, EPA) are fed, or if the milk or formula diet contains a high ratio of 22:6n-3 and 20:5n-3 to 20:4n-6.[100,101] This has important implications, because the effects of series 3 prostanoids and series 5 leukotrienes derived from eicosapentaenoic acid (20:5n-3) are often antagonistic to, or different from, the physiological effects of cyclooxygenase and lipoxygenase products of arachidonic acid (20:4n-6). Depression of normal tissue levels of arachidonic acid could also have important physiological consequences unrelated to n-3 fatty acid derived eicosanoids. For example, arachidonic acid is important in cell signaling systems, and its eicosanoid metabolites are involved in adipose tissue growth.

In addition to microsomal desaturation, linoleic acid (18:2n-6) and α-linolenic acid (18:3n-3) can be oxidized in mitochondria for energy production.[102] Linoleic acid is also incorporated into adipose tissue triglycerides in amounts proportional to the quantity provided in the infant's diet.[103-105] In contrast, arachidonic acid (20:4n-6) and docosahexaenoic acid (22:6n-3) are preferentially incorporated into membrane phospholipids, rather than being oxidized or acylated into triglycerides. Oxidation of carbon chain 20 and 22 polyunsaturated fatty acids is also different and may involve initial chain shortening and retroconversion in the peroxisomes, prior to mitochondrial β-oxidation. These differences in oxidation and acylation probably explain why only a portion of dietary linoleic acid (18:2n-6) and α-linolenic acid (18:3n-3) is converted to arachidonic acid (20:4n-6) and docosahexaenoic acid (22:6n-3), respectively. Because of this, linoleic acid and α-linolenic acid are considered to have lower biological activity as sources of membrane phospholipid LC-PUFA than dietary arachidonic acid or docosahexaenoic acid.

Linoleic Fatty Acid Deficiency

An inadeqate dietary supply of linoleic acid induces a specific deficiency syndrome with a dry, scaly dermatitis and a variety of other signs and symptoms (Table 2). Linoleic acid deficiency has been observed primarily in infants,[106,107] and a few adult patients given lipid-free parenteral nutrition. Infants are at a far higher risk of deficiency, presumably because of higher requirements for polyunsaturated fatty acids due to their rapid growth rate and limited body stores.

Biochemical indicators of linoleic acid deficiency include reduced linoleic acid levels in plasma and tissue lipids, as well as increased levels of palmitoleic acid (16:1n-9), eicosatrienoic acid (20:3n-9), and mead acid, a metabolite of oleic acid, (18:1n-9). Substrate affinity of the desaturase enzymes in the order of n-3>n-6>n-9 effectively limits desaturation of significant amounts of oleic acid (18:1n-9) to eicosatrienoic (20:3n-9) as long as there is a sufficient dietary intake of linoleic acid (18:2n-6) or α-linolenic acid (18:3n-3). Analyses of the proportion of eicosatrienoic acid (20:3n-9) in the plasma lipids, therefore, can be a useful diagnostic index of linoleic acid deficiency, particularly when considered in relation to the amount of the linoleic acid metabolite arachidonic acid (20:4n-6). The ratio of 20:3n-9 to 20:4n-6 (often referred to as the triene:tetraene ratio) in plasma lipids is usually <0.1 in healthy adults, children, and breast-fed infants, but increases to >0.2 in linoleic fatty acid deficiency.[108-109] This increase in the triene:tetraene ratio is explained by increased synthesis of eicosatrienoic acid (C20:3n-9) from oleic acid (18:1n-9) and decreased synthesis of arachidonic acid (20:4n-6) resulting from inadequate intake or absorption of linoleic acid (18:2n-6). Because desaturation of oleic acid (18:1n-9) to eicosatrienoic acid (20:3n-9) is inhibited by either linoleic acid (18:2n-6) or linolenic acid (18:3n-3), measurement of the triene:tetraene ratio is useful only for the diagnosis of inadequate intake or absorption of both linoleic and linolenic acid. It is not of value for diagnosing a deficiency of only n-6 fatty acids or only n-3 fatty acids, and it is not useful for judgments on the quality of the n-6 and n-3 fatty acid supply to the infant. Moreover, the increase of the triene:tetraene ratio may not be a sensitive indicator of linoleic acid deficiency in patients with protein-energy deficiency as observed in malnourished children.[110,111] In preterm infants, dietary intakes of linoleic acid (18:2n-6) below about 4.5% kcal have been reported to be associated with increased triene:tetraene ratios,[112] and linoleic acid intakes of >4.5% kcal have been recommended for LBW infants.[19]

Linolenic Fatty Acid Deficiency

Several reports of α-linolenic acid deficiency concerning adults and children maintained for long periods of time on parenteral lipids or powdered formulations without any n-3 fatty acids have been published.[113-116] Biochemical changes included a decrease in plasma docosahexaenoic acid (22:6n-3), which occurred with some neurological signs. These were resolved when α-linolenic acid was provided. While these reports are consistent with the importance of n-3 fatty acids, they provide no evidence for a specific metabolic role of α-linolenic acid rather

than its metabolites eicosapentenoic acid (20:5n-3) and docosahexaenoic acid (22:6n-3), and other confounding variables in the patients and their management limit interpretation of a specifc effect of n-3 fatty acids in the problems found.

Approaches to Define an Adequate PUFA Supply

Intrauterine PUFA supply

The requirement for incorporation of n-6 and n-3 fatty acids in tissue lipids may be estimated from data on the quantity of these fatty acids deposited in tissues at various stages of early development. Dietary requirements may then be extrapolated from the amounts needed for tissue growth if factors are available, or margins of safety are estimated, to account for losses in absorption, oxidation to energy, and incorporation into adipose tissue triglycerides. If the accretion of LC-PUFA in membranes and other structural lipids is to be achieved by the supply of the precursors linoleic acid (18:2n-6) and α-linolenic acid (18:3n-3), an estimate of the efficiency of conversion (bioequivalence) to arachidonic acid (20:4n-6) and docosahexaenoic acid (22:6n-3) would need to be included. The estimation of factors to account for conversion of linoleic acid to arachidonic acid and α-linolenic acid to docosahexaenoic acid is complex, since this rate of conversion will depend on the need to oxidize linoleic and α-linolenic acid for energy, and the amount of the two substrates, given that it is above requirement. The higher the amount of substrate given, the lower the relative percentage that may be converted into products.

The analysis of tissue composition from deceased infants and fetuses of different gestational ages has demonstrated the incorporation of relatively large amounts of long-chain polyunsaturated fatty acids (LC-PUFA), especially arachidonic acid (20:4n-6, AA) and docosahexaenoic acid (22:6n-3, DHA) into structural lipids of the brain, retina and other tissues during the latter part of gestation, as well as during postnatal growth.[117] High LC-PUFA concentrations are found in the phospholipids of brain grey matter membranes, such as synaptosomal membranes. DHA

	Triglycerides		Phospholipids	
	Maternal	**Cord**	**Maternal**	**Cord**
Total (mg/dl)	143.31 (63.73)	24.27 (12.43)*	172.22 (37.63)	62.55 (18.08)*
Linoleic (C18:2n-6)	11.91 (5.48)	10.05 (3.45)*	20.99 (3.38)	7.42 (1.37)*
Di-homo-γ-linolenic (C20:3n-6)	0.22 (0.07)	0.81 (0.43)*	3.37 (0.82)	4.82 (0.83)*
Arachidonic (C20:4n-6)	0.75 (0.29)	2.92 (1.11)*	7.68 (1.90)	16.14 (2.49)*
Total n-6-LC-PUFA	1.54 (0.41)	5.74 (2.20)*	12.37 (2.16)	22.55 (2.56)*
α-Linolenic (C18:3n-3)	0.52 (0.19)	0.20 (0.27)*	0.20 (0.10)	0.00 (0.03)*
Eicosapentaenoic (C20:5n-3)	0.06 (0.04)	0.00 (0.17)	0.35 (0.15)	0.20 (0.16)*
Docosahexaenoic (C22:6n-3)	0.32 (0.22)	1.33 (1.27)*	2.89 (0.99)	4.76 (1.70)*
Total n-3-LC-PUFA	0.51 (0.28)	1.59 (1.66)*	3.72 (1.24)	5.44 (2.12)*
	Cholesterol Esters		Non-esterified Fatty Acids	
	Maternal	**Cord**	**Maternal**	**Cord**
Total (mg/dl)	120.13 (48.99)	33.57 (17.85)*	25.21 (13.04)	9.60 (6.95)*
Linoleic (C18:2n-6)	48.75 (8.19)	15.28 (4.04)*	7.69 (4.28)	4.13 (2.94)*
Di-homo-γ-linolenic (C20:3n-6)	0.78 (0.30)	1.28 (0.39)*	0.33 (0.34)	0.41 (0.73)
Arachidonic (C20:4n-6)	5.66 (1.70)	11.39 (3.36)*	0.74 (0.56)	1.04 (1.27)*
Total n-6-LC-PUFA	6.69 (1.48)	14.75 (3.39)*	2.35 (3.47)	6.30 (7.22)*
α-Linolenic (C18:3n-3)	0.56 (0.31)	0.08 (0.15)*	0.15 (0.30)	0.00 (0.06)*
Eicosapentaenoic (C20:5n-3)	0.33 (0.20)	0.22 (0.34)*	0.00 (0.11)	0.00 (0.00)
Docosahexaenoic (C22:6n-3)	0.52 (0.38)	0.92 (0.52)*	0.18 (0.31)	0.00 (0.49)
Total n-3-LC-PUFA	0.93 (0.57)	1.26 (0.72)	0.29 (0.60)	0.00 (0.63)

Table 3: Comparison of n-6 and n-3 fatty acids in maternal and newborn infant cord plasma.
Total fatty acid concentration (mg/dl) and percentage contributions of major essential fatty acids (% wt/wt) in
plasma lipids in 41 pairs of mothers and their newborn infants at the time of birth (median [interquartile range];
* = p<0.05) show lower levels of the essential precursor fatty acids linoleic (18:2n-6) and α-linolenic (C18:3n-3)
acids in cord than in maternal blood. In contrast, the LC-PUFA metabolites di-homo-γ-linolenic (C20:3n-6),
arachidonic (C20:4n-6) and docosahexaenoic (C22:6n-3) acids are preferentially enriched in cord blood.[Modified from 222]

is also particularly high in retinal photoreceptor membranes. However, some 70% to 78% of the total n-6 and n-3 fatty acids accumulated by the fetus are accounted for by deposition in adipose tissue.[117-120] Third trimester weekly rates of accumulation have been estimated as follows: approximately 2.6 g n-6 fatty acid and 0.37 g n-3 fatty acids for adipose tissue; approximately 0.044 g n-6 and 0.022 g n-3 fatty acid

for the brain; and approximately 0.014 g n-6 and 0.004 g n-3 fatty acid for the liver. In brain and liver, almost all of the prenatal PUFA deposition is comprised of LC-PUFA. On average, the third trimester fetus accumulates an estimated 40 to 60 mg n-3 LC-PUFA per kg body weight per day.[121] Fetal liver, brain and adipose tissue growth seem to follow a sigmoidal (S-shaped) curve rather than a linear course

	Colostrum (5 days)	Transitional (10 days)	Mature (30 days)
Saturated fatty acids			
Total	43.65 (3.55)	43.05 (3.67)	44.30 (5.00)
Monounsaturated fatty acids			
C18:1n-9	32.1 (1.87)	32.10 (2.61)	31.50 (2.49)
Polyunsaturated fatty acids (PUFA)			
n-6 PUFA			
C18:2n-6	8.86 (1.30)	10.30 (2.15)	11.33 (2.17)
C18:3n-6	0.14 (0.31)	0.15 (0.08)	0.18 (0.10)
C20:2n-6	0.57 (0.12)	0.42 (0.06)	0.30 (0.07)
C20:3n-6	0.53 (0.13)	0.43 (0.11)	0.38 (0.08)
C20:4n-6	0.72 (0.07)	0.59 (0.09)	0.45 (0.07)
C22:4n-6	0.23 (6.00)	0.15 (0.03)	0.08 (0.02)
n-6 LC-PUFA	2.15 (0.34)	1.59 (0.20)	1.28 (0.19)
n-3 PUFA			
C18:3n-3	0.65 (0.07)	0.81 (0.17)	0.90 (0.20)
C20:3n-3	0.09 (0.03)	0.05 (0.03)	0.05 (0.04)
C20:5n-3	0.04 (0.08)	0.00 (0.03)	0.05 (0.07)
C22:5n-3	0.22 (0.05)	0.18 (0.04)	0.15 (0.03)
C22:6n-3	0.46 (0.08)	0.39 (0.06)	0.23 (0.06)
n-3 LC-PUFA	0.80 (0.21)	0.66 (0.11)	0.48 (0.16)

Table 4: Major fatty acids of human milk from omnivorous women consuming self-selected foods (% wt/wt, median values and interquartile ranges). [Adapted from 223]

during the last trimester. Calculations of average daily or weekly rates of fatty acid accretion that assume linear growth may, therefore, underestimate the tissue requirements at peak periods of growth. However, it is important to recognize that these autopsy data are based on a limited number of cases at specific ages, and the conditions resulting in death and time to autopsy and tissue sampling for analysis may have influenced the results.

The docosahexaenoic acid (DHA) content of the developing infant brain is more affected by the dietary intake of n-3 fatty acids than the brain AA content.[122] As noted, regardless of the gestational age at birth,

there appears to be considerable inter-individual variation in brain docosahexaenoic acid (DHA) content among human newborns. The variability may be due to differences in fatty acid supply or metabolism as well as other factors that influence development, or these apparent differences may reflect conditions surrounding fetal and infant death, delays in autopsy tissue recovery, or the small number of cases studied. There is little information as to what extent adipose triglyceride n-6 and n-3 fatty acids are of functional significance or provide a source for LC-PUFA deposition in brain or other tissues after birth. However, it is likely that a redistribution of

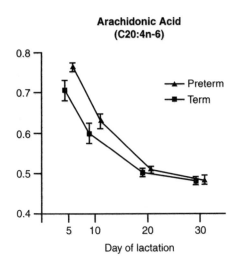 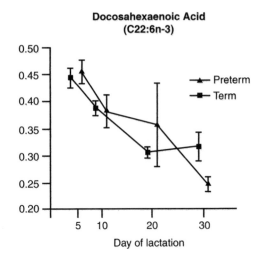

Figure 5: Changes in the percentage contents of arachidonic and docosahexaenoic (%wt/wt) in term and preterm milk during the first month of lactation.[Drawn from data of 223]

LC-PUFA from adipose tissue stores to other body pools occurs because infants fed a dietary source of LC-PUFA continue to have higher amounts of LC-PUFA in cells with rapid turnover, such as oral mucosal cells, even long after the end of the dietary LC-PUFA supply.[123]

The intrauterine supply of PUFA to the fetus depends entirely on placental transfer. Markedly lower levels of linoleic and α-linolenic acids, but much higher concentrations of arachidonic acid and docosahexaenoic acid are present in cord plasma than in maternal plasma lipids (Table 3).[124] This may indicate a preferential and selective maternofetal LC-PUFA transfer in utero. Alternative explanations include differences in transport and oxidation. Delta 5 desaturase has been found in the placenta,[125] but the contribution of placental desaturase activity to fetal LC-PUFA accretion is not known. LC-PUFA in the fetal circulation can also be derived from synthesis in fetal tissues, or from maternal stores, in addition to recent dietary intake. Preferential LC-PUFA transfer by the placenta, relative to the precursor PUFA, is supported by experimental studies in the perfused human placenta.[126,127] Furthermore, recent studies have described a specific placental fatty acid binding

protein which preferentially binds LC-PUFA and faciltates their selective placental transfer to the fetus.[128] Recent studies with stable isotope labeled fatty acids provide direct evidence for a preferential transfer of DHA accross the human placenta in vivo.[129]

PUFA Supply with Human Milk

Human milk is considered the ideal nutrition for healthy term infants and to generally meet the nutrient requirements during up to the first 6 months of life.[130] The composition of human milk lipids is variable and depends on the mother's diet, as well as other factors. Consequently, infant dietary or tissue requirements for particular fatty acids cannot be derived from simple extrapolation of the amounts supplied by human milk. Nonetheless, elucidation of the physiology of human milk feeding may provide some background that can help in understanding infant requirements.

During the course of lactation from colostrum to transitional and mature milk, the percentage of human milk lipids provided by the PUFA precursors linoleic and α-linolenic acid increases, whereas LC-PUFA values decrease (Table 4). However, human milk always contains LC-PUFA which includes arachidonic

Country	Australia	Canada	Congo	France	Germany	Italy	Norway	Spain
Reference	225	226	227	228	223	229	230	231
Linoleic acid	14.06	11.8	13.65	13.23	11.33	9.79	11.60	12.02
Arachidonic acid	0.41	0.4	0.44	0.50	0.45	0.47	0.40	0.50
α-Linolenic acid	0.97	1.5	1.19	0.57	0.90	0.36	0.93	0.78
Docosahexaenoic acid	0.21	0.3	0.55	0.38	0.23	0.12	0.46	0.34

Table 5: Contribution of linoleic acid (C18:2w-6), arachidonic acid (C20:4w-6), α-linolenic acid (C18:3w-3), and docosahexaenoic acid (C22:6w-3) to the fatty acid composition of mature human milk for women following their usual diets. Data are % weight/weight, medians or means from recently published studies using high-resolution capillary gas-liquid chromatography. Modified after 224

acid (AA) and docosahexaenoic acid (DHA). The percentage contributions of n-6 and n-3 LC-PUFA and their changes during the first months of lactation do not differ in the milk of mothers of term and of preterm infants (Figure 5).[131]

A review of some studies on the fatty acid composition of mature human milk lipids with modern analytical techniques (Table 5) indicates that linoleic acid contents vary with maternal dietary intake, with mean linoleic acid contents in the range of 10 to 15% of total fatty acids. In contrast, the milk contents of arachidonic acid appear to be relatively similar at 0.4-0.5% of total fatty acids, even in vegetarians who consume little preformed arachidonic acid[132] and in women consuming large amounts of marine lipids and hence eicosapentaenoic acid (20:5n-3)[133], a metabolic competitor of arachidonic acid. Recent careful studies using stable isotopes have investigated the transfer of specific fatty acids and their metabolites into human milk. Some 70% of milk linoleic acid originates not directly from the maternal diet, but from maternal body stores with slow turnover (Figure 6). An even higher proportion of arachidonic acid, more than 90% of the amount secreted in milk, is derived from maternal pools.[102,134] The contribution of maternal adipose and potentially other tissue lipid stores to the circulating plasma fatty acids taken up by the mammary gland for secretion in milk lipids might

be of biological benefit for the breast-fed infant, since it provides the infant with a relatively stable supply of PUFA even if maternal dietary intake changes over short periods of time.

In contrast, to arachidonic acid (AA), the milk concentration of docosahexaenoic acid (DHA) shows a considerably larger variation. Controlled trials supplementing n-3 LC-PUFA to lactating women show a direct effect on milk contents of docosahexaenoic acid (DHA).[135,136] Stable isotope measurements also demonstrate that n-3 LC-PUFA supplementation in lactation does not reduce the proportional docosahexaenoic acid (DHA) transfer from diet into milk.[135] Thus, the maternal consumption of n-3 LC-PUFA, for example from fatty fish such as herring, mackerel or salmon, directly influences the supply to the breastfed baby.

PUFA Sources for Infants Fed Infant Formula Milk: Diet, Body Stores and Endogenous Synthesis

LC-PUFA free formula. Until recently, the lipids in LBWI formula were based on vegetable oils containing linoleic and α-linolenic acids, but no LC-PUFA.[137-139] Feeding formula devoid of LC-PUFA results in a rapid decrease in LC-PUFA in the circulating plasma lipids,[140-143] and a somewhat slower decrease in red blood cells and oral mucosa cells of LBW

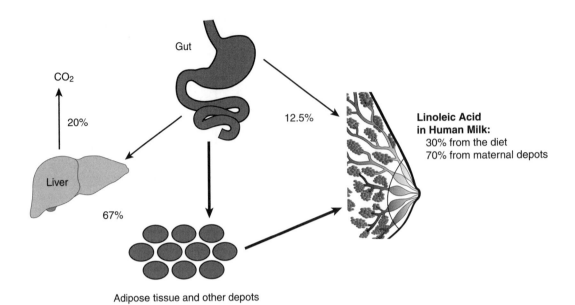

Figure 6: Linoleic acid turnover in breastfeeding women, based on results of a stable isotope study with oral application of 1 mg/kg bodyweight of U-¹³C-labeled linoleic acid and measurements of its oxidation from breath gas analyses and its transfer into milk by analysis of milk samples collected over 5 days.[102] Of the linoleic acid in the maternal diet, some 12.5% is transferred into milk, 20% is oxidized, and about 67% is deposited in maternal stores with slow turnover, such as adipose tissue. From the point of view of the recipient infant, only some 30% of milk linoleic acid is derived directly from the maternal diet, whereas 70% originate from maternal body depots with slow turnover. Thereby, the effects of short-term variation in maternal diet linoleic acid, for which there are large adipose tissue reserves, are buffered.

infants.[101,123,144] In many preterm infants, the rapid decrease in LC-PUFA status begins after birth with the initiation of parenteral nutrition, despite a small amount of LC-PUFA in the lipid emulsions.[145,146] In term infants, the lower blood lipid docosahexaenoic acid in infants fed formula continues for several months beyond the period of difference in dietary LC-PUFA intake.[147] The decrease in plasma and red blood cell docosahexaenoic acid (DHA) in infants fed formula when compared to breast fed infants tends to be more marked than the decrease in arachidonic acid (AA). Infants (mostly term born) who had been fed formula and had died from sudden infant death syndrome had lower DHA concentrations in brain, liver and adipose tissue than infants who been previously breast-fed.[104,122,148] These data illustrate

that the dietary supply of docosahexaenoic acid is important in supporting accretion of docosahexaenoic acid in the developing brain. This is likely to be even more important in the preterm, VLBW infant because these infants have much lower body stores of LC-PUFA than term infants, and they are at a much earlier and more vulnerable stage of neural and retinal development. For example, retinal accretion of docosahexaenoic acid is rapid during the third trimester of development but appears to be complete by 40 weeks of gestation.[117] A major component of brain lipid growth after term birth is myelinogenesis involving deposition of large amounts of saturated and monunstaurated fatty acids.

Endogenous synthesis of LC-PUFA. Early studies on the LC-PUFA status of LBWI postulated low activity of a putative delta 4 desaturase enzyme thought to be involved in the synthesis of DHA. Recent refinements of isotope techniques rendered it possible to investigate infant fatty acid metabolism in vivo.[15] With these techniques, endogenous synthesis of both AA and docosahexaenoic acid (DHA) has been demonstrated in term and in preterm infants, although the relative tracer enrichment in the products AA and DHA formed from linoleic acid and α-linolenic acid in plasma is very small.[149-152] There are some indications that the relative rate of conversion may be higher in preterm than in term infants.[150,152] The data obtained from these tracer studies do not allow any conclusions on the absolute rates of synthesis, tissue incorporation, or the relation between rates of synthesis and turnover. Thus, how much of the requirement for LC-PUFA for tissue growth can be met by endogenous synthesis from the linoleic acid and α-linolenic acid precursors is still unknown.

It has been proposed that AA synthesis in the formula fed infant might be increased by providing a dietary supply of γ-linolenic acid (18:3n-6), which is the product of D-6 desaturase which catalyzes the first, rate limiting step in the desaturation of linoleic acid (Figure 4). Clinical trials with preterm infants fed with formulas or with parenteral lipids show that γ-linolenic acid may increase the levels of its elongation product, di-homo-γ-linolenic acid (20:3n-6), although providing γ-linolenic acid does not support similar levels of arachidonic acid to those found in infants fed with human milk (143;153). An increased intake of α-linolenic acid (18.3n-3), with a concomitant decrease of the linoleic/α-linolenic acid ratio (18:2n-6/18.3n-3-ratio) has been explored as a possible way to increase docosahexaenoic acid status in infants fed formula. In term infants, 18:2n-6/18.3n-3-ratios below 4:1 increased DHA in red blood cells but did not result in DHA levels comparable to those of the breast-fed reference groups, and this was accompanied by low AA levels.[154] In another study, formula with 3.2% α-linolenic acid and a 18:2n-6/18:3n-3 ratio of 4.8 resulted in higher DHA, but lower AA in plasma lipids and lower weight gain in term infants than a formula with 0.4% 18:3n-3 and a 18:2n-6/18:3n-3 ratio of 9.8:1.[155,156] The provision of higher 18:3n-3 contents in formula does not result in similar plasma or red blood cell levels DHA in infants fed formula to those achieved in infants fed human milk with DHA. Since no evidence is available to document the efficacy and safety of α-linolenic acid intakes above 3-4% fatty acids in LBWI, and it is possible that high α-linolenic acid may reduce arachidonic acid synthesis, the inclusion of α-linolenic acid at levels greater than 3-4% fatty acids in formula for LBWI is not recommended.

Extensive data from clinical studies has clearly shown that feeding formula with α-linolenic acid does not support similar plasma and RBC levels of docosahexaenoic acid to that achieved when docosahexaenoic acid itself is provided either in the formula, or in human milk.[155-158] Data obtained from analyses of autopsy tissue also suggest that brain levels of docosahexaenoic acid are lower in infants fed formula without docosahexaenoic acid than in infants who were breast-fed.[122,148] This is explained by the oxidation of a large portion of dietary α-linolenic acid to carbon dioxide, rather than its desaturation to docosahexaenoic acid. The proportion of dietary α-linolenic acid converted to docosahexaenoic acid in infants is not yet known and may be influenced by dietary variables, such as the concurrent intake of n-6 fatty acids, docosahex-aenoic acid, and the total energy intake. Studies in pregnant baboons fed a diet with linoleic and α-linolenic acid in a ratio of 10:1 and given i.v. doses of U-^{13}C-labeled α-linolenic and docosahexaenoic acid found that docosahexaeoic acid was about 20 times effective in supporting docosahexaenoic acid accretion in the fetal baboon brain than the precursor α-linolenic acid.[159] Studies in neonatal piglets formula have also found that preformed docosaehxaenoic acid is at least 10 times more effective in supporting accretion of docosahexaenoic acid in the developing brain than dietary α-linolenic acid.[160]

Formula with preformed LC-PUFA. The addition of preformed LC-PUFA to LBWI formulas has been evaluated since the mid 1980s. In most studies, the sources of LC-PUFA were egg phospholipids or total lipids, egg triglycerides (that provide DHA and AA), fish oils (providing DHA and varying amounts of EPA) and single cell triglyceride oils from algae (providing docosahexaenoic acid) and fungi (providing arachidonic acid). Studies on the bioavailability of different sources of dietary LC-PUFA in preterm infants using balance studies have found that the absorption of n-3 LC-PUFA from phospholipid containing formula was higher (88.7%) than from formula with a single cell triglyceride (80.4%, p<0.05).[161] Recently, Wijendran and coworkers reported different brain incorporation of labeled LC-PUFA in the sn-2 position of dietary phospholipids and triglycerides: 4.0 ± 1.3% of phospholipid AA but only 2.1 ± 0.4% of triglyceride AA were incorporated into the brain of neonatal baboons.[162] These studies demonstrate that not only the amount but also the source of dietary LC-PUFA is of great importance for biological effects.

Supplementation of infant formula with docosahexaaenoic acid, and arachidonic acid, has been shown to induce a dose-related increase in infant plasma, red blood cells, and cheek mucosa cells DHA and AA, respectively.[141-143,163-167] Addition of both DHA and AA to formula can support similar plasma and RBC levels of DHA and AA in formula-fed LBWI to those found in comparable LBWI fed human milk.[142,165,167] Clandinin and coworkers compared the effects of feeding preterm infants of birthweight <2300 g with three infant formulas with AA ranging from 0.32 to 1.1% of fatty acids, and docosahexaenoic acid ranging from 0.24 to 0.75%.[168] Infants fed a formula with 0.49% arachidonic acid and 0.35% docosahexaenoic acid had similar AA and DHA in plasma lipoproteins to the infants fed human milk in this study.

Early studies that involved supplementation with n-3 LC-PUFA from fish oils with high eicosapentaenoic acid (EPA, 20:5n-3) without concomitant supplementation with AA, found lower growth, lower AA and an association between AA and growth.[101,169-172] These findings suggest that supplementation with n-3 LC-PUFA without AA, is not desirable for infant feeding. However, there is no

known reason for concern over small amounts of eicosapentaenoic acid found in human milk, which is always present together with arachidonic acid. Clinical trials involving a large number of preterm infants have shown that feeding with modern formulas containing both DHA and AA, in amounts and in a ratio within the usual range of human milk and with adequate antioxidant protection, is not associated with any adverse effects.[167,173,174]

A Cochrane review published in 2000 also concluded that the supplementation of formula with both n-3 and n-6 LC-PUFA does not impair the growth of preterm infants.[175] In Europe, LC-PUFA have been added to LBWI formulas since the beginning of the 1990s, and for many years all commercial LBWI formulas used in Europe have contained LC-PUFA, although in different amounts and relative compositions.[138] No untoward effects have become known. However, the growth of LBWI infants is often below that of their term gestation counterparts, and developmental problems are not infrequent, which suggests careful follow-up studies may be important to assess both positve and negative effects of LC-PUFA supplementation from different sources. Thus, all dietary products used for infant feeding, and their ingredients, need to be fully characterized with regard to their safety.[95]

LC-PUFA Metabolism and Early Human Growth

Birthweight, a major determinant of short- and long-term health, is influenced by genetic factors, maternal body size, and intrauterine substrate supply and metabolism.[176] Early observations studies demonstrated that a characteristic feature of n-6 fatty acid deficiency is growth failure.[177] A positive correlation between arachidonic acid and birthweight was first reported in preterm infants.[178] The absence of any correlation between birthweight and linoleic acid, or between arachidonic acid and gesational age in the latter studies suggests a possible specific relation of AA to growth. Other studies have also noted a positive association between arachidonic acid and growth in preterm infants.[100,101] Similarly, Elias et al[179] have reported a positive association between birthweight and arachidonic acid in cord plasma triglycerides and cholesteryl esters of term infants in Western Canada. Prospective clinical trials with preterm infants fed formulas supplemented with arachidonic acid and docosahexaenoic acid have also found a positive association between AA status and growth.[174,180] On the 10th day of life, red blood cell arachidonic acid was significantly and positively related to weight, length and head circumference in a group of 143 preterm infants fed five different infant formulas, including three without and two with dietary LC-PUFA. Red blood cell arachidonic acid values at 10 days of age was also significantly and positively related to birth weights, but there was no correlation between anthropometric data and red blood cell arachidonic acid at 42 days of age. The authors concluded that neonatal arachidonic acid status is related to intrauterine rather than to postnatal growth.

The observational data indicating a positive association between arachidonic acid and birthweight, together with early studies showing lower growth and lower arachidonic acid in LBWI fed formulas supplemented with fish oil providing n-3 LC-PUFA,[171] and with new data to suggest higher growth emerging from clinical trials with LBWI fed formulas with arachidonic acid raise important hypotheses on the possible relationships between n-6 fatty acid metabolism, and interrelations between n-6 and n-3 fatty acids and early human growth. In term infants, a low dietary linoleic acid to α-linolenic acid ratio of 3.8:1 was also associated with lower plasma arachidonic acid and lower growth in infants fed formula from birth to 120 days of age.[155] On a cellular and molecular level, eicosanoids derived from n-6 LC-PUFA, including PGE_2, TxA_2 and PGF_2, have been shown to stimulate cell growth, whereas PGI_2, PGA_2, and in some cell lines also PGE_2, inhibited cellular growth.[181] The cellular conversion of AA to PGE_2 induced the mitogenic response in mouse 3T3 fibroblasts, whereas n-3 LC-PUFA antagonized mitogenic stimulation with AA by reducing PGE_2 formation. Further understanding of the role of n-6 fatty acids and their metabolites in cell growth and

division may help to elucidate the effects of maternal and postnatal lipid intake and metabolism on pre- and postnatal growth.

LC-PUFA and Visual Function

Animal studies have clearly shown that the early development of the visual system function, as measured by electroretinography, visual evoked response potentials (VEP) and behavioural methods, is related to n-3 PUFA availability.[182-184] Prospective, randomized clinical trials have been published on preterm infants that report positive effects of the addition of docosahexaenoic acid to formula on the development of visual function.

- Uauy and coworkers[164] studied infants born at 27-33 weeks with an average birth weight of about 1300 g. The infants were randomized to feeding formulas with corn oil (very low in α-linolenic acid), soy oil (containing higher α-linolenic acid) or soy and fish oils (containing both α-linolenic acid and n-3 LC-PUFA, including 0.35% of fatty acids as DHA), or were part of a reference group fed human milk. At 36 weeks postconceptional age (PCA), infants fed the formula with soy and fish oil had similar rod electroretinogram (ERG)-thresholds and higher amplitudes than infants fed human milk, and lower ERG thresholds and higher amplitudes than infants fed the formula with corn oil. At 57 weeks, equivalent to about 4 months post-term, visual acuity assesed with transient visual evoked potential (VEP) and Teller acuity cards was higher in LBWI fed with human milk than the formula with fish oil than in the soy and corn oil groups.[185]

- Carlson and coworkers studied infants with an average gestational age of 29 weeks and birth weight of 1100 g who were randomized to be fed conventional formula or formula with fish oil (formula fat with 0.2% docosahexaenoic acid), until about 9 months post-term.[186] Visual acuity was significantly higher in infants fed the formula with fish oil at 2- and 4-months-corrected term age, but not at later ages.[187]

- In a subsequent study, Carlson and coworkers

randomized infants with a mean gestational age of 28.5 weeks and a birth weight of 1100 g to be fed either with formula supplemented with fish oil to provide 0.2% docosahexaenoic acid, or a conventional formula until 2 months post-term. Visual acuity was higher at 2-months-corrected age in the LBWI fed the fish oil supplemented rather than a control formula.[188] Visual acuity was not different at later time points. The subgroup of infants with chronic lung disease, however, showed no improvement of visual acuity with n-3 LC-PUFA with supplementation.

- Faldella and coworkers studied flash VEP at about 3 months post term in 58 preterm infants with an average gestational age of 31 weeks and birth weight of 1500 g who were fed breast milk or randomized to a control formula or a formula supplemented with LC-PUFA (with 0.23% docosahexaenoic acid).[189] VEP latencies were similar between infants fed human milk and those fed the LC-PUFA supplemented formula, but significantly delayed in infants fed the control formula.

- In a multi-center trial, O'Connor and coworkers studied 470 preterm infants with birth weights of 750-1800 g randomized to formulas without LC-PUFA, with 0.43% of fatty acids as arachidonic acid and 0.27% docosahexaenoic acid from fish and fungal oils, or with 0.41% arachidonic acid and 0.24% docosahexaenoic acid from fish and egg oils.[173] At term age, the infants were switched to formulas with the same oil sources, but only 0.15-0.16% docosahexaenoic acid. No adverse effects of any formula on growth or other side effects were found. Visual acuity measured by behavioral methods was not different. VEP acuity was higher in the two groups fed LC-PUFA supplemented formulas compared to the control group at 6-months-corrected-term age.

In summary, these trials support the efficacy of dietary docosahexaenoic acid in supporting the early development of the visual system in LBWI that is not achieved by providing α-linolenic acid as the source of n-3 fatty acids in formula. In a meta-analysis of the published results, SanGiovanni and coworkers concluded that the inclusion of docosahexaenoic acid in formula results in significant differences in visual resolution acuity, with combined estimates of behaviorally based visual resolution acuity of 0.47 ± 0.14 octaves and 0.28 ± 0.08 octaves at 2 and 4 months, respectively.[190] Similarly, a Cochrane review published in 2000 concluded there is evidence that docosahexaenoic acid supplementation of formula increases the early rate of visual maturation in preterm infants.[175]

LC-PUFA and Other Indices of Neural and Cognitive Development

A number of animal studies have shown that depletion of n-3 PUFA is associated with impaired learning ability, as well as other complex cognitive functions.[182] In infant rhesus monkeys, n-3 fatty acid deficiency resulted in a longer look duration in a test of visual attention, which could indicate a slower speed of information processing in the central nervous system.[183]

Bougle et al studied 40 preterm infants (<34 weeks postmenstrual age) fed for 30 days either with human milk or randomized to a control formula or a formula with 0.6% (of fatty acids) docosahexaenoic acid and 0.1% arachidonic acid.[191] Electrophysiological studies found no differences in auditory or visual evoked potentials during the 30 days of the study. However, the motor nerve conduction velocity recorded from the flexor hallucis brevis muscle increased significantly during the 30-day study in infants fed human milk or control formula, but was slower in infants fed the formula supplemented with docosaehexaenoic acid.[191]

Some studies have tested developmental outcomes in populations of breast and formula fed infants that differ in intakes of LC-PUFA as well as a large number of other factors. Anderson et al[169] performed a meta-analysis of 20 studies reporting on standard measures of developmental outcomes in more than 40,000 breast and formula fed infants. Overall, breast-feeding was associated with a 3.2 percentage point advantage of later cognitive development scores. There was a positive association between duration of breast feeding and extent of developmental advantage, and the benefit was greater in LBWI (5.2%) than in groups of infants with normal or mixed birth weight (2.7%). These observations are consistent with the hypothesis of beneficial effects of some critical substrates supplied with breast milk. In preterm infants with a birth weight <1850 g, Lucas and coworkers reported that the (mostly gavage) feeding of banked breast milk, when compared with preterm and term formula, provided a significant advantage in the Bayley Mental Developmental Index at the age of 18 months, which offset any deleterious effects of the low energy and protein content of the banked breast milk.[170] However, these observations do not provide any conclusive evidence on causal effects, since obviously breast feeding cannot be randomized and hence the possible effects of confounding factors cannot be fully excluded. Nonetheless, data such as these are consistent with a hypothesis that LC-PUFA in human milk might be beneficial in supporting cognitive development. However, many nutrient and non-nutrient components in human milk that are absent from formula, as well as unrecognized soci-demographic factors could be explain the findings of differences in outcome between groups of infants fed human milk and those fed formula. Randomized studies in term infants fed formulas with and without the addition of LC-PUFA have found either no developmental benefit[192-194] or have benefits on early mental development,[195] complex problem solving ability at the age of 10 months[196] and global development at the age of 18 months.[197]

Only very few data are available from randomized studies on LC-PUFA and cognitive development in LBWI. Carlson and coworkers[187] reported shorter look duration in the Fagan Test of Infant Intelligence in preterm infants fed a fish oil supplemented formula. The authors suggested this may indicate an advantage in the speed of processing of neural signals. Similar differences in looking behavior, with longer looking times were found in rhesus monkeys following prolonged dietary deficiency of n-3 fatty acids.[183] In a subsequent clinical study, Carlson and coworkers confirmed the shorter look duration during the Fagan Test in infants fed with a DHA containing formula.[198] Higher scores on the Bayley Scales of Infant Development were found among LBWI without bronchopulmonary dysplasia fed formula supplemented with fish oil low in eicosapentaenoic acid and high in docosahexaenoic acid, with no arachidonic acid.[188] More recently, a multi-center trial with LBWI fed formula with 0.25% docosahexaenoic acid and 0.4% arachidonic acid in hospital and 0.15% docosaehxaenoic acid and 0.4% arachidonic acid following hospital discharge from egg and fungal triglycerides found higher novelty preference at 6-months-corrected age than in infants fed unsupplemented formula.[173] Post hoc analysis also found that infants less than 1250 g birthweight who received formula supplemented with LC-PUFA from a combination of fish and fungal triglycerides had higher PDI scores on the Bayley Scales of Infant Development at 12-months-corrected age.

Effects of PUFA on the Immune System

There is accumulating evidence that lipids, and in particular the balance between n-6 and n-3 fatty acids, can influence immune function through mechanisms that involve changes in the balance of n-6 and n-3 fatty acid derived eicosanoids. For example, 5-lipoxygenase products derived from arachidonic acid act as proinflammatory mediators, whereas 5-lipoxygenase products synthesized from the n-3 fatty acid eicosapentaenoic acid are very inactive (Figure 7). Dietary supplementation with fish oils high in eicosapentaenoic acid can, therefore, exert antiinflammatory effects.[176,199,200] n-3 LC-PUFA also influence the production of NO and of cytokines, such as interleukin 1α and β, interleukin 2 and tumor necrosis factor.[201] The effects of n-3 fatty acids on immune function involve not only eicosanoid mediated pathways, but also effects on signal transduction and direct modulation of gene expression by regulating several transcription factors, including the nuclear factor κB and the peroxisome proliferator activated receptor.[202] Studies in premature infants have found that a dietary supply of arachidonic acid and docosahexaenoic acid either from human milk or supplemented formula resulted in an increased

	Preterm formula without LC-PUFA	Preterm formula with LC-PUFA	Human milk (with LC-PUFA)
CD4/CD8 ratio	4.1 ± 0.5[a]	2.9 ± 0.2[b]	2.9 ± 0.2[b]
CD4 + CD45RO⁺ (% total)	5.6 ± 0.4[a]	7.1 ± 1.0[b]	7.0 ± 0.7[b]
CD4 + CD45RA⁺ (% total)	85 ± 2[a]	77 ± 4[b]	72 ± 3[b]
IL10 (pg/ml)	11 ± 32[a]	167 ± 38[b]	296 ± 44[b]

Table 6: Immune phenotypes of infants fed formula without LC-PUFA differ significantly from those of infants receiving LC-PUFA from formula or from human milk. Peripheral blood cells were identified by monoclonal antibodies and IL-10 production following mitogen stimulation of peripheral lymphocytes measured by ELISA. Immune phenotypes at age 42 days were significantly different in infants fed formula without LC-PUFA than in infants who received preformed AA and DHA from either formula or human milk, with an increased proportion of mature (CD45RO+) CD4⁺ cells, enhanced IL-10 production and reduced IL-2 production. Modified from 203

proportion of mature (CD45RO+) CD4⁺cells, enhanced IL-10 production and reduced IL-2 production following ex vivo mitogen stimulation of peripheral blood lymphocytes, compared to infants fed formula without these LC-PUFA (Table 6).[203] The n-6 polyunsaturated fatty acid supply and the balance between n-6 and n-3 fatty acids, may also be linked to the risk of manifestation of atopic disease in term infants.[204] Specific intervention trials to address this, however, are not available. In view of the potential modulation of immune functions by LC-PUFA, further characterisation of clinically relevant effects in LBWI is desirable.

Recommendations on the Essential Fatty Acid and LC-PUFA Supply to Enterally Fed LBW Infants

Linoleic acid

Linoleic acid is an essential fatty acid that must be supplied with the diet. Expert groups have recommended intakes in the range of 500 - 1200 mg/100 kcal (4.5-10.8% of energy; E%)[19] and of 352-1425 mg/ 100 kcal (3.2-12.8 E%), which is equivalent to about 8-25% of the fatty acids in a preterm formula.[20] There is no evidence of linoleic acid deficiency or of adverse effects due to high intakes in infants

fed current preterm formulas. A range of intake of 352-1200mg/100 kcal is, therefore, considered reasonable.

Linoleic acid: 352-1425 mg/100 kcal (3.2-12.8 E%)

α-Linolenic acid

Current understanding suggests that the essential role of α-linolenic acid is due to its role as a precursor for synthesis of eicosapentaenoic acid and docosahexaenoic acid. Studies on the role of n-3 fatty acids in developing animals have compared animals fed diets with differing levels of α-linolenic acid and clearly shown that an α-linolenic acid deficient diet results in reduced retinal and visual function and altered behavior. Clinical trials in infants on the importance of a dietary supply of docosahexaenoic acid have involved supplementation of infant formulas containing α-linolenic acid. Definitive requirements for α-linolenic acid of preterm or term infants have not been established and may differ depending on the amount of docosahexaenoic acid in the milk or formula diet. In the absence of more information, a reasonable range for preterm infant formulas that do not supply preformed docosahexaenoic acid is regarded as 77-228 mg/ 100 kcal, or 0.7-2.1% of total energy, which is

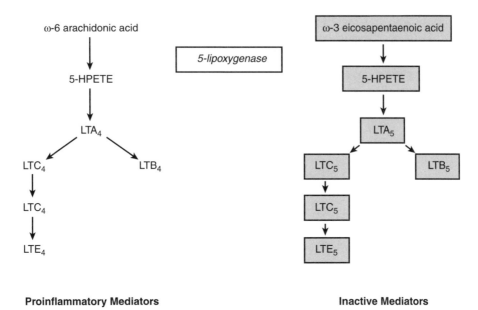

Proinflammatory Mediators   **Inactive Mediators**

Figure 7: N-6 and n-3 fatty acids are precurors of eicosanoids with different biological functions. Both arachidonic acid and eicosapentaenoic acid are substrates for 5-lipoxygenase. 5- lipoxygenase products of arachidonic acid, such as leukotriene B4, are potent proinflammatory mediators, wheres 5-lipoxygenase products of eicosapentaenoic acid are inactive. N-3-derived eicosanoids are also less potent in stimulating platelet aggregation and vessel wall constriction than n-6 derived eicosanoids. Supplementation with n-3 fatty acids, resulting in an increase of the n-6/n-3 balance, may thus suppress inflammatory processes, increase bleeding time and decrease blood pressure.

equivalent to about 1.75 to 4% of total fatty acids.[20] Lower ranges of intakes might also be adequate for formulas that provide preformed docosahexaenoic acid, but evidence to support this recommendation is missing.

α-Linolenic acid: 77-228 mg/100 kcal (0.7-2.1 E%)

Linoleic acid to α-Linolenic acid ratio
The ratio between linoleic and α-linolenic acids is important because these two fatty acids compete for the same desaturase enzymes. Because of this, high intakes of α-linolenic acid may suppress synthesis of arachidonic acid from linoleic acid, and conversely high intakes of linoleic acid could limit the synthesis of docosahexaenoic acid. The linoleic to α-linolenic acid ratio may be of greater importance for parenteral and enteral formulas that contain linoleic and α-linolenic

acid and provide no or very little LC-PUFA than for formulas supplemented with arachidonic acid and docosahexaenoic acid. Little clinical data is available for LBWI infants fed different ratios of linoleic and α-linolenic acid, although one study found lower growth among term and preterm infants fed formula with a ratio of of 4.8:1 when compared to a ratio of 16:1.[155] Based on these studies it seems reasonable to recommend that the linoleic acid to α-linolenic acid ratio should be in the range of 6-16[20] if no preformed arachidonic acid and docosahexaenoic acid are provided.

Linoleic acid/α-linolenic acid ratio: 6-16 (wt/wt)

Arachidonic Acid, Docosahexaenoic Acid, and Other Long Chain Polyunsaturated Fatty Acids
Recent clinical studies with LBWI fed formulas containing both arachidonic acid and docosahexaenoic

acid have shown beneficial effects on both the developing visual system and measures of cognitive development during the first year of life. These studies also found no evidence of adverse effects on growth or other problems among infants fed formulas containing docosahexaenoic acid at up to 0.35% and arachidonic acid at up to 0.7% of total formula fatty acids. Although the long-term implications of the early benefits on visual and neural development are not known, it is prudent to provide LBWI with a dietary source of these fatty acids. Lower growth has been observed in LBWI fed formulas supplemented with docosahexaaenoic acid and not archidonic acid. However, lower growth has not been found in subsequent clinical trials with LBW or term infants fed formulas with both docosahexaenoic acid and arachidonic acid, and even improved growth has been reported in LBWI fed formulas with AA. It is well-known that eicosapentaenoic acid antagonizes arachidonic acid, and that eicosapentaenoic acid levels are very low in human milk. These considerations allow a conclusion that both archidonic acid and docosahexaenoic acid should be included in preterm formulas, and that oils containing significant amounts of eicosapentaenoic acid should be avoided. Supplementation of infant formulas with arachidonic and docosahexaenoic acid requires the addition of oils, such as single cell oils, fish oils, or egg lipids containing these fatty acids. The upper range for arachidonic acid and docosahexaenoic acid, therefore, must be set consistent with the available data to establish safety of these oils, including all their constituents, when added to infant formulas. We choose to recommend intakes not higher than 0.5% DHA and 0.7% AA for which some clinical evaluations are available. It is possible that higher amounts of archidonic acid and docosahexaenoic acid might confer greater advantage for the growth and development of VLBWI. Clinical trials, to address this and to demonstrate safety of the oils used to provide these fatty acids at the higher amounts needed, are important. High levels of either arachidonic acid or docosahexaenoic acid might have adverse effects on the metabolism of the opposing series of polyunsaturated fatty acids, for example in

Outcome	Lipids <5 days	Lipids >5 days	RR (95% CI)
Death	53/265	50/257	1.01 (0.7-1.4)
CLD 28 d	104/265	99/257	1.03 (0.8-1.3)
CLD 36 wks	23/96	22/93	1.02 (0.6-1.7)

Table 7: Meta-analysis of 5 prospective, controlled clinical trials on the effects of early and later initiation of lipid infusion in LBWI on the risk of death and of chronic lung disease (CLD) at 28 days and at 36 weeks. Early lipid infusion is not associated with adverse outcomes. [Modified from 207]

eicosanoid-mediated pathways. To avoid this potential, a reasonable range for the balance between arachidonic acid and docosahexaenoic acid appears to be 1.2 to 2:1, which is similar to the ratio found in many studies on the fatty acid composition of human milk, and to limit the amount of eicosapentaenoic acid to no more than 30% of the amount of docosahexaenoic acid.[20]

Docosahexaenoic acid (22:6n-3):
0.2-0.5% of fatty acids
Arachidonic acid (20:4n-6):0.3-0.7%
of fatty acids AA/DHA-Ratio 1.2-2:1

Parenteral Nutrition with Intravenous Lipids
Metabolism of Intravenous Lipids
Lipid emulsions are indispensible for parenteral feeding of LBWI to meet their high energy needs for maintanance and growth. Moreover, lipid emulsions supply essential fatty acids and can carry lipid soluble vitamins. Concern over adverse effects, however, such as increased rates of chronic lung disease and mortality in LBWI has been raised.[205,206] Meta-analysis of the 5 prospective controlled trials in LBWI on this question has shown that lipid infusion within the first 5 days after birth is not associated with an increased risk of adverse outcomes (Table 7).[207]

Lipid emulsions consist of vegetable oil triglycerides

emulsified with egg yolk phospholipid, with glycerol to achieve isotonicity. The emulsion particles resemble endogenously produced chylomicrons in size, physico-chemical properties and metabolism. Triglycerides provided with the infused emulsion are hydrolyzed by lipoprotein lipase. Thus, the rate of clearance is determined by the available lipase activity, with the uptake of unesterified fatty acid products related to the adipose tissue mass and/or fatty acid oxidation in muscle. Heparin releases hepatic lipase and lipoprotein lipase from the capillary endothelium into the circulation and can lower circulating triglyceride concentrations. However, it also induces an increase in serum free fatty acids There is no evidence for an increase of lipid utilization or other clinical benefit of routine administration of heparin. No benefit of releasing fatty acids at rates in excess of the ability for adipose tissue or muscle uptake is apparent. In infants who simultaneously receive heparin together with a lipid emulsion and high calcium concentrations in the infusate, creaming of the lipid emulsion may occur.[208] Thus, the routine addition of heparin to lipid infusions is not recommended.

Adequate clearance of up to 2 g lipid/kg/day is found in most infants >28 weeks gestation and of up to 3 g lipid/kg/day in most infants >32 weeks gestation. However, very-low-birth-weight infants and small-for-gestational-age infants, as well as infants suffering from systemic infection, have lower lipoprotein lipase activity and are prone to develop plasma triglyceride levels greater than 100 mg/dL with lipid infusions between 2 and 3 g/kg/day.[209,210] Limited adipose tissue or muscle mass in infants <1000 g could also limit free fatty acid clearance leading to uptake by the liver resulting in secretion as VLDL triglyceride, thus contributing to the hypertriglyceridemia. Triglyceride concentrations >100 mg/dL are found regularly in enterally fed infants, and there is no evidence for adverse effects. However, it appears prudent to measure serum triglyceride concentrations in infants <1000 g or 28-weeks gestation that show signs of infection or other distress and adjust the lipid infusion to maintain serum triglyceride concentrations below 200 mg/dL.

Lipolysis of the emulsion triglyceride, without uptake of free fatty acids by adipose tissue or muscle, was once considered of concern because of possible displacement of bilirubin from albumin. Displacement depends on the relative concentrations of albumin, bilirubin, and unesterified fatty acids. It is now known that accumulation of free fatty acid sufficient to result in clinical problems is unlikely, because generation of free bilirubin does not occur until the molar ratio of free fatty acid to albumin exceeds 6. Infusion of 1 g IV lipid/kg per day to infants with a mean birthweight of 1.35 kg from the first morning after the infants were 24 hours old did result in a significant rise in free bilirubin in association with increased free fatty acids.[153] However, at no time and for no infant did the free fatty acid:albumin ratio remotely approach the range at which there may be some measurable risk of bilirubin encephalopathy. No reports of an increased incidence of kernicterus due to IV fat infusion in preterm infants have been published.

Dyslipoproteinemia, usually with hypercholesterolemia and hyperphospholipidemia, caused by infusion of 10% lipid emulsions is well known.[145] This occurs even in the absence of elevated triglycerides and is largely the result of accumulation of abnormal particles of free cholesterol and phospholipid, generally known as Lp X. Clearance probably involves the usual lipoprotein receptors, as well as the reticular endothelial system. The accumulation of cholesterol in the vascular compartment appears to be explained by the excess phospholipid emulsifier (mesophase phospholipid) in IV lipid emulsion products. When infused, this mesophase phospholipid causes efflux of unesterifed cholesterol from cell membranes, explained by movement of cholesterol down a concentration gradient to the cholesterol-free mesophase phospholipid particles. This in turn leads to increased intracellular cholesterol synthesis to replace cholesterol leached from the cell membrane. The amount of phospholipid present is constant in 10%, 20% and 30% intravenous lipid emulsions, thus the amount of phospholipid in mesophase, and not present in the triglyceride emulsion matrix, decreases with increasing triglyceride concentration.[145] Clinical studies have

Oils used	Soybean	Soybean/MCT	Olive/Soybean	Soybean/Fish
Product names	Intralipid, Ivelip, Lipofundin, Liposyn III Lipovenous	Lipofundin MCT	ClinOleic	Lipovenous + Omegavenous, 9 + 1 parts mix
Triglycerides (g/dL)	10 , 20 & 30%	20%	20%	10%
Ratio phospholipids/ triglycerides (mg/g)	120, 60 & 40	60	60	120
Glycerol (g/dL)	2.5	2.5	2.25	2.5
Energy (kcal/ml)	1.1-2.0	1.9	2.0	1.12
Fatty acid composition (% wt/wt)				
Medium chain (8:0+10:0)	n.d.	50	n.d.	n.d.
Palmitic (16:0)	9-11.2	5	13.5	10.8
Stearic (18:0)	4-4.2	2	2.9	3.7
Oleic (18:1n-9)	20.4-26	12	59.5	19.9
Linoleic (18:2n-6)	52.4-54.5	27	18.5	49.7
α-linolenic (18:3n-3)	8-8.5	4	2	6.5
γ-linolenic (18:3n-6)	-	-	-	-
Arachidonic (20:4n-6)	n.d.-0.2	n.d.	0.2	0.2
Eicosapentaenoic (20:5n-3)	n.d.	n.d.	n.d.	2.4
Docosahexaenoic (22:6n-3)	n.d.-0.1	n.d.	0.1	2.3

Table 8: Commercial intravenous lipid emulsions currently used in preterm infants. [Modified from 145]

confirmed that problems of hypercholesterolemia and hyperphospholipidemia are substantially lower when lipid emulsions with a low PL/TG ratio (standard 20% emulsions or some 10% emulsions) are infused rather than triglyceride emulsions with a high PL/TG ratio (conventional 10% emulsions).[211] The use of 30% emulsions would offer further advantages, but the small amounts required by some very small VLBWI may be problematic for infusions given over 24 hours.

Intravenous (IV) lipid emulsions provide high calorie, isotonic solutions of linoleic acid (18:2n-6) and α-linolenic acid (18:3n-3), as well as other fatty acids, which can be given through peripheral lines. The lipid infusions most commonly used previously in Europe, and still today in North America, are prepared from soybean oil triglycerides emulsified with egg yolk phospholipids. Soybean oil contains 45% to 55% linoleic acid (18:2n-6) and 6% to 9% α-linolenic acid (18:3n-3), but very little saturated or monounsaturated fat (Table 8). There are considerable concerns over the effect of this unphysiological, highly polyunsaturated fatty acid supply, which differs markedly from the relative fatty acid composition of human milk or most enteral diets, on the composition of fatty acids deposited in the developing tissues of LBWI. More recently, alternative and less highly unsaturated fat blends have become available (Table 8), and these deserve careful evaluation.

Emulsions containing mixtures of MCT with soy or other vegetable oils (Table 8) offer potential advantages due to more rapid rates of clearance of MCT, which could be of benefit for infants with low lipase activity.[153] Dyslipoproteinemia with lipid accumulation in the LDL region of plasma is not improved. Studies of parenterally fed septic rats have not confirmed a benefit of mixed MCT-long-chain fatty acid emulsions. Further, the margin between safety and toxicity was narrow leading to greater mortality in previously starved animals infused with MCT-long-chain fatty acid emulsions compared with 100% long-chain fatty acid emulsions. Intravenous lipid emulsions containing eicosapentaenoic acid and docosahexaenoic acid from fish oil have also been developed (Table 8). The amount of arachidonic acid present is an order of magnitude lower than the amount of either eicosapentaenoic acid or docosahexaenoic acid, which raises concern with respect to growth and support of normal developmental and physiological functions related to arachidonic acid and its eicosanoid products.

Emulsions containing a mixture of soybean oil and olive oil offer potential advantages due to lower amounts of polyunsaturated fatty acids and higher monounsaturated fatty acids, which were shown to reduce oxidative stress and may improve docosahexaenoic status.[145] A recent study evaluated a new parenteral lipid emulsion based on olive and soybean oils (ratio 4:1) with less polyunsaturated fatty acids (PUFA) and more α-tocopherol, relative to a standard soybean oil emulsion, in premature infants. Infants with a mean gestational age of about 220 days and a mean birth weight of about 1.6 kg were randomized to receive either the olive/soybean oil emulsion or a standard soybean oil emulsion for 7 days. At study end, the olive oil group showed higher values of the PUFA intermediates C18:3n-6 (0.19 ± 0.01 vs 0.13 ± 0.02%, p<0.05) and C20:3n-6 (2.92 ± 0.12 vs 2.21 ± 0.17%, p=0.005). Moreover, the plasma α-tocopherol/total lipid ratio was higher in the olive oil group (2.45 ± 0.27 vs 1.90 ± 0.08 mmol/mmol, p=0.001), whereas urinary MDA excretion did not differ.[212] Thus, the lower PUFA supply with the olive/soybean oil emulsion appears to enhance linoleic acid conversion. The reduced PUFA content, combined with a higher antioxidant intake in the olive oil group results in an improved Vitamin E status. The olive oil based emulsion appears as a valuable alternative for parenteral feeding of preterm infants who are often exposed to oxidative stress, while their antioxidative defense is weak. Other new emulsions are also considered for use in parenteral feeding of premature infants. However, detailed characterization of any new emulsions in well-controlled trials to document their suitability and safety is required before endorsing routine administration to VLBWI.

Fat Administration and Requirements

Even short delays in addition of fat to the intravenous diet of preterm infants leads to biochemical essential fatty acid deficiency, evident as a rise in the plasma triene:tetraene ratio within 72 hours after birth.[108,213] These changes extend to the lung and most likely to other organs as well.[214] The clinical implications of short-term essential fatty acid deficiency are not well understood. Abnormalities in platelet function, which could have implications for clinical bleeding, have been described.[213] Essential fatty acid deficiency is avoided by infusions of 0.5 to 1.0 g lipid per kg per day.

The absence of an elevated triene:tetraene ratio does not provide assurance of adequate formation of arachidonic acid (20:4n-6) and/or docosahexaenoic acid (22:6n-3) in very small infants. If the total kcal supply is less than approximately 80 kcal/kg/day, it is likely that linoleic acid (18:2n-6) and linolenic acid (18:3n-3) will be oxidized to provide energy for essential metabolic and physiological functions, rather than being desaturated.[215] Negative energy balance is also accompanied by mobilization of limited tissue n-6 and n-3 fatty acids, further compromising tissue status. The duration of parenteral nutrition with inadequate energy for anabolic metabolism is an important criterion in determining the extent of arachidonic acid (20:4n-6) and docosahexaenoic acid (22:6n-3) depletion. Since it is important to preserve functional and anatomical development of the CNS, parenteral lipid must be fed with sufficient energy intake to allow prompt postnatal resumption of growth and utilization of fatty acids for essential functions, rather than energy. In order to facilitate this, lipid infusion from a 20% emulsion should preferably proceed from the first 1 to 2 days after birth, increasing as tolerated in increments of 0.5 g/day to 3.0 g/day unless contraindicated.

Infusion of IV lipid, using a 20% long-chain fatty acid emulsion, should commence within 24 hours of birth for infants >28-weeks gestation and >1000 g. The dose should be increased, as tolerated, in increments of 0.5 g every 2 to 3 days to a maximum of 3 g/kg/day. In all cases, the triglyceride infusion dose should be adjusted to maintain a serum lipid not above 200 mg/dL. Infants <28-weeks gestation or <1000 g may have low lipase activity or limited adipose mass for clearance of free fatty acids. A more cautious approach should be taken with assessment of serum lipid clearance in these infants throughout the infusion period. Lipid clearance should also be monitored in all infants as the infusion approaches and exceeds 3 g/kg/day. Infants with sepsis, or in whom there is a severe compromise in oxygenation, should be carefully monitored and the lipid infusion restricted to 0.5 to 1.0 g/kg/day, sufficient to prevent essential fatty acid deficiency if acceptable triglyceride concentrations are exceeded.

Carnitine

The need to provide a source of carnitine for parenterally fed infants is not yet clear. Arguments for this are based on information that led to inclusion of carnitine in soy protein and semi-elemental formulas, as well as a few published studies on carnitine supplementation during parenteral nutrition of preterm infants.[216]

The best known function of carnitine is to facilitate the transport of long-chain fatty acids across the mitochondrial membrane, which would otherwise be impermeable to them.[216] This function gives carnitine an essential role in oxidation of fatty acids for energy, particularly in heart and skeletal muscle, and in ketogenesis in the liver. The precursor of carnitine, γ-butyrobetaine, is synthesized in the kidney from the essential amino acids lysine and methionine, and then hydroxylated to form carnitine in the liver. The activity of γ-butyrobetaine hydroxylase is much lower in infant than adult liver, increasing from about 12% of usual adult values during the first months of life to 100% of adult activity by 15 years of age.[216] Studies conducted prior to routine addition of carnitine to soy-protein or protein hydrolysate formulas found that plasma carnitine concentrations decreased over prolonged feeding, whereas blood carnitine levels were maintained and urinary carnitine increased with age in small preterm infants fed their mother's milk. This, together with the very low tissue carnitine contents and limited ability of preterm and term infants to produce ketone bodies even in the presence of hypoglycemia,[217] suggests a need for dietary carnitine. Despite these considerations, there does not seem to be any definitive evidence of metabolic or physiologic benefit following carnitine supplementation in infants.[218,219]

Several studies have shown that plasma and tissue carnitine and ketone body concentrations are low in preterm infants receiving parenteral lipid without carnitine. Supplementation with approximately 10 mg L-carnitine/kg per day may increase fat oxidation, as indicated by decreased serum-plasma free fatty acid concentrations and increased ketones,[220] while higher doses result in increased protein and fat oxidation with loss of potential metabolic energy. For example, supplementation with 48 mg L-carnitine/kg per day (about 300μmol/kg/day) increased the metabolic rate, decreased fat and protein accretion, and prolonged the time to regain birth weight in preterm infants receiving parenteral nutrition with lipid.[219]

The carnitine content of human milk is approximately 9 to 10 μmol/dL in the first 2 weeks postpartum, decreasing to approximately 6 μmol/dL in mature milk and is not different in milk from women delivering prematurely. Similar amounts are now provided by all formulas, either as a component of the bovine milk protein, or by supplementation of soy protein or semi-elemental products prepared from hydrolysates of bovine milk protein.[221] The Committee on Nutrition of the European Society of Paediatric Gastroenterology and Nutrition recommended that infant formulas contain at least 7.5 μmol/100 kcal.[19] Calculations based on intrauterine carnitine accretion have predicted tissue accretion of carnitine equivalent to approximately 13 μmol/day.

In summary, it is recognized that carnitine plays an essential role in metabolism and is provided in human milk in amounts that should cover the needs of the growing, fully enterally fed LBWI for in utero rates of tissue accretion, but may have undesirable effects if given in high doses. There seems to be no convincing evidence of metabolic or physiologic benefit in preterm infants following addition of carnitine to parenteral lipid infusions. However, if parenterally nourished infants are supplemented with carnitine (approximately 15 μmol/100 kcal), which is similar to the amount provided by 200 mL/day human milk and enough to support in utero rates of tissue accretion, would seem appropriate.

References

1. Ziegler EE, O'Donnell AM, Nelson SE, Fomon SJ. Body composition of the reference fetus. *Growth* 1976; 40(4):329-341.

2. Usher R, MacLean F. Intrauterine growth of life-born Caucasian infants at sea level: standards obtained from measurments in 7 dimensions of infants born between 25 and 44 weeks of gestation. *J Pediatr* 1969; 74:901.

3. Shaw JCL. Parenteral nutrition in the management of sick low birthweight infants. *Ped Clin North Am* 1973; 20:333.

4. Reichman B, Chessex P, Putet G, Verellen G, Smith JM, Heim T, et al. Diet, fat accretion, and growth in premature infants. *N Engl J Med* 1981; 305(25):1495-1500.

5. Pieltain C, De Curtis M, Gerard P, Rigo J. Weight gain composition in preterm infants with dual energy X-ray absorptiometry. *Pediatr Res* 20; 49(1):120-124.

6. Fomon SJ, Haschke F, Ziegler E, Nelson SE. Body composition of reference children from birth to age 10 years. *Am J Clin Nutr* 1982;1169-1175.

7. Michaelsen KF, Skafte L, Badsberg JH, Jorgensen M. Variation in macronutrients in human bank milk: influencing factors and implications for human milk banking. *J Pediatr Gastroenterol Nutr* 1990; 11(2): 229-239.

8. Jensen RG. *Handbook of Milk Composition.* San Diego: Academic Press; 1995.

9. Rodriguez PM, Koletzko B, Kunz C, Jensen R. Nutritional and biochemical properties of human milk: II. Lipids, micronutrients, and bioactive factors. *Clin Perinatol* 1999; 26(2):335-359.

10. Hellerstein MK, Christiansen M, Kaempfer S, Kletke C, Wu K, Reid JS, et al. Measurement of *de novo* hepatic lipogenesis in humans using stable isotopes. *J Clin Invest* 1991; 87(5):1841-1852.

11. Flatt JP, Ravussin E, Acheson KJ, Jéquier E. Effects of dietary fat on postprandial substrate oxidation and on carbohydrate and fat balance. *J Clin Invest* 1985; 76(1019):1024.

12. Dauncey MJ, Bingham SA. Dependence of 24 hour energy expenditure in man on the composition of nutrient intake. *Br J Nutr* 1983; 50:1-13.

13. Lean MEJ, James PT. Metabolic effects of isoenergetic nutrient exchange over 24 hours in relation to obesity in women. *Int J Obes* 1988; 12:15-27.

14. Van-Aerde JE, Sauer PJ, Pencharz PB, Smith JM, Heim T, Swyer PR. Metabolic consequences of increasing energy intake by adding lipid to parenteral nutrition in full-term infants. *Am J Clin Nutr* 1994; 59(3):659-662.

15. Koletzko B. Lipid supply and metabolism in infancy. *Current Opinion in Clinical Nutrition and Metabolic Care.* 1998;1:171-177.

16. Valentine CJ, Hurst NM, Schanler RJ. Hindmilk improves weight gain in low-birthweight infants fed human milk. *J Pediatr Gastroenterol Nutr* 1994;18: 474-477.

17. Boehm G, Muller DM, Senger H, Borte M, Moro G. Nitrogen and fat balances in very low birth weight infants fed human milk fortified with human milk or bovine milk protein. *Eur J Pediatr* 1993; 152(3): 236-239.

18. Flatt JP. Use and storage of carbohydrate and fat.

Am J Clin Nutr 1995; 61(4 Suppl):952S-959S.

19. ESPGAN Committee on Nutrition, Aggett PJ, Haschke F, Heine W, Hernell O, Koletzko B, et al. Committee report. Comment on the content and composition of lipids in infant formulas. *Acta Paediatr Scand* 1991; 80:887-896.

20. Klein CJ. Nutrient requirements for preterm infant formulas. *J Nutr* 2002; 132:1395S-1577S.

21. Russell DW. Cholesterol biosynthesis and metabolism. *Cardiovasc Drugs Ther* 1992; 6:103-110.

22. Rudney H, Panini SR. Cholesterol biosynthesis. *Curr Opinion Lipidol* 1993; 4:230-237.

23. Wong WW, Hachey DL, Insull W, Opekun AR, Klein PD. Effect of dietary cholesterol on cholesterol synthesis in breast-fed and formula-fed infants. *J Lipid Res* 1993; 34:1403-1411.

24. Wong WW, Hachey DL, Clarke LL, Zhang S. Cholesterol synthesis and absorption by ^2H_2O and ^{18}O-cholesterol and hypocholesterolemic effect of soy protein. *J Nutr* 1995; 125:612S-618S.

25. Tint GS, Salen G, Batta AK, Shefer S, Irons M, Elias ER, et al. Correlation of severity and outcome with plasma sterol levels in variants of the Smith-Lemli-Opitz syndrome. *J Pediatr* 1995; 127:82-87.

26. Abuelo DN, Tint GS, Kelley R, Batta AK, Shefer S, Salen G. Prenatal detection of the cholesterol biosynthetic defect in the Smith-Lemli-Opitz syndrome by the analysis of amniotic fluid sterols. *Am J Med Genet* 1995; 56:281-285.

27. Edmond J, Higa TA, Korsak RA, Bergner EA, Lee WN. Fatty acid transport and utilization for the developing brain. *J Neurochem* 1998; 70:1227-12234.

28. Carlson SE, Montalto MB, Ponder DL, Werkman SH, Korones SB. Lower incidence of necrotizing enterocolitis in infants fed a preterm formula with egg phospholipids. *Pediatr Res* 1998; 44(4):491-498.

29. Caplan MS, Russell T, Xiao Y, Amer M, Kaup S, Jilling T. Effect of polyunsaturated fatty acid (PUFA) supplementation on intestinal inflammation and necrotizing enterocolitis (NEC) in a neonatal rat model. *Pediatr Res* 2001; 49(5):647-652.

30. Hernell O, Bläckberg L, Chen Q, Sternby B, Nilsson A. Does the bile salt-stimulated lipase of human milk have a role in the use of the milk long-chain polyunsaturated

fatty acids? *J Pediatr Gastroenterol Nutr* 1993;16: 426-431.

31. Chen Q, Blackberg L, Nilsson A, Sternby B, Hernell O. Digestion of triacylglycerols containing long-chain polyenoic fatty acids in vitro by colipase-dependent pancreatic lipase and human milk bile salt-stimulated lipase. *Biochim Biophys Acta* 1994 Jan 3; 1210:2-43.

32. Hamosh M. Lingual and Gastric Lipases: Their Role in Fat Digestion. Boca Raton, FL: CRC Press; 1990.

33. Hernell O, Bläckberg L, Bernbäck S. Digestion of human milk fat in early human infancy. *Acta Paediatr Scand* 1989; 351 (Suppl):57-62.

34. Shiau YF. Lipid digestion and absorption. In: Johnson LR, editor. *Physiology of the Gastrointestinal Tract*. New York: 1987: 1527-1556.

35. Tso P. General aspects of intestinal lipid digestion and absorption. *Adv Lipid Res* 1985; 21:144-186.

36. Menard D, Monfils S, Tremblay E. Ontogenity of human gastric lipase and pepsin activities. *Gastroenterology* 1995; 108:1650-1656.

37. Hamosh M. Digestion in the premature infant: the effects of human milk. *Semin Perinatol* 1994; 18(6):485-494.

38. Armand M, Hamosh M, Mehta NR, Angelus PA, Philpott JR, Henderson TR et al. Effect of human milk or formula on gastric function and fat digestion in the premature infant. *Pediar Res* 1996; 40:429-437.

39. Bernback S, Blackberg L, Hernell O. The complete digestion of human milk triacylglycerol in vitro requires gastric lipase, pancreatic co-lipase-dependent lipase, and bile salt stimulated lipase. *J Clin Invest* 1990; 85: 1221-1226.

40. Nilsson J, Blackberg L, Carlsson P, Enerback S, Hernell O, Bjursell G. cDNA cloning of human-milk bile-salt-stimulated lipase and evidence for its identity to pancreatic carboxylic ester hydrolase. *Eur J Biochem* 1990; 192(2):543-550.

41. Lowe ME. Properties and function of pancreatic lipase related protein 2. *Biochimie* 2000; 82:997-1004.

42. Boehm G, Muller MD, Senger H, Melichar V. Influence of postnatal age on nitrogen metabolism in very low birth weight infants appropriate for gestational age. *Acta Paediatr Hung* 1990; 30(3-4):423-433.

43. Chappell JE, Clandinin MT, Kearney-Volpe C,

Reichman B, Swyer PW. Fatty acid balance studies in premature infants fed human milk or formula: effect of calcium supplementation. *J Pediatr* 1986; 108(3): 439-447.

44. Ikeda I, Tomari Y, Sugano M, Watanabe S, Nagata J. Lymphatic absorption of structured glycerolipids containing medium-chain fatty acids and linoleic acid, and their effect on cholesterol absorption in rats. *Lipids* 1991; 26(5):369-373.

45. Mahan JT, Heda GT, Rao RH, Mansbach CM. The intestine expresses pancreatic triacylglycerol lipase: regulation by dietary lipid. *Am J Physiol Gastrointest Liver Physiol* 2001; 280:G1187-G1196.

46. Rao RH, Mansbach CM. Alkaline lipase in rat intestinal mucosa: physiological parameters. *Arch Biochem Biophys* 1993; 304:483-489.

47. McDonald GB, Weidman M. Partitioning of polar fatty acids into lymph and portal vein after intestinal absorption in the rat. *Q J Exp Physiol* 1987; 72(2): 153-159.

48. Swift LL, Hill JO, Peters JC, Greene HL. Medium-chain fatty acids: evidence for incorporation into chylomicron triglycerides in humans. *Am J Clin Nutr* 1990; 52(5):834-836.

49. Dhanireddy R, Hamosh M, Sivasubramanian KN, Chowdhry P, Scanlon JW, Hamosh P. Postheparin lipolytic activity and intralipid clearance in very low-birthweight infants. *J Pediatr* 1981; 98:617-622.

50. Berkow SE, Spear ML, Stahl GE, Gutman A, Polin RA, Pereira GR et al. total parenteral nutrition with intralipid in premature infants receiving TPN with heparin: effect on plasma lipolytic enzymes, lipids, and glucose. *J Pediatr Gastroenerol Nutr* 1987; 6:581-588.

51. Bach AC, Babayan V. Medium-chain triglycerides: an update. *Am J Clin Nutr* 1982; 36:950-962.

52. Sulkers EJ, von-Goudoever JB, Leunisse C, Wattimena JL, Sauer PJ. Comparison of two preterm formulas with or without addition of medium-chain triglycerides (MCTs). I: Effects on nitrogen and fat balance and body composition changes. *J Pediatr Gastroenterol Nutr* 1992; 15(1):34-41.

53. Hamosh M, Mehta NR, Fink CS, Coleman J, Hamosh P. Fat absorption in premature infants: medium-chain triglycerides and long-chain triglycerides

are absorbed from formula at similar rates. *J Pediatr Gastroenterol Nutr* 1991; 13(2):143-149.

54. Brooke OG. Energy balance and metabolic rate in preterm infants fed standard and high-energy formulas. *Br J Nutr* 1980; 44:13-23.

55. Huston RK, Reynolds JW, Jensen C, Buist NR. Nutrient and mineral retention and Vitamin D absorption in low-birth-weight infants: effect of medium-chain triglycerides. *Ped* 1983; 72(1):44-48.

56. Okamoto E, Muttart CR, Zucker CL, Heird WC. Use of medium-chain triglycerides in feeding the low-birthweight infant. *Am J Dis Child* 1982; 136(5): 428-431.

57. Tantibhedhyangkul P, Hashim SA. Clinical and physiologic aspects of medium-chain triglycerides: allviation of steatorrhea in premature infants. *Bull N Y Acad Med* 1971; 47(1):17-33.

58. Baba N, Bracco EF, Hashim SA. Enhanced thermogenesis and diminished deposition of fat in response to overfeeding with diet containing medium chain triglyceride. *Am J Clin Nutr* 1982; 35(4):678-682.

59. Seaton TB, Welle SL, Warenko MK, Campbell RG. Thermic effect of medium-chain and long-chain triglycerides in man. *Am J Clin Nutr* 1986; 44:630-634.

60. Borum PR. Medium-chain triglycerides in formula for preterm neonates: Implications for hepatic and extrahepatic metabolism. *J Ped* 1992; 120:S139-S145.

61. Rossle C, Carpentier YA, Richelle M, Dahlan W, D'Attellis NP, Furst P, et al. Medium-chain triglycerides induce alterations in carnitine metabolism. *Am J Physiol* 1990; 258(6 Pt 1):E944-E947.

62. Rebouche CJ, Panagides DD, Nelson SE. Role of carnitine in utilization of dietary medium-chain triglycerides by term infants. *Am J Clin Nutr* 1990; 52:820-824.

63. Whyte RK, Campbell D, Stanhope R, Bayley HS, Sinclair JC. Energy balance in low birth weight infants fed formula of high or low medium-chain triglyceride content. *J Pediatr* 1986; 108:964-971.

64. Henderson MJ, Dear PR. Dicarboxylic aciduria and medium chain triglyceride supplemented milk. *Arch Dis Child* 1986; 61(6):610-611.

65. Shigematsu Y, Momoi T, Sudo M, Suzuki Y. (omega-1)-Hydroxymonocarboxylic acids in urine of infants fed

medium-chain triglycerides. *Clin Chem* 1981; 27(10):1661-1664.

66. Sulkers EJ, Lafeber HN, Sauer PJ. Quantitation of oxidation of medium-chain triglycerides in preterm infants. *Pediatr Res* 1989; 26(4):294-297.

67. Whyte RK, Whelan D, Hill R, McClorry S. Excretion of dicarboxylic and omega-1 hydroxy fatty acids by low birth weight infants fed with medium-chain triglycerides. *Pediatr Res* 1986; 20(2):122-125.

68. Dupont C, Rocchiccioli F, Bougneres PF. Urinary excretion of dicarboxylic acids in term newborns fed with 5% medium-chain triglycerides-enriched formula. *J Pediatr Gastroenterol Nutr* 1987; 6(2):313-314.

69. Roe CR, Ding J. Mitochondrial fatty acid oxidation disorders. In: Scriver CR, Beaudet AL, Sly WS, Valle D, editors. *The Metabolic and Molecular Basis of Inherited Disease.* New York: Mac Graw Hill, 2001: 2297-2326.

70. Kraus H, Schlenker S, Schwedesky D. Developmental changes of cerebral ketone body utilization in human infants. *Hoppe Seylers Z Physiol Chem* 1974; 355(2): 164-170.

71. Bossi E, Kohler E, Herschkowitz N. Utilization of D-beta-hydroxybutyrate and oleate as alternate energy fuels in brain cell cultures of newborn mice after hypoxia at different glucose concentrations. *Pediatr Res* 1989; 26(5):478-481.

72. Sarda P, Lepage G, Roy CC, Chessex P. Storage of medium-chain triglycerides in adipose tissue of orally fed infants. *Am J Clin Nutr* 1987; 45:399-405.

73. Carnielli V, Sulkers EJ, Moretti C, Wattimena JL, van Goudoever JB, Degenhart HJ, et al. Conversion of octanoic acid into long-chain saturated fatty acids in premature infants fed a formula containing medium-chain triglycerides. *Metabolism* 1994; 43:1287-1292.

74. Lucas A, Quinlan P, Abrams S, Ryan S, Meah S, Lucas PJ. Randomised controlled trial of a synthetic triglyceride milk formula for preterm infants. *Arch Dis Child Fetal Neonatal Ed* 1997; 77(3):F178-F184.

75. Koletzko B, Tangermann R, von Kries R, Stannigel H, Willberg B, Radde I, et al. Intestinal milkbolus-obstruction in formula fed premature infants given high doses of calcium. *J Pediatr Gastro Nutr* 1988; 7:548-553.

76. Sulkers EJ, Lafeber HN, van-Goudoever JB,

Kalhan SC, Beaufrere B, Sauer PJ. Decreased glucose oxidation in preterm infants fed a formula containing medium-chain triglycerides. *Pediatr Res* 1993; 33(2):101-105.

77. Sann L, Mathieu M, Lasne Y, Ruitton A. Effect of oral administration of lipids with 67% medium chain triglycerides on glucose homeostasis in preterm neonates. *Metabolism* 1981; 30(7):712-716.

78. Rodriguez M, Funke S, Fink M, Demmelmair H, Turini M, Crozier G, et al. Plasma fatty acids and [^{13}C]linoleic acid metabolism in preterm infants fed a formula with medium-chain triglycerides. *J Lipid Res* 2003; 44:41-48.

79. Tantibhedhyangkul P, Hashim SA. Medium-chain triglyceride feeding in premature infants: effects on calcium and magnesium absorption. *Ped* 1978; 61(4):537-545.

80. Sauerwald TU, Demmelmair H, Koletzko B. Polyunsaturated fatty acid supply with human milk. *Lipids* 2001; 36:991-996.

81. Innis SM, Dyer R, Nelson CM. Evidenced that palmitic acid is absorbed as sn-2 monoacylglycerol from human milk by breast fed-fed infants. *Lipids* 1994; 29:541-545.

82. Carnielli VP, Luijendijk IH, van-Goudoever JB, Sulkers EJ, Boerlage AA, Degenhart HJ, et al. Feeding premature newborn infants palmitic acid in amounts and stereoisomeric position similar to that of human milk: effects on fat and mineral balance. *Am J Clin Nutr* 1995; 61(5):1037-1042.

83. Vochem M, Hamprecht K, Jahn G, Speer CP. Transmission of cytomegalovirus to preterm infants through breast milk. *Pediatr Infect Dis J* 1998; 17(1):53-58.

84. Hamprecht K, Witzel S, Maschmann J, Speer CP, Jahn G. Transmission of cytomegalovirus infection through breast milk in term and preterm infants. In: Koletzko B, Michaelsen KF, Hernell O, editors. *Short and Long Term Effects of Breast Feeding on Child Health.* New York: Kluwer Academic/Plenum Publishers; 2000: 231-239.

85. Wardell JM, Wright AJ, Bardsley WG, D'Souza SW. Bile salt-stimulated lipase and esterase activity in human milk after collection, storage, and heating: nutritional

implications. *Pediatr Res* 1984; 18(4):382-386.

86. Henderson TR, Fay TN, Hamosh M. Effect of pasteurization on long chain polyunsaturated fatty acid levels and enzyme activities of human milk. *J Pediatr* 1998; 132(5):876-878.

87. Soderhjelm L. Fat absorption studies in children. 1. Influence of heat treatment on milk fat retention in premature infants. *Acta Paediatr Scand* 2001; 41: 207-211.

88. Lepri L, Del-Bubba M, Maggini R, Donzelli GP, Galvan P. Effect of pasteurization and storage on some components of pooled human milk. *J Chromatogr B Biomed Sci Appl* 1997; 704(1-2):1-10.

89. Fidler N, Sauerwald TU, Koletzko B, Demmelmair H. Effects of human milk pasteurization and sterilization on available fat content and fatty acid composition. *J Pediatr Gastroenterol Nutr* 1998; 27(3):317-322.

90. Christie DL, Cleverly DR, O'Connor CJ. Human milk bile-salt stimulated lipase. Sequence similarity with rat lysophospholipase and homology with the active site region of cholinesterases. *FEBS Lett* 1991; 278(2): 190-194.

91. Hui DY, Kissel JA. Sequence identity between human pancreatic cholesterol esterase and bile salt-stimulated milk lipase. *FEBS Lett* 1990; 276(1-2):131-134.

92. Stromqvist M, Tornell J, Edlund M, Edlund A, Johansson T, Lindgren K, et al. Recombinant human bile salt-stimulated lipase: an example of defective O-glycosylation of a protein produced in milk of transgenic mice. *Transgenic Res* 1996; 5(6):475-485.

93. Hansson L, Blackberg L, Edlund M, Lundberg L, Stromqvist M, Hernell O. Recombinant human milk bile salt-stimulated lipase. Catalytic activity is retained in the absence of glycosylation and the unique prolinerich repeats. *J Biol Chem* 1993; 268(35): 26692-26698.

94. DiPersio LP, Kissel JA, Hui DY. Purification of pancreatic cholesterol esterase expressed in recombinant baculovirus-infected Sf9 cells. *Protein Expr Purif* 1992; 3(2):114-120.

95. ESPGHAN Committee on Nutrition, Aggett P, Agostoni C, Goulet O, Hernell O, Koletzko B, et al. The Nutritional and Safety Assessment of Breast Milk Substitutes and other dietary products for infants: A

commentary by the ESPGHAN Committee on Nutrition. *J Ped Gastro Nutr* 2001; 32:256-258.

96. Koletzko B, Ashwell M, Beck B, Bronner A, Mathioudakis B. Characterisation of infant food modifications in the European Union. *Ann Nutr Metab* 2002; 46:231-242.

97. de-Urquiza AM, Liu S, Sjoberg M, Zetterstrom RH, Griffiths W, Sjovall J, et al. Docosahexaenoic acid, a ligand for the retinoid X receptor in mouse brain. *Science* 2000; 290(5499):2140-2144.

98. Innis SM. Essential fatty acid requirements in human nutrition. *Can J Physiol Pharmacol* 1993; 71(9): 699-706.

99. Innis SM. The role of dietary n-6 and n-3 fatty acids in the developing brain. *Dev Neurosci* 2000; 22(5-6): 474-480.

100. Lapillonne A, Picaud JC, Chirouze V, Goudable J, Reygrobellet B, Claris O, et al. The use of low-EPA fish oil for long-chain polyunsaturated fatty acid supplementation of preterm infants. *Pediatr Res* 2000; 48(6):835-841.

101. Carlson SE. Arachidonic acid status of human infants: influence of gestational age at birth and diets with very long chain n-3 and n-6 fatty acids. *J Nutr* 1996; 126(4 Suppl):1092S-1098S.

102. Demmelmair H, Baumheuer M, Koletzko B, Dokoupil K, Kratl G. Metabolism of U^{13}C-labelled linoleic acid in lactating women. *J Lipid Res* 1998; 39:1389-1396.

103. Harant I, Ghisolfi J, Couvaras O, Garcia J, Vaysse P, Thouvenot J. Fatty acid composition of adipocyte membrane phospholipids and stored triglycerides in infants receiving total parenteral nutrition. *J Parenter Enter Nutr* 1990; 14(1):42-46.

104. Farquharson J, Cockburn F, Patrick WA, Jamieson EC, Logan RW. Effect of diet on infant subcutaneous tissue triglyceride fatty acids. *Arch Dis Child* 1993; 69(5):589-593.

105. Widdowson EM, Dauncey MJ, Gairdner DM, Jonxis JH, Pelikan-Filipkova M. Body fat of British and Dutch infants. *Br Med J* 1975; 1(5959):653-655.

106. von Gröer F. Zur Frage der praktischen Bedeutung des Nährwertbegriffes nebst einigen Bemerkungen über das Fettminimum des menschlichen Säuglings.

Biochem Z 1919; 97:311-329.

107. Koletzko B. Essentielle Fettsäuren: Bedeutung für Medizin und Ernährung. *Akt Endokr Stoffw* 1986; 7:18-27.

108. Koletzko B. Importance of dietary lipids. In: Tsang R, Zlotkin SH, Nichols B, Hansen JW, editors. *Nutrition During Infancy. Principles and Practice.* Cincinnati: Digital Educational Publishing; 1997: 123-153.

109. Food and Agriculture Organization of the United Nations. *Dietary Fats and Oils in Human Nutrition.* Rome: FAO, Publications Division; 1980.

110. Koletzko B, Abiodun PO, Laryea MD, Bremer HJ. Fatty acid composition of plasma lipids in Nigerian children with protein-energy malnutrition. *Eur J Pediatr* 1986; 145:109-115.

111. Decsi T, Zaknun D, Zaknun J, Sperl W, Koletzko B. Long-chain polyunsaturated fatty acids in children with severe protein-energy malnutrition with and without human immunodeficiency virus-1 infection. *Am J Clin Nutr* 1995; 62(6):1283-1288.

112. Farrell PM, Gutcher GR, Palta M, DeMets D. Essential fatty acid deficiency in premature infants. *Am J Clin Nutr* 1988; 48:220-229.

113. Bjerve KS, Mostad IL, Thoresen L. Alpha-linolenic acid deficiency in patients on long-term gastric tube feeding: estimation of linolenic and long-chain unsaturated n-3 fatty acid requirement in man. *Am J Clin Nutr* 1987; 45:66-77.

114. Holman RT, Johnson SB. Linolenic acid deficiency in man. *Nutr Rev* 1982; 40:144-147.

115. Bjerve KS, Fischer S, Wammer F, Egeland T. Alpha-Linolenic acid and long-chain omega-3 fatty acid supplementation in three patients with omega-3 fatty acid deficiency: effect on lymphocyte function, plasma and red cell lipids, and prostanoid formation. *Am J Clin Nutr* 1989; 49:290-300.

116. Bjerve KS, Mostad IL, Thoresen L. Alpha-linolenic acid deficiency in patients on long-term gastric-tube feeding: estimation of linolenci and long-chain unsaturated n-3 fatty acid requirement in man. *Am J Clin Nutr* 1987; 45:66-77.

117. Martinez M. Tissue levels of polyunsaturated fatty acids during early human development. *J Pediatr*

1992; 120:S129-S138.

118. Clandinin MT, Chappell JE, Leong S, Heim T, Swyer PR, Chance GW. Intrauterine fatty acid accretion in human brain: implications for fatty acid requirements. *Early Hum Dev* 1980; 4:121-129.

119. Clandinin MT, Chapell JE, Leong S, Heim T, Swyer P, Chance GW. Extrauterine fatty acid accretion in human brain: implications for fatty acid requirements. *Early Hum Dev* 1980; 4:131-138.

120. Innis SM. n-3 Fatty Acid Requirements of the newborn. *Lipids* 1992; 27(11):879-885.

121. Koletzko B, Agostoni C, Carlson SE, Clandinin MT, Hornstra G, Neuringer M, et al. Long chain polyunsaturated fatty acids (LC-PUFA) and perinatal development. *Acta Paediatr* 2001; 90:460-464.

122. Farquharson J, Cockburn F, Patrick WA, Jamieson EC, Logan RW. Infant cerebral cortex phospholipid fatty-acid composition and diet. *Lancet* 1992; 340:810-813.

123. Koletzko B, Knoppke B, von Schenck U, Demmelmair H, Damli A. Non-invasive assessment of essential fatty acid status by cheek cell analysis. *J Pediatr Gastroenterol Nutr* 1999; 29:467-474.

124. Koletzko B, Müller L. Cis- and transisomeric fatty acids in plasma lipids of newborn infants and their mothers. *Biol Neonate* 1990; 57:172-178.

125. Cho HP, Nakamura MT, Clarke SD. Cloning, expression, and fatty acid regulation of the human delta-5 desaturase. *J Biol Chem* 1999; 274: 37335-37339.

126. Kuhn DC, Crawford MA, Stevens P. Transport and metabolism of essential fatty acids by the human placenta. *Contr Gynec Obstetr* 1985; 13:139-140.

127. Haggarty P, Page K, Abramovich DR, Ashton J, Brown D. Long-chain polyunsaturated fatty acid transport across the perfused human placenta. *Placenta* 1997; 18(8):635-642.

128. Dutta-Roy AK. Transport mechanisms for long-chain polyunsaturated fatty acids in the human placenta. *Am J Clin Nutr* 2000; 71:315S-322S.

129. Larque E, Hasbargen U, Koletzko B. In vivo investigation of the placental transfer of 13C-labeled fatty acids in humans. *J Lipid Res* 2003; 44:in press.

130. Kunz C, Rodriguez PM, Koletzko B, Jensen R.

Clin Perinatol 1999; 26(2):307-333.

131. Genzel-Boroviczeny O, Wahle J, Koletzko B. Fatty acid composition of human milk during the first month after term and preterm delivery. *Eur J Ped* 1997; 156:142-147.

132. Sanders TAB, Reddy S. The influence of a vegetarian diet on the fatty acid composition of human milk and the essential fatty acid status of the infant. *J Ped* 1992; 120:S71-S77.

133. Innis SM, Kuhnlein HV. Long chain omega-3 fatty acids in breast milk of Inuit women consuming traditional foods. *Early Hum Dev* 1988; 18:185-189.

134. Del-Prado M, Villalpando S, Elizondo A, Rodriguez M, Demmelmair H, Koletzko B. Contribution of dietary and newly formed arachidonic acid to human milk lipids in women eating a low-fat diet. *Am J Clin Nutr* 2001; 74(2):242-247.

135. Fidler N, Sauerwald T, Pohl A, Demmelmair H, Koletzko B. Docosahexaenoic acid transfer into human milk after dietary supplementation: a randomised clinical trial. *J Lipid Res* 2000; 41: 1376-1383.

136. Jensen CL, Maude M, Anderson RE, Heird WC. Effect of docosahexaenoic acid supplementation of lactating women on the fatty acid composition of breast milk lipids and maternal and infant plasma phospholipids. *Am J Clin Nutr* 2000; 71 (1 Suppl):292S-299S.

137. Koletzko B, Bremer HJ. Fat content and fatty acid composition of infant formulae. *Acta Paediatr Scand* 1989; 78:513-521.

138. Koletzko B, Sinclair A. Long-chain polyunsaturated fatty acids in diets for infants: choices for recommending and regulating bodies and for manufacturers of dietary products. *Lipids* 1999; 34(2):215-220.

139. Decsi T, Behrendt E, Koletzko B. Fatty acid composition of Hungarian infant formulae revisited. *Acta Paediatr Hung* 1994; 34:107-116.

140. Carlson SE, Rhodes PG, Ferguson MG. Docosahexaenoic acid status of preterm infants at birth and following feeding with human milk or formula. *Am J Clin Nutr* 1986; 44:798-804.

141. Koletzko B, Schmidt E, Bremer HJ, Haug M, Harzer G. Effects of dietary long-chain polyunsaturated fatty acids on the essential fatty acid status of premature infants. *Eur J Pediatr* 1989; 148:669-675.

142. Vanderhoof J, Gross S, Hegyi T, Clandinin T, Porcelli P, DeCristofaro J, et al. Evaluation of a long-chain polyunsaturated fatty acid supplemented formula on growth, tolerance, and plasma lipids in preterm infants up to 48 weeks postconceptional age. *J Pediatr Gastroenterol Nutr* 1999; 29(3):318-326.

143. Demmelmair H, Feldl F, Horvath I, Niederland T, Ruszinko V, Raederstorff D, et al. Influence of formulas with borage oil or borage oil plus fish oil on the arachidonic acid status in premature infants. *Lipids* 2001; 36:555-566.

144. Hoffman DR, Birch EE, Birch DG, Uauy R. Fatty acid profile of buccal cheek cell phospholipids as an index for dietary intake of docosahexaenoic acid in preterm infants. *Lipids* 1999; 34(4):337-342.

145. Koletzko B. Intravenous lipid infusion in infancy - physiological aspects and clinical relevance. *Clin Nutr* 2002; 21:S53-S65.

146. Innis SM. Essential fatty acids in growth and development. *Prog Lipid Res* 1991; 30:39-103.

147. Decsi T, Kelemen B, Minda H, Burus I, Kohn G. Effect of type of early infant feeding on fatty acid composition of plasma lipid classes in full-term infants during the second 6 months of life. *J Pediatr Gastroenterol Nutr* 2000; 30(5):547-551.

148. Makrides M, Neumann MA, Byard RW, Simmer K, Gibson RA. Fatty acid composition of brain, retina, and erythrocytes in breast- and formula-fed infants. Am J Clin Nutr 1994; 60:189-194.

149. Carnielli VP, Wattimena DJ, Luijendijk IH, Boerlage A, Degenhart HJ, Sauer PJ. The very low birthweight premature infant is capable of synthesizing arachidonic and docosahexaenoic acids from linoleic and linolenic acids. *Pediatr Res* 1996; 40(1):169-174.

150. Sauerwald T, Hachey DL, Jensen CL, Chen H, Anderson RE, Heird WC. Intermediates in endogenous synthesis of C22:6w3 and C20:4w6 by term and preterm infants. *Ped Res* 1997; 41:183-187.

151. Salem N, Wegher B, Mena P, Uauy R. Arachidonic

and docosahexaenoic acids are biosynthesized from their 18-carbon precursors in human infants. *Proc Natl Acad Sci USA* 1996; 93(1):49-54.

152. Uauy R, Mena P, Wegher B, Nieto S, Salem N. Long chain polyunsaturated fatty acid formation in neonates: effect of gestational age and intrauterine growth. *Pediatr Res* 2000; 47(1):127-135.

153. Rubin M, Harell D, Naor N, Moser A, Wielunsky E, Merlob P, et al. Lipid infusion with different triglyceride cores (long-chain vs. medium-chain/long-chain triglycerides): effect on plasma lipids and bilirubin binding in premature infants. *J Parent Ent Nutr* 1991; 15:642-646.

154. Clark KJ, Makrides M, Neumann MA, Gibson RA. Determination of the optimal ratio of linoleic to alpha-linolenic acid in infant formulas. *J Pediatr* 1992; 120:S151-S158.

155. Jensen CL, Prager TC, Fraley JK, Chen H, Anderson RE, Heird WC. Effect of dietary linoleic/alpha-linolenic acid ratio on growth and visual function of term infants [see comments]. *J Pediatr* 1997; 131(2):200-209.

156. Jensen CL, Chen H, Fraley JK, Anderson RE, Heird WC. Biochemical effects of dietary linoleic/alpha-linolenic acid ratio in term infants. *Lipids* 1996; 31(1):107-113.

157. Ponder DL, Innis SM, Benson JD, Siegman JS. Docosahexaenoic acid status of term infants fed breast milk or infant formula containing soy oil or corn oil. *Pediatr Res* 1992; 32:683-688.

158. Putnam JC, Carlson SE, DeVoe P, Barness LA. The effect of variations in dietary fatty acids on the fatty acid composition of erythrocyte phosphatidylcholine and phosphatidylethanolamine in human infants. *Am J Clin Nutr* 1982; 36:106-114.

159. Greiner RC, Winter J, Nathanielsz PW, Brenna JT. Brain docosahexaenoate accretion in fetal baboons: bioequivalence of dietary alpha-linolenic and docosahexaenoic acids. *Pediatr Res* 1997; 42(6): 826-834.

160. De la Presa Owens S, Innis SM. Docosahexaenoic and arachidonic acid prevent a decrease in dopaminergic and serotoninergic neurotransmitters in frontal cortex caused by linoleic and alpha-linolenic acid deficient

diet in formula fed piglets. *J Nutr* 1999; 129: 2088-2093.

161. Carnielli VP, Verlato G, Pederzini F, Luijendijk I, Boerlage A, Pedrotti D, et al. Intestinal absorption of long-chain polyunsaturated fatty acids in preterm infants fed breast milk or formula. *Am J Clin Nutr* 1998; 67(1):97-103.

162. Wijendran V, Huang MC, Diau GY, Boehm G, Nathanielsz PW, Brenna JT. Efficacy of dietary arachidonic acid provided as triglyceride or as substrates for brain arachidonic acid accretion in baboon neonates. *Pediatr Res* 2002; 51:265-272.

163. Carlson SE, Rhodes PG, Rao VS, Goldgar DE. Effect of fish oil supplementation on the n-3 fatty acid content of red blood cell membranes of preterm infants. *Pediatr Res* 1987; 21:507-510.

164. Uauy R, Birch DG, Birch EE, Tyson JE, Hoffman DR. Effect of dietary omega-3 fatty acids on retinal function of very-low-birth-weight neonates. *Pediatr Res* 1990; 28:485-492.

165. Koletzko B, Edenhofer S, Lipowsky G, Reinhardt D. Effects of a low birthweight infant formula containing docosahexaenoic and arachidonic acids at human milk levels. *J Pediatr Gastro Nutr* 1995; 21:200-208.

166. Uauy R, Hoffman DR, Birch EE, Birch DG, Jameson DM, Tyson J. Safety and efficacy of omega-3 fatty acids in the nutrition of very low birth weight infants: soy oil and marine oil supplementation of formula. *J Pediatr* 1994; 124:612-620.

167. Carlson SE, Wilson WW. Docosahexaenoic acid (DHA) supplementation of preterm (PT) infants: effect on the 12-month Bayley mental developmental index (MDI). *Pediatric Research* 1994; 35:20A. Ref Type: Abstract.

168. Clandinin MT, Van Aerde JE, Parrott A, Field CJ, Euler AR, Lien E. Assessment of feeding different amounts of arachidonic and docosahexaenoic acids in preterm infant formulas on the fatty acid content of lipoprotein lipids. *Acta Paediatr* 1999; 88(8):890-896.

169. Anderson JW, Johnstone BM, Remley DT. Breast-feeding and cognitive development: a meta-analysis. *Am J Clin Nutr* 1999; 70(4):525-535.

170. Lucas A, Morley R, Cole TJ, Gore SM. A randomised multicentre study of human milk versus formula and

later development in preterm infants. *Arch Dis Child Fetal Neonatal Ed* 1994; 70(2):F141-F146.

171. Carlson SE, Werkman SH, Peeples JM, Cooke RJ, Tolley EA. Arachidonic acid status correlates with first year growth in preterm infants. *Proc Natl Acad Sci USA* 1993; 90(3):1073-1077.

172. Ryan AS, Montalto MB, Groh-Wargo S, Mimouni F, Sentipal-Walerius J, Doyle J et al. Effect of DHA-containing formula on growth of preterm infants to 59 weeks postmenstrual age. *Am J Human Biol* 1999; 11:457-467.

173. O'Connor DL, Hall R, Adamkin D, Auestad N, Castillo M, Connor WE, et al. Growth and development in preterm infants fed long-chain polyunsaturated fatty acids: a prospective, randomized controlled trial. *Ped* 2001; 108(2):359-371.

174. Innis SM, Adamkin D, Hall RT, Kalhan SC, Lair C, Lim M et al. Docosahexaenoic acid and arachidonic acid enhance growth with no adverse effects in preterm infants fed formula. *J Pediatr* 2002; 140: 547-554.

175. Simmer K. Longchain polyunsaturated fatty acid supplementation in preterm infants. Cochrane Database Syst Rev 2000;(2):CD000375.

176. Koletzko B, Aggett PJ, Bindels JG, Bung P, Ferre P, Gil A, et al. Growth, development and differentiation: a functional food science approach. *Br J Nutr* 1998; 80 (Suppl) 1:S5-45.

177. von Gröer F. Zur Frage der praktischen Bedeutung des Nährwertbegriffes nebst einigen Bemerkungen über das Fettminimum des menschlichen Säuglings. *Biochem Z* 1919; 97:311-329.

178. Koletzko B, Braun M. Arachidonic acid and early human growth: is there a relation? *Ann Nutr Metab* 1991; 35:128-131.

179. Elias SL, Innis SM. Infant plasma trans, n-6, and n-3 fatty acids and conjugated linoleic acids are related to maternal plasma fatty acids, length of gestation, and birth weight and length. *Am J Clin Nutr* 2001; 73(4):807-814.

180. Woltil HA, van-Beusekom CM, Schaafsma A, Muskiet FA, Okken A. Long-chain polyunsaturated fatty acid status and early growth of low birthweight infants. *Eur J Pediatr* 1998; 157(2):146-152.

181. Sellmayer A, Koletzko B. Polyunsaturated fatty acids and eicosanoids in infants: physiological and pathophysiological aspects and open questions. *Lipids* 1999; 34(2):199-205.

182. Lauritzen L, Hansen HS, Jorgensen MH, Michaelsen KF. The essentiality of long chain n-3 fatty acids in relation to development and function of the brain and retina. *Progr Lipid Res* 2001; 40:1-94.

183. Neuringer M. Infant vision and retinal function in studies of dietary long-chain polyunsaturated fatty acids: methods, results, and implications. *Am J Clin Nutr* 2000; 71(1 Suppl):256S-267S.

184. Neuringer M, Reisbick S, Janowsky J. The role of n-3 fatty acids in visual and cognitive development: current evidence and methods of assessment. *J Pediatr* 1994; 125(5 Pt 2):S39-S47.

185. Birch EE, Birch DG, Hoffman DR, Uauy R. Dietary essential fatty acid supply and visual acuity development. *Invest Ophthalmol Vis Sci* 1992; 33(11):3242-3253.

186. Carlson SE, Werkman SH, Rhodes PG, Tolley EA. Visual-acuity development in healthy preterm infants: effect of marine-oil supplementation. *Am J Clin Nutr* 1993; 58(1):35-42.

187. Carlson SE, Werkman SH. A randomized trial of visual attention of preterm infants fed docosahexaenoic acid until two months. *Lipids* 1996; 31(1):85-90.

188. Carlson SE, Werkman SH, Tolley EA. Effect of long-chain n-3 fatty acid supplementation on visual acuity and growth of preterm infants with and without bronchopulmonary dysplasia. *Am J Clin Nutr* 1996; 63(5):687-697.

189. Faldella G, Govoni M, Alessandroni R, Marchiani E, Salvioli GP, Biagi PL, et al. Visual evoked potentials and dietary long chain polyunsaturated fatty acids in preterm infants. *Arch Dis Child Fetal Neonatal Ed* 1996; 75(2):F108-F112.

190. SanGiovanni JP, Parra CS, Colditz GA, Berkey CS, Dwyer JT. Meta-analysis of dietary essential fatty acids and long-chain polyunsaturated fatty acids as they relate to visual resolution acuity in healthy preterm infants. *Ped* 2000; 105/6(1292-1298):-1298.

191. Bougle D, Denise P, Vimard F, Nouvelot A,

Penneillo MJ, Guillois B. Early neurological and neuropsychological development of the preterm infant and polyunsaturated fatty acids supply. *Clin Neurophysiol* 1999; 110(8):1363-1370.

192. Lucas A, Stafford M, Morley R, Abbott R, Stephenson T, MacFadyen U, et al. Efficacy and safety of long-chain polyunsaturated fatty acid supplementation of infant-formula milk: a randomised trial. *Lancet* 1999; 354(9194): 1948-1954.

193. Auestad N, Montalto MB, Hall RT, Fitzgerald KM, Wheeler RE, Connor WE, et al. Visual acuity, erythrocyte fatty acid composition, and growth in term infants fed formulas with long chain polyunsaturated fatty acids for one year. Ross Pediatric Lipid Study. *Pediatr Res* 1997; 41(1):1-10.

194. Makrides M, Neumann A, Simmer K, Gibson RA. A critical appraisal of the role of dietary long-chain polyunsaturated fatty acids on neural indices of term infants: a randomized, controlled trial. *Ped* 2000; 105:32-38.

195. Agostoni C, Trojan S, Bellu R, Riva E, Giovannini M. Neurodevelopmental quotient of healthy term infants at 4 months and feeding practice: the role of long-chain polyunsaturated fatty acids. *Ped Res* 1995; 38:262-266.

196. Willatts P, Forsyth JS, DiModugno MK, Varma S, Colvin M. Effect of long-chain polyunsaturated fatty acids in infant formula on problem solving at 10 months of age. *Lancet* 1998; 352(9129):688-691.

197. Birch EE, Garfield S, Hoffman DR, Uauy R, Birch DG. A randomized controlled trial of early dietary supply of long-chain polyunsaturated fatty acids and mental development in term infants. *Devel Med Child Neurol* 2000; 42:174-181.

198. Carlson SE, Werkman SH, Peeples JM, Wilson WM. Growth and development of premature infants in relation to n-3 and n-6 fatty acid status. In: Galli C, Simopoulos AP, Tremoli E, editors. *Fatty Acids and Lipids: Biological Aspects.* Basel: S. Karger AG; 1994: 63-69.

199. Keicher U, Koletzko B, Reinhardt D. Omega-3 fatty acids suppress the enhanced production of 5-lipoxygenase products from polymorph neutrophil

granulocytes in cystic fibrosis. *European Journal of Clinical Investigation* 1995; 25:915-919.

200. Calder PC. Dietary fatty acids and the immune system. *Lipids* 1999; 34 Suppl:S137-S140.

201. Endres S, Ghorbani R, Kelley VE, Georgilis K, Lonnemann G, Van der Meer JWM et al. The effect of dietary supplementation with n-3 polyunsaturated fatty acids on the synthesis of interleukin-1 and tumor necrosis factor by mononuclear cells. *N Engl J Med* 1989; 320:265-271.

202. Miles EA, Calder PC. Modulation of immune function by dietary fatty acids. *Proc Nutr Soc* 1998; 57(2):277-292.

203. Field CJ, Thomson CA, van Aerde JE, Parrott A, Euler A, Lien E et al. Lower proportion of CD45R0+ cells and deficient interleukin-10 production by formula fed infants, compared with human-fed, is corrected with supplementation of long-chain polyunsaturated fatty acids. *J Pediatr Gastroenterol Nutr* 2000; 31:291-299.

204. Yu G, Bjorksten B. Serum levels of phospholipid fatty acids in mothers and their babies in relation to allergic disease. *Eur J Pediatr* 1998; 157(4):298-303.

205. Hammerman C, Aramburo MJ. Decreased lipid intake reduces morbidity in sick premature neonates. *J Pediatr* 1988; 113:1083-1088.

206. Cooke RWI. Factors associated with chronic lung disease in preterm infants. *Arch Dis Child* 1991; 66:776-779.

207. Wilson DC, Fox GF, Ohlsson A. Meta-analyses of effects of early or late introduction of intravenous lipids to preterm infants on mortality and chronic lung disease (abstract). *Journal of Pediatric Gastroenterology and Nutrition* 1998; 26:599. Ref Type: Abstract.

208. Raupp P, von Kries R, Schmidt E, Pfahl HG, Günther O. Incompatibility between fat emulsion and calcium plus heparin in parenteral nutrition of premature babies. *Lancet* 1988; 1:700.

209. Rovamo LM, Nikkila EA, Raivio KO. Lipoprotein lipase, hepatic lipase, and carnitine in premature infants. *Arch Dis Child* 1988; 63:140-147.

210. Rovamo LM, Nikkila EA, Taskinen MR, Raivio KO. Postheparin plasma lipoprotein and hepatic lipases in

preterm neonates. *Pediatr Res* 1984; 18:1104-1107.

211. Haumont D, Deckelbaum RJ, Richelle M, Dahlan W, Coussaert E, Bihain BE et al. Plasma lipid and plasma lipoprotein concentrations in low birth weight infnats given parenteral nutrition with twenty or ten percent lipid emulsion. *J Pediatr* 1989; 115:787-793.

212. Göbel Y, Koletzko B, Engelberger I, Forget D, Le Brun A, Peters J, et al. Parenteral fat emulsions based on olive and soybean oils: a randomized clinical trial in preterm infants. *J Pediatr Gastroenterol Nutr* 2003; in press.

213. Friedman Z, Danon A, Stahlman MT, Oates JA. Rapid onset of essential fatty acid deficiency in the newborn. *Ped* 1976; 58(5):640-649.

214. Friedman Z, Rosenberg A. Abnormal lung surfactant related to essential fatty acid deficiency in a neonate. *Pediatrics* 1979; 63(6):855-859.

215. Innis SM. Essential fatty acids in growth and development. *Prog Lipid Res* 1991; 30(1):39-103.

216. Borum PR. Carnitine in neonatal nutrition. *J Child Neurol* 1995; 10 Suppl 2S25-31:-31.

217. Sann L, Divry P, Cartier B, Vianey-Laud C, Maire I. Ketogenesis in hypoglycemic neonates. Carnitine and dicarboxylic acids in neonatal hypoglycemia. *Biol Neonate* 1987; 52(2):80-85.

218. Magnusson G, Boberg M, Cederblad G, Meurling S. Plasma and tissue levels of lipids, fatty acids and plasma carnitine in neonates receiving a new fat emulsion. *Acta Paediatr* 1997; 86(6):638-644.

219. Sulkers EJ, Lafeber HN, Degenhart HJ, Przyrembel H, Schlotzer E, Sauer PJ. Effects of high carnitine supplementation on substrate utilization in low-birth-weight infants receiving total parenteral nutrition. *Am J Clin Nutr* 1990; 52(5):889-894.

220. Penn D, Schmidt-Sommerfeld E, Wolf H. Carnitine deficiency in premature infants receiving total parenteral nutrition. *Early Hum Dev* 1980; 4(1): 23-34.

221. Penn D, Dolderer M, Schmidt-Sommerfeld E. Carnitine concentrations in the milk of different species and infant formulas. *Biol Neonate* 1987; 52(2):70-79.

222. Berghaus TM, Demmelmair H, Koletzko B. Fatty acid composition of lipid classes in maternal and cord

plasma at birth. *Eur J Pediatr* 1998; 157(9):763-768.

223. Genzel BO, Wahle J, Koletzko B. Fatty acid composition of human milk during the 1st month after term and preterm delivery. *Eur J Pediatr* 1997; 156(2):142-147.

224. Decsi T, Koletzko B. Role of long-chain polyunsaturated fatty acids in early human neurodevelopment. *Nutr Neurosci* 2000; 3:293-306.

225. Makrides M, Neumann MA, Gibson RA. Effect of maternal docosahexaenoic acid (DHA) supplementation on breast milk composition. *Eur J Clin Nutr* 1996; 50(6):352-357.

226. Cherian G, Sim JS. Changes in the breast milk fatty acids and plasma lipids of nursing mothers following consumption of n-3 polyunsaturated fatty acid enriched eggs. *Nutrition* 1996; 12(1):8-12.

227. Rocquelin G, Tapsoba S, Dop MC, Mbemba F, Traissac P, Martin PY. Lipid content and essential fatty acid (EFA) composition of mature Congolese breast milk are influenced by mothers' nutritional status: impact on infants' EFA supply. *Eur J Clin Nutr* 1998; 52(3):164-171.

228. Guesnet P, Antoine JM, Rochette-de LJ, Galent A, Durand G. Polyunsaturated fatty acid composition of human milk in France: changes during the course of lactation and regional differences. *Eur J Clin Nutr* 1993; 47(10):700-710.

229. Serra G, Marletta A, Bonacci W, Campone F, Bertini I, Lantieri PB et al. Fatty acid composition of human milk in Italy. *Biol Neonate* 1997; 72(1):1-8.

230. Helland IB, Saarem K, Saugstad OD, Drevon CA. Fatty acid composition in maternal milk and plasma during supplementation with cod liver oil. *Eur J Clin Nutr* 1998; 52:839-845.

231. de-la-Presa OS, Lopez SM, Rivero UM. Fatty acid composition of human milk in Spain. *J Pediatr Gastroenterol Nutr* 1996; 22(2):180-185.

Vitamins A, E, and K
Frank R. Greer, M.D.

Reviewed by Manuel Moya, M.D., and Hiroshi Tamai, M.D.

Vitamin A
Introduction

The term Vitamin A refers to a number of compounds that includes both the naturally occurring and synthetically derived retinoids. Its biologic activity is diverse. It is essential for vision, growth, healing, reproduction, cell differentiation, and immunocompetency. This multiplicity of effects led to the proposal that its mechanism of action was through gene regulation. The molecular biology of retinoids in regulating gene expression at specific body sites has been the major thrust of recent retinoid research. Vitamin A's action is similar to that of steroid hormones in that a specific retinoic-acid-receptor protein complex becomes bound to nuclear DNA, resulting in regulation of specific genes (Figure 1). This subject is reviewed in detail elsewhere.[1] By convention, the amount of Vitamin A from all sources in the diet is converted into a single unit, a "retinol equivalent" (RE), which equals 1 µg of all trans-retinol.[2] One International Unit (IU) is equivalent to 0.3 µg of preformed retinol, or 0.3 RE. Retinol is the naturally occurring alcohol formed in vivo from its precursor ß-carotene, found in plants. Other metabolic forms of importance include retinaldehyde (retinal), retinoic acid, and retinyl esters. Vitamin A is transported in plasma as retinol, bound to a specific carrier protein synthesized in the liver, retinol-binding protein (RBP).

Physiology and Metabolism
Maternal – Fetal Relationship

The mechanism and regulation of retinol transport from the maternal circulation to the fetus through the human placenta is not well described. In animals, pregnant mice and rats receiving a liberal supply of retinol transfer an adequate portion of the vitamin to the fetus. In animals, transplacental transfer of retinol to the fetus is maintained regardless of maternal retinol status. Even when maternal intake of retinol is restricted, the amount of retinol in fetal liver is similar to that of fetuses from mothers with ample retinol stores.[3] Fetal RBP appears coincident with retinol and blood concentration increases with the growth of the fetus during midgestation in the rat (11-14 days), probably reflecting transplacental transport of RBP-bound retinol.[4] A further increase in fetal liver retinol occurs later, and another rise in blood RBP concentration is attributed to the onset of fetal RBP synthesis. In humans, significant correlations between maternal and cord blood RBP concentrations have not been reported consistently.[5,6] Cord blood concentrations of Vitamin A are generally lower in preterm than term infants, and also appear to be lower in multiple gestations.[7] The ratio of maternal to fetal concentrations of plasma Vitamin A in healthy pregnancies is approximately 2:1.[8-12] Fetal plasma Vitamin A concentrations appear to be maintained within a normal range despite variations in the maternal Vitamin A status and intake.[8,13] Hence, the RDA during pregnancy for Vitamin A is the same as in the nonpregnant state.[14]

It has been known for years that excess maternal Vitamin A may cause congenital anomalies in animal fetuses,[15,16] and retinoic acid seems especially teratogenic.[17] A recent warning about the potential

141

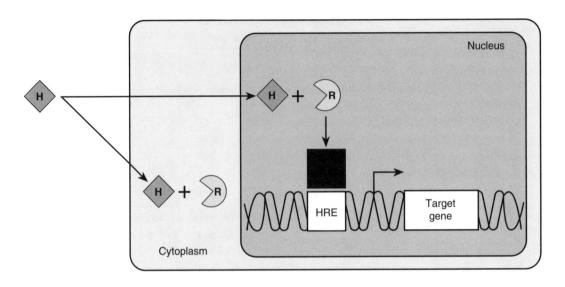

Figure 1: Nuclear hormone receptor signaling. Retinoic acid is known to function in a manner analogous to the other lipid-soluble hormones such as steroids, thyroid hormone and Vitamin D. Because of its hydrophobic character, the hormone (H) is able to penetrate the cell membrane and bind to an intracellular receptor (R). Most steroid hormone receptors are in the cytoplasm and translocated to the nucleus after binding hormone. All other receptors, including those for thyroid hormone, Vitamin D and retinoic acid, are nuclear proteins even in the absence of hormone. Unlike membrane receptor second messenger systems, in this pathway the ligand receptor complex becomes the signal to the nucleus where it directly interacts with hormone-specific response elements (HREs) in the target gene promoter and thereby elicits a transcriptional response. (From Mangelsdorf DJ, Vitamin A Receptors. Nutr Rev 1994: 52: 532-544).

teratogenic effect of retinoids comes from a clinical study in which babies born to women who took more than 10,000 IU (approximately 3000 RE) of Vitamin A per day as a supplement had an increased frequency of birth defects. The highest frequency of defects was related to high consumption before the 7th week of gestation.[18] The defects (mostly craniofacial, cardiac, and thymic) resulted in a high mortality rate.[19-21]

Both retinol and RBP have been found in amniotic fluid,[22,23] but not retinyl esters. Although based on few observations, it appears that the concentration of amniotic fluid retinol decreases close to term gestation (≥ 36 weeks), and is approximately 10-20% of that found in the mother's serum or in cord blood.

Intestinal Absorption, Transport, Storage and Excretion (Figure 2)

Ingested carotene and dietary retinyl esters are converted to free retinol in the proximal small intestine after the action of hydrolases from the pancreas and intestinal brush border. These enzymes may have low activity in the premature infant in the early days of life. After solubilization with bile salts into mixed micelles, retinol is absorbed into the intestinal cells, reesterified, and incorporated into chylomicrons that are transported via lymph (thoracic duct) into the circulation, as with all fat soluble vitamins. Intraluminal bile acid, important for this process, is decreased in premature infants and may lead to inadequate micelle formation and affect retinol absorption.[24] The absorption process is facilitated by type II cellular retinol-binding protein (CRBP-II) which is found almost exclusively in the microvilli of the mucosal cells of the small intestine and is distinctly different from the other cellular retinol-binding protein (CRBP) found in nearly all other tissues.[25,26]

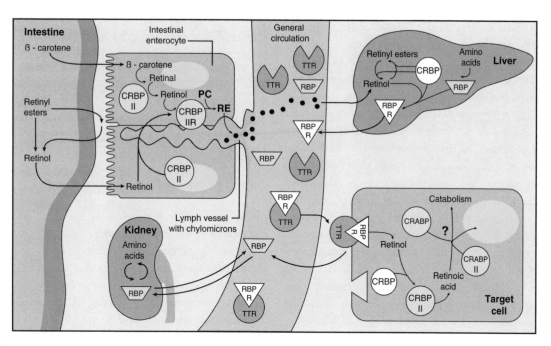

Figure 2: Vitamin A movement and metabolism in the body with possible participation of the cellular retinoid-binding proteins indicated. CRBP = cellular retinol binding protein; CRABP = cellular retinoic acid binding protein; RBP= retinol binding protein (circulating); TTR = transthyretin; RE = retinyl ester; R = retinol. (Ong DE. Cellular transport and metabolism of Vitamin A: Roles of the cellular retinoid-binding proteins. Nutr Rev. 1994;52:S24-S31).

The absorption of Vitamin A from the intestine seems inefficient in the preterm infant, and as enteral feedings are often delayed, parenteral administration may be preferred to increase Vitamin A intake.

After absorption, chylomicrons, containing lipoprotein-bound retinyl esters, are taken up by the liver. The liver is the main storage organ for retinol (90% of body stores), predominantly in the form of retinyl esters (retinyl palmitate, retinyl stearate).[2] Fetal retinol stores can be influenced somewhat by maternal retinol supplementation. Fetal and neonatal liver retinol stores can be increased fourfold after a large dose of retinyl acetate to the pregnant mouse.[27] The absolute amount and concentration of hepatic retinol storage increases during the perinatal period in the rat pup.[4,28,29] Maternal intake of retinol may explain the exponential rise in liver Vitamin A described in Swedish fetuses during the second and third trimester.[30] The normal liver Vitamin A

concentration in healthy human adults ranges from 100-300 µg/g.[31] Many premature infants are born with low or marginal liver Vitamin A stores of less than 20 µg/g of liver tissue.[32,33] In one study of 25 preterm infants who died within the first 24 hours of life, 37% had liver concentrations less than 20 µg/g.[32] Thus, the ability of many preterm infants to offset an inadequate intake of Vitamin A from liver stores would be limited. Other organs, including the developing lung in fetal rats, are capable of storing Vitamin A.[34,35] In the rat pup, there is a marked fall in the pulmonary content of retinyl ester shortly after birth, even if birth is premature.[29,34,35] Furthermore, Vitamin A content of the fetal rat lung can be increased by large doses of intragastric Vitamin A to the pregnant rat.[36] Whether the developing lung of humans is capable of Vitamin A uptake and storage is not known.

A highly regulated process subsequently liberates free retinol from the liver for delivery to peripheral target tissues (Figure 2). Retinyl esters must be hydrolyzed by the enzyme retinyl ester hydrolase (REH) as the first step in mobilization from the liver. REH has not been studied in the human fetus or neonate. Following retinol hydrolysis, the subsequent transport of retinol from the liver to other tissues for metabolism is dependent on liver RBP synthesis and secretion.[37] After secretion of the RBP-retinol complex, RBP binds in a 1:1 molar ratio with plasma transthyretin, reducing the chance for glomerular filtration and renal catabolism of RBP. At the time of birth, plasma RBP concentration was lower in a group of 39 preterm infants (gestational age 24-36 wks) compared to a group of 32 term infants (2.8 ± 1.2 µg/dL vs 3.6 ± 1.1 µg/dL, mean ± SD, p < 0.001).[38] In this same study, mean plasma Vitamin A was also lower in preterm compared to full term infants (16.0 ± 6.2 µg/dL vs 23.9 ± 10.2 µg/dL , mean ± SD, p < 0.001). One can make the argument that premature infants are Vitamin A deficient due to decreased placental delivery of Vitamin A. Furthermore, given the lower protein and calorie intakes in many sick, premature infants, the low RBP at the time of birth may significantly affect the delivery of retinol to target tissues, as RBP synthesis or release in preterm infants may be altered by protein and calorie deprivation. One study observed that blood RBP declined from day 0 to day 3 in premature infants with neonatal respiratory distress syndrome (RDS) but increased in a control group of premature neonates without RDS.[6] At present there is no explanation for this observation. However, premature neonates with RDS characteristically have a diuresis on days 3-5, which in conjunction with immature renal tubular function may increase RBP turnover through renal losses.

The circulating retinol-RBP-transthyretin complex is delivered to target tissues (Figure 2). Target tissue cytoplasm contains CRBP-I and CRBP-II (intestine), cellular retinoic acid binding protein (CRABP-I and –II) and other tissue-specific proteins.[25,39] Roles for these various proteins are still being identified. After the circulating complex delivers retinol to target tissues, free RBP is rapidly excreted by the kidney, and

	Colostrum	Mature	Preterm
Vitamin A IU/dL	400-600	60-200	50-400 (36days)
Vitamin E mg/dL	1.0 ± 0.5	0.2-0.3	0.29-1.45 (36days)
Vitamin K µg/dL	0.18-0.52	0.12-0.92	0.30 ± 0.23

From references

Table 1: Vitamins A, E and K in human milk.

transthyretin is largely degraded by the liver. Various metabolites of Vitamin A appear in the urine, though the enterohepatic circulation of retinoic acid serves to conserve the biologically active form of Vitamin A.[40]

Adrenocortical hormones may accelerate retinol mobilization from the liver.[41] Dexamethasone stimulates the release of RBP from cultured rat liver cells.[42] Since antenatal steroids are used in many human mothers in premature labor to accelerate fetal lung surfactant maturation, an effect on RBP metabolism by antenatal steroids seems possible. In a study of pregnant rhesus monkeys receiving intramuscular dexamethasone to stimulate fetal lung maturation, both maternal and fetal serum concentrations of RBP increased in those that had received antenatal steroids.[43] The increase in fetal serum RBP was dose-dependent. A similar effect of steroids on RBP was found in premature human neonates whose mothers were treated with prenatal steroids.[44] Cord blood transthyretin in premature neonates is also elevated by antenatal steroids.[45] It is unclear whether these changes of RBP and transthyretin observed as a result of antenatal steroids are useful or detrimental to retinol metabolism and function in the human premature neonate. The effects of postnatal dexamethasone on Vitamin A metabolism in premature infants will be discussed below.

Beta-Carotene

For β-carotene there is little specific information on its uptake or its metabolism to Vitamin A during the perinatal period. However, it has been known for years that β-carotene can meet the fetal and

	Vitamin A IU/dL	Vitamin E mg/dL	Vitamin K µg/dL
Enfamil Premature 24 Liquid (Mead Johnson, Evansville, Ind)	1015	5.1	6.5
Similac Special Care 24 Liquid (Ross, Columbus, OH)	1015	3.2	10.0
Infacare 22 cal Liquid (Mead Johnson, Evansville, IN)	333	3.0	5.9
Neosure 22 cal Liquid (Ross, Columbus, OH)	342	2.7	8.2
Enfamil Human Milk Fortifier (4 pkt per 100 ml)	950	4.6	4.4
Similac Human Milk Fortifier (4 pkt per 100 ml)	620	3.2	8.3
Similac Natural Care Fortifier (Liquid, 100ml*)	552	3.2	10.0

*Similac Natural Care is to be diluted 1:1 with human milk which will decrease concentrations by 50% in the feedings.

Table 2: Vitamins A, E, K in formulas and human milk fortifiers for premature infants.

newborn growth requirements for Vitamin A. There is β-carotene in human cord blood, and there is a weakly positive correlation with gestational age and maternal serum β-carotene concentration.[46] In addition, human breast milk contains β-carotene, but the relatively high concentration on day one declines by 80% by day five of lactation. One perinatal role of carotenoids that should be investigated further is their role as antioxidants. Since β-carotene can be metabolized to retinol, retinyl palmitate, and retinoic acid (all potential antioxidants) in isolated rat lung type II cells,[47] studies on the effect of carotene supplementation on developing or injured neonatal lung would be of interest.

Vitamin A and the Premature Infant
Vitamin A in Human Milk (Table 1)
The Vitamin A content of human milk varies somewhat, depending on postpartum age and the volume and fat content of the milk. 90% or more of the Vitamin A in human milk is in the form of retinyl esters contained in milk fat globules.[48] Most of the remainder is present as free retinol.[49,50]

Vitamin A is higher in colostrum (400-600 IU/dL) and decreases to a range of 60 to 200 IU/dL in mature human milk.[51] The Vitamin A content of preterm human milk reported is quite variable, but generally is comparable to that of mature milk, particularly after the first few weeks of lactation.[52] However, there is not enough Vitamin A in human milk to supply the recommended intakes for the premature infant.

Vitamin A in Formula and Oral Supplements
Though standard formulas for term infants contain approximately 200 IU/dL of Vitamin A, there is considerably more in special formulas for preterm infants, both for use in hospital (about 1000 IU/dL) and after discharge (340 IU/dL)

Vitamin preparation	Vitamin A IU	Vitamin E Mg	Vitamin K μg
MVI Pediatric* 2 ml	920	2.8	80
Vita-lipid	920	2.8	80
Cernevit	-	-	-
Infuvit** 2 ml	1125	3.5	100
Poly-Vi-Sol	1500	5	0
Vi-Daylin	1500	5	0
Tri-Vi-Sol	1500	0	0

Table 3: Vitamins A, E, K concentrations in multivitamin preparations used for TPN solutions or oral vitamin supplementation.

(Table 2). The vitamin is in the form of retinyl esters in these products.

The Vitamin A content of a typical multi-vitamin oral supplement used for preterm infants is 1500 IU/mL. At present, there are no single compound preparations of Vitamin A suitable for oral-gastric use in premature infants available in the US.

Thus, the recommended intake for the orally fed preterm infant can be met with preterm infant formula and/or multivitamin preparations (Table 3).

Vitamin A and Parenteral Nutrition

Using either of two standard multivitamin preparations for TPN solutions provides 920 IU to 1125 IU of Vitamin A per 2 ml (Table 3). However, administration of Vitamin A by this method is very inefficient because of loss of Vitamin A due to photodegradation and binding to intravenous tubing.[53,54] Net losses of Vitamin A by an in vitro study in this system estimated Vitamin A losses between 62% and 89%.[55,56] Thus, the Vitamin A intake in an infant receiving 120 ml/kg day of TPN solution would approximate 400-500 IU/kg/day, assuming a 62% loss in the delivery process. For intramuscular supplementation, a water-miscible

preparation (Aquasol A Parenteral, Astrazeneca, Wilmington, DE) containing 50,000 IU/ml of Vitamin A as retinyl palmitate can be used. It is unstable if diluted for administration purposes. Thus the preparation should be "unit dosed" from the hospital pharmacy and shielded from light prior to use.

Another method of parenteral supplementation of retinol in TPN solutions is to add retinol to lipid solutions.[54,57,58] Greene et al have reported that delivery of retinol can be increased to 90% by adding a multivitamin preparation to an intravenous lipid emulsion.[58] In one randomized control trial, a dose of Aquasol A Parenteral (Astrazeneca, Wilmington, DE) intended for intramuscular injection was diluted in a commercial lipid emulsion to a concentration of 26,000 IU/dL, with maintenance of serum retinol levels of ≥ 0.70 μmol/L.[57] However, the manufacturer does not recommend direct intravenous use of the undiluted product because of the high concentration of retinyl palmitate and the danger of Vitamin A toxicity.

High Dose Vitamin A Supplements for Premature Infants

Experimental supplementation of premature infants

	Enteral	**Parenteral**
Vitamin A	700-1500 IU/kg/day	700-1500 IU/kg/day
Vitamin E	6-12 IU/kg/day	2.8-3.5 IU/kg/day
Vitamin K*	8-10 µg/kg/day	10 µg/kg/day

*Infants >1000g at birth should receive 1 mg intramuscularly.
Infants <1000g at birth should receive 0.3 mg/kg intramuscularly
as a one time dose.

Table 4: Recommended intakes of Vitamins A, E and K.

with 1500 IU/kg/day results in "normalization" of serum retinol and RBP.[59,60] In clinical practice, this intake of Vitamin A generally is not achieved with standard preterm formulas or TPN solutions as discussed above. One of the more controversial neonatal issues is whether or not this level of supplementation, or even a higher one, may prevent bronchopulmonary dysplasia.[59-63] Studies are confounded in premature infants, and especially the extremely low-birth-weight infant (birth weight less than 1000g), by the frequent use of dexamethasone in this population. When given to the human neonate, dexamethasone results in a transient rise followed by a decrease in serum retinol and RBP, though it is not known what is happening to liver stores of Vitamin A.[64] It is also clear that intramuscular Vitamin A is more effective than the enteral route in premature infants for delivering these large doses.[66,67] A recent study reported that a daily oral supplement of 5000 IU/day was equivalent to a parenteral intake of 2000 IU/day in preterm infants whose birth weight was less than 1500g.[65] Pertinent to the use of Vitamin A for the prevention of bronchopulmonary dysplasia, in addition to its tissue healing effects, is that retinol, retinyl palmitate, and retinoic acid are all potential antioxidants as has been demonstrated in rat lungs.[47] A recent report, utilizing a decrease in lipid peroxidation quantified by the ethane content of expired air, demonstrated that Vitamin A had significant anitoxidant effect in premature infants < 30-weeks gestation.[67] These investigators gave oral supplements of 4354 ± 225 IU/day (more than triple the recommended intake in Table 4) beginning at one week of age.[67]

Randomized trials using large doses of parenteral Vitamin A to prevent chronic lung disease have recently been reviewed.[68] To date, six randomized trials have been published,[51,59,61,69-71] though one of these[71] has a sample size four times larger than all the others combined and enrolled the smallest and most premature infants (birth weights 401-1000g). A total of 554 infants treated with Vitamin A have been compared to 543 control infants in a recent meta-analysis.[68]

All studies except that of Werkman et al gave a supplement of Vitamin A (water soluble retinyl palmitate) by the intramuscular route shortly after birth (usually by day 4). The supplement was continued for at least 28 days.[57] Injections of 4000 IU were given three times a week in the study by Bental,[69] on alternate days in the study by Papagaroufalis et al,[70] and 2000 IU on alternate days in the studies by Pearson[61] and Shenai.[59] Tyson gave injections of 5000 IU three days a week for four weeks.[71] In the study by Werkman, Vitamin A was given as retinyl palmitate in a lipid emulsion over 16 hours, and study infants received 1300 to 3300 IU/kg/d of Vitamin A in the first two weeks.[57]

The amount of Vitamin A in standard therapy, and hence received by control groups, varied between studies. When on parenteral nutrition in the study by Shenai, control infants received 400 IU/100ml of Vitamin A in protein-dextrose infusion and usually < 700 IU/kg/d from all sources.[59] Control infants in the study by Pearson received 1200-1500 IU/day of Vitamin A in the protein-dextrose solution.[61] In the study by Bental, control infants on TPN received no Vitamin A but some received 1500-3000 IU/day after one week when fed orally.[69] In the study by Papagaroufalis, the amount of standard Vitamin A is not stated.[70] In Werkman's study, standard Vitamin A was added to the protein-dextrose solution, control infants <1000g receiving 700 IU/day and infants >1000g receiving 1580 IU/day.[57] In the study by Tyson, infants on standard therapy received approximately 700 IU/kg/day during the first week in the TPN solution and approximately 1000 IU/kg/day in weeks two to four from all sources.[71]

Overall, the results of these studies were mixed. Five studies reported death by one month of age as an endpoint, and none showed a difference between Vitamin A and the control groups.[59,61,69-71] Six studies reported oxygen use at one month in survivors and one of these[59] reported a significant reduction of oxygen needs in Vitamin A treated infants. The pooled data for all six studies showed a trend towards reduction in oxygen use at one month in survivors that does not reach statistical significance[68] (RR 0.93 (0.86,1.01). Five studies reported combined outcomes of death and oxygen use at one month.[59,61,69-71] Only one of these found a significant difference in this outcome[59] in Vitamin A treated infants, though in the meta-analysis of these studies there is a trend towards reduction in death or oxygen use at one month of age that is of borderline statistical significance [RR 0.93 (0.86, 1.00)]. Only one study reported death by 36-weeks-post-menstrual age and found no differences between Vitamin A and control groups.[71] This study reported no significant difference in the combined outcomes of death and oxygen use at 36 weeks [RR 0.89, 0.79, 1.0)]. However, there was a significant reduction of oxygen use in the Vitamin A group at 36 weeks [RR 0.85 (0.73,0.98)]. The need for supplemental oxygen at 36-weeks-post-menstrual age declined from 62% in the unsupplemented controls to 55% in the supplemented infants. Thus, it would require treatment of 14.5 infants with supplemental Vitamin A to benefit one patient.[71]

There has been concern about the invasiveness of repeated intramuscular injections of Vitamin A in return for a very modest benefit. A very recent study used an oro-gastric rather than a parenteral supplement of 5000 IU day of Vitamin A, beginning on the first day of life and continuing for 28 days in infants with a birth weight of < 1000g.[72] 154 infants were randomized. The study found no differences in mortality or oxygen requirement at 28 days or 36 weeks between the controls and Vitamin A group. There were also no differences in the incidence of retinopathy of prematurity (ROP), patent ductus arteriosus, necrotizing enterocolitis, intraventricular hemorrhage, or sepsis. However, at 7 and 28 days into therapy, there were no differences in the plasma retinol concentrations in the two groups. Furthermore, in 50% of the Vitamin A treated infants in whom retinol concentrations were measured (about half of those randomized), 50% had concentrations that were considered deficient at less than 20 µg/dl at 28 days of age, implying that even larger oral supplements may be needed. The variation in the serum concentrations was very large, however.[72]

Two studies reported on ROP.[59,61] One noted a trend towards a reduced incidence of ROP in the Vitamin A supplemented infants,[59] though pooled data from both studies showed no significant difference in incidence of ROP.[68] Two studies also reported on culture proven nosocomial sepsis.[69,71] The pooled data showed a non-significant trend toward a reduction in sepsis in Vitamin A supplemented infants [RR 0.89 (0.75,1.05)].[68]

It is important to note that no side effects from the high dose Vitamin A supplements were reported from any of these studies. These included clinical monitoring of anterior fontanel pressure and biochemical evidence of Vitamin A toxicity.

One can conclude from these studies, that the data would support a statistically significant reduction in the use of oxygen supplementation at one month of age and 36-weeks-post-menstrual ages, in infants treated with parenteral Vitamin A. These results are not clinically dramatic however, as the number of infants treated to achieve the benefits at 36 weeks in one infant is 14.5.[71] It is important to note that studies did not find any differences in days on ventilation or length of hospital stay.

Assessment of Vitamin A Adequacy

The "adequate" concentration of Vitamin A in very low-birth-weight infants is not known. Serum concentrations below 20.0 µg/dL (0.70 µmol/L) have been considered as deficient in premature infants and concentrations below 10.0 µg/dL (0.35 µmol/L) as indicating severe deficiency and depleted liver stores. Unfortunately, a single plasma retinol value does not correlate well with liver stores until it becomes very low [<10.0 mg/dL (<0.35 mmol/L)][33,41,73-75] or extremely low [< 5 mg/dL (< 0.17 mmol/L)].[76] Many authors have noted this problem but the use of a single plasma retinol concentration continues in the evaluation of premature infants.

Mean plasma RBP concentration at birth is lower in preterm infants than in term infants (2.8 ± 1.2 versus 3.6 ± 1.1 µg/dL).[38] A high percentage of preterm infants, up to 77%, had plasma RBP below 3.0 µg/dL, [38] which maybe indicative of Vitamin A deficiency.[77] Both the plasma RBP response[60] and the relative rise in serum retinol concentration[64] following intramuscular Vitamin A administration have been described as useful tests to assess functional Vitamin A status. This is a better method of confirming actual low Vitamin A storage than random plasma concentrations.[64] The obvious disadvantages of these methods are the need for a baseline plasma retinol, and injection of Vitamin A followed by a second plasma sample 5 hours later. A less invasive method of tissue retinoid assessment, such as the modified RDR (relative dose response),[78-80] might be more useful in this premature population if parenteral administration could be standardized. This remains an area that needs further study.

In the very large study by Tyson, 25% of infants receiving supplemental Vitamin A and 54% of controls had Vitamin A concentrations below 20.0 µg/dL on day 28.[71] Similar percentages, 22% of those receiving supplemental Vitamin A and 45% of controls, had a relative dose response (change in the serum retinol concentration divided by the pre-injection concentration) of > 10% following an intramuscular dose of 2000 IU. From these data it was suggested than an even higher dose of Vitamin A may be required to achieve Vitamin A sufficiency in very premature infants (birth weights < 1000g). Furthermore, the modest benefits of supplemental Vitamin A must be weighed against the discomfort of repeated intramuscular injections.

This is an area in need of more study given that the potential toxicity of higher doses of Vitamin A in the premature infant has not been determined.

Recommendations

Recommended supplements for the very-low-birth-weight infant are in the 700-1500 IU/kg/day range, whether enteral or parenteral, with 1500 IU/kg/d being preferable (Table 4). Most infant formulas for the very-low-birth-weight infant will easily supply this amount of intake (Table 2). However, preterm human milk, with a Vitamin A concentration of about 300 IU/dl, would supply only 450 IU/kg day assuming a 150 ml/kg/day intake.[52] These recommended intakes for the preterm infant are much higher than the RDA for term neonates — 330 IU/kg/day — which is based on the Vitamin A content of mature human milk. M.V.I. Pediatric or Infuvit supplied at 2 ml/kg to infants on TPN will generally supply closer to 1000 IU/kg/day than 1500 IU/kg/day (Table 3).

For premature infants with significant lung disease, recommendations for a larger intake of Vitamin A can be justified at this time from the available clinical trials. Thus, a parenteral or enteral dose of 2000-3000 IU per kg per day is recommended, with 3000 IU being preferred (Table 4). However, it should be noted that there is no satisfactory preparation for administering this dose enterally at this time, and an intramuscular injection is required.

It is clear that Vitamin A supplementation of the neonate by the enteral route is not as effective as that by intramuscular administration.[65,66,72] With the practice of increasing supplements in preterm infants at risk for BPD, there is also an increased concern for Vitamin A toxicity. The studies reviewed above, with high dose Vitamin K supplements, did not report any Vitamin A toxicity as noted.[59,61,69-72] Dosages used in these studies were roughly twice the recommended RDA for premature infants. Another report states that one oral dose of 50,000 IU (15,000 mg) given to newborns was associated only with an asymptomatic bulging anterior fontanel in 4-5% of the infants.[81] However, clinical assessment of toxicity in preterm infants has not been really studied, so guidelines in this area must be made carefully.

Vitamin E

Introduction

The term Vitamin E refers to eight naturally occurring

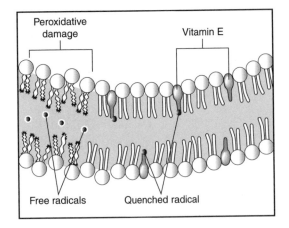

Figure 3: Biological role of Vitamin E as a membrane antioxidant, protecting polyunsaturated fatty acids that are esterified in the phospholipid bilayer by halting the chain reactions that can lead to peroxidative damage. Adapted from Greer et al, 1991.[184]

compounds with characteristic biological activities. Though the biological activities of E vitamers vary considerably, they all show antioxidant capability with the ability to protect cellular and subcellular membranes from oxidative destruction initiated at the molecular level by lipid peroxidation.[82] It is generally believed that all tocopherols function as free radical scavengers in membranes. As illustrated in Figure 3, phospholipids in cellular and subcellular membranes contain polyunsaturated fatty acids (PUFA) that are susceptible to peroxidation.[83] To be effective, tocopherol must be localized in membrane sites exposed to free radicals. The most abundant and active isomer is alpha-tocopherol. Despite growing interest, the vitamin remains somewhat of an enigma in regard to its precise subcellular role(s), although it clearly can function in animals as a biological antioxidant to prevent disease.

Studies during the 1940s and 1950s revealed that premature neonates as well as patients with malabsorption have a low concentration of blood tocopherol and abnormal hemolysis of erythrocytes incubated in the presence of hydrogen peroxide.[84,85] These studies indicated that cellular and subcellular membranes of humans are susceptible to oxidative

degeneration in the absence of Vitamin E. Subsequently, the vitamin was officially recognized in 1968 as an essential nutrient for humans by inclusion in the Recommended Dietary Allowances table of the National Academy of Sciences.[85]

The original international standard of Vitamin E, synthesized from natural phytol and initially designated dl-α-tocopherol acetate, is defined as having 1 IU/mg. The corresponding value for naturally occurring α-tocopherol is 1.49 IU/mg. On the basis of in vivo bioassays, the approximate relative potencies of the other Vitamin E isomers compared to dl-α-tocopherol are β 40-50%, γ 10-30%, Δ about 1%.

Physiology and Metabolism
Maternal-Fetal Relationship

A relatively low concentration of vitamin E is found in fetal tissues until body fat increases in late gestation. Total body content of tocopherol in the human fetus increases from about 1 mg at 5 months gestation to approximately 20 mg at term.[86] Although pregnancy is associated with a high maternal concentration of circulating Vitamin E proportional to rising plasma lipids, transplacental delivery of tocopherols to the fetus is limited. Administering large doses of Vitamin E to women in the last weeks of pregnancy has little effect on cord Vitamin E levels.[87,88] The ratio of maternal to fetal tocopherol concentration in blood is approximately 4:1, with the former concentration averaging 1.5 mg/dl and the latter 0.38 mg/dl in five studies.[89] Similarly, neonatal tissues show a relative paucity of Vitamin E isomers. In premature neonates the low proportion of adipose tissue further limits the total body Vitamin E content.

Vitamin E and PUFA

Several biochemical interactions have been identified between Vitamin E and other nutrients. It is clear that the intake of PUFA (polyunsaturated fatty acids) markedly influences the Vitamin E requirements of animals. There is good evidence that this tocopherol to PUFA relationship is also true in humans.[90-94] When determining tocopherol-PUFA requirements, not only

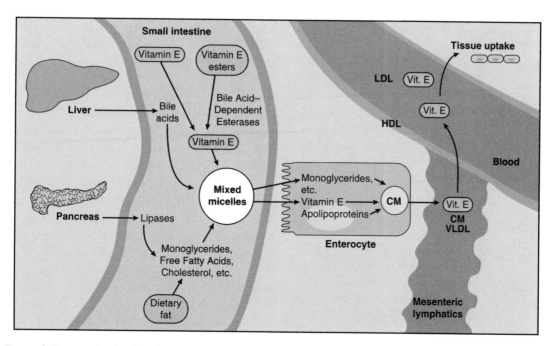

Figure 4: Processes involved in the intestinal absorption of Vitamin E in humans. CM = chylomicron. Adapted from Hdydishi and Mino. (Hdydishi O, Mino M, eds. Clinical and Nutritional Aspects of Vitamin E. New York: Elsevier; 1987:169-181.)

the amount of PUFA consumed affects this ratio, but also the degree of unsaturation of the fatty acids has an influence. In human diets where the primary fatty acid is linoleic, an α-tocopherol/PUFA ratio of 0.4 mg/g is considered nutritionally adequate, though a higher ratio is probably required for premature infants (see below).

Intestinal Absorption, Transport, Storage, and Excretion (Figure 4)

Vitamin E must be absorbed, transported, and delivered to cells. The absorption of tocopherols is variable depending on total lipid absorption as with the other fat-soluble vitamins.[95] Bile salts and pancreatic enzymes are essential to the absorption process.[90,96] In general the efficiency of absorption decreases as larger amounts of tocopherol are consumed.[97] Decreased absorption of fat, as seen in the premature neonate, results in a parallel lloss of tocopherols.[95] Factors important in the absorption of Vitamin E by the neonate include gestational age, the fat component of the diet, and the preparation of Vitamin E given.

Little is known about passage of Vitamin E through the absorptive cells of the mucosa as no intestinal transfer proteins have been identified for tocopherol. After micelle formation with bile salts, Vitamin E is absorbed, incorporated into chylomicrons and transported with fat along with the other fat-soluble vitamins via lymphatic vessels into the venous system. The concentration of tocopherol in plasma varies depending on the amount of associated lipoproteins. How Vitamin E compounds are liberated from chylomicrons and joined with the various lipoproteins is not exactly known. The enzyme lipoprotein lipase found on the endothelial surfaces of capillaries is thought to be important. During the catabolism of chylomicrons to remnant particles, various forms of Vitamin E are distributed to the circulating lipoproteins and ultimately to tissues. It is thought that chylomicron remnant uptake directly by the liver may account for a major portion of absorbed tocopherols, just as it is important for retinol.

Liver, adipose tissue, and skeletal muscle are the

major storage organs for Vitamin E. At the cellular level, it must be integrated into lipid droplets, cellular membranes, and organelles to be effective. It is concentrated wherever there is abundant fatty acid, especially in phospholipid membrane-containing structures (eg, mitochondrial, microsomal, and plasma membranes). Fat accumulates α-tocopherol and can sequester it.[98] When the intake of Vitamin E is high, the liver is a major repository, but the tocopherol pool in adipose tissue is much larger. Although adipose tissue is sometimes considered a "store" of Vitamin E, the tocopherol present in adipocytes is not readily available to other tissues.[99]

In the liver, newly absorbed lipids are incorporated into very low-density lipoproteins (VLDL), and VLDL particles secreted by the liver are preferentially enriched with α-tocopherol. The liver is responsible for the control and release of α-tocopherol into human plasma.[100-106] The function of the liver in maintaining plasma Vitamin E concentrations, and its discrimination of the various forms of tocopherol, are dependent upon the hepatic cytosolic α-tocopherol transfer protein(TTP).[107] Originally identified[108] in rat liver cytosol, TTP has now been isolated from human liver cytosol[109] and its complementary DNA sequence reported.[110] The human protein has a 94% homology with the rat protein and the gene has been localized to the 8q13.1-13.3 region of chromosome 8.[110,111] Furthermore, human deficiencies of this protein have now been reported which present as progressive peripheral neuropathy and ataxia.[112-115]

The metabolism and turnover of a-tocopherol have been investigated only to a limited extent in humans and have not been adequately quantitated in any species. The major route of excretion of tocopherol metabolites appears to be fecal elimination, possibly in association with bile secretion and also due to the fact that many forms of tocopherol in the diet are poorly absorbed. Also, with increasing intakes of tocopherol, more appears in the urine. When a Vitamin E-deficient diet is fed to animals, plasma and liver concentrations of α-tocopherol decrease rapidly. There seem to be two tocopherol pools present, at least in rats: a rapidly metabolized pool (liver, plasma red cells), and a component that is retained for longer periods primarily present in adipose tissue, skeletal muscle, and neural tissue.[99]

Vitamin E and the Premature Infant
Vitamin E in Human Milk (Table 1)
There is a large inter-individual variation in the human milk content of Vitamin E. Colostrum contains relatively high concentrations of tocopherol isomers averaging 1.0 ± 0.5 mg/dl.[116] (Table 1)   After two weeks of lactation, the Vitamin E concentration of human milk declines. Mature human milk contains all the expected isomers of tocopherol, but the vitamers other than α-tocopherol account for only about 2% of the Vitamin E activity.[117] Generally, mature human milk contains 0.2-0.3 mg/dl of α-tocopherol (Table 1).[116] It is appropriate to examine milk Vitamin E concentration in relation to PUFA. Although the lipid composition of human milk is influenced by maternal diet, it may be assumed that, on average, human milk provides approximately 6% of calories as linoleic acid. The amount of Vitamin E concurrently ingested daily (approximately 2 mg of α-tocopherol equivalents in 750 ml of mature milk) appears to be adequate to prevent antioxidant deficiency in the term neonate. For the preterm infant, however, with lower initial stores and reduced intestinal absorption, human milk may not provide sufficient Vitamin E. Some investigators have suggested that preterm infants receiving "preterm" breast milk may not need Vitamin E supplements.[119] However, given that the Vitamin E stores are very low at birth in very premature infants with increased risk of oxidative stresses, it seems prudent to supplement these infants with additional Vitamin E.

Vitamin E in Formulas and Oral and Parenteral Supplemental Vitamins
Though standard formulas for term infants contain 1.3 to 2.5 IU/dL of Vitamin E, there is considerably more in special formulas for preterm infants both for use in the hospital (3.2-5.1 IU/dL) and after discharge (2.7-3.0 IU/dL (Table 2). The vitamin is in the form of α-tocopherol in these products.

The Vitamin E content of a typical multivitamin oral supplement used for preterm infants is 5 IU/ml (Table 3). Using one of two multivitamin solutions available for pediatric TPN solutions, 2.8 to 3.5 IU of Vitamin E (α-tocopherol) per 2ml of the multivitamin solution are provided (Table 3).

Vitamin E Deficiency in Neonates

Several adverse consequences potentially attributable to Vitamin E deficiency have been described in the medical literature regarding infants and children.[85,92,120-132] Unfortunately, controversy has surrounded almost all of the conditions attributed to human Vitamin E deficiency or those claimed to be favorably responsive to Vitamin E therapy. Two lines of evidence have accumulated suggesting a role for tocopherol in human disease states: (1) signs and symptoms of a disorder potentially attributable to Vitamin E deficiency have been documented and a corrective or preventative effect of Vitamin E demonstrated (eg, hemolytic anemia in premature infants); and (2) Vitamin E supplementation, usually in pharmacological amounts well above the recommended dietary allowance, has been utilized in clinical research protocols, and a lower incidence or severity of bronchopulmonary dysplasia and retinopathy of prematurity was initially reported. Despite numerous studies of this type, there have been relatively few clinical trials with adequate randomization and controlled conditions of study.

There have been three eras of investigation concerning Vitamin E in neonates. From 1949 to 1967, generally stable neonates on enteral feedings were studied and their blood levels of tocopherol were described along with some of the consequences of Vitamin E deficiency (eg, hemolysis).[84,85,120,133,134] When neonatal intensive care became routine during the 1970s, investigations were pursued on the Vitamin E status of critically ill premature neonates leading to a better description of low Vitamin E concentration and some of the associated clinical consequences and nutrient interactions.[93,135] During the 1980s, more comprehensive investigations were performed on Vitamin E status using sensitive

microanalytical methods, and the interrelations between Vitamin E and other nutrients were more fully characterized.[126-140] The more recent studies have demonstrated that Vitamin E deficiency is common among premature neonates receiving intensive care.[118,137-140] Some of these investigations have defined methods of correcting or preventing Vitamin E deficiency in the critically ill, low-birth-weight neonate,[141-147] but they have also identified toxicity associated with excess doses of tocopherol preparations.[148]

The crisis in neonatal care associated with an alarming increase in retrolental fibroplasia during the late 1940s, provided the occasion for the first demonstration that neonates are low in Vitamin E. Owens and Owens first called attention to this state of potential malnutrition in 1949 when they reported that a group of 46 premature infants, 2 to 8 weeks old, had serum total tocopherol concentration averaging 0.2 mg/dl, about one-half the mean value for adults.[133] Shortly thereafter, this observation was confirmed.[134] In a series of 53 term and 32 premature neonates, all of whom had an uncomplicated hospital course, it was noted on the day of delivery that no significant differences were present in the serum tocopherol concentrations of the two groups. However, whereas term neonates showed a significant increase in blood tocopherol concentration during the first week of life, the concentration in low-birth-weight infants did not rise until after 3 months of age.[134]

The absorption of Vitamin E in premature neonates has been studied primarily by the technique of administering large single dosages and measuring the blood concentration sequentially. From these results, it appears that neonates less than 32 weeks gestation have significant malabsorption of tocopherol compared to term neonates and older children.[135] Prematurely delivered neonates may show evidence of Vitamin E deficiency owing to several factors, including limited tissue storage at birth, intestinal malabsorption, and rapid growth rates that increase nutritional requirements in general. Many premature neonates may not be given enteral or even parenteral Vitamin E for several days because of respiratory disorders requiring ventilatory assistance. Even when they are given tocopherol supplements, premature neonates with respiratory distress syndrome may have a low blood tocopherol concentration.[135-139]

Oski and Barness have incriminated tocopherol deficiency as a responsible factor in hemolytic anemia of prematurity.[120] As described in detail elsewhere, the conclusions from hematological studies of Vitamin E supplementation in premature neonates differ depending on other variables that influence Vitamin E status and requirements.[85,140] Nevertheless, the careful investigations of Gross and Melhorn indicated the following: (1) an abnormal degree of hemolysis occurs in association with Vitamin E deficiency; (2) supplementation of premature neonates with 25 IU of α-tocopherol acetate per day decreases the hemolysis and leads to a modest but significant increase in blood hemoglobin content; and (3) the hemolytic anemia associated with Vitamin E deficiency is aggravated by ingestion of iron in iron-fortified formulas.[149] It has been established that Vitamin E deficiency under certain nutritional dietary conditions contributes to accelerated hemolysis and causes prolonged anemia in premature neonates.

Assessment of Vitamin E Adequacy

In clinical studies, assessment for Vitamin E status has depended on biochemical analysis of plasma or serum, erythrocytes, adipose tissue biopsies, and organs obtained at autopsy. In practice, serum or plasma samples have been used most commonly to evaluate total tocopherol concentration. A concentration of at least 0.5 mg/dl indicates adequate nutritional status.[85] 90% or more of the circulating Vitamin E is normally α-tocopherol. Most would agree that Vitamin E concentration in tissue is the most appropriate parameter to measure in order to assess Vitamin E status, though in premature infants, only a blood concentration is usually available.

Vitamin E concentrations depend on plasma lipid concentrations, and in adults the Vitamin E-total lipid ratio is considered to be a more appropriate test. Because of the marked influence of plasma lipids on circulating Vitamin E concentration, tocopherol data have been expressed as a function of lipid concentration in many studies.[150-152] These investigations have demonstrated that, although children have significantly lower levels of plasma Vitamin E than adults, a tocopherol:total lipid ratio of 0.6-0.8 mg/g indicates adequate nutritional status.[150,151] This ratio would be important to measure in the very premature infant in whom marked changes in lipid levels occur, ranging from very low at birth to high during intravenous feedings of fatty acids. However, this ratio requires measurement of cholesterol, triglycerides, and phospholipids and requires considerable amounts of blood for a very small premature infant. Part of the explanation for low circulating tocopherol in premature infants relates to decreased plasma lipids compared to the lipid concentration in adults.

To characterize the apparent Vitamin E deficiency of premature neonates, a comprehensive analysis of Vitamin E status was performed by analyzing tocopherol isomers, plasma lipids, and erythrocyte hemolysis in a group of 62 infants who received varied nutritional support over a 21-day study period.[137] The group of infants studied had a mean gestational age of 31.2 ± 2.5 weeks (± SD) (range 27-36 weeks) and a birth weight of 1475 ± 407g (± SD) (range 720-2240 g). There were no correlations between maternal and cord blood concentrations of β-and γ-tocopherol. However, for α-tocopherol there was a correlation (r = 0.675, p <0.01) with neonates having about one-fourth of the maternal level, as has been described by others. During the first 24 hours after delivery, in regard to total tocopherol and α-tocopherol concentrations, 95% and 98% of the neonates were "abnormal" (ie, below the lower limit of the adult normal range) respectively. The hydrogen peroxide hemolysis test confirmed this Vitamin E deficiency in 79% of those patients. Measures of Vitamin E status rose during the 21-day study period. By using a well-established lower limit of normal hemolysis value to discriminate antioxidant status as a biological index of Vitamin E activity, and mathematical or statistical modeling techniques, it was shown that the critical plasma tocopherol values are close to the 0.5 mg/dl level, a level conventionally accepted as the discriminator of Vitamin E adequacy or inadequacy in adults.[96,150]

Another method is the functional assessment of Vitamin E status using the hydrogen peroxide hemolysis test. In addition to measuring tocopherol concentration in blood, the hydrogen peroxide hemolysis test is helpful in providing an index of antioxidant potential and Vitamin E status. Although this test is not entirely specific, a normal result (< 5% hemolysis during a 3-hours incubation in 2% H_2O_2) can be assumed to rule out Vitamin E deficiency.[150] This test has limitations in babies, where unlike adults, hemoglobin release from hemolysis does not correlate with plasma Vitamin E levels.[153,154] Many studies have detected abnormally high rates of peroxide induced erythrocyte hemolysis in premature infants.

A very recent study in premature infants (mean 33 weeks gestation) compared plasma and erythrocyte Vitamin E levels, Vitamin E to lipid ratios, and two variations of the hydrogen peroxide hemolysis test. The investigators concluded that there was no satisfactory method for the clinical assessment of Vitamin E deficiency in the premature infant.[154] Yet, it is important to differentiate between tocopherol-sufficient and tocopherol-deficient premature neonates, particularly as parenteral Vitamin E is being advocated in high doses for prophylaxis against neonatal disorders associated with oxygen toxicity.

High Dose Vitamin E Therapy

A potential role of Vitamin E supplementation in preventing or ameliorating retinopathy of prematurity was proposed in 1949 by Owens and Owens and has remained controversial.[133] It is difficult to interpret many clinical studies on this issue because of the predominant role of oxygen in injuring the immature retina and the fact that numerous variables have influenced every study. The assessment of retinopathy of prematurity has varied and often is subjective. The rationale for Vitamin E therapy for this condition seems logical. The disease is characterized by a disorder of the control of retinal vascularization, leading to excessive proliferation of poorly organized fibrovascular tissue. In its severe form, retinopathy of prematurity causes retinal scarring, detachment, and blindness. Tocopherols are concentrated in the retinal tissue,

where lipid concentrations are high and clearly can interrupt oxidation reactions that conceivably initiate the injury process. It has been proposed that Vitamin E at a high concentration can suppress retinal neovascularization by inhibition of gap junction formation by spindle cells, the mesenchymal precursors of the inner retinal capillaries and putative inducers of neovascularization in this disease.[125,126]

Hittner et al[124,125] were among proponents of mega-supplementation with Vitamin E in premature neonates susceptible to retinopathy of prematurity. Their investigations, including a double-blind clinical trial, have shown an apparent beneficial effect when oral doses of tocopherol as high as 100 IU/kg/day are given. The benefit is a reduced severity of the disease in susceptible neonates rather than its prevention. Another report has also supported the use of Vitamin E administration in high dosages.[123] In addition, a negative controlled clinical trial was reported[131] in which the investigators were unable to demonstrate prevention or amelioration of retinopathy of prematurity by Vitamin E in large doses given intravenously. A recent meta-analysis[155] of 6 randomized controlled trials with a total sample of 704 VLBW infants treated with Vitamin E and 714 VLBW controls,[123,124,131,156-158] found no difference in the overall incidence of ROP between the two groups. However, there was a significant difference in the incidence of Grade III ROP between the two groups, 2.4% in the Vitamin E versus 5.5% in the controls (pooled odds ratio 0.44, 95% CI 0.21,0.81, p<0.02). However, the total number of infants with severe ROP was very small and the authors recommended that further studies be done on the smallest infants (birth weight below 1000g). It must be concluded that at present there is no clear benefit of giving large doses of Vitamin E for the intended purpose of preventing severe retinal disease.

Bronchopulmonary dysplasia is another condition of premature neonates that was reported to be preventable by Vitamin E therapy.[122] Further investigation of the role of Vitamin E in bronchopulmonary dysplasia did not lead to confirmation of the original data, by either the same investigators[130] or others.[159,160] The rationale for this proposed effect is again logical, as tocopherols prevent oxidation-related injury of pulmonary membrane systems. In fact, Vitamin E-deficient animals show an increased susceptibility to pulmonary oxygen toxicity. However, it cannot be claimed that Vitamin E in large doses prevents bronchopulmonary dysplasia in preterm infants.

There are also data supporting the suggestion that Vitamin E supplementation, if given in the first 12 hours of life, can reduce the incidence of intraventricular hemorrhage.[128,129,161,162] The hypothesis is that the effect is related to the vitamin's ability to scavenge free radicals, which then protects brain matrix capillary endothelial cells from hypoxic-ischemic injury. However, Vitamin E in large doses cannot be recommended to prevent intraventricular hemorrhage at this time. Further study is required.[163]

Serious toxicity has been associated with mega Vitamin E supplement in premature neonates.[148] As reviewed elsewhere,[140] the adverse effects may be attributable to the vehicle used for mega Vitamin E supplementation rather than the tocopherol preparation per se. Doses of Vitamin E exceeding 3.5 IU/kg/day by the parenteral route or 25 IU/kg/day by the enteral route should be regarded as experimental and having potentially more risk than benefit for premature neonates at this time. It must be emphasized there is no compelling evidence to treat the premature infant with pharmacologic doses of Vitamin E to prevent any condition.

Vitamin E Requirements and Therapy (Table 4)
Because the neonate, especially the premature neonate, is born with low stores of α-tocopherol in addition to a decreased blood concentration, early provision of Vitamin E is necessary to correct the depleted state and prevent adverse consequences attributable to insufficient antioxidants. In the term neonate with normal intestinal absorption, it has been calculated from data obtained in studies of milk-fed neonates that 2 IU/day is sufficient to raise blood and tissue levels. The amount is higher per kilogram than the 10-15 IU recommended for older children and adults.[164] It is

clear that normal blood and tissue concentrations of tocopherol can be achieved promptly in term neonates fed the usual volume of either breast milk or commercial formula.

The situation is different for premature neonates. A variety of studies have been pursued to determine the Vitamin E requirement of the premature neonate. Two kinds of investigation have been performed, the first dealing with neonates who received only parenteral nutritional support and the second investigating enterally fed neonates. The results in intravenously nourished neonates indicates that 1 IU/kg/day eventually corrects the Vitamin E deficiency state, but up to 7-10 days may be required.[163,165,166] Parenteral α-tocopherol acetate at 3 IU/kg/day rapidly corrects low Vitamin E levels and abnormal peroxide hemolysis tests within 24 hours.[139,141] Once a normal blood concentration of Vitamin E is achieved, 1-2 IU/kg/day can be given to maintain Vitamin E sufficiency,[217] but without continued provision of tocopherol in the parenterally fed infant, insufficiency quickly develops.[141]

The pharmacokinetics of intravenously administered tocopherol preparations have been carefully studied.[147] Interestingly, it has been demonstrated that the acetate ester of α-tocopherol may not be adequately hydrolyzed when given intravenously. Accumulation of the acetate ester has been demonstrated in lung tissue. It is more likely that hydrolysis occurs in the intestine when preparations such as α-tocopherol acetate are provided by the enteral route.

In studies of enteral nutrition, it has been shown that a daily dose of 10-25 IU of water-miscible α-tocopherol acetate given to 0.6- to 1.5-kg neonates may be required to produce and maintain normal Vitamin E status.[95,118,140,142,144,145] Even some premature neonates on this regimen (10-25 IU/day) may not maintain a plasma tocopherol concentration above 0.5 mg/dl, especially if they receive iron-fortified formula. Six IU/kg/day may be insufficient.[138] Data from studies of enterally fed neonates are generally more difficult to interpret in relation to the dose and time required to correct a low blood Vitamin E concentration. This point may be attributable to the variable intestinal absorption of tocopherol preparations in premature neonates, although some authors dispute this.[167]

From studies of parenterally and enterally nourished premature neonates, it is reasonable to conclude that the immediate requirement of such neonates for absorbed Vitamin E is 2-3 IU/kg/day and that 1 IU/kg/day suffices once the initial deficiency state is corrected and tissue stores are established. The decreased intestinal absorption that has been well demonstrated makes it necessary to give larger amounts (ie, 6-12 IU/kg/day) when Vitamin E supplements are provided enterally.

Recommendations (Table 4)

It is recommended that premature infants receive 2.8-3.5 IU/kg/day Vitamin E parenterally and 6-12 IU/kg day enterally.[168] These intakes are approximated with the present formulas and multivitamin preparations (Tables 2 and 3).

The American Academy of Pediatrics Committee on Nutrition has recommended that formulas provide a minimum of 1 IU of Vitamin E per gram of linoleic acid and 0.7 IU per 100 kcal, though the special formulas with iron for premature infants contain 4-6 IU/100 kcal, because of the higher requirement for Vitamin E with these formulas.[169]

Clinical Case Report

A male infant is born at 28 weeks gestation weighing 1,050g. He suffers from severe respiratory distress, requiring mechanical ventilation for the first week of life. Enteral feeds are started on day 7 of life with proprietary formula. During the next 3 weeks, the infant has recurrent episodes of abdominal distention necessitating temporary discontinuance of enteral feeds on three occasions. He receives dextrose and electrolyte fluids intravenously.

At 4 weeks of age, the infant is tolerating 15cc of formula (110 cc/kg/day) every 3 hours. He is receiving no iron or vitamin supplements. Routine laboratory testing reveals a hematocrit of 24% and a reticulocyte count of 10%. What is the cause of this infant's anemia?

In light of the fact that the infant has received no

vitamin supplementation and has had poor enteral intake, Vitamin E deficiency should be considered. Further studies reveal a peripheral blood smear showing red blood cell fragments and moderate poikilocytes, a serum tocopherol concentration of 0.3 mg/dL and a serum tocopherol to total lipid ratio of 0.5. Erythrocyte hemolysis in hydrogen peroxide is 30%.

This infant is subsequently begun on oral tocopherol supplementation (25 IU/kg/day), resulting in a resolution of his hemolytic anemia. Three weeks later, hematocrit is 32% and reticulocyte count is 3%.

Vitamin K

Introduction

Of the fat soluble vitamins, for vitamin K there is the least specific information regarding the requirements for the premature infant. It is also the only vitamin routinely administered in large quantities at the time of birth. Its concentration in cord blood is not reliably detectable by present assay techniques at any gestational age. The Vitamin K concentration of human milk is very low, and for the newborn breastfeeding infant, a deficiency state has been described. There is not a "gold standard" for assessing the nutritional needs of this vitamin in infants. It is only very recently that even longitudinal serum levels have been determined in term and preterm infants.

Overview of Physiology and Metabolism

Vitamin K exists in two forms: 1) Vitamin K_1 or phylloquinone which is the plant form of the vitamin, and 2) Vitamin K_2, a series of compounds with unsaturated side chains of varying length, synthesized by bacteria and collectively referred to as menaquinones. Menquinones are often designated by the repeated number of "prenyl units," hence MK-4, MK-8, etc.

The vitamin functions post-ribosomally as a cofactor in the metabolic conversion of intracellular precursors of Vitamin K-dependent proteins to active forms. The coagulation factors II (prothrombin), VII, IX, and X were the first of these proteins to be described. Other Vitamin K dependent proteins in plasma include proteins C, S, and Z. Vitamin K

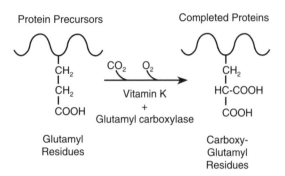

Figure 5: Vitamin K functions as a cofactor with the microsomal enzyme glutamyl carboxylase to convert glutamyl residues to gamma-carboxy-glutamic acid residues on precursor proteins (ie, prothrombin).

dependent proteins have been identified in nearly all tissues of the body. These include osteocalcin or bone Gla protein as well as matrix Gla protein of the skeleton, and kidney Gla protein.[170]

All of the known Vitamin K dependent proteins have in common gamma-carboxyglutamic acid (Gla), the unique amino acid formed by the postribosomal action of Vitamin K dependent carboxylase. These Gla residues, located in the homologous amino-terminal domain with a high degree of amino acid sequence identity seen in all Vitamin K dependent proteins,[171] are required for the calcium mediated interaction of these proteins and are the location of specific calcium binding sites. An overview of the current knowledge of Vitamin K metabolism can be found in more detail elsewhere.[170]

The conversion of glutamyl residues to gamma-carboxyglutamic acid residues on the Vitamin K-dependent protein molecule requires a microsomal Vitamin K-dependent carboxylase (Figure 5). It is apparent that during the posttranslational conversion of glutamyl to gamma-carboxylglutamyl residues on the Vitamin K-dependent peptides by carboxylase, Vitamin K is converted to its 2,3-epoxide form (Figure 6).[172] Subsequently, the epoxide form of Vitamin K is reduced to the quinone form by an

epoxide reductase and to the active coenzyme form, the hydroquinone, by various microsomal quinone reductases. It is hypothesized that the role of Vitamin K is to abstract the hydrogen of a glutamyl (Gla) residue as a proton from a Vitamin K-dependent protein, leaving a carbon ion, which is attacked by free CO_2 to form a gamman-carboxyglutamic acid (Figure 6).[172] Coumarin anticoagulants, such as warfarin apparently antagonize Vitamin K action by inhibiting the epoxide reductase and quinone reductase activities of liver. These actions increase the concentration of Vitamin K epoxide and result in an insufficient amount of reduced Vitamin K required for the action of carboxylase, resulting a clinical Vitamin K deficiency. The mechanism of action of Vitamin K is reviewed in more detail elsewhere.[173]

Menaquinones

Menaquiones can exhibit Vitamin K activity in both in vitro systems and in animals, and can participate in the Vitamin K metabolic cycle such as that seen in Figure 6. There is very little information on menaquinones in the perinatal period. Most of the bacteria comprising the normal intestinal flora of human milk fed infants do not produce menaquinones, including Bifidobacterium, Lactobacillus and Clostridium species. Bacteria which produce menaquinones include Bacteroides fragilis and Escherichia coli which are more common in formula-fed infants. Both phylloquinone and menaquinone are actually more prevalent in the stools of formula-fed infants (all formulas in the US are fortified with phylloquinone) compared to breast-fed infants.[174,175] In the newborn liver, unlike adults, phylloquinone predominates over menaquinones (81 ± 73 vs 9 ± 2 pmol/g/liver).[176] Menaquinones are not readily available compared to phylloquinone from the hepatic pool.[177] Little is known about their absorption from the intestinal tract, plasma transport, or clearance from circulation. Most of the gut bacterial pool of menaquinones, located within bacterial membranes, is probably not available for absorption.

Of considerable research interest is menaquinone-4 (MK-4), which is not a bacterial product. It is the

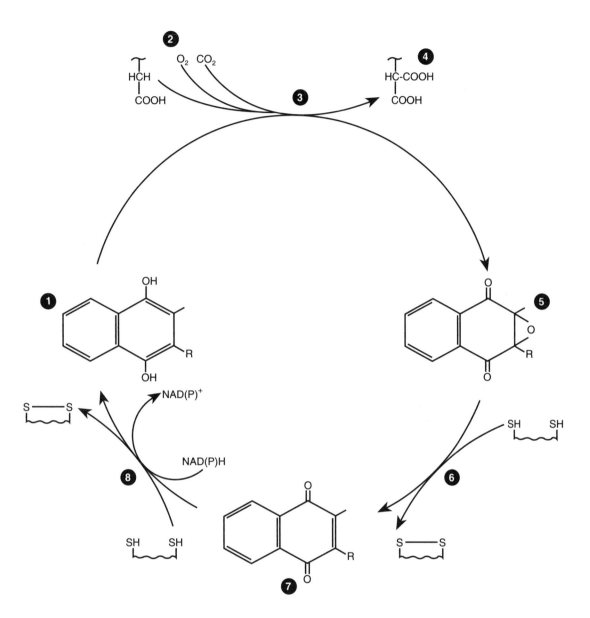

Figure 6: Metabolism of Vitamin K₁ (1) in the liver. The conversion of a glutamyl residue on a Vitamin K-dependent protein (2) to a gamma-carboxyglutamyl (gla) residue (4) by the enzyme glutamyl carboxylase (3), is dependent on the reduced Vitamin K (1) and is coupled to the formation of Vitamin K epoxide (5). The regeneration of Vitamin K₁ from the epoxide form requires a dithio (-SH) dependent enzyme, epoxide reductase (6) to form the quinone form (7) of Vitamin K and further reduction by a second dithiol dependent enzyme (8), quinone reductase, to the hydroquinone, Vitamin K₁ (1). In this proposed Vitamin K cycle, the two dithiol-dependent steps in Vitamin K metabolism are blocked by the commonly used oral anticoagulants.

major form of supplemental Vitamin K utilized for infants in Japan. Most organs have detectable levels of MK-4. In adults with the exception of the liver, organ MK-4 concentration is higher than that of phylloquinone. It has been proposed that this MK-4 accumulation is due to synthesis rather than uptake. This would mean that organs contain an enzyme capable of converting phylloquinone to MK-4. This is viewed by some to be very likely.[178-180] However, it is apparent that MK-4 can replace phylloquinone in the diet of infants. There will be no further discussion of menaquinones in preterm infants as there is almost no specific information available.

Vitamin K and the Preterm Infant

Maternal-Fetal Relationship

Vitamin K_1 has been reported to be present in low (<2 µg/ml) to undetectable concentrations in cord blood.[175,181-183] Our own recent data has shown that out of 156 cord bloods in term infants, none had measurable Vitamin K.[184] Thus, there is no correlation between maternal and cord blood levels. From all of the available evidence it appears that only very small quantities of Vitamin K cross the placenta from mother to fetus. Indeed, even maternal pharmacological doses of Vitamin K have unpredictable effects on cord blood concentration.[175,181-183] In rats, though physiological concentrations are transported across the placenta, maternal pharmacological doses do not increase placental transport proportionally.[185,186]

Absorption, Transport, Storage and Excretion

Similar to all fat soluble vitamins, Vitamin K is absorbed from the intestine into the lymphatic system, requiring the presence of both bile salts and pancreatic secretions.[187] The lymphatic system is the major route of intestinal transport of absorbed phylloquinone in association with chylomicrons. Little is known of the existence of carrier proteins. There is little specific information about the intestinal absorption of Vitamin K in humans. In the neonate, 29% of an oral dose of Vitamin K_1 is reportedly absorbed from the intestine.[188] The importance of the enterohepatic circulation of Vitamin K in the human is unknown. Compared to other fat soluble vitamins, relatively small amounts of Vitamin K have been reported in the liver of the neonate.

Vitamin K is found in relatively high concentrations in liver, heart and bone.[178,189] Other organs such as brain, have a low concentration. After the injection of Vitamin K in the rat, Vitamin K_1 is rapidly concentrated in liver but has a short half-life (17 hours) consistent with little long-term storage by this organ.[190] In adult humans it has been demonstrated with labeled Vitamin K_1 that the total body pool of Vitamin K is replaced approximately every 2.5 hours.[191]

Assessment of Deficiency

In the neonate the concentrations of the Vitamin K-dependent clotting factors (factors II, VII, IX, and X) are generally 25-70% of normal adult concentrations, and there is little difference at the time of birth between 30- and 40-weeks-gestational-age infants.[192,193] Normal adult concentrations of these factors are not achieved until 6 months of age, and if anything, premature infants show an accelerated postnatal maturation towards adult levels compared to term infants. The prothrombin time shows a wider range and variablity in the newborn at birth (11-16 seconds) compared to the adult (11-14 seconds), and this persists through the first six months of life. The activated partial thromboplastin time shows a similar pattern compared to adults through the first six months of life.[192,193] Interestingly enough, in the neonate, injections of Vitamin K_1 do not significantly alter these tests or the measurements of the individual clotting factors.[183,194] Thus, the differences in coagulation between adults and newborns cannot totally be ascribed to Vitamin K "deficiency." The coagulation differences may be limited by the availability of precursor proteins for the synthesis of Vitamin K dependent carboxylase enzyme of the Vitamin K cycle (Figure 6) rather than the availability of Vitamin K_1.

Human Vitamin K deficiency results in the secretion of partially carboxylated prothrombin into the plasma, referred to as abnormal prothrombin, or PIVKA-II (protein induced by Vitamin K absence or antagonism).[195] PIVKA-II is a heterogeneous molecule. It consists of a pool of partially carboxylated prothrombin, as well as some completely acarboxylated prothrombin.[196] The number of acarboxylated sites (up to 10) per individual prothrombin molecule and the specific sites involved remain an area of investigation. Likewise, the degree of physiologic activity may vary with the number of carboxylated sites. A preparation lacking 20% of the gamma-carboxylated sites, primarily at the more carboxy-terminal sites on the molecule, has been demonstrated to have near-normal physiologic activity.[196] PIVKA-II can be detected with a murine monoclonal antibody that is subsequently utilized in an ELISA. A number of such specific antibodies have now been described, which makes comparisons of clinical studies difficult.[197-200] Detection rates of PIVKA-II in cord blood using this assay have ranged from 10% to 30%.[199-202] We have recently reported PIVKA-II values in a large series of full term newborn infants in the US at the time of birth. Of 148 cord bloods, 49/148 (33%) were positive for PIVKA-II (≥0.2 AU/ml).[184] Similarly, in another study of 13 premature infants (27-36 weeks gestation) and 46 term infants (37-41 weeks), there was no correlation between gestation age and PIVKA-II values in cord blood.[203] Thirty-one infants (52%) had elevated PIVKA-II in cord blood. Finally, in a recent report in premature infants (24-36 weeks gestation), PIVKA-II levels were elevated in cord blood in 19/69 samples (27.5%).[204]

The usefulness of this measurement for showing a subclinical Vitamin K deficiency is a point of controversy. A number of studies have shown that prophylactic Vitamin K administered to the newborn results in near elimination of the positive PIVKA-II values that were present in cord blood.[205-208] In a recent study of exclusively breast feeding infants who received Vitamin K prophylaxis at birth (either orally or intramuscularly), we did not find a significant correlation between measurable PIVKA-II levels and low plasma Vitamin K levels during the first three months of life.[184]

Vitamin K and Human Milk (Table 1)
Vitamin K is found in the milk fat globules. Human

milk generally contains less than 1 µg/dL, and there is no significant difference between mature milk and colostrum (Table 1).[51] A recent report found a concentration 0.30 ± 0.23 µg/dL (SD) in six mothers delivering between 26- and 30-weeks-gestation.[209] By supplementing these mothers with 2.5 mg phylloquinone a day orally for two weeks the Vitamin K concentration of the milk was increased to 6.42 ± 3.14 µg/dL (SD).[209] Without this maternal supplementation, it would not be possible to supply these infants with even the minimal recommended Vitamin K intake for very-low-birth-weight infants of 2 µg /kg day (Table 4). However, there are no long-term studies of preterm infants maintained on unfortified human milk, and the available human milk fortifiers all contain Vitamin K (Table 2).

Vitamin K in Formula, Supplemental Vitamins, and Parenteral Nutrition
As all infant formulas for low-birth-weight-infants contain large amounts of Vitamin K (65-100 µg/L) (Table 2), 150 ml/kg per day for the 1000g infant would supply 9.6 to 15.0 µg/kg/day. For the very-low- birth-weight infant on Vitamin K supplemented formula, no additional Vitamin K is needed. The available human milk fortifiers for the very-low-birth-weight infants in the US all contain Vitamin K (Table 2). Premature infants on formula or fortified human milk by 40-weeks-postconceptional age have plasma Vitamin K concentrations and intakes comparable to those of term infants on fortified formula.[204]

For preterm infants maintained on TPN, those receiving 2 ml of M.V.I. Pediatric or Infuvite will receive 80 µg and 100 µg of Vitamin K respectively (Table 3). No additional Vitamin K supplements are necessary. Also, it is of note that 20% Intralipid contains about 70 µg/dl of Vitamin K.[210]

A recent study has measured longitudinal plasma Vitamin K concentrations in premature infants during hospitalization in the intensive care nursery.[204] All infants received 1 mg of Vitamin K at birth, followed by 60 µg/day (weight < 1000g) or 130 µg/day (weight ≥ 1000g) via TPN. After TPN, infants continued

	Group I = 28 wk	Group II 29-32 wk	Group III 33-36 wk
Vitamin K (2 wk) (ng/ml)	130.7±125.6[*‡]	60.8±52.9[‡]	27.2±24.4[*‡]
Vitamin K (6 wk) (ng/ml)	13.8±10.7[‡]	14.0±19.5	[†]
Vitamin K (40 wk) (ng/ml)	5.4 ±3.8[‡]	5.9±3.9[‡]	9.3±8.5[‡]

[*]p < 0.05 (Group I vs III)

[†]By six weeks of age, infants were 40-weeks-post-conceptional age

[‡]p <0.05 (Intra group differences from 2-40 wk)

Table 5: Plasma Vitamin K concentrations in premature infants.

to receive Vitamin K fortified enteral feedings. Very high plasma concentrations of Vitamin K were measured on these high Vitamin K intakes at 2 weeks (see Table 5) at which time 60-80% of the infants were still receiving TPN. By six weeks, intakes and plasma Vitamin K concentrations had decreased and only 14-30% of the infants were still receiving TPN, the remainder receiving Vitamin K supplemented enteral feedings (formula or fortified human milk) (Table 5). No PIVKA-II's were measurable at 2 or 6 weeks. Plasma values continued to fall and by 40 weeks gestation age Vitamin K intakes were 10-15 µg/kg/day and plasma levels were comparable to those found in formula fed term infants (5-6ng/ml).[204] It is apparent from the very high levels of plasma Vitamin K seen while on TPN, that the Vitamin K concentration should be reduced in the intravenous multivitamin supplements.

High Dose Vitamin K for Preterm Infants

A number of studies have tried to associate periventricular-intraventricular hemorrhage (PIVH) in the very-low-birth-weight infant with Vitamin K deficiency.[211-216] Maternal supplements of Vitamin K have been given as a result.[217-219] However, given the very low transfer rate of Vitamin K across the placenta even when given in large doses to the mother, and the mixed results of these studies, one cannot conclude that PIVH in the premature infant is secondary to Vitamin K deficiency at birth. In fact, it is clear that many cases of PIVH occur in infants 3 or

more days after receiving the customary prophylactic dose of phylloquinone at birth, implying that Vitamin K does not prevent PIVH. To date, toxicity from Vitamin K has not been reported in the premature infant.

Recommendations (Table 4)

Though the official RDA for infants is 1 µg/kg/day, it seems prudent to continue 1 mg of phylloquinone intramuscularly at birth in the premature infant greater than 1000g birthweight. For those with birth weights < 1000g, 0.3mg/kg intramuscularly would be sufficient. This amount of Vitamin K should sustain the premature infant at least through the first two weeks of life.

For infants on TPN, it is likely that they will receive approximately 10µg/kg/day if they are receiving 3g/kg/day of Intralipid. Though 10µg/kg/day (comparable to what formula fed infants receive, see below) would seem adequate for these infants, presently available multivitamin solutions would provide 80-100 µg per day if used according to recommended doses of these vitamin preparations (Table 3). This would approximate the intake recommended by Greene et al of 100µg/kg/day for infants on TPN solutions,[168] though there is no justification for such large quantities of Vitamin K.

Finally, during the periods of stabilization and post-hospital discharge for up to 6 months, fortified formulas will supply 7-9 µg/kg/day of Vitamin K. No additional supplements of Vitamin K are needed during this period.

References

1. Mangelsdorf DJ, Umesono K, Evans RM. The retinoid receptors. In: Sporn MB, Roberts AB, Goodman DS, eds. The Retinoids, 2nd Ed. Orlando. Academic Press, 1994;319-350.

2. Blomhoff R. Transport and metabolism of vitamin A. *Nutr Rev* 1994;52:513-523.

3. Moore T. Vitamin A transfer from mother to offspring in mice and rats. *Int J Vitam Nutr Res* 1971;41: 301-306.

4. Takahashi YI, Smith JE, Goodman DS. Vitamin A and retinol binding protein metabolism during fetal development in the rat. *Am J Physiol* 1977;233: E263-E272.

5. Dostalova L. Correlation of the vitamin status between mother and newborn at delivery. *Dev Pharmacol Ther* 1982;4:45-47.

6. Hustead VA, Gutcher GR, Anderson SA, et al. Relationship of vitamin A (retinol) status to lung disease in the preterm infant. *J Pediatr* 1984;105: 610-615.

7. Tammela O, Aitola M, Ikonen S. Cord blood concentrations of Vitamin A in preterm infants. *Early Hum Dev* 1999;56:39-47.

8. Lund CJ, Kimble MS. Plasma Vitamin A and carotene of the newborn infant with consideration of fetal-maternal relationships. *Am J Obstet Gynecol* 1943;46:207-221.

9. Baker H, Thompson FO, Langer AD, Munves A, DeAngelis ED, Kaminetzky HA. Vitamin profile of 174 mothers and newborns at parturition. *Am J Clin Nutr* 1975;28:59-65.

10. Baker H, Thind IS, Frank O, De Angelis B, Caterini H, Louria DB. Vitamin levels in low birth-weight newborn infants and their mothers. *J Obstet Gynecol* 1977; 129:521524.

11. Vahlquist A, Rask L, Peterson PA, Berg T. The concentrations of retinol-binding protein, prealbumin, and transferrin in sera of newly delivered mothers and children of various ages. *Scand J Clin Lab Invest* 1975;35:569-575.

12. Jansson L, Nilsson B. Serum retinol and retinol-

binding protein in mothers and infants at delivery. *Biol Neonate* 1983;43:269-271.

13. Barnes AC. The placental metabolism of vitamin A. *Am J Obstet Gynecol* 1951;61:368-372.

14. Underwood BA. Maternal vitamin A status and its importance in infancy and early childhood. *Am J Clin Nutr* 1994;59(suppl):517S-524S.

15. Robens JR. Teratogenic effects of hypervitaminosis A in the hamster and guinea pig. *Toxicol Appl Pharmacol* 1970;16;88-94.

16. Geelan JCA. Hypervitaminosis A-induced teratogensis. *CRC Crit Rev Toxicol* 1979;6:351-375.

17. Shenefelt RE. Morphogenesis of malformations in hamsters caused by retinoic acid: relation to dose and stage at treatment. *Teratology* 1972;5:103-118.

18. Rothman KJ, Moore LL, Singer MR, et al. Teratogenicity of high vitamin A intake. *N Engl J Med* 1995; 333:1369-1373.

19. Lammer EJ, Chen DT, Hoar RM, et al. Retinoic acid embryopathy. *N Engl J Med* 1985;313:837-841.

20. Benke PJ. The isotretinoin teratogen syndrome. *JAMA* 1984;251:3267-3269.

21. Lott IT, Bocian M, Pribram HW, et al. Fetal hydrocephalus and ear anomalies associated with maternal use of isotretinoin. *J Pediatr* 1984;105: 597-602.

22. Sklan D, Shalit I, Lasebnik N, et al. Retinol transport proteins and concentrations in human amniotic fluid, placenta, and fetal and maternal sera. *Br J Nutr* 1985;54:577-583.

23. Wallingford JC, Milunsky A, Underwood BA. Vitamin A and retinol binding protein in amniotic fluid. *Am J Clin Nutr* 1983;38:377-381.

24. Ong DE. Absorption of Vitamin A. In: Blomhoff R ed. *Vitamin A in Health and Disease.* New York: Marcel Dekker, Inc; 1994;37-72.

25. Ong DE, Newcomer ME, Chytil F. Cellular retinol-binding proteins. In: Sporn MB, Roberts AB, Goodman DS, eds: *The Retinoids*, 2nd Ed. Orlando: Academic Press, 1994;283-318.

26. Crow JA, Ong DE. Cell-specific immunohistochemical localization of cellular retinol-binding protein (type two) in the small intestine of rat. *Proc Natl Acad Sci USA* 1985;82:4707-4711.

27. Matsumoto E, Hirosawa K, Abe K, et al. Development of the Vitamin A storing cell in mouse liver during late fetal and neonatal periods. *Anat Embryol* 1984;169:249-259.

28. Ismadi SD, Olson JA. Dynamics of the fetal distribution and transfer of vitamin A between rat fetuses and their mother. *Int J Vitam Nutr Res* 1982;52:111-118.

29. Zachman RD, Kakkad B, Chytil F. Perinatal rat lung retinol (vitamin A) and retinyl palmitate. *Pediatr Res* 1984;18:1297-1299.

30. Gehre-Medhin M, Vahlquist A. Vitamin A nutrition in the human fetus. *Acta Paediatr Scand* 1984;73:333-340.

31. Hugue T. A survey of human liver reserves of retinol in London. *Br J Nutr* 1982;47:165-172.

32. Shenai JP, Chytil F, Stahlman MT. Liver vitamin A reserves of very low birth weight neonates. *Pediatr Res* 1985;19:892-893.

33. Olson JA, Gunning DB, Tilton RA. Liver concentrations of vitamin A and carotenoids, as a function of age and other parameters of American children who died of various causes. *Am J Clin Nutr* 1984;39:903-910.

34. Shenai JP, Chytil F. Vitamin A storage in lungs during perinatal development in the rat. *Biol Neonate* 1990;57:126-132.

35. Zachman RD, Valceschini G. Effect of premature delivery on rat lung retinol (vitamin A) and retinyl ester stores. *Biol Neonate* 1988;54:285-288.

36. Shenai JP, Chytil F. Effect of maternal Vitamin A administration on fetal lung Vitamin A stores in the perinatal rat. *Biol Neonate* 1990;58:318-325.

37. Soprano DR, Blaner WS. Plasma retinol-binding proteins. In: Sporn MB, Roberts AB, Goodman DS, eds: *The Retinoids*, 2nd Ed. Orlando: Academic Press; 1994: 257-282.

38. Shenai JP, Chytil F, Jhaveri A, et al. Plasma Vitamin A and retinol binding protein in premature and term neonates. *J Pediatr* 1981;99:302-305.

39. Saari JC. Retinoids in photosensitive systems. In: Sporn MB, Roberts AB, Goodman DS, eds: *The Retinoids*, 2nd Ed. Orlando: Academic Press; 1994: 351-386.

40. Zile MH, Inhorn RC, DeLuca HF. The biological activity of 5,6-epoxyretinoic acid. *J Nutr* 1980; 110:2225-2230.

41. Zachman RD. Retinol (Vitamin A) and the neonates: special problem of the human premature infant. *Am J Clin Nutr* 1989;50:413-424.

42. Borek C, Smith JE, Soprano DR, et al. Regulation of retinol-binding protein metabolism by glucocorticoid hormones in cultured H4IIEC3 liver cells. *Endocrinology* 1981;109:386-391.

43. Hustead VA, Zachman RD. The effect of antenatal dexamethasone on maternal and fetal retinol-binding protein. *Am J Obstet Gynecol* 1986;154:203-205.

44. Georgieff MK, Chockalingam UM, Sasanow SR, et al. The effect of antenatal betamethasone on cord blood concentrations of retinol-binding protein, transthyretin, transferrin, retinol and Vitamin E. *J Pediatr Gastroenterol Nutr* 1988;7:713-718.

45. Georgieff MK, Susanow SR, Mammal MC, et al. Cord prealbumin values in newborn infants: effect of prenatal steroids, pulmonary maturity, and size for dates. *J Pediatr* 1986;108:972-976.

46. Ostrea EM Jr, Balum JE, Winkler R, et al. Influence of breastfeeding on the restoration of the low serum concentration of Vitamin E and β-carotene in the newborn infant. *Am J Obstet Gynecol* 1986;154:1014-1017.

47. Zachman RD, Grummer MA. Uptake and metabolism of β-carotene in isolated rat lung type II cells. *Pediatr Res* 1989;25:333A.

48. Thompson SY, Kon SK, Mawson EH. The application of chromotagraphy to the study of carotenoids of human and cow's milk. *Biochem J* 1942;36:17-18.

49. Gebre-Medhin M, Vahlquist A, Hofvander Y, Uppsall L, Valquist B. Breast milk composition in Ethiopian and Swedish mothers: I, Vitamin A and β-carotene. *Am J Clin Nutr* 1976;29:441-451.

50. Valhquist A, Nilsson S. Mechanisms for Vitamin A transfer from blood to milk in rhesus monkeys. *J Nutr* 1979;109:1456-1463.

51. Canfield LM, Giuliano AR, Graver EJ. Carotenoids, retinoids, and vitamin K in human milk. In: Jensen RG, ed; *Handbook of Milk Composition*. San Diego: Academic Press; 1995:693-705.

52. Atkinson SA. Effects of gestational stage at delivery on human milk components. In: Jensen RG, ed;

Handbook of Milk Composition. San Diego: Academic Press; 1995:222-237.

53. Howard L, Chu R, Feman S, Mintz H, Ovesen L, Worf B. Vitamin A deficiency from long-term parenteral nutrition. *Ann Intern Med* 1980; 93: 576-577.

54. Silvers KM, Sluis KB, Darlow BA, McGill F, Stocker R, Winterbourn CC. Limiting light-induced lipid peroxidation and vitamin loss in infant parenteral nutrition by adding multivitamin preparations to intralipid. *Acta Paediatr* 2001;90:242-249.

55. Shenai JP, Stahlman MT, Chytil F. Vitamin A delivery from parenteral alimentation solution. *J Pediatr* 1981;99:661-663.

56. Gillis J, Jones G, Pencharz P. Delivery of Vitamins A, D, and E in total parenteral nutrition solutions. *J Parenterol Enteral Nutr* 1983;7:11-14.

57. Werkman SH, Peeples JM, Cooke RJ, Tolley EA, Carlson SE. Effect of Vitamin A supplementation of intravenous lipids on early Vitamin A intake and status of premature infants. *Am J Clin Nutr* 1994;59:586-592.

58. Greene HL, Phillips BL, Franck L, et al. Persistently low blood retinol levels during and after parenteral feeding of very low birth weight infants: examination of losses into intravenous administration sets and a method of prevention by addition to a lipid emulsion. *Pediatrics* 1987;79:894-900.

59. Shenai JP, Kennedy KA, Chytil F, et al. Clinical trial of vitamin A supplementation in infants susceptible to bronchopulmonary dysplasia. *J Pediatr* 1987;111: 269-277.

60. Shenai JP, Rush MG, Stahlman MT, et al. Plasma retinol binding protein response to Vitamin A administration in infants susceptible to bronchopulmonary dysplasia. *J Pediatr* 1990;116: 607-614.

61. Pearson E, Bose C, Snidow T, et al. Trial of Vitamin A supplementation in very low birth weight infants at risk for bronchopulmonary dysplasia. *J Pediatr* 1992; 121:420-427.

62. Shenai JP, Rush MG, Stahlman MT, Chytil F Vitamin A supplementation and bronchopulmonary dysplasia - revisited. *J Pediatr* 1992;121:399-401.

63. Robbins ST, Fletcher AB. Early vs. delayed Vitamin A supplementation in very-low-birth-weight infants. *J Parenter Enteral Nutr* 1993;17:220-225.

64. Zachman RD, Samuels DP, Brand JM, et al. Use of the intramuscular relative dose response test to predict bronchopulmonary dysplasia in premature infants. *Am J Clin Nutr* 1996;63:123-129.

65. Landman J, Sive A, Heise HD, et al. Comparison of enteral and intramuscular Vitamin A supplementation in preterm infants. *Early Human Development* 1992;30:163-170.

66. Rush MG, Shenai JP, Parker RA, et al. Intramuscular versus enteral Vitamin A supplementation in very low birth weight neonates. *J Pediatr* 1994;125:458-462.

67. Schwartz KB, Cox JM, Clement L, Humphrey J, Gleason C, Abbey H, Sehnert SS, Risby TH. Possible antioxidant effect of Vitamin A supplementation in premature infants. *J Pediatr Gastro Nutr* 25:408-414, 1997.

68. Darlow BA, Graham PJ. Vitamin A supplementation for preventing morbidity and mortality in very low birthweight infants (Cochrane Review). In: The Cochrane Library, Issue 2,2001. Oxford: Update Software.

69. Bental RY, Cooper PA, Cummins RR, et al. Vitamin A therapy-effects on the incidence of bronchopulmonary dysplasia. *S Afr J Food Sci Nutr* 1994;6:141-145.

70. Paragaroufalis C, Cairis M, Pantazatou E, et al. A trial of Vitamin A supplementation in infants susceptible to bronchopulmonary dysplasia (abstract). *Pediatr Res* 1988;23:518A.

71. Tyson JE, Wright LL, Oh W, et al. Vitamin A supplementation for extremely-low-birth-weight infants. *N Engl J Med* 1999;340:1962-1968.

72. Wardle SP, Hughes A, Chen S, et al. Randomized controlled trial of oral Vitamin A supplementation in preterm infants to prevent chronic lung disease. *Arch Dis Child Fetal Neonatal Ed* 2001;84:F9-F13.

73. Underwood BA. Vitamin A in animal and human nutrition. In: Sporn MG, Goodman DS, eds. *The Retinoids.* Vol I. New York: Academic Press; 1984: 281-392.

74. Meyer KA, Popper H, Steigmann F, et al. Comparison of Vitamin A of liver biopsy specimens with plasma Vitamin A in man. *Proc Soc Exp Biol Med* 1942;49:

589-591.

75. Olson JA. Serum levels of Vitamin A and carotenoids as reflectors of nutritional status. *J Natl Cancer Inst* 1984;73:1439-1444.

76. Montreewasuwat N, Olson JA. Serum and liver concentrations of Vitamin A in Thai fetuses as a function of gestational age. *Am J Clin Nutr* 1979;32:601-606.

77. Shenai JP, Chytil F, Jhaveri A., et al. Plasma Vitamin A and retinol binding protein in premature and term neonates. *J Pediatr* 99:302-305,1981.

78. Tanumihardjo SA, Olson JA. A modified relative dose response assay employing 3,4-didehydroretinol (Vitamin A2) in rats. *J Nutr* 1988;118:598-603.

79. Tanumihardjo SA, Koellner PG, Olson JA. The modified relative-dose-response assay as an indicator of Vitamin A status in a population of well-nourished American children. *Am J Clin Nutr* 1990;52: 1064-1067.

80. Tanumihardjo SA, Permaesih D, Dahro AM, et al. Comparison of Vitamin A status assessment techniques in children form two Indonesian villages. *Am J Clin Nutr* 1994;60:136-141.

81. Agaoestina T, Humphrey JH, Taylor GA, et al. Safety of one 52-mmol (50,000 IU) oral dose of Vitamin A administered to neonates. *Bull World Health Org* 1994;72:859-868.

82. Burton GW, Traber GW. Vitamin E: antioxidant activity, biokinetics and bioavailability. *Annu Rev Nutr* 1990; 10:357-382.

83. McCay PB, King M. Biochemical function. In: Machlin LJ, ed. *Vitamin E. A Comprehensive Treatise.* New York: Marcel Dekker; 1980:289-317.

84. Nitowsky HM, Cornblath M, Gordon HH. Studies of tocopherol deficiency in infants and children. II. Plasma tocopherol and erythrocyte hemolysis in hydrogen peroxide. *Am J Dis Child* 1956;92:164-174.

85. Farrell PM. Vitamin E. A comprehensive treatise. In: Machlin LJ, ed. *Human Health and Disease.* New York: Marcel Dekker; 1980:519-620.

86. Dju MY, Mason KI, Filer LI. Vitamin E (tocopherol) in human fetuses and placentae. *Etudes Neonatales* 1952;1:46-62.

87. Cruz CS, Wimberley PD, Johansen K, Friis-Hansen B.

The effect of Vitamin E on erythrocyte hemolysis and lipid peroxidation in newborn premature infants. *Acta Paediatr Scand* 1983;72:823-826.

88. Mino M, Nishimo H. Fetal and maternal relationship in serum Vitamin E level. *J Nutr Sci Vitaminol* 1973; 19:475-482.

89. Farrell PM. Vitamin E. In: Shils M, Young V, eds: *Modern Nutrition in Health and Disease.* Philadelphia: Lea & Febeger; 1988:340-354.

90. Bieri JG, Farrell PM. Vitamin E. *Vitam Horm* 1976; 34:31-75.

91. Farquhar JW, Ahrens EH. Effects of dietary fats on human erythrocyte fatty acid patterns. *J Clin Invest* 1963;5:675-685.

92. Witting LA. The role of polyunsaturated fatty acids in determining Vitamin E requirements. *Ann NY Acad Sci* 1972;203:192-198.

93. Williams ML, Shott RJ, O'Neal PL, et al. Role of dietary iron and fat on Vitamin E deficiency anemia of infancy. *N Engl J Med* 1975;292:887-890.

94. Horwitt MK. Vitamin E and lipid metabolism in man. *Am J Clin Nutr* 1960;8:451-461.

95. Farrell PM, Zachman RD, Gutcher GR. Fat soluble Vitamins A, E, and K in the premature infant. In: Tsang RC, ed. *Vitamin and Mineral Requirements in Preterm Infants.* New York: Marcel Dekker; 1985:63-98.

96. Farrell PM, Bieri JG, Fratantoni JF, et al. The occurrence and effects of human Vitamin E deficiency: a study in patients with cystic fibrosis. *J Clin Invest* 1977;60:233-241.

97. Losowky MS, Kelleher J, Walker BE. Intake and absorption of tocopherol. *Ann NY Acad Sci* 1972; 203:212-222.

98. Bieri JG, Evarts RP. Effect of plasma lipid levels and obesity on tissue stores of α-tocopherol. *Proc Soc Exp Biol Med* 1975;149:500-502.

99. Bieri JG. Kinetics of tissue α-tocopherol depletion and repletion. *Ann NY Acad Sci* 1972;203:181-191.

100. Traber MG, Burton GW, Hughes L, et al. Discrimination between forms of Vitamin E by humans with and without genetic abnormalities of lipoprotein metabolism. *J Lipid Res* 1992;33: 1171-1182.

101. Traber MG, Burton GW, Ingold KU, et al. *RRR-*

and *SRR*-α-tocopherols are secreted without discrimination in human chylomicrons, but *RRR*-α-tocopherol is preferentially secreted in very low density lipoproteins. *J Lipid Res* 1990;31:675-685.

102. Traber MG, Ingold KU, Burton GW, et al. Absorption and transport of deuterium-substituted 2R,4'R,8'R-α-tocopherol in human lipoproteins. *Lipids* 1988;23:791-797.

103. Traber MG, Kayden HJ. Preferential incorporation of α-toxopherol vs. γ-tocopherol in human lipoproteins. *Am J Clin Nutr* 1989;49:517-526.

104. Traber MG, Kayden HJ. α-tocopherol as compared with γ-tocopherol is preferentially secreted in human lipoproteins. *Ann NY Acad Sci* 1989;570:95-108.

105. Traber MG, Sokol RJH, Burton GW, Ingold KU, Papas AM, et al. Impaired ability of patients with familial isolated Vitamin E deficiency to incorporate α-tocopherol into lipoproteins secreted by the liver. *J Clin Invest* 1990;85:397-407.

106. Traber MG, Sokol RJ, Kohlschutter A, et al. Impaired discrimination between stereoisomers of α-tocopherol in patients with familial isolated Vitamin E deficiency. *J Lipid Res* 1993;34:201-210.

107. Traber MG. Determinants of plasma Vitamin E concentrations. *Free Rad Biol Med* 1994;16:229-239.

108. Catignani GL, Bieri JG. Rat liver α-tocopherol binding protein. *Biochim Biophys Acta* 1977;497;349-357.

109. Kuhlenkamp J, Ronk M, Yusin M, et al. Identification and purification of a human liver cytosolic tocopherol binding protein. *Prot Exp Purif* 1993;4:382-389.

110. Arita M, Sato Y, Miyata A, et al. Human α-tocopherol transfer protein: cDNA cloning, expression and chromosomal localization. *Biochem J* 1995;306:437-443.

111. Doerfllinger N, Linder C, Puahchi K, et al. Ataxia with Vitamin E deficiency: refinement of genetic localization and analysis of linkage disequilibrium by using new markers in 14 families. *Am J Hum Genet* 1995;56:1116-1124.

112. Sokol RJ, Kayden HJ, Bettis DB, et al. Isolated Vitamin E deficiency in the absence of fat malabsorption--familial and sporadic cases:

characterization and investigation of causes. *J Lab Clin Med* 1988;111:548-559.

113. Ben Hamida C, Doerflilnger N, Belal S, et al. Localization of Friedreich ataxia phenotype with selective Vitamin E deficiency to chromosome 8q by homozygosity mapping. *Nature Genet* 1993;5:195-200.

114. Ben Hamida M, Belal S, Sirugo G, et al. Friedreich's ataxia phenotype not linked to chromosome 9 and associated with selective autosomal recessive Vitamin E deficiency in two inbred Tunisian families. *Neurology* 1993;43:2179-2183.

115. Ouahchi K, Arita M, Kayden H, et al. Ataxia with isolated Vitamin E deficiency is caused by mutations in the α-toxopherol transfer protein. *Nature Genet* 1995;9:141-145.

116. Lammi-Keefe CJ. Vitamin D and E in human milk. In: Jensen RG, ed. *Handbook of Milk Composition* San Diego:Academic Press;1995;706-717.

117. Kobayaski H, Kanno C, Yamauchi K, et al. Identification of α-, β-, γ-, and δ-tocopherols and their contents in human milk. *Biochim Biophys Acta* 1975;380:282-290.

118. Gross SJ, Gabriel E. Vitamin E status in preterm infants fed human milk or infant formula. *J Pediatr* 1985;106:634-640.

119. Kaempf D, Linderkamp O. Do healthy premature infants fed breast milk need Vitamin E supplementation: α- and γ-tocopherol levels in blood components and buccal mucosal cells. *Pediatr Res* 1998;44:54-59.

120. Oski FA, Barness LA. Vitamin E deficiency: a previously unrecognized cause of hemolytic anemia in the premature infant. *J Pediatr* 1967;70:211-220.

121. Horwitt MK, Bailey P. Cerebellar pathology in an infant resembling chick nutritional encephalomalacia. *Arch Neural Psychiatr* 1959;95:869-872.

122. Ehrenkranz RA, Bonta BW, Ablow RC, et al. Amelioration of bronchopulmonary dysplasia after Vitamin E administration: A preliminary report. *N Engl J Med* 1978;229:564-569.

123. Johnson L, Schaffer D, Quinn G, et al. Vitamin E supplementation and the retinopathy of prematurity. *Ann NY Acad Sci* 1982;393:473-484.

124. Hittner HM, Godio LB, Rudolph AJ, et al. Retrolental

fibroplasia: Efficacy of Vitamin E in a double-blind clinical study of preterm infants. *N Engl J Med* 1981;305:1365-1371.

125. Hittner HM, Godio LB, Speer MI, et al. Retrolental fibroplasia: further clinical evidence and ultrastructural support for efficacy of Vitamin E in the preterm infants. *Pediatrics* 1983;71:423-432.

126. Kretzer FL, Hittner JM, Johnson AT, et al. Vitamin E and retrolental fibroplasia: ultrastructural support of clinical efficacy. *Ann NY Acad Sci* 1982;393:145-164.

127. Sokol RJ. Vitamin E deficiency and neurologic disease. *Am Rev Nutr* 1988;8:351-373.

128. Chiswick ML, Johnson M, Woodhall C, et al. Protective effect of vitamin E (dl-alpha-tocopherol) against intraventricular hemorrhage in premature babies. *Br Med J* 1983;287:81-84.

129. Speer ME, Blifeld C, Rudolph AJ, et al. Intraventricular hemorrhage and Vitamin E in the very low-birth-weight infant: evidence of efficacy of early intramuscular Vitamin E administration. *Pediatrics* 1984;74:1107-1112.

130. Ehrenkranz RA, Ablow RC, Warshaw JB. Effect of Vitamin E on the development of oxygen-induced lung injury in neonates. *Ann NY Acad Sci* 1982; 393:452-465.

131. Phelps DL, Rosenbaum AL, Isenberg SJ, et al. Tocopherol efficacy and safety for preventing retinopathy of prematurity: a randomized, controlled, double-masked trial. *Pediatrics* 1987;79:489-500.

132. Bell EF. Prevention of bronchopulmonary dysplasia: Vitamin E and other antioxidants. In: Farrell PM, Tausing LM, eds. *Bronchopulmonary Dysplasia and Related Chronic Respiratory Disorders.* Report of the Ninetieth Ross Conference on Pediatric Research. Columbus, OH: Ross Laboratories; 1986:77-82.

133. Owens WC, Owens EU. Retrolental fibroplasia in premature infants. *Am J Ophthalmol* 1949;32: 1631-1637.

134. Moyer WT. Vitamin E levels in term and premature newborn infants. *Pediatrics* 1950;6:893-896.

135. Melhorn DK, Gross S. Vitamin E-dependent anemia in the premature infant. II. Relationships between gestational age and absorption of Vitamin E. *Pediatrics* 1971;79:581-588.

136. Gutcher GR, Lax AM, Farrell PM. Tocopherol

isomers in intravenous lipid emulsions and resultant plasma concentrations. *J Parent Enteral Nutr* 1984;8:269-273.

137. Gutcher GR, Raynor WJ, Farrell PM. An evaluation of Vitamin E status in premature infants. *Am J Clin Nutr* 1984;40:1078-1089.

138. Huijbers WAR, Schrijver J, Speek AJ, et al. Persistent low plasma Vitamin E levels in premature infants surviving respiratory distress syndrome. *Eur J Pediatr* 1986;145:170-171.

139. Phillips B, Franck LS, Greene HL. Vitamin E levels in premature infants during and after intravenous multivitamin supplementation. *Pediatrics* 1987; 80:680-683.

140. Slagle TA, Gross SJ. Vitamin E. In: Tsang RC, Nichols BL, eds. *Nutrition During Infancy.* Philadelphia: Hanley & Belfus; 1988:277-288.

141. Gutcher GR, Farrell PJM. Early intravenous correction of Vitamin E deficiency in premature infants. *J Pediatr Gastroenterol Nutr* 1985;4:604-609.

142. Hittner HM, Speer ME, Rudolph AJ, et al. Retrolental fibroplasia and vitamin E in the preterm infant - comparison of oral versus intramuscular administration. *Pediatrics* 1984;73:238-249.

143. Greene HL, Moore MEC, Phillips B, et al. Evaluation of a pediatric multiple vitamin preparation for total parenteral nutrition. II. Blood levels of Vitamins A, D, and E. *Pediatrics* 1986;77:539-547.

144. Ronnholm KAR, Dostalova L, Simes MA. Vitamin E supplementation in very-low-birth-weight infants: Long-term follow-up at two different levels of Vitamin E supplementation. *Am J Clin Nutr* 1989; 49:121-126.

145. Friedman CA, Wender DF, Temple DM, et al. Serum α-tocopherol concentrations in preterm infants receiving less than 25 mg/kg/day α-tocopherol acetate supplements. *Dev Pharmacol Ther* 1988;11:273-280.

146. Bougle D, Boutroy MJ, Heng J, et al. Plasma kinetics of parenteral tocopherol in premature infants. *Dev Pharmacol Ther* 1986;9:310-316.

147. Knight ME, Roberts RJ. Disposition of intravenously administered pharmacologic doses of Vitamin E in newborn rabbits. *J Pediatr* 1986;108:145-150.

148. Balistreri WF, Farrell MK, Bove KE. Lessons from the E-ferol tragedy. *Pediatrics* 1986;78:503-506.

149. Gross S, Melhorn DK. Vitamin E, red cell lipids and red cell stability in prematurity. *Ann NY Acad Sci* 1972;203:141-162.

150. Farrell PM, Levine SL, Murphy MD, et al. Plasma tocopherol levels and tocopherol-lipid relationships in a normal population of children as compared to healthy adults. *Am J Clin Nutr* 1978;31:1720-1726.

151. Horwitt MK, Harvey CC, Dahm CH, Jr, et al. Relationship between tocopherol and serum lipid levels for determination of nutritional adequacy. *Ann NY Acad Sci* 1972;203:223-226.

152. Sokol RJ, Heubi JE, Iannacone ST, et al. Vitamin E deficiency with normal serum Vitamin E concentrations in children with chronic cholestasis. *N Engl J Med* 1984;310:1209-1212.

153. Cynamon HA, Isenberg JN. Characterization of Vitamin E status in cholestatic children by conventional laboratory standards and a new functional assay. *J Pediatr Gastroenterol Nutr* 1987;6:46-50.

154. Van Zoeren-Grobben D, Jacobs NJM, Houdkamp E, Lindeman JHN, Drejer DF, Berger HM. Vitamin E status in preterm infants: Assessment by plasma and erythrocyte Vitamin E-lipid ratios and hemolysis tests. *J Pediatr Gastro Nutr* 1998;26:73-79.

155. Taju TNK, Langenberg P, Bhutani V, Quinn GE. Vitamin E prophylaxis to reduce retinopathy of prematurity: A reappraisal of published trials. *J Pediatr* 1997;131:844-50.

156. Milner RA, Watts JL, Paes B, Zipursky A. RLF in <1500 gram neonates. Part of a randomized clinical trial of the effectiveness of Vitamin E. Retinopathy of Prematurity Conference. Columbus, OH: Ross Laboratories;1981:703-716.

157. Finer NN, Schindler RF, Grant G, Hill GB, Peters KL. Effect of intramuscular Vitamin E on frequency and severity of retrolental fibroplasia. A controlled trial. *Lancet* 1982;1:1087-1091.

158. Puklin JE, Simon RM, Ehrenkranz RA. Influence on retrolental fibroplasia of intramuscular Vitamin E administration during respiratory distress syndrome. *Ophthalmology* 1982;89;96-103.

159. Saldanha RL, Cepeda EE, Poland RL. The effect of Vitamin E prophylaxis on the incidence and severity of bronchopulmonary dysplasia. *J Pediatr* 1982;

101:89-93.

160. Watts JL, Milner R, Zipursky A, et al. Failure of supplementation with vitamin E to prevent bronchopulmonary dysplasia in infants <1500 g birthweight. *Eur Respir J* 1991;4:188-190.

161. Chiswick M, Gladman G, Sinba S, et al. Vitamin E supplementation and periventricular hemorrhage in the newborn. *Am J Clin Nutr* 1991;53:370S-372S.

162. Fish WH, Cohen M, Franzek E, et al. Effect of intramuscular vitamin E on mortality and intracranial hemorrhage in neonates of 1,000 grams or less. *Pediatrics* 1990;85;578-584.

163. Laro MR, Wojewardine K, Wald NJ. Is routine Vitamin E administration justified in very low-birth-weight infants? *Dev Med Child Neurol* 1990;32: 442-450.

164. Food and Nutrition Board, Institute of Medicine, Dietary Reference Intakes for Vitamin C, Vitamin E, Selinium, and Carotinoids. Washington DC: National Academy Press; 2000:186-283.

165. Farrell PM. Vitamin E deficiency in premature infants. *J Pediatr* 1979;95:869-872.

166. Banagale RC, Bray JJ, Erenberg AP. Serum free tocopherol levels in premature infants (PI) receiving total parenteral nutrition (TPN). *Pediatr Res* 1981; 15:492A.

167. Bell EF, Brown EJ, Milner R, et al. Vitamin E absorption in small premature infants. *Pediatrics* 1979;63:830-832.

168. Greene HL, Hambridge KM, Schanler R, Tsang RC. Guidelines for the use of vitamins, trace elements, calcium, magnesium, and phosphorus in infants and children receiving total parenteral nutrition: report of the Subcommittee on Pediatric Parenteral Nutrient Requirements from the Committee on Clinical Practice Issues of The American Society for Clinical Nutrition. *Am J Clin Nutr* 1988;48:1324-1342.

169. American Academy of Pediatrics, Committee on Nutrition. Nutritional needs of preterm infants. In: *Pediatric Nutrition Handbook*, 1998;55-87.

170. Greer FR, Zachman RD. Neonatal vitamin metabolism. Fat soluble. In: Cowett RM, ed. *Principles of Perinatal-Neonatal Metabolism.* New York: Springer; 1998;943-975.

171. Suttie JW. Synthesis of Vitamin K-dependent

proteins. *FASEB J* 1993;7:445-452.

172. Suttie JW. Vitamin K-dependent carboxylase. *Ann Rev Biochem* 1985;54:459-477.

173. Dowd P, Ham SW, Naganathan S, Hershline R. The mechanism of action of Vitamin K. *Ann Rev Nutr* 1995;15:419-440.

174. Fujita K, Kakuya F, Ito S. Vitamin K_1 and K_2 status and fecal flora in breast fed and formula fed 1-month-old infants. *Eur J Pediatr* 1993;152:852-855.

175. Greer FR, Mummah-Schendel LL, Marshall S, Suttie JW. Vitamin K_1 (phylloquinone) and Vitamin K_2 (menaquinone) status in newborn during the first week of life. *Pediatrics* 1988;81:137-140.

176. Kayata S, Kindberg C, Greer FR, et al. Vitamin K_1 and K_2 in infant human liver. *J Pediatr Gastroenterol Nutr* 1989;8:304-307.

177. Suttie JW. The importance of menaquinones in human nutrition. *Annu Rev Nutr* 1995;15:399-417.

178. Thijssen JW, Drittij-Reijnders MJ, Fischer MAJG. Phylloquinoine and menaquinone-4 distribution in rats: Synthesis rather than uptake determines menaquinone-4 organ concentrations. *J Nutr* 1996; 126:537-543.

179. Will BH, Usui Y, Suttie JW. Comparative metabolism and requirement of Vitamin K in chicks and rats. *J Nutr* 1992;122:2354-2360.

180. Guillaumont M, Weiser H, Sann L, Vignal B, Ledercq M, Frederich A. Hepatic concentration of Vitamin K active compounds after application of phylloquinone to chickens on a Vitamin K deficient or adequate diet. *Int J Vitam Nutr Res* 1992;62:15-20.

181. Pietersma-deBruyn ALJM, Van Haard PMM. Vitamin K_1 in the newborn. *Clin Chim Acta* 1985; 150:95-101.

182. Shearer MJ, Barkhan P, Rahim S, et al. Plasma Vitamin K_1 in mothers and their newborn babies. *Lancet* 1982;2:460-463.

183. Mandelbrot L, Guillaumont M, Leclercq M, et al. Placental transfer of Vitamin K_1 and its implication in fetal hemostasis. *Thromb Haemost* 1988;60:39-43.

184. Greer FR, Marshall SP, Severson RR, Smith DA, Shearer MJ, Pace DG, Joubert PH. A new mixed-micellar preparation for oral Vitamin K prophylaxis. Comparisons with an intramuscular formulation in

breast-fed infants. *Arch Dis Child* 1998;79:300-305.

185. Hamulyak K, DeBoer-van den Berg MAG, Thijssen HHW, et al. The placental transport of [^{3}H] Vitamin K_1 in rats. *Br J Haematol* 1987;65:335-338.

186. Guillaumont MJ, Durr FM, Combet JM, et al. Vitamin K_1 diffusion across the placental barrier in the gravid female rat. *Dev Pharmacol Ther* 1988; 11:57-64.

187. Blomstrand R, Forsgren L. Vitamin K_1 ^{3}H in man: its intestinal absorption and transport in the thoracic duct lymph. *Int Z Vitam Forschung* 1968;38:45-64.

188. Sann L, Leclercq M, Guillaumont M, et al. Serum Vitamin K_1 concentrations after oral administration of Vitamin K_1 in low birth weight infants. *J Pediatr* 1985;107:608-611.

189. Hodges SJ, Bejui J, Leclercq M, et al. Detection and measurement of Vitamins K_1 and K_2 in human cortical and trabecular bone. *J Bone Miner Res* 1993;8:1005-1008.

190. Thierry MJ, Hermodson MA, Suttie JW. Vitamin K and warfarin distribution and metabolism in the warfarin-resistant rat. *Am J Physiol* 1970;219: 854-859.

191. Bjornsson TD, Meffin PG, Swezey SE, et al. Disposition and turnover of Vitamin K_1 in man. In: Suttie JW, ed. *Vitamin K Metabolism and Vitamin K-Dependent Proteins*. Baltimore: University Park Press, 1980; 328-332.

192. Andrew M, Paes B, Milner R, et al. Development of the human coagulation system in the full-term infant. *Blood* 1987;70:165-172.

193. Andrew M, Paes B, Milner R, et al. Development of the human coagulation system in the healthy premature infant. *Blood* 1988;72:1651-1657.

194. Göbel U, Sonnenschein-Kosenow S, Petrich C, et al. Vitamin K deficiency in the newborn. *Lancet* 1977; 2:187-188.

195. Von Kries R, Greer FP, Suttie JW. Assessment of Vitamin K status of the newborn infant. *J Pediatric Gastroenterol Nutr* 1993;16:231-238.

196. Liska DJ, Sutie JW. Location of γ-carboxyglutamy residues in partially carboxylated prothrombin preparations. *Biochemistry* 1988;27:8636-8641.

197. Amiral J, Grosley M, Plassart V, et al. Development of

a monoclonal immunoassay for the direct measurement of decarboxyprothrombin on plasma (abstract). *Thromb Haemost* 1991;65:10.

198. Belle M, Breband R, Guinet R, et al. Detection of human plasmatic des-gamma-carboxyprothrombins by enzyme-linked immunosorbent assay using a new monoclonal antibody, in press.

199. Bovill EG, Soll RF, Lynch M, et al. Vitamin K_1 metabolism and the production of descarboxypro-thrombin and protein C in the term and premature neonate. *Blood* 1993;81:77-83.

200. Motahara K, Endo F, Matsuda I. Effect of Vitamin K administration on a carboxyprothrombin (PIVKA-II) levels in newborns. *Lancet* 1985;2:242-244.

201. Motohara K, Takayi S, Endo F, et al. Oral supplementation of Vitamin K for pregnant women and effects on levels of plasma Vitamin K and PIVKA-II in the neonate. *J Pediatr Gastroenterol Nutr* 1990;11:32-36.

202. Von Kries R, Shearer MJ, Widdershoven J, et al. Des-gamma-carboxyprothrombin (PIVKA-II) and plasma Vitamin K_1 in newborns and their mothers. *Thromb Haemost* 1992;68:383-387.

203. Greer FR, Costakos DT, Suttie JW. Determination of des-gamma-carboxy-prothrombin (PIVKA II) in cord blood of various gestational ages with the STAGO antibody-a marker of Vitamin K deficiency. *Pediatric Research*, 1999;45:283A. (Abstract)

204. Kumar D, Greer FR, Super DM, Suttie JW, Moore JJ. Vitamin K status of premature infants. Implications for current recommendations. *Pediatrics*, 2001; 108:1117-1122.

205. Widdershoven J, Lambert W, Motohara K, et al. Plasma concentrations of Vitamin K_1 and PIVKA-II in bottle-fed and breast-fed infants with and without Vitamin K prophylaxis at birth. *Eur J Pediatr* 1988; 148:139-142.

206. Cornelissen E, Kollée L, DeAbreu R, et al. Effects of oral and intramuscular Vitamin K prophylaxis on Vitamin K_1, PIVKA-II and clotting factors in breast-fed infants. *Arch Dis Child* 1992;67:1250-1254.

207. Cornelissen E, Kollée L, DeAbreu R, et al. Prevention of Vitamin K deficiency in infancy by weekly administration of Vitamin K. *Acta Pediatr*

1983;82:656-659.

208. Cornelissen E, Kollée L, van Lith T, et al. Evaluation of a daily dose of 25 mg Vitamin K_1 to prevent Vitamin K deficiency in breast-fed infants. *J Pediatr Gastroenterol Nutr* 1993;16:301-305.

209. Bolisetty S, Gupta GG, Salonikas C, Naidoo D. Vitamin K in preterm breastmilk with maternal supplementation. *Acta Paediatr* 1998;87:960-962.

210. Lennon C, Davidson KW, Sadowski JA, Mason JB. The Vitamin K content of intravenous lipid emulsions. *J Parenteral Enteral Nutr* 1993;17: 142-144.

211. Gray OP, Ackerman A, Fraser AJ. Intracranial hemorrhage and clotting defects in low-birth-weight infants. *Lancet* 1968;1:545-548.

212. Cole VA, Durbin M, Olaffson A, Reynolds EOR, Rivers RPA, Smith JF. Pathogenesis of intraventricular hemorrhage in newborn infants. *Arch Dis Child* 1974;49:722-728.

213. Setzer ES, Webb IB, Wassenaar JW, Reeder JD. Mehta PS, Eitzman DV. Platelet dysfunction and coagulopathy in intraventricular hemorrhage in the premature infant. *J Pediatr* 1982;100:599-605.

214. MacDonald MM, Johnson ML, Rumack CM, Koops BL, Guggenheim MA, Babb C, Hathaway WE. Role of coagulopathy in newborn intracranial hemorrhage. *Pediatrics* 1984;74:26-31.

215. Beverly DW, Chance GW, Inwood MJ, Shaus M, O'Keefe B. Intraventricular hemorrhage and haemostasis defects. *Arch Dis Child* 1984;59: 444-448.

216. Van de Bor M, Van Bel F, Lineman R, Ruys JH. Perinatal factors and periventricular haemorrhage in preterm infants. *Am J Dis Child* 1986;140: 1125-1130.

217. Pomerance JJ, Teal JG, Gogolok JF, Brown S, Stewart ME. Maternally administered antenatal Vitamin K_1: effect on neonatal prothrombin activity, partial thromboplastin time, and intraventricular hemorrhage. *Obstet Gynecol* 1987;70:235-241.

218. Morales WJ, Angel JL, O'Brien WF, Knuppel RA, Marsalis F. The use of antenatal Vitamin K in the prevention of early neonatal intraventricular hemorrhage. *Am J Obstet Gynecol* 1988;159:774-779.

219. Kazzi NJ, Ilagan NB, Liang KC, Kazzi GM,
     Poland RL, Grietsel LA, Fujii Y, Brans YW.
     Maternal administration of vitamin K does not
     improve coagulation profile of preterm infants.
     Pediatrics 1989;84:1045-1050.

Water-Soluble Vitamins for Premature Infants
Richard J. Schanler, M.D.

Reviewed by Hans Boehles, M.D., and Harry Greene, M.D.

Introduction

Water-soluble vitamins play key roles in the developing infant. Water-soluble vitamins function as cofactors for enzyme reactions in intermediary metabolism, and as such, are dependent upon energy and protein contents of the diets, as well as on rates of growth and energy utilization of the infant. The necessity of water-soluble vitamins was reiterated during the early development of artificial diets and parenteral feeding.

Active transport of water-soluble vitamins during pregnancy results in concentration gradients favoring the fetus.[1] Maternal vitamin supplementation during pregnancy prevents vitamin deficiency. At birth, the concentration of water-soluble vitamins is greater in the neonate than in the mother.

In human milk there is a general relationship between water-soluble vitamin concentration and maternal dietary intake, but this association exists primarily when intake is deficient (Table 1). Only in occasional circumstances does pharmacologic vitamin supplementation affect milk content (Figure 1).

Prematurity

It is difficult to establish vitamin needs for the premature infant as classic deficiency syndromes are not described and little data exist describing dose-response relationships. Furthermore, defined water-soluble vitamin toxicity data also are lacking in premature infants. Yet, in some respects the premature infant is protected from excessive intakes because the water-soluble vitamins are excreted by the kidney. However, the premature infant may be at risk for deficiency because of the immaturity of the organs needed for digesting and excreting the vitamins, the low tissue stores of these vitamins, and the potential effects of their associated diseases on increasing vitamin needs or complicating vitamin absorption and excretion. With the exception of Vitamin B_{12}, water-soluble vitamins are not stored in the body to any great extent and are rapidly depleted if intake is marginal. Thus, because of the rapid growth of the premature infant, and their increased energy and protein needs, they require a constant supply of water-soluble vitamins.

Parenteral water-soluble vitamins, even more than enteral vitamins, may be degraded by exposure to light, oxidation, and interaction with the delivery tubing. Environmental effects have only recently been studied. There is some suggestion that parenteral water-soluble vitamin mixtures also contribute to the oxidant stress of the premature infant.[2,3]

Maternal and full-term newborn plasma water-soluble vitamin indices are correlated significantly.[4,5] This may be particularly important in assessing the needs of the premature infant. Some investigators suggest that the full-term infant's cord blood vitamin concentration be used as a reference for establishing adequate intakes in premature infants. The use of cord blood values as a reference has not been investigated in premature infants.

Given that the vitamin needs of premature infants are incompletely understood, there are additional concerns because human milk may not provide adequate amounts of many water-soluble vitamins (Table 2). Commercial formulas and fortifiers for human milk designed for premature infants contain larger quantities of water-soluble vitamins than do

	Change from Early to Mature Milk	Maternal Supplementation	Term vs Preterm Milk
Thiamin (µg)	I	+	T
Riboflavin (µg)	I	++	=
Niacin (mg)	I	+	=
Vitamin B$_6$ (µg)	I	++	T
Folate (µg)	I	+	=
Vitamin B$_{12}$ (µg)	D	+	P
Pantothenic acid (mg)	I	+	P
Biotin (µg)	I	+	=
Vitamin C (mg)	I	+	P

I - Increases from early lactation (1-5 days) to later lactation (> 1 mo).
D - Decreases from early lactation (1-5 days) to later lactation (> 1 mo).

+ - Maternal supplementation can affect milk content if mother is malnourished or vitamin deficient.
++ - Maternal supplementation can affect milk content even if vitamin status of mother is adequate.

P - Vitamin content is greater in preterm milk than full-term milk.
T - Vitamin content is greater in full-term milk than preterm milk.
= - Vitamin content similar in full-term and preterm milk.

Table 1: Human milk water-soluble vitamin content and effect of stage of lactation, maternal supplementation, and preterm delivery. Adapted from Picciano.[12]

enriched, post-discharge formulas, and standard infant formulas, perhaps even in excess of needs (Table 3).

This chapter addresses the physiologic role and dietary adequacy pertinent to the premature infant for each of the water-soluble vitamins: thiamin, riboflavin, niacin, Vitamin B$_6$, folate, Vitamin B$_{12}$, pantothenic acid, biotin, and Vitamin C.

Thiamin (Vitamin B$_1$)

General Metabolism

Thiamin is absorbed in the proximal small intestine by both active and passive mechanisms and phosphorylated in the mucosal cells to yield the functional form of the vitamin, coenzyme thiamin pyrophosphate (TPP).[6,7] Thiamin pyrophosphate functions, with magnesium as a cofactor, in biochemical reactions related to carbohydrate metabolism, ie, active aldehyde transfer of two general types.[6,8,9] The first type, catalyzed by dehydrogenases, is the oxidative decarboxylation of α-keto acids (pyruvate to acetyl CoA, α-ketoglutarate to succinate, and the keto analogues of branched-chain amino acids). The second type of general reaction requiring TPP is the formation of α-ketols catalyzed by the enzyme transketolase. That enzyme reaction supplies reduced nicotinamide adenine dinucleotide phosphate (NADPH) needed for biosynthetic reactions in the pentose phosphate pathway. In addition to its coenzyme functions, thiamin is thought to play a specific role in neurophysiology. The coenzyme forms are located in peripheral nerve membranes and may function to facilitate nerve conduction.[9,10]

Sources

The thiamin concentration in human milk increases from 20 µg/L during the first five days of lactation to

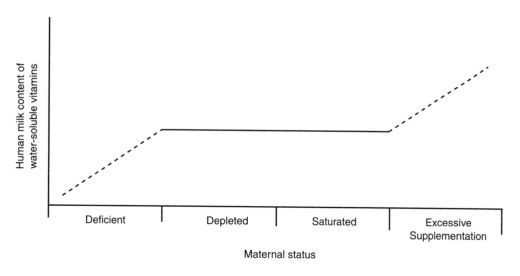

Figure 1: Effect of maternal water-soluble vitamin status on the content of water-soluble vitamins in human milk. Modified from Picciano.[12]

210 μg/L in mature milk (Table 2).[11,12] Milk thiamin can be increased by increasing dietary intake but only from the malnourished to the usual range of milk concentrations.[13] Thiamin is destroyed or inactivated by heat (cooking, pasteurization), alkaline solutions, and ionizing radiation.[8,14,15]

Laboratory Assessment

The classic test for thiamin deficiency is the erythrocyte transketolase assay. In this assay, transketolase activity is measured before and after the addition of thiamin pyrophosphate. The "TPP effect" refers to the increase in transketolase activity. In deficiency states, there is a low baseline activity of the enzyme and so the incremental response to thiamin is enhanced. Severe thiamin deficiency exists when this value is >25%, mild deficiency occurs when the value is 15% to 25%, and adequate status is suggested by a value of <15%.[8] The concentration of thiamin in whole blood or cerebrospinal fluid is a more quantitative measure of vitamin excess.[16,17] Urinary excretion of thiamin parallels dietary intake except at low levels of intake.[8,18]

Deficiency

Thiamin deficiency occurs most frequently in areas of the world where the diet consists of unenriched white rice or flour. Because of its association with intermediary metabolism, thiamin deficiency usually manifests by abnormalities of carbohydrate metabolism, eg, elevation of plasma pyruvate and lactate.[19] Marginal thiamin deficiency may be unmasked, therefore, by the administration of large carbohydrate diets.[20] Deficiency may be detected biochemically one week after removal of dietary thiamin. Thus, thiamin deficiency might be considered in an infant receiving high quantities of glucose who has signs of lactic acidosis. Although not documented in infants, thiamin deficiency in adults has been associated with malabsorption syndromes, prolonged antacid therapy, renal dialysis, folate deficiency, chronic malnutrition, chronic alcoholism, and potentially following the use of diuretics.[8,14]

The deficiency of thiamin results in beriberi. The signs of this disease relate to the chronicity of the depletion, its severity, and associated stresses.[16] In adults, symptoms may include weakness, confusion, anorexia, peripheral neuropathy, and paresthesias. The illness has been described as "wet" or "dry" depending on the presence of edema or muscle wasting, respectively. In addition to neurologic manifestations, severe deficiency will cause cardiovascular changes which may progress to fulminant cardiac

	Mature Human Human Milk* (units/L)	Enfamil Human Milk Fortifier (units/4 packs)	Similac Human Milk Fortifier (units/4 packs)
Thiamin (μg)	210 (165-220)	150	233
Riboflavin (μg)	350 (350-575)	220	417
Niacin (mg)	2.0 (1.8-2.5)	3.0	3.57
Vitamin B$_6$ (μg)	140 (130-310**)	115	211
Folate (μg)	85 (80-135)	25	23
Vitamin B$_{12}$ (μg)	0.6 (0.2-1.0)	0.18	0.64
Pantothenic acid (mg)	2.0 (2.0-2.5)	0.73	1.5
Biotin (μg)	6.0 (5.0-9.0)	2.7	26
Vitamin C (mg)	50 (35-85)	11.6	25

* References[11,12,36,56,69,91,110,123,127,140]
** Values significantly greater with maternal B$_6$ supplementation
Enfamil (Mead Johnson Nutritionals, Evansville, IN)
Similac (Ross Laboratories, Columbus, OH)

Table 2: Milk concentrations of water-soluble vitamins.

failure ("cardiac beriberi").[14,21]

The Wernicke-Korsakoff syndrome results from severe, acute thiamin deficiency often observed in alcoholics and in pregnancies associated with severe vomiting. The high intake of calories solely derived from carbohydrate is associated with neuropsychiatric manifestations, including confusion, coma, ophthalmoplegia, nystagmus, ataxia, psychosis, and emotional disturbances.

Although thiamin deficiency in infants may be either acute or chronic, the acute cardiac symptoms and signs generally predominate.[14] Anorexia, apathy, vomiting, restlessness, and pallor progress to dyspnea and cyanosis from cardiomegaly and congestive heart failure causing death in 24 to 48 hours. Acute cardiac failure at 4 days of age was the presenting sign in one infant whose mother was thiamin deficient.[22] Cardiac beriberi also has been reported in an adolescent girl who received an inadequate dose of thiamin while receiving TPN.[20]

"Infantile" beriberi may occur between one and four months of age in breastfed infants whose mothers have a deficient thiamin intake.[21] Maternal signs of thiamin deficiency, however, may not be apparent. Infantile beriberi also has been associated with maternal alcoholism and with improperly prepared or inadequately supplemented formula.[23-25] Symptoms generally include weak swallowing, nuchal rigidity, apnea, spasticity, ophthalmoplegia, hypothermia, and coma. The infant with beriberi may have a characteristically aphonic cry because of paralysis of the recurrent laryngeal nerve. A pseudomeningitic phase characterized by bulging fontanelle, seizures, and coma also has been reported.[6,23,24]

Large doses of thiamin have been included in treatments for metabolic disorders, including a variant of maple syrup urine disease, Leigh's encephalopathy, thiamin-responsive megaloblastic anemia, and an abnormality in pyruvate decarboxylase characterized clinically by severe lactic acidosis.[6]

	Premature Infant Formula	Postdischarge Formula	Term Infant Formula
Energy (kcal)	810	730	670
Thiamin (µg)	1600-2000	1500-1600	500-700
Riboflavin (µg)	2400-5000	1100-1500	940-1010
Niacin (mg)	32-40	15	6.7-7.0
Vitamin B_6 (µg)	1200-2000	730-750	400
Folate (µg)	280-300	190	100
Vitamin B_{12} (µg)	2-4	2-3	1.7-2.0
Pantothenic acid (mg)	10-15	6	3.0-3.3
Biotin (µg)	32-300	45-70	20-30
Vitamin C (mg)	160-300	110-120	60-80
Based on: Enfamil (Mead Johnson Nutritionals, Evansville, IN) Similac (Ross Laboratories, Columbus, OH)			

Table 3: Milk concentrations of water-soluble vitamins (units/L).

Recommended Intakes

The need for thiamin is directly related to the amount of metabolizable carbohydrate consumed. The minimum intake of the vitamin, 140 to 200 µg/day, was proposed because marked decreases in the urinary excretion of thiamin occurred in infants at intakes below this level.[26]

The thiamin intake of full-term breastfed infants appears satisfactory, and thiamin deficiency in breast-fed infants of well-nourished mothers has not been reported.[27] An Adequate Intake (AI) is used as a goal for intake by infants (Table 4).[11] The AI has the following assumptions: a reference milk intake of 780 ml/day and body weight of 7 kg. Based on the content of thiamin in human milk, the AI for infants 0 to 6 months is 200 µg/day or approximately 30 µg/kg/day.

Because of the variability in milk composition, the potential need for milk banking (which may include heat-treatment of the milk), and the greater energy needs for growth, the available thiamin in human milk may be inadequate for premature infants. The intakes of thiamin from fortified human milk or preterm formula are approximately 8-fold greater than from unfortified human milk (Table 5). It appears that a reasonable enteral intake of thiamin for premature infants of approximately 300 µg/kg/day will maintain normal thiamin status.[28 29]

Full-term infants and children are thiamin sufficient during parenteral nutrition (TPN) following parenteral thiamin hydrochloride intakes of 1200 µg/day (130 µg/100 kcal).[30] Elevated whole blood thiamin concentrations after 50 and 115 days of TPN are reported in children receiving 1500 to 4500 µg/day.[31] Premature infants receiving 780 µg/day thiamin hydrochloride (970 µg/100 kcal, 720 µg/kg/day) were thiamin-sufficient as assessed by the transketolase assay, although that method of assessment does not distinguish sufficient from excessive concentrations.[30] In one study, an intake of 510 µg/kg/day was associated with 1/16 infants manifesting biochemical thiamin deficiency by the transketolase assay.[28] However, other studies with intakes of approximately 500 µg/kg/day were not

	Units/day*	Units/kg/day**
Thiamin (μg)	200	30
Riboflavin (μg)	300	40
Niacin, preformed (mg)	2	0.2
Vitamin B₆ (μg)	100	14
Folate (μg)	65	9.4
Vitamin B₁₂ (μg)	0.4	0.05
Pantothenic acid (mg)	1.7	0.2
Biotin (μg)	5	0.7
Vitamin C (mg)	40	6

* Based on average human milk content between 0 and 6 months and a milk intake of 780 ml/day.[11]
** Based on a 7 kg body weight.[11]

Table 4: Adequate Intakes (AI) of water-soluble vitamins for full-term infants.[11,36,56,69,91,110,123,127,140]

associated with any evidence of deficiency.[32]

The American Medical Association Nutritional Advisory Group recommendation for full-term infants, 1.2 mg/day, appears appropriate (Table 6).[33,34] A practical dose for premature infants (based on 2 ml/kg/d of either MVI-Pediatric or Infuvite, Tables 6-7) is 480 μg/kg/day, but a reasonable parenteral intake of thiamin (if there are reformulations of the current vitamin mixtures) is as low as 350 μg/kg/day.[32,34]

Toxicity

Thiamin toxicity is rare. Excess parenteral doses in adults, however, have been reported to produce respiratory depression.[35] Anaphylaxis may occur with rapid intravenous administration.

Riboflavin (Vitamin B₂)

General Metabolism

The coenzymes of riboflavin, flavin mononucleotide (FMN) and flavin adenine dinucleotide (FAD), function as electron donors and acceptors in biological oxidation-reduction systems. They are intimately involved with a number of enzymatic reactions affecting the metabolism of glucose, fatty acids, and amino acids. In the intestinal mucosa, riboflavin is phosphorylated to riboflavin-5'-phosphate (also known as FMN) and further phosphorylated and adenylated to FAD. Vitamin absorption is reduced in biliary obstruction and in conditions that decrease intestinal transit time.[15] The predominant mode of excretion is via the kidney, with secondary excretion through the biliary tract.

Sources

The riboflavin concentration increases slightly during lactation (Tables 1, 2).[36,12] Vitamin supplementation is reflected in a greater milk riboflavin concentration than when deficiency exists.[19,37-39] The riboflavin contents of full-term and preterm human milk are similar. Earlier analyses of human milk reported higher values for riboflavin content because the total flavin was measured, only 67% of which is riboflavin.[36] Thus, latest estimates suggest that 350 μg/L be used for average milk content in the first 6 months of lactation.[36]

Riboflavin and its phosphates are decomposed by exposure to light and in strong alkaline solutions.[40,41] The concentration of riboflavin is reduced by 50% after 8 hours of indirect sunlight.[42] Since parenteral MVI-Pediatric (Astra Pharmaceuticals) contains riboflavin-5-phosphate, photodegradation reportedly is less of a problem. However, during parenteral administration, the compound is dephosphorylated to riboflavin and, therefore, becomes susceptible to photodegradation.[43] Riboflavin is resistant to heat, acid, and oxidation. The processes of pasteurization, evaporation, and condensation of milk do not destroy the vitamin.[44]

Laboratory Assessment

The classic method for assessment of riboflavin deficiency is the activity of the enzyme erythrocyte glutathione reductase (EGR) before and after FAD administration. An activation coefficient of 1.2 or greater (20% increase) strongly suggests a deficient state.[45] The urinary excretion of riboflavin decreases in

Component (units/kg/day)	Unfortified Human Milk	Fortified Human Milk or Preterm Formula
Intake (ml)	200	150
Thiamin (µg)	30 - 45	250 - 350
Riboflavin (µg)	70 - 115	350 - 750
Niacin (mg)	0.4 - 0.5	4.5 - 6.0
Vitamin B_6 (µg)	25 - 65	180 - 300
Folate (µg)	15 - 30	40 - 50
Vitamin B_{12} (µg)	0.05 - 0.20	0.3 - 1.0
Pantothenic acid (mg)	0.4 - 0.5	1.5 - 2.5
Biotin (µg)	1 - 2	4 - 45
Vitamin C (mg)	5 - 20	25 - 45

Table 5: Water-soluble vitamin intakes from unfortified human milk and fortified human milk or preterm formula.

the early stages of deficiency. Plasma and red blood cell riboflavin, FMN, and FAD concentrations, however, may be preferable to distinguish deficiency from toxicity states.[17,46]

Deficiency

Generally, a deficiency of riboflavin occurs in conjunction with more generalized malnutrition and deficiencies of other vitamins. Ariboflavinosis is characterized by angular stomatitis, glossitis, cheilosis, seborrheic dermatitis around the nose and mouth, and eye changes which include reduced tearing, photophobia, corneal vascularization, and cataracts. Because these coenzymes are involved in the metabolism of Vitamin B_6, the conversion of tryptophan to niacin is impaired in their absence.

Overt signs of deficiency are rare in inhabitants of developed countries. However, the biochemical evidence of subclinical riboflavin deficiency has been identified in infants undergoing phototherapy for hyperbilirubinemia and in children with chronic cardiac disease.[44,47-49] Phototherapy treatment for hyperbilirubinemia especially in breastfed newborn infants has been associated with subclinical biochemical riboflavin deficiency.[40-42,50-52] As xanthine oxidase is a riboflavin-dependant enzyme, low uric acid concentrations also may be observed in phototherapy-induced riboflavin deficiency.

Recommended Intakes

Riboflavin is interrelated with protein metabolism, but riboflavin needs are based on caloric intake because of practical considerations, such as the close relationship between protein and calories and the similarity to the estimation of thiamin needs.[14] Healthy, breastfed full-term infants have satisfactory riboflavin status.[27,47] Based on the content of riboflavin in human milk, the AI for infants 0 to 6 months is 300 µg/day or approximately 40 µg/kg/day.[36]

Premature infants may have greater riboflavin needs due to their frequent need for phototherapy. Exposure of stored milk to light also may reduce the amount of the vitamin available to the infant. For these reasons, as

	Full-term infants and children (units/day)	Premature infants (units/kg/day)*	Premature infants Best estimate (units/kg/day)**
Thiamin (μg)	1200	80	350
Riboflavin (μg)	1400	560	150
Niacin (mg)	17	6.8	5
Vitamin B₆ (μg)	1000	400	180
Folate (μg)	140	56	56
Vitamin B₁₂ (μg)	1.0	0.4	0.30
Pantothenic acid (mg)	5	2.0	2.0
Biotin (μg)	20	8.0	6.0
Vitamin C (mg)	80	32	25

* Based on 2 ml/kg/d of either MVI-Pediatric or Infuvite, Table 7, not to exceed full-term infant dose.

** A more realistic dose of multivitamin mixtures are reformulated, not to exceed full-term infant dose.

Table 6: Parenteral intakes of water-soluble vitamins for infants and children.[34]

well as their greater energy needs for growth, the riboflavin intake for the premature infant fed human milk is inadequate.[48,51,52] The intakes of riboflavin from fortified human milk or preterm formula are nearly 6-fold greater than from unfortified human milk (Table 5). Urinary riboflavin excretion is diminished in very low birth weight infants and the plasma half-life is prolonged even at 28 days of age.[53] For these reasons some investigators have suggested that enteral intakes of riboflavin be 150 to 300 μg/kg/day.[53] However, other investigators have demonstrated that urinary riboflavin increases with postnatal age and that a reasonable enteral riboflavin intake of 450 (range 300 to 700) μg/kg/day is appropriate.[28,29,32]

Full-term infants and children receiving TPN are riboflavin sufficient if they receive 1400 μg/day (150 μg/100 kcal) of the vitamin.[30] Whole blood riboflavin concentrations after 50 and 115 days of TPN are adequate in children receiving 1800 to 5400 μg/day.[31]

Premature infants who received 900 μg/day (1180 μg/100 kcal, 830 μg/kg/day) had elevated riboflavin concentrations, especially if less than 1 kg birth weight.[30,46] The high plasma concentrations may result in renal accumulation and renal toxicity.[46] Despite potential photodegradation, it has been suggested that that dose is excessive. The markedly elevated concentrations probably reflect excessive intake and poor renal clearance of riboflavin by premature infants.[43]

The recommendation for the riboflavin content of TPN for full-term infants is 1400 μg/day.[52] A practical dose for premature infants (based on 2 ml/kg/d of either MVI-Pediatric or Infuvite) (Tables 6 & 7) is 560 μg/kg/day, but a more reasonable parenteral riboflavin intake (if there are reformulations of the current vitamin mixtures) is 150 μg/kg/day.[32,34,43]

	MVI-Pediatric*	Infuvite-Pediatric**	Cernivite***
Volume (ml)	5	4+1	5
Thiamin (μg)	1200	1200[4]	3520
Riboflavin (μg)	1400	1400[4]	4140
Niacin (mg)	17	17[4]	46
Vitamin B_6 (μg)	1000	1000[4]	4520
Folate (μg)	140	140[1]	420
Vitamin B_{12} (μg)	1.0	1.0[1]	6
Pantothenic acid (mg)	5	5[4]	17.2
Biotin (μg)	20	20[1]	69
Vitamin C (mg)	80	80[4]	125

* Astra Pharmaceuticals, Wayne, PA.
** Baxter (Deerfield, IL): Provides 2 vials, 4 ml and 1 ml; [4]amount per 4 ml vial; [1]amount per 1 ml vial.
*** Baxter (Maurepaul, France).

Table 7: Commercial preparations of water-soluble vitamins for parenteral nutrition in infants.

Toxicity

There are no clearly defined toxic effects of riboflavin. Riboflavin does produce a yellow coloration of the urine.[35] A potentially toxic effect of excess parenteral riboflavin intake was reported in a premature infant. Precipitation of riboflavin and obstructive uropathy were observed in an infant who had plasma riboflavin concentrations 100-fold greater than cord blood concentrations.[46] This complication is similar to what is described as the toxicity of riboflavin in rats.

Niacin

General Metabolism

The term niacin refers to the compound nicotinic acid and its amide form, nicotinamide (niacinamide). The vitamin is biologically active as a component of the coenzymes nicotinamide adenine dinucleotide (NAD) and nicotinamide adenine dinucleotide phosphate (NADP). The coenzymes are important in two-electron transfers and are involved in multiple metabolic processes, including fat synthesis, intracellular respiratory metabolism, and glycolysis.[54,55] The physiologic need for niacin is related to energy expenditure, because of the involvement of NAD and NADP in the respiratory chain.

Because dietary tryptophan is converted to niacin, the tryptophan content of the diet also must be considered when describing the needs for niacin. Tryptophan pyrrolase converts tryptophan eventually to kynurenine and after multiple additional conversions to niacin. The conversion is catalyzed by riboflavin and Vitamin B_6. Generally, niacin needs are described as niacin equivalents (NE). One niacin equivalent (NE) equals 60 mg tryptophan or 1 mg niacin.[19,54] Tryptophan accounts for 1.5% of the amino acids in milk protein.[54]

Sources

The concentration of niacin in human milk remains stable throughout lactation (Table 2).[12,56] If the mother is malnourished, niacin supplementation will increase the concentration in the milk.[39] Approximately 70% of the total niacin equivalents (NE) in human milk are derived from tryptophan. The tryptophan content of human milk, 220 mg/L provides 3.8 NE/L. The sum of preformed niacin and niacin equivalents derived from tryptophan in human milk is approximately 5.7 NE/L.[19] Most commercial formulas tabulate the content of preformed niacin. Niacin is stable in foods and can withstand heating and prolonged storage.[55]

Laboratory Assessment

Niacin is converted in the liver to multiple metabolites prior to its excretion in the urine. The measurement of the urinary excretion of niacin metabolites, N^1-methylniacinamide and N^1-methyl-6-pyridone-3-carboxamide ("pyridone"), is considered a good method for diagnosing niacin deficiency.[14,55,57] Although the excretion of the pyridone decreases earlier in niacin deficiency, it is the most difficult to assay. The ratio of N^1-methylniacinamide to creatinine in random urine samples is an easier tool for assessment.[14] Serum N^1-metabolites and nicotinamide can be assayed fluorimetrically.[55]

Deficiency

Corn contains a poorly absorbed form of niacin and its tryptophan content is low. A deficiency of niacin results in the clinical syndrome pellagra, a disease endemic to areas where corn is the primary staple.[54,55,57,58] The deficiency disease is characterized by weakness, lassitude, dermatitis, inflammation of mucous membranes, diarrhea, vomiting, dysphagia, and in severe cases, dementia, and death (the "4 Ds"). Initially, cutaneous inflammation looks like a sunburn because only areas exposed to light are affected. Alkaline treatment of corn (eg, the addition of lime water to corn in the preparation of corn tortillas as practiced in Mexico and Central America) will make niacin more bioavailable.[59]

A familial disorder of tryptophan-niacin metabolism, Hartnup's disease, is an impaired absorption of monoamino/monocarboxylic acids, including tryptophan, which responds to niacin supplementation. This entity has been characterized as a pellagra-like photosensitive skin rash, cerebellar ataxia, emotional instability, and aminoaciduria.[14,15,55,57,58,60]

Recommended Intakes

In infants, niacin status, as assessed by urinary excretion of niacin metabolites, was normal when fed 6 NE/day but not 4 NE/day.[61] The distribution of preformed niacin vs. tryptophan-derived niacin in milks for infant has not been studied in relation to the estimated needs of this vitamin. For infants in the first 6 months after birth, the AI is based on the intake of preformed niacin. Based on the content of preformed niacin in human milk, the AI for infants 0 to 6 months is 2 mg/day or approximately 0.2 mg/kg/day.[56] For premature infants, the intakes of niacin from fortified human milk or preterm formula are 10-fold greater than from unfortified human milk (Table 5). A reasonable range of enteral niacin intakes is 4.5 to 6.0 mg/kg/day.

Full-term infants and children who receive 17 to 60 mg/day of nicotinamide in TPN have adequate niacin status.[30,31] Premature infants receiving 11 mg/day were niacin-sufficient.[30] Although exogenous niacin needs may decrease if dietary tryptophan is excessive, the small amount of tryptophan available in pediatric parenteral nutrition formulations probably would not alter recommendations.

The recommendation for parenteral niacin intake in full-term infants and children is 17 mg/day.[34] A practical dose for premature infants (based on 2 ml/kg/d of either MVI-Pediatric or Infuvite) (Tables 6 & 7) is 6.8 mg/kg/day, but a more reasonable parenteral niacin intake (if there are reformulations of the current vitamin mixtures) is 5 mg/kg/day.[34]

Toxicity

Excessive intakes of nicotinic acid in adults (which has been used as a pharmacologic agent to lower blood lipid concentrations) can cause cutaneous vasodilation, flushing, headache, pruritus, liver disease, skin rash, hyperuricemia, gastrointestinal ulcers, and impaired glucose tolerance.[33,62] However, nicotinamide (niacinamide) is not a cholesterol-lowering agent and does not have the same side effects. It is the latter form that is used in pediatric preparations.

Pyridoxine (Vitamin B$_6$)

General Information

"Pyridoxine," or Vitamin B$_6$, refers collectively to three naturally occurring pyridines--pyridoxine (PN, pyridoxol), pyridoxal (PL), and pyridoxamine (PM)--and their phosphorylated derivatives.[63] The vitamin is phosphorylated in the liver where conversion of pyridoxine to pyridoxal and 4-pyridoxic acid (4-PA), the major excretory product, occurs. In the blood, the dominant forms of the vitamin are PL, PN, PLP (pyridoxal-5-phosphate), and 4-PA.

In the phosphorylated form (primarily PLP), Vitamin B$_6$ plays a key role in metabolism by acting as a coenzyme in interconversion reactions of amino acids, conversion of tryptophan to niacin and serotonin, neurotransmitter synthesis and metabolic reactions in the brain, carbohydrate metabolism, immune system development, and the biosynthesis of heme and prostaglandins.[63] There is a relationship between Vitamin B$_6$ and protein metabolism, so it has been customary to consider the ratio of the vitamin/protein when assessing needs. The usual ratio of Vitamin B$_6$/protein is 15 µg/g; the two standard deviation lower limit is 11 µg/g.[64] In adults with Vitamin B$_6$ deficient diets, abnormalities of tryptophan and methionine metabolism develop faster and Vitamin B$_6$ concentrations decline more rapidly when protein intakes are high.[64] During repletion studies, tryptophan and methionine metabolism and plasma vitamin concentrations normalize faster at low protein intakes. Similarly, infants with B$_6$ deficiency and seizures have some relief of symptoms with high carbohydrate diets and have exacerbations of symptoms with high protein diets.[64]

High dietary protein intakes and the destruction of Vitamin B$_6$ by light both increase Vitamin B$_6$ needs. Heat destruction of the PL and PM vitamers probably was responsible for Vitamin B$_6$ deficiency in infants

fed improperly processed formulas.[65] The heat-stable vitamer, pyridoxine hydrochloride, is used for the fortification of commercial infant formulas.

The intake of Vitamin B$_6$ during the last trimester of pregnancy determines the nutritional state of the infant with respect to this vitamin.[66-68]

Sources

The Vitamin B$_6$ content of human milk reflects the Vitamin B$_6$ nutritional status of the mother (Table 1).[12,69] Milk Vitamin B$_6$ content of women not receiving vitamin supplements is approximately 140 µg/L (Table 2). Greater milk Vitamin B$_6$ concentrations are reported in mothers who take Vitamin B$_6$ supplements.[12] The Vitamin B$_6$/protein ratio in milk, 8.5 to 30 µg/g, depends upon the maternal intake of Vitamin B$_6$.[70-75]

Laboratory Assessment

Quantitative assays for total Vitamin B$_6$ generally employ the microbiological assay of *Saccharomyces uvarum*.[71-73,76] Methods for the assessment of Vitamin B$_6$ nutritional status include the plasma PLP concentration, the tryptophan load test, the measurement of 4-PA excretion, and the measurement of erythrocyte activity of aspartate aminotransferase (glutamic-oxalacetic transaminase) and alanine aminotransferase (glutamic-pyruvic transaminase).[17,67] The erythrocyte glutamic-pyruvic transaminase index (EGPT) measures the enzyme activity before and after the addition of PLP. Normal individuals have an index of less than 1.25.[67,73]

Deficiency

In infants, dietary deprivation or malabsorption of Vitamin B$_6$ results in hypochromic microcytic anemia, vomiting, diarrhea, failure to thrive, listlessness, hyperirritability, and seizures. In adults, Vitamin B$_6$ deficiency may result in depression, confusion, peripheral neuritis, electroencephalograph abnormalities, and seizures.[65-67,71,72] As protein intake increases, the onset of vitamin deficiency becomes more rapid.

Clinical Vitamin B$_6$-deficiency, manifested by seizures, has been reported in infants who were fed an improperly sterilized milk, which partially destroyed the vitamin.[77,78] Seizures were noted when Vitamin B_6 intakes were 60 μg/day.[64] A dose of Vitamin B_6, 260 μg/day, cured the seizure disorder, but 300 μg/day normalized tryptophan metabolism.[64,77] Whether the higher dose is beneficial for all infants is unclear, because intakes of milk with Vitamin B_6 concentrations of 100 μg/L did not result in any deficiency symptoms.[79]

Several conditions are associated with abnormalities in Vitamin B_6 metabolism that require pharmacologic doses of the vitamin for adequate function. These Vitamin B_6-dependency syndromes include the following conditions: pyridoxine-dependent seizures in the neonate, pyridoxine-responsive hypochromic microcytic anemia, xanthurenic aciduria, cystathioninuria, and homocystinuria. For these conditions, massive doses of the vitamin, 200 to 600 mg/day, have been given.[62] Routine Vitamin B_6 supplementation is recommended for infants and children receiving isoniazid and for breastfed infants whose mothers receive isoniazid.[6]

Recommended Intakes

If the Vitamin B_6 intake of a mother is adequate, the healthy breastfed full-term infant has sufficient stores of the vitamin to meet its needs during the first weeks of life. Based on the content of Vitamin B_6 in human milk, the AI for infants 0 to 6 months is 100 μg/day or approximately 14 μg/kg/day.[69] The human milk-fed premature infant would not receive adequate Vitamin B_6.[80] The intakes of Vitamin B_6 from fortified human milk and preterm formula are approximately 5-fold greater than from unfortified human milk (Table 5). A reasonable range of enteral Vitamin B_6 intakes is 180 to 300 μg/kg/day.

No deficiency of Vitamin B_6 was observed in full-term infants and children receiving 1000 to 3000 μg/day of pyridoxine hydrochloride in TPN.[30,31] When premature infants received 650 μg/day or 850 mg/100 kcal, no deficiencies were observed.[30,81] However, as computed based on energy intakes, it is unclear whether the doses for premature infants are excessive. Although there is a concern that premature infants <30-weeks gestation may be unable to convert parenterally administered pyridoxine to PLP, when given parenteral pyridoxine at doses of 300 to 700 μg/day, conversion of pyridoxine to other B_6 vitamers is observed.[82] Therefore, it is suggested that PLP may not be the appropriate indicator for vitamin B6 status in premature infants < 30 weeks gestation.[83]

The recommended parenteral intake of Vitamin B_6 in full-term infants is 1000 μg/day.[34] A practical intake for premature infants (based on 2 ml/kg/d of either MVI-Pediatric or Infuvite) (Tables 6 & 7) is 400 μg/kg/day, but a more reasonable parenteral Vitamin B_6 intake (if there are reformulations of the current vitamin mixtures) is 180 μg/kg/day.[34]

Toxicity

Toxicity from large doses of the vitamin is rare. A sensory neuropathy occurs in adults taking large doses of the vitamin for a long period of time.[84]

Folate

General Metabolism

Folate is the general term that describes compounds having nutritional and chemical properties similar to folic acid (pteroylglutamic acid, PGA). The parent compound is a pteridine moiety joined to para-aminobenzoic acid. Reduction of the pyrazine ring to yield tetrahydrofolate, addition of multiple glutamyl residues, and acquisition of one-carbon fragments result in activation of the vitamin. The coenzyme participates in the biosynthesis of purines and pyrimidines, the metabolism of some amino acids, and the catabolism of histidine.[85,86]

Dietary folate occurs predominantly as polyglutamate, usually as 5-methyl or 10-formyl pteroylpolyglutamate, which is hydrolyzed to the monoglutamate by the intestinal mucosa prior to absorption.[86] Zinc deficiency will decrease the conjugase activity, resulting in decreased folate uptake.[87] Folate homeostasis is regulated, at least in part, by the enterohepatic cycle.[88] Because the biliary folate content is large, enterohepatic recirculation results in a long half-life of the vitamin.[85,89,90] The vitamin is synthesized by colonic bacteria.[19]

Sources

The folate content of human milk increases through lactation, but an average value of 85 µg/L is used.[12,91] Folate supplementation will increase the concentration of the vitamin in the milk of women who are malnourished.[39,74,92] Differences in folate concentrations between fore- and hindmilk have been reported.[93] Goat milk, containing 6 µg/L, is an inadequate source of folate.[86,89] The vitamin is inactivated by heat, canning, and light exposure.[45]

Laboratory Assessment

Folate status is assessed by evaluating concentrations of the vitamin in serum and red blood cells. Erythrocyte folate is less variable and is useful for assessing adequacy of long-term intake. Urinary excretion of FIGLU (formiminoglutamate), an intermediate in the metabolism of histidine to glutamic acid, is an indicator of folate deficiency. Mean red blood cell volume (MCV) and the degree of granulocyte nuclear segmentation also are used to assess status.

Deficiency

Nutritional folate deficiency results in growth retardation, anemia, and abnormalities in neurological status and small intestinal morphology.[94] In a population of infants who consumed boiled and pasteurized bovine milk, which has a low folate concentration, supplementation of the vitamin was shown to improve growth at 4 to 6 months of age despite the absence of hematologic markers of deficiency.[95] Folate deficiency has been identified more commonly in small-for-gestational-age infants.[96] Correction of a folate-deficient maternal diet resulted in a 50% decrease in the incidence of small-for-gestational age infants in India.[89] The fall in serum folate observed in the neonatal period reflects an increased need for folate for DNA and RNA synthesis.[97] Certain medications, eg, phenobarbital, phenytoin, and sulfasalazine may increase the need for the vitamin. Requirements for folate increase during pregnancy, periods of intense hematopoiesis, and growth.[45] The premature infant appears to have several risk factors for folate deficiency: diminished hepatic stores, rapid growth, increased

erythropoeisis, use of antibiotics, use of anticonvulsants, and potential for malabsorption.[98] Data from three randomized trials of folate vs no folate intakes in premature infants indicated that supplementation was associated with an increase in red cell folate concentration and an increase in hemoglobin by 1 g%, but no increase in the incidence of anemia.[98]

Low folate concentrations are encountered in Vitamin B_{12} deficiency. Treatment with folate may improve the hematologic manifestations of Vitamin B_{12} deficiency, but will not affect the progressive neurologic degeneration associated with that deficiency state. Iron deficiency may lead to decreased utilization of folate.[99] Folic acid therapy may inhibit zinc absorption.[100]

The hematological manifestations of folate deficiency include hypersegmentation of neutrophils (more than 5% of granulocytes have more than 5 segments), megaloblastosis, and anemia.[86,89,96] The sequential changes due to ingestion of a folate-deficient diet have been described in adults.[89] The earliest finding, after three weeks of a deficient intake, is a low serum folate concentration. Continued deficient intake results in hypersegmentation of neutrophils by 5 weeks. At 13 weeks, there is increased urinary FIGLU excretion. A diminished red cell folate concentration is noted by 17 weeks, and megaloblastosis and anemia are evidenced by 20 weeks. Although megaloblastic anemia is reported in premature infants, anemia is a late sign of folate deficiency. Other more subtle changes in red cells and neutrophils are more sensitive indicators of deficiency in premature infants.

The incidence of congenital neural tube defects may be associated with preconceptional folate deficiency.[101,102] Significantly lower concentrations of red cell folate in mothers delivering infants with neural tube defects compared with control mothers have been reported.[103] Women who took multivitamin preparations during the periconceptional period appear to have a lower risk of delivering an infant with a neural tube defect than women who did not take multivitamins.[104] Folate supplementation even before conception is advisable.[91]

Recommended Intakes

Folate doses as low as 5 mg/kg/day will produce a hematologic response in folate-deficient children and daily doses of 1 to 5 mg are needed for maintenance.[62]

The folate status of healthy breastfed full-term infants appears adequate.[91] Based on the content of folate in human milk, the AI for full-term infants 0 to 6 months is 65 µg/day or approximately 9.4 µg/kg/day.[91] There are conflicting opinions regarding the folate recommendations for the premature infant.[45,94,96,105] No differences in rate of growth and hematological indices were reported in premature infants given folate doses of either 100 µg/day or 3.5 µg/day.[105] Formula-fed premature infants given folate in doses of 65 µg/day for one year have differences in plasma and red cell folate concentrations at 2 to 6 months of age but no differences in growth and hematological indices compared with doses of 15 µg/day.[106] Intakes of approximately 45 to 50 µg/kg/day were associated with adequate plasma folate indices.[29,32] The unfortified human milk-fed premature infant probably would not receive adequate folate.[80] The intakes of folate from fortified human milk and preterm formula are 2- to 3-fold greater than from unfortified human milk (Table 5). A reasonable range for enteral folate intakes is 45 to 50 µg/kg/day.

Folate has been administered in TPN formulations to full-term infants in doses of 140 µg/day (15 µg/ 100 kcal).[30] At those intakes, red blood cell folate concentrations remained unchanged for 7 days, but increased at days 14 and 21. In children who received long-term TPN, red cell folate concentrations remained stable for 5 months. An increase in plasma folate concentrations was observed from 0 to 90 days and with increases in intakes from 200 to 600 µg/day.[31] Red cell and/or plasma folate concentrations in premature infants were somewhat elevated while receiving parenteral doses of 70 to 85 µg/kg/day.[30,32] Parenteral doses of approximately 40 µg/kg/day appeared to correspond with plasma folate concentrations similar to enteral feeding in premature infants.[32]

The recommended TPN folate intake in full-term infants and children is 140 µg/day.[34] A reasonable recommended parenteral folate intake for premature infants is 56 µg/kg/day.[34]

Toxicity

Large doses of folate are infrequent because the vitamin has not been present in large quantities in over-the-counter preparations.[35] Folate may mask Vitamin B_{12} deficiency and depress zinc absorption.[100]

Vitamin B_{12}
General Metabolism

Vitamin B_{12} consists of a corrin ring which is a macrocyclic ring formed by the linkage of four reduced pyrrol rings. In the case of Vitamin B_{12}, the center of the ring is cobalt. Perpendicular to the ring is a nucleotide (5-6 dimethylbenzimidazole) linked to the ring by D-1-amino-2-propanol. "Cobalamin" is used to describe Vitamin B_{12} regardless of the moiety attached to the cobalt. Cyanocobalamin is the synthetic compound used in commercial preparations containing the vitamin. It is not found in significant amounts in food or in the human body and is not metabolically active until the cyanide moiety is removed.

Upon ingestion, Vitamin B_{12} is released from food at gastric pH. It is then complexed with salivary R binder which has greater affinity than intrinsic factor.[107] At the alkaline pH of the upper small bowel, pancreatic enzymes digest the R binder and release Vitamin B_{12}. Intrinsic factor then binds Vitamin B_{12} to facilitate Ca-dependent absorption, at alkaline pH, across ileal mucosa. Within the mucosa, intrinsic factor is replaced by a plasma transport protein.[108] One to three percent of Vitamin B_{12} is absorbed passively. An effective enterohepatic circulation of Vitamin B_{12} accounts for its long half-life.[108] Therefore, unlike other water-soluble vitamins, there is storage of Vitamin B_{12} which may last an adult 3 to 5 years. Hepatic storage of Vitamin B_{12} does relate to the duration of pregnancy, with those infants delivering prematurely having less than one-half of the stores of a full-term infant.[29]

Vitamin B_{12} is active in metabolism in two forms: methylcobalamin and 5-deoxyadenosylcobalamin (coenzyme B_{12}).[109] The methylated version is involved in one-carbon transfers. In particular, Vitamin B_{12}

transfers a methyl group from tetrahydrofolate to homocysteine for the synthesis of methionine. Vitamin B_{12} is necessary for the regeneration of tetrahydrofolate. In Vitamin B_{12} deficiency, folate may be trapped in its demethylated form, and as such it is unavailable for pyrimidine synthesis. This role of Vitamin B_{12} in folate metabolism is responsible for the cellular folate deficiency.

Adenosylcobalamin participates in the reduction of purine and pyrimidine ribonucleotides to their corresponding deoxyribonucleotides necessary for DNA synthesis. The adenosyl form also is necessary for the conversion of methylmalonyl-coenzyme A to succinyl-CoA. In this role, Vitamin B_{12} is a key factor in the metabolism of fat, branched-chain amino acids, and carbohydrate.[109] A lack of Vitamin B_{12} will result in an accumulation of methylmalonic acid with subsequent excretion in the urine.

Sources

The Vitamin B_{12} content of human milk declines from 1.2 µg/L at 1 week to 0.5 µg/L at 6 months of lactation (Table 1). The average concentration in the first 6 months of lactation is approximately 0.6 µg/L Table 2).[12,110] Maternal supplementation with Vitamin B_{12} tends to increase the vitamin content in the milk from the malnourished to the normal state.[39,73,74,111,112] The concentration of Vitamin B_{12} in milk from strict vegetarian women is lower than that reported from women eating a usual diet.[12]

Laboratory Assessment

The most commonly used test for the adequacy of Vitamin B_{12} is serum concentration.[113] Red cell concentrations are less reliable because they overlap between normal and deficient subjects and because they are low in folate and iron deficiency, despite adequate total body stores of Vitamin B_{12}.[114] A functional test of Vitamin B_{12} adequacy is the measurement of methylmalonic acid excretion with or without a loading dose of valine or isoleucine, but this test is less reliable and more complex.[113] The Schilling test also is used in the evaluation of Vitamin B_{12} deficiency. Radiolabeled Vitamin B_{12} is given orally

and urinary excretion of labeled vitamin is measured both in the presence and absence of intrinsic factor. The test measures Vitamin B_{12} absorption and the contribution of intrinsic factor to vitamin malabsorption.[115]

Deficiency

The result of Vitamin B_{12} deficiency is ineffective DNA synthesis, which is evident clinically as megaloblastic anemia and hypersegmentation of neutrophils. In addition, demyelination of the spinal cord is a characteristic feature.[29] The sequential stages in the development of Vitamin B_{12} deficiency have been described.[107]

An association between Vitamin B_{12} and osteoblast-specific proteins has been reported.[116] Vitamin B_{12} deficient adults had lower skeletal alkaline phosphatase activity and lower osteocalcin concentrations in plasma compared with those in control subjects. Changes in the concentrations of those proteins were reported following Vitamin B_{12} therapy.[116]

Because cobalamin stores greatly exceed daily needs, deficiency of this vitamin is encountered rarely. Clinical circumstances which produce Vitamin B_{12} deficiency include lack of intrinsic factor (pernicious anemia, post-gastrectomy, destruction of gastric mucosa), small bowel bacterial overgrowth, specific intestinal mucosal defects leading to malabsorption (celiac disease, ileal resection), inborn errors of metabolism, and drug interactions. Inadequate Vitamin B_{12} status may result from a vegan diet.[108,117-119]

In adults, the deficiency state is characterized by weakness, anemia, congestive heart failure, glossitis, lemon-colored skin, and neurological conditions: paresthesias, degeneration of posterior and lateral columns of the spinal cord, and peripheral neuritis.[117-119]

Vitamin B_{12} deficiency is reported in exclusively breastfed infants whose mothers are strict vegans and take no vitamin supplements.[117] Delayed developmental milestones, coma, and hematologic findings (megaloblastic anemia, neutropenia, and thrombocytopenia) are the presenting findings. Urinary excretion of methylmalonic acid, glycine, methylcitric acid, and homocystine are elevated. A dramatic response to intramuscular Vitamin B_{12} is reported.[117] Elevated urinary methylmalonic acid concentrations in lactating vegan women and in their infants decline following Vitamin B_{12} therapy in infants and mothers.[119] Oral doses as little as 0.1 µg/day, however, will correct or prevent a deficiency state in the breastfed infant of a vegan.[108]

Resection of the terminal ileum, such as may occur as a result of necrotizing enterocolitis, may impair Vitamin B_{12} absorption. Six of 14 children who had undergone ileal resection for necrotizing enterocolitis had evidence of malabsorption of the vitamin.[120] In these circumstances, therapy with parenteral Vitamin B_{12} is needed every 1 to 3 months.[62]

Recommended Intakes

Unless the maternal diet is deficient or conditions exist which impair maternal vitamin absorption, the breastfed infant will have an adequate Vitamin B_{12} status. Based on the content of Vitamin B_{12} in human milk, the AI for infants 0 to 6 months is 0.4 µg/day or approximately 0.05 µg/kg/day.[110] No deficiencies have been reported in preterm infants fed human milk. The intakes of Vitamin B_{12} from fortified human milk and preterm formula are 5-fold greater than from unfortified human milk (Table 5). Vitamin B_{12} intakes of 0.6 µg/kg/day have been associated with elevated plasma concentrations of the vitamin.[29] Despite the lack of data demonstrating any toxicity of the vitamin, it has been suggested that a reasonable enteral intake for premature infants is approximately 0.3 µg/kg/day to avoid excessive plasma concentrations.[29,32]

Vitamin B_{12} status during TPN has been reported for full-term infants receiving 1 µg/day (0.1 µg/100 kcal).[30] Those infants maintained Vitamin B_{12} concentrations above reference controls, but these values tended to decline toward baseline cord blood values after 21 days of therapy. During the long-term administration of TPN in children, Vitamin B_{12} concentrations remained above reference controls, especially while receiving doses of 2.5 to 7.5 µg/day.[30,31] The serum Vitamin B_{12} concentration of premature infants receiving 0.65 µg/day (0.85 µg/100 kcal, 0.6 µg/kg/day) remained elevated

throughout a 28-day study.[30] In a short-term study, parenteral intakes of 0.35 µg/kg/day were associated with elevated plasma vitamin concentrations in 40% of premature infants.[32]

The recommended parenteral intake of Vitamin B_{12} in full-term infants and children of 1 µg/day possibly is excessive, and a dose of 0.75 µg/day may be more appropriate.[34] The practical intake of Vitamin B_{12} (based on 2 ml/kg/d of either MVI-Pediatric or Infuvite) (Tables 6 & 7) is 0.40 µg/kg/day, but a more reasonable parenteral Vitamin B_{12} intake (if there are reformulations of the vitamin mixtures) is 0.3 µg/kg/day.[32,34]

Toxicity

There are no reports of Vitamin B_{12} toxicity.

Pantothenic Acid
General Metabolism

The pantothenic acid molecule consists of β-alanine joined to pantoic acid (2,4-dihydroxy-3, 3-dimethyl-butyric acid) by an amide bond. It serves as an integral part of coenzyme A, which functions in acyl group transfers in the synthesis of fatty acids, cholesterol, and steroids; the oxidation of fatty acids, pyruvate, and α-ketoglutarate; and in other acetylation reactions.[19,60,121,122] The plasma concentration of pantothenic acid in cord blood is several-fold greater than maternal blood.[121]

Sources

The concentration of pantothenic acid in mature human milk is approximately 2.0 mg/L (Table 2).[12,123] Supplementation of malnourished women or consumption of extremely large quantities of the vitamin results in increases in the milk content of pantothenic acid.[39,124,125]

Laboratory Assessment

Plasma concentrations may be measured.[34]

Deficiency

Because of the ubiquitous distribution of this vitamin, a specific clinical deficiency syndrome has not been reported.[122] The essential biologic role of pantothenic acid was defined in animal experiments, but extraordinary circumstances were required to produce the deficiency in man. For example, experimental deficiency has been produced in volunteers fed the antagonist ω-methyl-pantothenic acid as part of a pantothenic acid-deficient diet.[122] Subjects developed burning feet, gastrointestinal disturbances, headache, insomnia, fatigue, and muscle weakness. A deficiency of pantothenic acid also is observed in severe malnutrition. Pantothenic deficiency is considered to have caused the "burning feet syndrome" described in World War II prisoners in the Far East.[122]

Recommended Intakes

Pantothenic acid status has not been a problem in full-term and premature infants fed human milk. Based on the content of pantothenic acid in human milk, the AI for infants 0 to 6 months is 1.7 mg/day or approximately 0.2 mg/kg/day.[123] The intakes of pantothenic acid from fortified human milk and preterm formula are 4- to 5-fold greater than from unfortified human milk. A reasonable enteral pantothenic acid intake for premature infants is approximately 2 mg/kg/day.

The vitamin needs during TPN have been evaluated in a small number of children.[30] Full-term infants and children who received 5 mg/day maintained stable plasma concentrations for 21 days; premature infants who received 3.2 mg/day (2.9 mg/kg/day) demonstrated slightly elevated plasma concentrations relative to their baseline and to controls.

The recommendation for parenteral pantothenic acid, 5 mg/day, is appropriate for full-term infants and children.[34] A reasonable parenteral pantothenic acid intake of 2.0 mg/kg/day would provide adequate vitamin status for premature infants.[34]

Toxicity

Pantothenic acid toxicity has not been reported. High doses may be associated with water retention and diarrhea.[35] Anorexia, vomiting, hypotension, personality changes, and increased deep tendon reflexes also have been associated with ingestion of high doses of the vitamin.[62]

Biotin
General Metabolism

Biotin functions as a coenzyme for carboxylation, decarboxylation, and transcarboxylation reactions. As such, it plays an important role in the biosynthesis of amino and fatty acids and as a cofactor in gluconeogenesis. Urinary excretion reflects dietary intake; fecal excretion, generally unaffected by intake, indicates enteric synthesis.[19,126]

Sources

The average biotin content of human milk rises from the first week of lactation to later lactation (Table 1).[12] The average biotin concentration in mature human milk is 6.0 µg/L (Table 2).[12,127] Dietary supplementation of malnourished women will result in a rise in the biotin content of the milk.[6]

Laboratory Assessment

Plasma biotin concentration commonly is assayed by microbiological methods and by competitive binding assays using avidin.[115]

Deficiency

In individuals fed normal diets, a deficiency of biotin is unlikely to occur. A deficiency state is observed, however, when gastrointestinal flora is suppressed or when biotin absorption is diminished, such as occurs in diets consisting of raw eggs.[126,128] Symptoms of biotin deficiency include anorexia, nausea, glossitis, pallor, mental changes, alopecia, and a fine maculosquamous dermatitis which becomes exfoliative.[60,129,130] Biotin deficiency has been reported in patients with short gut syndrome when the vitamin was omitted from TPN solutions.[128-131] A young girl receiving TPN for six months reportedly developed a scaly dermatitis, alopecia, pallor, irritability, lethargy, and markedly reduced urinary excretion and plasma concentration of biotin.[130] Administration of biotin corrected the abnormalities. Biotin-dependent carboxylase deficiency states have been described. The multiple carboxylase defect (pyruvate carboxylase, propionyl carboxylase, acetyl-CoA-carboxylase, and methylcrotonyl CoA carboxylase) has been shown to be biotin responsive.[60] Antibiotics may affect biotin status by decreasing enteric synthesis of the vitamin.[128]

Recommended Intakes

Biotin deficiency has not been reported in infants fed either human milk or formulas despite a wide range of intakes. Based on the content of biotin in human milk, the AI for infants 0 to 6 months is 5 µg/day or approximately 0.7 µg/kg/day.[127] The intakes of biotin from fortified human milk and preterm formula are 4 to 20-fold greater than from unfortified human milk (Table 5). A reasonable range of enteral biotin intakes for premature infants is 4 to 40 µg/kg/day.

The vitamin needs during TPN have been investigated.[30,31] Full-term infants and children receiving 20 to 90 µg/day maintained stable, adequate plasma biotin concentrations for as long as 90 days. Premature infants receiving 13 µg/day (12 µg/kg/day) had elevated plasma biotin concentrations, tenfold greater than controls, during sampling intervals over a 28-day period.

The recommendation for TPN biotin intake for full-term infants and children is 20 µg/day.[34] A practical recommendation for parenteral biotin intake is 8.0 µg/kg/day, but a more reasonable parenteral biotin intake is 6.0 µg/kg/day for premature infants.[34]

Toxicity

There are no reports of biotin toxicity.

Vitamin C

General Information

The two principal forms of Vitamin C are L-ascorbic acid and the oxidized form, dehydroascorbic acid. L-ascorbic acid, the biologically more active form of the vitamin, is an antioxidant and accelerates hydroxylation reactions in many biosynthetic processes.[132] Vitamin C functions in the hydroxylation of lysine and methionine to carnitine, the synthesis of norepinephrine from dopamine, the conversion of tryptophan in serotonin metabolism, and the catabolism of tyrosine. The latter action particularly is important to the premature infant because Vitamin C enhances the activity of the immature hepatic enzyme, p-hydroxyphenylpyruvic acid oxidase, which increases the catabolism of tyrosine.[132-134] Transient tyrosinemia resulting from Vitamin C deficiency and/or high tyrosine or protein intakes was a common problem for premature infants in the past.[60,134,135]

Vitamin C is involved in the synthesis of neurotransmitters. The human fetal brain contains 4 to 11 times the content of Vitamin C found in the adult brain.[136] The brain Vitamin C content declines with increasing gestational age, but the content remains three-fold greater than that in adults even after four weeks of age. The significance of the brain Vitamin C concentration is unclear, but suggests that the provision of adequate Vitamin C to the premature infant may be important. The rise in serum Vitamin C concentrations reported after intraventricular hemorrhage in premature infants may be a marker of the disruption of the blood brain barrier.[15,137] As an antioxidant, Vitamin C may be important to the high-risk premature infant exposed to hyperoxic environments and mechanical ventilation.[15,132,133] Vitamin C also acts as a pro-oxidant under certain conditions, such as if free iron is available.[3] Exposure of milk to copper, iron, and oxygen will reduce Vitamin C concentrations. The plasma Vitamin C concentration is reported to decline during febrile and gastrointestinal illnesses.

Placental transfer results in a greater concentration of Vitamin C in the fetus and in cord blood than in the mother.[134] Vitamin C deficiency has been reported, however, in the offspring of mothers who were clinically Vitamin C deficient.[138]

Vitamin C is excreted in the urine primarily as oxalic acid. At moderate intakes, urinary excretion is the main source of elimination. At high intakes, the urinary excretion of the vitamin increases, and with intakes above 3 g/day, the fecal excretion of the vitamin rises and protects against excessive intakes.[132,139]

Sources

The Vitamin C concentration of human milk generally is stable during lactation, averaging 50 mg/L.[12,140] A 20% decline in milk concentration is reported after 6 to 25 months of lactation.[141,142] When the diet of a lactating mother is supplemented with Vitamin C, an increase in milk concentration of the vitamin occurs if her diet had been deficient in Vitamin C.[39,143,144] The availability of Vitamin C is influenced by its physical characteristics. The Vitamin C content of human milk is reduced 90% by pasteurization.[132,145] Storage time, temperature, and oxidation affect Vitamin C concentrations. The Vitamin C content of pooled human milk is 50% lower than that of fresh milk.[145]

Laboratory Assessment

Plasma and leukocyte Vitamin C concentrations reflect recent intake of the vitamin and are reported most often in assessments of vitamin status. Acceptable plasma Vitamin C values are >0.6 mg/dL; values below 0.2 mg/dL are observed in scurvy.[132,134] Subclinical Vitamin C deficiency is likely when the concentration of Vitamin C in leucocytes is below 100 µg/g.[45]

Deficiency

A deficiency of Vitamin C results in scurvy. Scurvy, the first dietary deficiency disease to be recognized, was not a matter of concern for infants until the end of the 19th century when the use of pasteurized milk and commercial formulas became prevalent. Infantile scurvy was observed in affluent families who purchased prepared infant formulas. The initial description of scurvy in premature infants was associated with the exclusive feeding of pooled, pasteurized human milk.[145]

The earliest clinical manifestation of scurvy in adults is petechial hemorrhage, which indicates increased capillary fragility.[134] A classical manifestation of scurvy in adults is failure of wound healing. In that situation, collagen fibrils and intercellular cement are deposited improperly, and bone growth ceases. Infantile scurvy is manifested by irritability and tenderness, swelling, and pseudoparalysis of the lower extremities. Enlargement of the costochondral junction (scorbutic rosary) is observed in scurvy and may be confused with rickets.[60]

Characteristic radiologic abnormalities indicating a cessation of osteogenesis and marked bony changes, hyperkeratosis of hair follicles, and mental status changes characterize the progression of the illness.[60,146] Hemorrhagic manifestations in children include bleeding at the site of tooth eruption, bloody diarrhea, epistaxis, ocular bleeding, and petechiae at pressure points. Anemia, secondary to bleeding, decreased iron absorption, and abnormal folate metabolism, is a common finding.[133] Sepsis and failure to thrive are characteristics of premature infants reported with scurvy.

Recommended Intakes

The Vitamin C needs of full-term infants are obtained from estimates of the availability of the vitamin from human milk. Breastfed full-term infants appear to be saturated with respect to their Vitamin C needs.[134,141] Formula-fed, full-term infants require a minimum Vitamin C supplement of 10 mg/day to prevent scurvy.[132,134] Based on the content of Vitamin C in human milk, the AI for infants 0 to 6 months is 40 mg/day or approximately 6.0 mg/kg/day.[140]

Vitamin C intakes in premature infants of less than 5 mg/kg/day result in a marked decline of plasma concentrations, from 1.56 to 0.48 mg/dL during the first fourteen days.[147] Normal plasma concentrations are maintained in premature infants, however, when enteral feedings supplemented with Vitamin C (5 to 10 mg/kg/day) are begun by five days of age.[147] The Vitamin C needs of the premature infant may be similar to the full-term infant unless large quantities of tyrosine and/or protein (>5 g/kg/day) are administered. To prevent hypertyrosinemia a daily intake of 75 to 100 mg of Vitamin C has been suggested for premature infants who receive high protein intakes.[134,135] Because protein intakes of 5 to 6 g/kg/day are no longer recommended, this problem is of less significance today than in the past.[27] Furthermore, serum tyrosine concentrations in premature infants fed human milk and whey-dominant formulas are lower than those of similar infants fed casein-dominant formulas, which are not used for feeding premature infants today.[148] The intakes of Vitamin C from fortified human milk and preterm formula are 2- to 5-fold greater than unfortified human milk. There are theoretical reasons to support greater intakes of Vitamin C in premature infants because they: require a greater protein intake; may have reduced Vitamin C stores due to limited placental transfer early in the last trimester; have a rapid rate of growth; and need a greater intake of antioxidants. Intakes of approximately 30 mg/kg/day were associated with adequate plasma Vitamin C concentrations.[28] A reasonable enteral intake of Vitamin C for premature infants is 30 to 40 mg/kg/day.

Parenteral Vitamin C needs have been evaluated. Plasma Vitamin C concentrations were maintained in an adequate range in full-term infants and children who received 80 mg Vitamin C daily in TPN.[30] Premature infants, however, who received 52 mg of Vitamin C daily (48 mg/kg/day) for 28 days had plasma concentrations two- to three-fold greater (3.2 to 2.6 mg/dL) than their baseline and those of full-term infants.[30,137] Plasma values were highest in the infants with birthweights <1 kg. However, other investigators found that parenteral Vitamin C intakes of approximately 30 mg/kg/day were associated with borderline low plasma Vitamin C concentrations in infants whose average birthweight was 1.3 kg and postnatal age 2 weeks.[28]

The recommended parenteral Vitamin C intake for full-term infants and children is 80 mg/day.[34] The practical parenteral Vitamin C intake for premature infants (based on 2 ml/kg/d of either MVI-Pediatric or Infuvite) (Tables 6 & 7) is 32 mg/kg/day.[34] A more reasonable parenteral Vitamin C intake is 25 mg/kg/day, half the dose used in the above evaluations.[30,34] This dose, however, is not available with current parenteral vitamin preparations, without significantly affecting the intakes of other vitamins.

Toxicity

Prolonged intakes of Vitamin C in adults, >1.0 g/day, may cause oxaluria, uricosuria, and acidification of the urine.[33] Theoretically, renal calculi may result from these changes. High doses may result in false positive tests for urinary glucose, occult blood in feces, exacerbations of glucose-6-phosphate deficiency, and alterations in the bactericidal functions of white blood cells. The phenomenon of rebound scurvy has been reported in adults who reduce their high vitamin intakes abruptly.[35,133,139] The rebound effect also has been reported in infants born to mothers who took large doses of the vitamin during pregnancy.[33,60,132] Large doses of Vitamin C may decrease the absorption of Vitamin B_{12} and copper and increase the absorption of iron. Vitamin C also functions as a pro-oxidant, increasing free radical formation.

Conclusion

The best assessment of water-soluble vitamin needs for full-term infants is based on the human milk-fed infant in whom deficiencies of water-soluble vitamins are rare. The deficiencies that arise in human milk-fed infants generally result from inadequacies in the maternal diet.

When we consider the variability in the concentrations of vitamins in human milk, it is curious that the human milk-fed infant is protected from deficiencies of water-soluble vitamins.[149] Because we employ human milk as a model, the lack of consistency in vitamin concentrations makes precise recommendations difficult. For these reasons, ample allowances are given for infant formula guidelines.

Unfortunately, adequate data are lacking to assess the water-soluble vitamin needs for the premature infant. Indeed, the doses administered are extraordinarily high compared with body weight adjusted doses for full-term infants. Although there are newer parenteral vitamin formulations (Table 7) no preparation meets the best, and lower, estimate for the premature infant.

Acknowledgments

I appreciate the secretarial assistance of Idelle Tapper. This work is a publication of the US Department of Agriculture (USDA)/Agricultural Research Service (ARS) Children's Nutrition Research Center, Department of Pediatrics, Baylor College of Medicine and Texas Children's Hospital, Houston, TX. The contents of this publication do not necessarily reflect the views or policies of the U.S. Department of Agriculture, nor does mention of trade names, commercial products, or organizations imply endorsement by the U.S. Government.

References

1. King JC. Vitamin requirements during pregnancy. In: Campbell DM, Billmer MDG (eds): *Nutrition in Pregnancy*. London, The Royal College of Obstetricians and Gynaecologists 1983; 33-45.

2. Chessex P, Lavoie J-C, Laborie S, Rouleau T. Parenteral multivitamin supplementation induces both oxidant and antioxidant responses in the liver of newborn guinea pigs. *J Pediatr Gastroenterol Nutr* 2001;32: 316-321.

3. Chessex P, Laborie S, Lavoie J-C, Rouleau T. Photoprotection of solutions of parenteral nutrition decreases the infused load as well as the urinary excretion of peroxides in premature infants. *Semin Perinatol* 2001;25:55-59.

4. Dostalova L. Correlation of the vitamin status between mother and newborn during delivery. *Dev Pharmacol Ther* 1982;4:45-57.

5. Link G, Zempleni J. Intrauterine elimination of pyridoxal 5'-phosphate in full-term and preterm infants. *Am J Clin Nutr* 1996;64:184-189.

6. Moran JR, Greene HL. The B Vitamins and Vitamin C in human nutrition I. General considerations and "obligatory" B Vitamins. *Am J Dis Child* 1979;l33: l92-l99.

7. Rindi G, Venura U. Thiamine intestinal transport. *Physiol Rev* 1972;52:821-827.

8. Gubler CJ. Thiamin. In: Machlin LJ ed *Handbook of Vitamins*. New York, NY: Marcel Dekker, Inc.; 1991; 233-282.

9. Davis RE, Icke GC. Clinical chemistry of thiamin. *Adv Clin Chem* 1983;23:93-140.

10. Itokawa Y, Cooper JR. Ion movements and thiamin. II. Release of the vitamin from membrane fragments. *Acta Biochim Biophys* 1970;196:274-284.

11. Institute of Medicine. Thiamin. In: Panel on folate - other B Vitamins and choline (ed): *Dietary Reference Intakes for Thiamin, Riboflavin, Niacin, Vitamin B6, Folate, Vitamin B12, Pantothenic Acid, Biotin, and*

12. Picciano MF. Vitamins in Milk. A. Water-soluble vitamins in human milk. In: Jensen RG ed: *Handbook of Milk Composition*. San Diego, Academic Press; 1995; 675-688.

13. Pratt JP, Hamil BM, Moyer EZ, Kaucher M, Roderuck C, Coryell MN, Miller S, Williams HH, Macy IG. Metabolism of women during the reproductive cycle. XVIII. The effect of multi-vitamin supplements on the secretion of B vitamins in human milk. *J Nutr* 1951;44:141-157.

14. Goldsmith GA. Vitamin B complex. Thiamine, riboflavin, niacin, folic acid (folacin), Vitamin B_{12}, biotin. *Prog Food Nutr Sci* 1975;1:559-609.

15. Schanler RJ, Nichols BL. The water soluble Vitamins C, B_1, B_2, B_6, and niacin. In: Tsang RC (ed): *Vitamin and Mineral Requirements in Preterm Infants*. New York, Marcel Dekker, Inc; 1985; 39-62.

16. McCormick DB. Thiamin. In: Shils ME, Young VR (eds): *Modern Nutrition in Health and Disease*. Philadelphia, PA: Lea and Febiger; 1988; 355-361.

17. Powers JS, Zimmer J, Meurer K, Manske E, Collins JC, Greene HL. Direct assay of vitamins B_1, B_2, and B_6 in hospitalized patients: relationship to level of intake. *JPEN* 1993;17:315-316.

18. Heller S, Salkeld RM, Korner WF. Vitamin B_1 status in pregnancy. *Am J Clin Nutr* 1974;27:1221-1224.

19. National Research Council (U.S), Subcommittee on the Tenth Edition of the RDAs. *Recommended Dietary Allowances*, Tenth ed. Washington, DC, National Academy Press, 1989.

20. La Selve P, Demolin P, Holzapfel L, Blanc PL, Teyssier G, Robert D. Shoshin beriberi: an unusual complication of prolonged parenteral nutrition. *J Parenter Enteral Nutr* 1986;10:102-103.

21. Rascoff H. Beriberi heart in a 4 month old infant. *JAMA* 1942;120:1292-1293.

22. King EQ. Acute cardiac failure in the newborn due to thiamine deficiency. *Exp Med Surg* 1967;25:173-177.

23. Wyatt DT, Noetzel MJ, Hillman RE. Infantile beriberi presenting as subacute necrotizing encephalomyelopathy. *J Pediatr* 1987;110:888-891.

24. Van Gelder DW, Darby FU. Congenital and infantile

beriberi. *J Pediatr* 1944;25:226-235.

25. Cochrane WA, Collins-Williams C, Donohue WL. Superior hemorrhagic polioencephalitis (Wernicke's Disease) occurring in an infant--probably due to thiamine deficiency from use of a soya bean product. *Pediatrics* 1961;28:771-777.

26. Holt LE, Jr., Nemir RL, Snyderman SE, Albanese AA, Ketron KC, Guy LP, Carretero R. The thiamine requirement of the normal infant. *J Nutr* 1949;37: 53-66.

27. American Academy of Pediatrics, Committee on Nutrition. Nutritional needs of low-birth-weight infants. *Pediatrics* 1985;75:976-986.

28. Friel JK, Bessie JC, Belkhode SL, Edgecombe C, Steele-Rodway M, Downton G, Kwa PG, Aziz K. Thiamine, riboflavin, pyridoxine, and Vitamin C status in premature infants receiving parenteral and enteral nutrition. *J Pediatr Gastroenterol Nutr* 2001;33:64-69.

29. Friel JK, Andrews WL, Long DR, Herzberg G, Levy R. Thiamine, riboflavin, folate, and Vitamin B$_{12}$ status of infants with low birth weights receiving enteral nutrition. *J Pediatr Gastroenterol Nutr* 1996;22: 289-295.

30. Moore MC, Greene HL, Phillips B, Franck L, Shulman RJ, Murrell JE, Ament ME. Evaluation of a pediatrics multiple vitamin preparation for total parenteral nutrition in infants and children. I. Blood levels of water-soluble vitamins. *Pediatrics* 1986;77:530-538.

31. Marinier E, Gorski AM, Potier de Courcy G, Criqui C, Bunodiere M, Christides JP, Bourgeay, Causse M, Brion F, Ricour C, Navarro J. Blood levels of water soluble vitamins in pediatric patients on total parenteral nutrition using a multiple vitamin preparation. *J Parenter Enteral Nutr* 1989;13:176-184.

32. Levy R, Herzberg GR, Andrews WL, Sutradhar B, Friel JK. Thiamine, riboflavin, folate, and Vitamin B$_{12}$ status of low birth weight infants receiving parenteral and enteral nutrition. *J Parenter Enteral Nutr* 1992;16:241-247.

33. American Medical Association, Council on Scientific Affairs. Vitamin preparations as dietary supplements and therapeutic agents. *JAMA* 1987;257:1929-1936.

34. Greene HL, Hambidge KM, Schanler RJ, Tsang RC. Guidelines for the use of vitamins, trace elements, calcium, magnesium, and phosphorus in infants and children receiving total parenteral nutrition: report of the Subcommittee on Pediatric Parenteral Nutrient Requirements from the Committee on Clinical Practice Issues of The American Society for Clinical Nutrition. *Am J Clin Nutr* 1988;48:1324-1342.

35. Alhadeff L, Gualtieri CT, Lipton M. Toxic effects of water soluble vitamins. *Nutr Rev* 1984;42:33-40.

36. Institute of Medicine. Riboflavin. In: Panel on folate - other B vitamins and choline (ed): *Dietary Reference Intakes for Thiamin, Riboflavin, Niacin, Vitamin B6, Folate, Vitamin B12, Pantothenic Acid, Biotin, and Choline.* Washington DC, National Academy Press; 1998; 87-122.

37. Nail PA, Thomas MR, Eakin R. The effect of thiamin and riboflavin supplementation on the level of those vitamins in human breast milk and urine. *Am J Clin Nutr* 1980;33:198-204.

38. Hughes J, Sanders TAB. Riboflavin levels in the diet and breast milk of vegans and omnivores. *Proc Nutr Soc* 1979;38:95A.

39. Deodhar AD, Rajalakshmi R, Ramakrishnan CV. Studies on human lactation - Part III: Effect of dietary vitamin supplementation on vitamin contents of breast milk. *Acta Paediatr* 1964;53:42-48.

40. Bates CJ, Liu DS, Fuller NJ, Lucas A. Susceptibility of riboflavin and vitamin A in breast milk to photodegradation and its implications for the use of banked breast milk in infant feeding. *Acta Paediatr Scand* 1985;74: 40-44.

41. Fritz I, Said H, Harris C, Murrell J, Greene HL. A new sensitive assay for plasma riboflavin using high performance liquid chromatography. *J Am Coll Nutr* 1987;6:449-449.

42. Chen MF, Boyce HW, Triplett L. Stability of the B vitamins in mixed parenteral nutrition solution. *J Parenter Enteral Nutr* 1983;7:462-464.

43. Porcelli PJ, Greene HL, Adcock EW. Retinol (vitamin A) and riboflavin (vitamin B2) administration and metabolism in very low birth weight infants. *Semin Perinatol* 1992;16:170-180.

44. Cooperman JM, Lopez R. Riboflavin. In: Machlin LJ (ed): *Handbook of Vitamins.* New York, Marcel Dekker, Inc.; 1991; 283-310.

45. Wharton BA. Nutrition and feeding of preterm infants. Oxford, Blackwell Scientific Publications, 1987.

46. Baeckert PA, Greene HL, Fritz I, Oelberg DG, Adcock EW. Vitamin concentrations in very low birth weight infants given vitamins intravenously in a lipid emulsion: measurement of vitamins A, D, E, and riboflavin. *J Pediatr* 1988;113:1057-1065.

47. Hovi L, Hekali R, Siimes MA. Evidence of riboflavin depletion in breast-fed newborns and its further acceleration during treatment of hyperbilirubinemia by phototherapy. *Acta Paediatr Scand* 1979;68:567-570.

48. Sisson TR. Photodegradation of riboflavin in neonates. *Fed Proc* 1987;46:1883-1885.

49. Lopez R, Cole HS, Montoya F, Cooperman JM. Riboflavin deficiency in a pediatric population of low socioeconomic status in New York City. *J Pediatr* 1975;105:420-422.

50. Horwitt MK. Interpretations of requirements for thiamin, riboflavin, niacin- tryptophan, and vitamin E plus comments on balance studies and vitamin B6. *Am J Clin Nutr* 1986;44:973-86.

51. Ronnholm KAR. Need for riboflavin supplementation in small preterms fed with human milk. *Am J Clin Nutr* 1986;43:1-6.

52. Lucas A, Bates C. Transient riboflavin depletion in preterm infants. *Arch Dis Child* 1984;59:837-841.

53. Porcelli PJ, Rosser ML, DelPaggio D, Adcock EW, Swift L, Greene H. Plasma and urine riboflavin during riboflavin-free nutrition in very-low-birth-weight infants. *J Pediatr Gastroenterol Nutr* 2000;31:142-148.

54. McCormick DB. Niacin. In: Shils ME, Young VR (eds): *Modern Nutrition in Health and Disease.* Philadelphia, Lea and Febiger; 1988; 370-375.

55. Hankes LV. Nicotinic acid and nicotinamide. In: Machlin LJ (ed): *Handbook of Vitamins.* New York, Marcel Dekker, Inc. pp 329-377, 1984.

56. Institute of Medicine. Niacin. In: Panel on folate - other B vitamins and choline (ed): *Dietary Reference Intakes for Thiamin, Riboflavin, Niacin, Vitamin B6, Folate, Vitamin B12, Pantothenic Acid, Biotin, and Choline.* Washington DC, National Academy Press; 1998; 123-149.

57. Darby WJ, McNutt KW, Todhunter EN. Niacin. *Nutr Rev* 1975;33:289-97.

58. Spivak JL, Jackson DL. Pellagra: an analysis of 18 patients and a review of the literature. *Johns Hopkins Med J* 1977;140:295-309.

59. Moran JR, Greene HL. Nutritional biochemistry of water-soluble vitamins. In: Grand RJ, Sutphen JL, Dietz WH, Jr. (eds): *Pediatric Nutrition Theory and Practice.* Stoneham, Butterworth Pub.; 1987; 51-67.

60. Moran JR, Greene HL. The B Vitamins and Vitamin C in human nutrition. II: 'Conditional' B Vitamins and Vitamin C. *Am J Dis Child* 1979;133:308-314.

61. Holt LE, Jr. The adolescence of nutrition. *Arch Dis Child* 1956;31:427-438.

62. Udall JN, Jr., Greene HL. Vitamin update. *Pediatr Rev* 1992;13:185-194.

63. Lumeng L, Li TK, Lui A. The interorgan transport and metabolism of Vitamin B6. In: Reynolds RD, Leklem JE (eds): *Vitamin B6: Its Role in Health and Disease.* New York, Alan R. Liss, Inc.; 1985; 35-54.

64. Bender DA. Vitamin B6 requirements and recommendations. *Eur J Clin Nutr* 1989;43:289-309.

65. Fomon SJ. *Nutrition of Normal Infants.* St. Louis, Mosby-Year Book, Inc., 1993.

66. Contractor SF, Shane B. Blood and urine levels of Vitamin B6 in the mother and fetus before and after loading of the mother with Vitamin B6. *Am J Obstet Gynecol* 1970;107:635-640.

67. Driskell JA. Vitamin B6. In: Machlin LJ (ed): *Handbook of Vitamins.* New York, Marcel Dekker, Inc.; 1984; 379-401.

68. Heiskanen K, Siimes MA, Perheentupa J, Salmenpera L. Risk of low Vitamin B6 status in infants breast-fed exclusively beyond six months. *J Pediatr Gastroenterol Nutr* 1996;23:38-44.

69. Institute of Medicine. Vitamin B6. In: Panel on folate - other B Vitamins and choline (ed): *Dietary Reference Intakes for Thiamin, Riboflavin, Niacin, Vitamin B6, Folate, Vitamin B12, Pantothenic Acid, Biotin, and Choline.* Washington DC, National Academy Press; 1998; 150-195.

70. Thomas MR, Sneed SM, Wei C. The effects of Vitamin C, Vitamin B6, Vitamin B12, folic acid, riboflavin, and thiamin on the breast milk and maternal status of well-nourished women at 6 months postpartum. *Am J Clin Nutr* 1980;33:2151-2156.

71. Styslinger L, Kirksey A. Effects of different levels of Vitamin B_6 supplementation on Vitamin B_6 concentrations in human milk and Vitamin B_6 intakes of breastfed infants. *Am J Clin Nutr* 1985;41:21-31.

72. Borschel MW, Kirksey A, Hannemann RE. Effects of Vitamin B_6 intake on nutriture and growth of young infants. *Am J Clin Nutr* 1986;43:7-15.

73. Thomas MR, Kawamoto J, Sneed SM, Eakin R. The effects of Vitamin C, Vitamin B_6, and Vitamin B_{12} supplementation on the breast milk and maternal status of well- nourished women. *Am J Clin Nutr* 1979;32:1679-1685.

74. Sneed SM, Zane C, Thomas MR. The effects of ascorbic acid, Vitamin B_6, Vitamin B_{12}, and folic acid supplementation on the breast milk and maternal nutritional status of low socioeconomic lactating women. *Am J Clin Nutr* 1981;34:1338-1346.

75. West KD, Kirksey A. Influence of Vitamin B_6 intake on the content of the vitamin in human milk. *Am J Clin Nutr* 1976;29:961-969.

76. Kirksey A, Udipi SA. Vitamin B_6 in human pregnancy and lactation. In: Reynolds RD, Leklem JE (eds): *Vitamin B_6: Its Role in Health and Disease*. New York, Alan R. Liss, Inc.; 1985; 57-77.

77. Bessey OA, Adam DJD, Hansen AE. Intake of Vitamin B_6 and infantile convulsions: A first approximation of requirements of pyridoxine in infants. *Pediatrics* 1957;20:33-44.

78. Molony CJ, Parmelee AH. Convulsions in young infants as a result of pyridoxine (Vitamin B_6) deficiency. *J Am Med Assoc* 1954;154:405-406.

79. Borschel MW. Vitamin B_6 in infancy: requirements and current feeding practices. In: Raiten DJ (ed): *Vitamin B_6 Metabolism in Pregnancy, Lactation, and Infancy*. Boca Raton, CRC Press; 1995; 109-124.

80. McCoy E, Strynadka K, Brunet K. Vitamin B_6 intake and whole blood levels of breast and formula fed infants: serial whole blood Vitamin B_6 levels in premature infants. In: Reynolds RD, Leklem JE (eds): *Vitamin B_6: Its Role in Health and Disease*. New York, Alan R. Liss, Inc.; 1985; 79-96.

81. Bank MR, Kirksey A, West K, Giacoia G. Effect of storage time and temperature on folacin and Vitamin C levels in term and preterm human milk. *Am J Clin Nutr* 1985;41:235-242.

82. Andon MB, Reynolds RD, Moser PB, Raiten D, Robbins S. Impaired ability of premature infants 29 wks gestational age to convert pyridoxine to pyridoxal phosphate. *Fed Proc* 1987;46:1016.

83. Raiten DJ, Reynolds RD, Andon MB, Robbins ST, Fletcher AB. Vitamin B_6 metabolism in premature infants. *Am J Clin Nutr* 1991;53:78-83.

84. Schaumburg H, Kaplan J, Windebank A, Vick N, Rasmus S, Pleasure D, Brown MJ. Sensory neuropathy from pyridoxine abuse - A new megavitamin syndrome. *N Engl J Med* 1983;309:445-448.

85. Brody T. Folic acid. In: Machlin LJ (ed): *Handbook of Vitamins*. New York, Marcel Dekker, Inc.; 1991; 453-489.

86. Davis RE. Clinical chemistry of folic acid. *Adv Clin Chem* 1986;25:233-94.

87. Tamura T, Shane B, Baer MT, King JC, Margen S, Stokstad ELR. Absorption of mono- and polyglutamyl folates in zinc-depleted man. *Am J Clin Nutr* 1978;31:1984-1987.

88. Hillman RS, McGuffin R, Campbell C. Alcohol interference with the folate enterohepatic cycle. *Trans Assoc Am Phys* 1977;90:145-156.

89. Herbert V. Recommended dietary intakes (RDI) of folate in humans. *Am J Clin Nutr* 1987;45:661-70.

90. Herbert V, Das KC. The role of Vitamin B_{12} and folic acid in hemato- and other cell-poiesis. *Vitam Horm* 1976;34:1-30.

91. Institute of Medicine. Folate. In: Panel on folate - other B Vitamins and choline (ed): *Dietary Reference Intakes for Thiamin, Riboflavin, Niacin, Vitamin B_6, Folate, Vitamin B_{12}, Pantothenic Acid, Biotin, and Choline*. Washington DC, National Academy Press; 1998; 196-305.

92. Metz J, Zalusky R, Herbert V. Folic acid binding by serum and milk. *Am J Clin Nutr* 1968;21:289-297.

93. Brown CM, Smith AM, Picciano MF. Forms of human milk folacin and variation patterns. *J Pediatr Gastroenterol Nutr* 1986;5:278-82.

94. Ek J. Folic acid and Vitamin B_{12} requirements in premature infants. In: Tsang RC (ed): *Vitamin and Mineral Requirements in Preterm Infants*. New York, Marcel Dekker, Inc.; 1985: 23-38.

95. Matoth Y, Zehavi E, Topper E, Klein T. Folate nutrition and growth in infancy. *Arch Dis Child* 1979;54:699-702.

96. Strelling MK, Blackledge DG, Goodall HB. Diagnosis and management of folate deficiency in low birthweight infants. *Arch Dis Child* 1979;54:271-277.

97. Shojania AM, Hornady G. Folate metabolism in newborns and during early infancy. *Pediatr Res* 1970;4:422-426.

98. Specker BL, Demarini S, Tsang RC. Vitamin and mineral supplementation. In: Sinclair JC, Bracken MB (eds): *Effective Care of the Newborn Infant.* Oxford, Oxford University Press; 1992; 161-176.

99. Rodriguez MS. A conspectus of research on folacin requirements of man. *J Nutr* 1978;108:1983-2075.

100. Newman V, Lyon RB, Anderson PO. Evaluation of prenatal vitamin-mineral supplements. *Clin Pharm* 1987;6:770-777.

101. Edwards JH, Holmes-Siedle M, Lindenbaum RH. Vitamin supplementation and neural tube defects. *Lancet* 1982;1:275-276.

102. Rush D. Periconceptional folate and neural tube defect. *Am J Clin Nutr* 1994;59:511S-516S.

103. Smithells RW, Shepard S, Schorah CJ. Vitamin deficiencies and neural tube defects. *Arch Dis Child* 1976;51:944-950.

104. Mulinare J, Cordero JF, Erickson JD, Berry RJ. Periconceptional use of multivitamins and the occurrence of neural tube defects. *J Am Med Assoc* 1988;260:3141-3145.

105. Stevens D, Burman D, Strelling K, Morris A. Folic acid supplementation in low birth weight infants. *Pediatrics* 1979;64:333-5.

106. Ek J, Behneke L, Halvorsen KS, Magnus E. Plasma and red cell folate values and folate requirements in formula-fed premature infants. *Eur J Pediatr* 1984;142:78-82.

107. Herbert V. The 1986 Herman Award Lecture. Nutrition science as a continually unfolding story: the folate and Vitamin B_{12} paradigm. *Am J Clin Nutr* 1987;46:387-402.

108. Herbert V. Recommended dietary intakes (RDI) of Vitamin B_{12} in humans. *Am J Clin Nutr* 1987; 45:671-678.

109. Herbert VD, Colman N. Folic acid and Vitamin B_{12}. In: Shils ME, Young VR (eds): *Modern Nutrition in Health and Disease.* Philadelphia, Lea and Febiger; 1988; 388-416.

110. Institute of Medicine. Vitamin B_{12}. In: Panel on folate - other B Vitamins and choline (ed): *Dietary Reference Intakes for Thiamin, Riboflavin, Niacin, Vitamin B_6, Folate, Vitamin B_{12}, Pantothenic Acid, Biotin, and Choline.* Washington DC, National Academy Press; 1998; 306-356.

111. Sandberg DP, Begley JA, Hall CA. The content, binding, and forms of Vitamin B_{12} in milk. *Am J Clin Nutr* 1981;34:1717-1724.

112. Johnson PR, Jr., Roloff JS. Vitamin B_{12} deficiency in an infant strictly breast-fed by a mother with latent pernicious anemia. *J Pediatr* 1982;100:917-919.

113. Herbert V. Vitamin B_{12}. In: Hegsted DM, Chichester CO, Darby WJ, McNutt KW, Stalvey RM, Stotz EH (eds): *Nutrition Review's Present Knowledge in Nutrition.* New York, Nutrition Foundation; 1976; 191-203.

114. Harrison RJ. Vitamin B_{12} levels in erythrocytes in hypochromic anaemia. *J Clin Path* 1971;24:698-700.

115. Riedel BD, Greene HL. Vitamins. In: Hay WW, Jr. (ed): *Neonatal Nutrition and Metabolism.* St. Louis, Mosby Year Book ; 1991; 143-170.

116. Carmel R, Lau K-HW, Baylink DJ, Saxena S, Singer FR. Cobalamin and osteoblast-specific proteins. *N Engl J Med* 1988;319:70-75.

117. Higginbottom MC, Sweetman L, Nyhan WL. A syndrome of methylmalonic aciduria, homocystinuria, megaloblastic anemia and neurologic abnormalities in a Vitamin B_{12}-deficient breast-fed infant of a strict vegetarian. *N Engl J Med* 1978;299:317-323.

118. Stollhoff K, Schulte FJ. Vitamin B_{12} and brain development. *Eur J Pediatr* 1987;146:201-205.

119. Specker BL, Miller D, Norman EJ, Greene H, Hayes KC. Increased urinary methylmalonic acid excretion in breast-fed infants of vegetarian mothers and identification of an acceptable dietary source of Vitamin B_{12}. *Am J Clin Nutr* 1988;47:89-92.

120. Collins JE, Rolles CJ, Sutton H, Ackery D. B_{12} absorption after necrotizing enterocolitis. *Arch Dis Child* 1984;59:731-734.

121. Gross SJ. Choline, pantothenic acid, and biotin. In: Tsang RC (ed): *Vitamin and Mineral Requirements in Preterm Infants.* New York, Marcel Dekker, Inc.; 1985; 191-201.

122. Fox HM. Pantothenic acid. In: Machlin LJ (ed): *Handbook of Vitamins.* New York, Marcel Dekker, Inc.; 1984; 437-458.

123. Institute of Medicine. Pantothenic Acid. In: Panel on folate - other B Vitamins and choline (ed): *Dietary Reference Intakes for Thiamin, Riboflavin, Niacin, Vitamin B$_6$, Folate, Vitamin B$_{12}$, Pantothenic Acid, Biotin, and Choline.* Washington DC, National Academy Press; 1998; 357-373.

124. Song WO, Chan GM, Wyse BW, Hansen RG. Effect of pantothenic acid status on the content of the vitamin in human milk. *Am J Clin Nutr* 1984;40: 317-324.

125. Johnston L, Vaughn L, Fox HM. Pantothenic acid content of human milk. *Am J Clin Nutr* 1981;34:2205-9.

126. Roth KS. Biotin in clinical medicine-a review. *Am J Clin Nutr* 1981;34:1967-1974.

127. Institute of Medicine. Biotin. In: Panel on folate - other B Vitamins and choline (ed): *Dietary Reference Intakes for Thiamin, Riboflavin, Niacin, Vitamin B$_6$, Folate, Vitamin B$_{12}$, Pantothenic Acid, Biotin, and Choline.* Washington DC, National American Press; 1998; 374-389.

128. Bonjour JP. Biotin in man's nutrition and therapy-a review. *Int J Vitam Nutr Res* 1977;47:107-118.

129. Hamil BM, Coryell M, Roderuck C, Kaucher M, Moyer EZ, Harris ME, Williams HH. Thiamine, riboflavin, nicotinic acid, pantothenic acid and biotin in the urine of newborn infants. *Am J Dis Child* 1947;74:434-446.

130. Mock DM, DeLorimer AA, Liebman WM, Sweetman L, Baker H. Biotin deficiency: an unusual complication of parenteral alimentation. *N Engl J Med* 1981;304:820-823.

131. Goldsmith SJ, Eitenmiller RR, Feeley RM, Barnhart HM, Maddox FC. Biotin content of human milk during early lactational stages. *Nutr Res* 1982;2:579-583.

132. Olson JA, Hodges RE. Recommended dietary intakes (RDI) of vitamin C in humans. *Am J Clin Nutr* 1987;45:693-703.

133. Levine M. New concepts in the biology and biochemisty of ascorbic acid. *N Engl J Med* 1986;314:892-902.

134. Irwin MI, Hutchins BK. A conspectus of research vitamin C requirements of man (2). *J Nutr* 1976;106:823-879.

135. Light IJ, Berry HK, Sutherland JM. Aminoacidemia of prematurity. *Am J Dis Child* 1966;112:229-236.

136. Adlard BPF, De Souza SW, Moon S. Ascorbic acid in the fetal human brain. *Arch Dis Child* 1974;49: 278-282.

137. Arad ID, Eyal FG. High plasma ascorbic acid levels in preterm neonates with intraventricular hemorrhage. *Am J Dis Child* 1983;137:949-951.

138. Malone JI. Vitamin passage across the placenta. *Clin Perinatol* 1975;2:295-307.

139. Jaffe GM. Vitamin C. In: Machlin LJ (ed): *Handbook of Vitamins.* New York, Marcel Dekker, Inc.; 1984; 199-244.

140. Institute of Medicine. Vitamin C. In: Panel on Dietary Antioxidants and Related Compounds (ed): *Dietary Reference Intakes for Vitamin C, Vitamin E, Selenium, and Carotenoids.* Washington DC, National Academy Press; 2000; 95-185.

141. Salmenpera L. Vitamin C nutrition during prolonged lactation: optimal in infants while marginal in some mothers. *Am J Clin Nutr* 1984;40:1050-1056.

142. Karra MV, Udipi SA, Kirksey A, Roepke JLB. Changes in specific nutrients in breast milk during extended lactation. *Am J Clin Nutr* 1986;43:495-503.

143. Selleg I, King CG. The Vitamin C content of human milk and its variation with diet. *J Nutr* 1936;11: 599-606.

144. Bates CJ, Prentice AM, Prentice A, Lamb WH, Whitehead RG. The effect of Vitamin C supplementation on lactating women in Keneba, a West African rural community. *Int J Vitam Nutr Res* 1983;53:68-76.

145. Ingalls TH. Ascorbic acid requirements in early infancy. *N Engl J Med* 1938;218:872-5.

146. Grewar D. Scurvy and its prevention by Vitamin C fortified evaporated milk. *Can Med Assoc J*

1959;80:977-979.

147. Arad ID, Sagi E, Eyal FG. Plasma ascorbic acid levels
     in preterm infants. *Int J Vitam Nutr Res* 1982;52:
     50-57.

148. Rassin DK, Gaull GE, Raiha NCR, Heinonen K. Milk
     protein quantity and quality in low-birth-weight
     infants. IV. Effects on tyrosine and phenylalanine in
     plasma and urine. *J Pediatr* 1977;90:356-360.

149. Packard VS. Vitamins. In: Packard VS (ed): *Human
     Milk and Infant Formula.* New York, Academic Press
     pp 29-49, 1982.

150. Nutrition Committee, Canadian Paediatric Society.
     Nutrient needs and feeding of premature infants.
     Can Med Assoc J 1995;152:1765-1785.

Water, Sodium, Potassium and Chloride

Ch. Fusch, M.D. and F. Jochum, M.D.

Reviewed by Stephen Baumgart, M.D.

Preface

In the first edition, the nutrients "water, sodium and electrolytes" have been discussed in separate chapters (Chapter 1 "water" and Chapter 8 "sodium and electrolytes"). Because metabolism of electrolytes is closely linked to that of water, both topics are now treated in one chapter. Andrew T. Costarino, Stephen Baumgart and Billy S. Arant were the authors who wrote these two chapters of the previous edition. Their pioneer work is gratefully acknowledged. Some parts of their work have been incorporated into this second edition.

The data and recommendations given in this chapter are based on a literature search using the "Medline" database covering the period from January 1966 until October 2001. Search items used were: "water"; "sodium"; "potassium"; "newborn"; "neonate"; "preterm"; "BPD"; and "PDA", as well as some of their boolean combinations.

Introduction

"Water – the major nutrient" is the title of a review in the "Journal of Pediatrics" that was published by Bent Friis-Hansen in 1982.[84]

Although since then many "new" nutrients have been identified that have an impact on fetal and postnatal growth and well-being (eg, oligosaccharides and nucleotides) water represents the major component of the human body (50-90% of body weight).[83] It is also the major compound of enteral and parenteral nutrition. The "overall" metabolic homeostasis of a mammalian organism depends on intact water metabolism. Water is integral to all life functions. It carries nutrients to the body's cells, removes waste products, and makes up the physico-chemical milieu that allows cellular work to occur. Different from most other nutrients, the human body has no major physiological water stores and therefore needs continuous supply with water to assure the integrity of basal metabolic processes.

Compared with the "state of the art" of neonatology at the period when the first edition of this textbook was written (in 1991), treatment of VLBW preterm infants has further improved during the last decade. The more mature VLBW infants (> 28 weeks of gestational age eg) are today usually in a better condition at birth and experience less aggressive and less compromising support during their adaptation to extrauterine life. Also, very immature infants (gestational age of 24 weeks and below) may now be successfully treated– at least in terms of survival rates.[139]

Water physiology and homeostasis show the highest variation when compared with all other nutritional "ingredients" discussed in this textbook, and depend upon the maturational status (mostly reflected by gestational age) and postnatal age. A VLBW infant at 32 gestational weeks with a birth weight of 1450 gm shows a different physiological behaviour than a 24-week fetus weighing 550 gm. This is caused by differences in body size, proportion, body surface, and skin properties, as well as conditions occuring during the transitional period itself (ie, degree of immaturity and intensity of support needed: like mechanical ventilation vs. nasal continuous positive airways pressure [nCPAP] etc.).

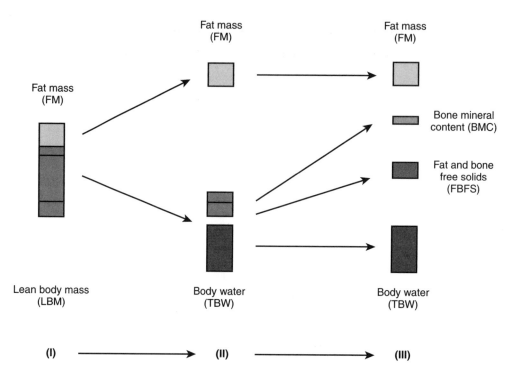

Figure 1: Compartmental models of body composition (I –III). The body may be divided into fat and lean mass (I). Lean mass consists of total body water and the compartment of solids (II). This may be further divided into bone mass (mainly minerals) and the compartment of fat- and bone-free solids (protein, glycogen, DNA etc.) (III).

Knowledge about the physiology of water and electrolyte metabolism is needed for safe administration of fluids and electrolytes, and to adjust these to the actual needs of an infant in order to avoid harm: too low administration may lead to cardiovascular/pulmonary insufficiency and/or metabolic compromise: inappropriate high intake of fluid or electrolytes may lead to or promote conditions like patent ductus arteriosus, bronchopulmonary dysplasia, etc.

Moreover, infants exposed to different intrauterine conditions may have different needs concerning water physiology (polycythemia, impaired renal circulation, and renal function).

It will be the aim of the second edition of this chapter to focus on these developmental aspects of water and electrolyte metabolism and homeostasis.

Body Composition

The human body may be divided in two main compartments: fat mass (FM) and lean body mass (LBM) (Figure 1).

Fat mass (Figures 1 and 2) represents the energy stores of the body. FM is the compartment that is basically free from water and is mainly metabolically "inactive." Energy metabolism occurs only in the cytoplasm of the adipocyte; here, energy is consumed to maintain intracellular adipocyte homeostasis, to store and release triglycerides, as well as to produce hormones like leptin. The major part of the adipocyte is the triglyceride-containing vacuole. The triglyceride moiety is assumed to be free from water. Fat mass is the compartment that shows the highest inter- and intra-individual variation: the fat content of prematurely born infants is approximately 8% as measured with dual energy x-ray absorptiometry and up to 25% at term.[86,88] During later infancy, fat mass accounts for up to 23% of body weight[96]; during adult life mean fat mass is 30% in males and 36% in females.

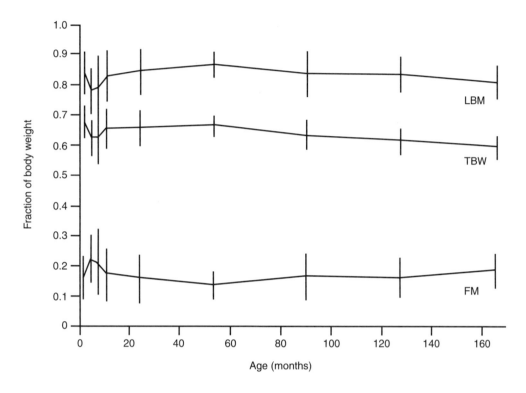

Figure 2: Age-dependent variations of body compartments. Mean and standard deviations of total body water (TBW), lean body (LBM) and fat mass (FM) for different age groups from infancy to adolescence.[87]

Lean body mass (Figure 1) represents the active metabolic cell mass. Here, the major part of body energy is consumed either by substrate oxidation or by mechanisms linked to protein synthesis. The amount of protein synthesis is the sum of newly-synthesized protein needed during periods of growth and protein needed to maintain a steady-state of body cell mass during the regular turnover of body cells.

Water is found only in the lean tissue. The refined body composition model therefore divides the lean mass into the compartment of total body water (TBW) and that containing the fat-free solids (FFS). FFS may be further divided in the compartments of bone minerals (BMC) and of the fat-and bone-free solids (FBFS). This compartment mainly contains protein, glycogen, DNA, etc. (Figure 1).

Metabolism of water and electrolytes is correlated closer with lean mass than with total body mass (or weight). This must be taken into account when subjects with different body composition (eg, percent body fat) are compared (as in SGA versus LGA neonates).

The time course of the water content of the human body during the entire life span is given in the following paragraph.

Note: FM is mainly free from water: the major part of energy-consuming and water-requiring processes occur in LBM. In VLBW infants, FM stores are reduced when compared with that of term newborns, leading to a higher percentage of LBM, and of water in body composition of premature infants.

Total Body Water (TBW)

The amount of body water decreases remarkably from intrauterine life to adulthood (Figure 3). At the age of 24 weeks, the fetus contains about 90% water.[82,226] TBW declines during fetal life to about 75% at 40 weeks of gestational age.[82,226]

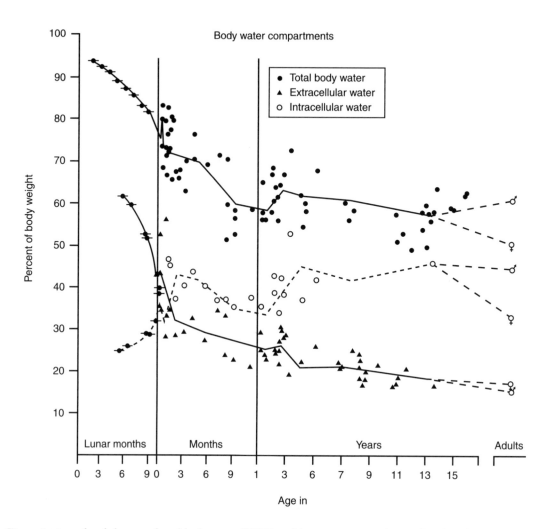

Figure 3: Age-related changes of total body water (TBW) and its compartments (intra- (ICV) and extracellular (ECV) volume) from fetal life until adolescence.[83]

This decrease occurs because fat mass is continuously accumulated during the third trimester of intrauterine development, and because the water content of lean body mass drops.[88]

Until the onset of puberty there are no major differences between male and female subjects. With differences in body composition that develop between genders during sexual maturation (ie, usually more fat mass in females), TBW content shows sex-specific patterns, with a lower water content in females. In later adult life (70 - 80 yrs), TBW of males and females decreases further, down to <60% and 50%, respectively.[212]

Note: The rapid decrease in % TBW observed during intrauterine and early postnatal life is mainly caused by accumulation of new tissues and structural proteins during the phase of organogenesis and body growth. It is also due to the accumulation of fat mass, which has a low water content in relation to other tissues and therefore leads to a lower % TBW.

Body Water Compartments

In order to enhance further understanding of water metabolism and its physiology, one should have a closer look at the different body water pools, because

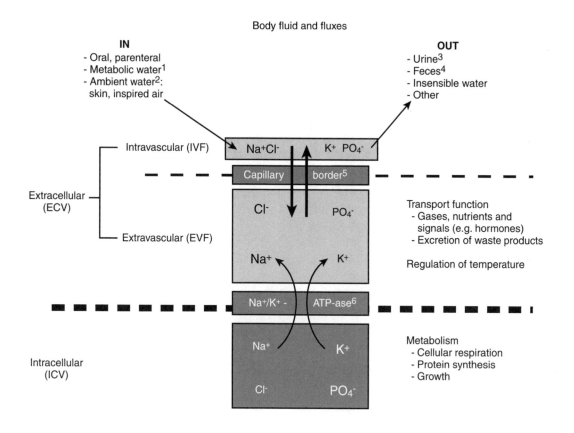

Figure 4: Water and electrolytes: fluxes between body water compartments.
Explanations: 1) Metabolic water production depending on exact intake of carbohydrates, protein and fat (approximately 15 ml water/kg/day), 2) input via skin and inspired air (see page 105), 3) volume depending upon need for excretion of fixed acids and urea and desired urine osmolarity, 4) fecal water losses: quantities are negligibly small in healthy subjects, but considerable in diarrhea and/or in presence of ileostoma (e.g. NEC surgery), 5) oncotic pressure, 6) activity of Na+/K+-ATPase defines the long-term ratio of ECV / ICV; short-term changes are subject to short-term variation of ECV; content of water and electro-/osmolytes: any change in either ICV or ECV osmolarity will result in movement of water into the compartment with the higher osmolarity.

they play different physiological roles and experience different physiological conditions and regulatory mechanisms (Figure 4, Table 1).

Intracellular Fluid (ICF)

The intracellular fluid is that part of body water located within the cellular cytoplasm. It is enveloped by the double-lipid cellular membrane. The leading ion of the ICF is potassium (K^+) (see Figures 4 and 5); it is pumped via the Na^+/K^+-ATPase (see next

paragraph) from the extracellular space into the cytoplasm. Water passively follows ion movements and gradients across compartmental membranes.

The Na^+/K^+-ATPase is one of the major enzyme systems necessary for maintenance of water and electrolyte homeostasis. It establishes the transmembranal Na^+/K^+ gradient, by pumping Na^+ out from cytoplasm, thus keeping intracellular space almost free of Na^+. The enzyme pumps K^+ into the cytoplasm, making cells potentially vulnerable to

	Plasma		Extracellular fluid		Intracellular fluid	
	mval/l	mmol/l	mval/l	mmol/l	mval/l	mmol/l
Na^+	141	141	143	143	10	10
K^+	4	4	4	4	155	155
Ca^{2+}	5	2.5	2.6	1.3	<0.001	<0.0005
Mg^{2+}	2	1	1.4	0.7	30	15
Sum of cations	152					
Cl^-	103	103	115	115	8	8
HCO_3^-	25	25	28	28	10	10
HPO_4^{2-}	2	1	2	1	95	65
SO_4^{2-}	1	0.5	1	0.5	20	10
Organic acids	4	4	5	5	2	2
Proteins	17	2	<1	<1	60	6
Sum of anions	152		151		195	

Table 1: Electrolyte concentrations in different body water compartments.[34]

extracellular excess of K^+-ions. Apart from general factors like temperature, oxygen pressure, pH, and excessive deviations from normal electrolyte concentrations, other regulatory mechanisms of this enzyme are poorly understood. *In vitro* studies in endothelial cells show that Na^+/K^+-ATPase consumes about 5 - 15% of resting energy expenditure of the cell.[94]

The total amount of intracellular water increases with the number and size of body cells during body growth. Because different body tissues have different water contents (fat mass versus bone versus muscle mass), there are sex differences detectable after puberty (see Figures 2 and 3).

Extracellular Fluid (ECF): Intravascular Fluid (IVF), Extravascular Fluid (EVF) and Third Space

Extracellular fluid (ECF) represents water volume that is located outside cell membranes. This compartment is subdivided into intravascular (IVF) and extravascular (EVF) components, as well as a "third space" which characterizes free fluid in preformed body compartments under physiological (like urine in the bladder, cerebral spinal fluid [CSF] etc.) and pathological conditions (like ascites, or pleural effusions). Like total body water, ECF decreases during growth. Its leading ion is sodium. Intravascular volume also decreases during growth. In preterm and term infants total blood volume is 85 - 100 ml/kg body weight compared to 60 - 70 ml blood volume/kg body weight in adults.[158,173,186]

In a multi-tracer study (deuterium oxide, Evans blue, sucrose), water compartments in healthy term infants on day one of life were: extracellular fluid 31 ± 6%; intracellular fluid 44 ± 8%; total body water 75 ± 5%; intravascular fluid 10 ± 1% of body weight.[159] In infants with birth weight < 1000 gm, Shaffer et al found the extracellular volume to be 48 ± 11 % of body weight.[199]

Note: The relative contribution of ICF on total body water increases after birth and during infancy because ECF contracts and body cell mass grows. After puberty, the long-term ratio of ICF/ECF remains essentially constant.[179]

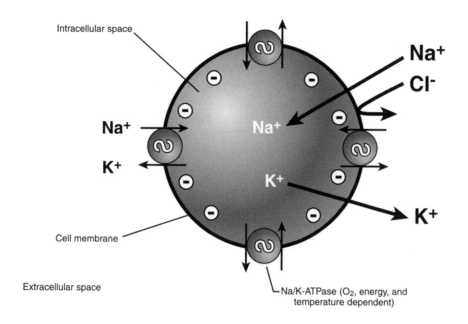

Figure 5: Na⁺/K⁺-ATPase regulates active transcellular Na⁺ and K⁺ transport between the intra- and extra-cellular compartments.

Mechanisms that Regulate Body Fluids
Control of Body Water

Whole body water homeostasis is effected via the extracellular fluid (ECF), which communicates as an "interface" with the environment. ECF regulation (intake, absorption, excretion etc.) is mainly achieved via intravascular fluid volume. Usually, the amount of water and sodium is independently regulated, within certain limits. The inset No. 1 gives details on components of the ECF control system and highlights the limitations of the system present in the critically ill and premature infant. The following paragraph gives a summary.

While the ECF limits the range of osmolalities that confront the ICF, a whole-organism system of water volume and concentration regulation is needed to regulate ECF. Changes in water balance associated with an infant's interaction with the environment and energy production are reflected in changes in size of the ECF. The ECF regulatory response should: 1) assure the integrity of the circulation (vascular pressure); and 2) keep the osmolality of the ECF

compartment within 3% of the osmolar set point (280 to 290 mOsm).[4,34,180] Regulation is achieved through changes in gastrointestinal intake (thirst); vascular tone, heart rate and contractility; and renal excretion of water and electrolytes. In critically ill newborns, intake is completely controlled by others, making the thirst effector nonfunctional. The system is modulated through hormonal effects on renal excretion of water and solutes, including the renin-angiotensin-aldosterone axis, arginine-vasopressin, and atrial natriuretic peptide (see insert No. 1).

The ECF control mechanism functions as follows: an increase in ECF is reflected in an increase in intravascular volume, which in turn increases blood flow and pressure. Increased vascular pressure leads to an increase in urinary flow, which returns the ECF volume to baseline.[97,180] If the perturbation-increasing ECF volume lowers plasma osmolality, a dilute urine is produced. Conversely, a decrease in the ECF volume results in decreased cardiac output and glomerular filtration pressure, leading to decreased urinary flow that lasts until intake replenishes the lost volume.

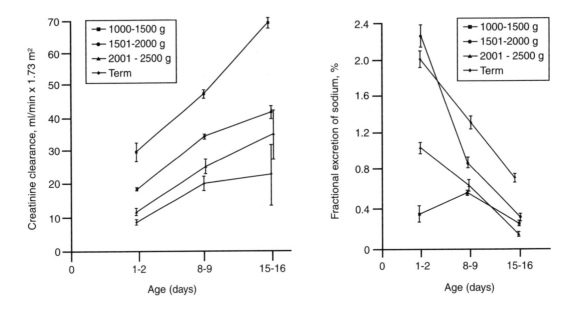

Figure 6: Renal maturation: changes of creatinine clearance and fractional sodium excretion with birth weight and postnatal age.[47]

Hypertonicity, which accompanies many low-volume states, stimulates thirst and renal resorption of water (see Figure 4).[144]

Regulation of ICF and ECF: The Na^+/K^+-ATPase pump clears the cytoplasm almost completely of sodium, therefore the cellular membranes appear to be relatively impermeable to sodium. The Na^+/K^+-ATPase pump is therefore the most important regulator of the ICF:ECF ratio.[137,142] As a consequence, the intracellular water space is shielded from direct interface with the external environment, preventing most tissues from sudden and large changes in solute or water concentration.

The different electrolyte content of different body pools (see Table 1) is achieved by the energy-dependent active transport mechanism of the Na^+/K^+-ATPase pump. This enzyme is the major agonist for cellular homeostasis and is located inside the membranes that divide ICF from ECF. The Na^+/K^+-ATPase establishes the transmembranal Na^+/K^+ gradient by continuously shuffling Na^+-ions out of, and K^+-ions into, the cell thereby making ICF vulnerable to extracellular excess

of K^+-ions. Like other enzymes, the Na^+/K^+-ATPase pump depends on pH and temperature optima and is disturbed in cases when the supply of oxygen and energy is insufficient. In the case of impairment of active sodium/potassium transport, an osmotic sodium shift from extracellular to the intracellular compartment occurs. This can produce intracellular edema, compromising cell integrity. This might happen if body temperature is low, or energy or oxygen supply is deficient (see Figure 5).

Note: Neonates are vulnerable to imbalances between intra- and extracellular compartments because of their temperature instability (large body surface in combination with a small body volume).

Insert No. 1: Mechanisms for regulation IVF

1. Renal factors (Figure 6): The number of nephrons in the fetal kidney is completed at 34 to 36 weeks of gestational age.[181,182] *Therefore the glomerular surface area available for filtration is smaller in preterm infants below 35 gestational weeks compared to that in older infants and adults.*[124] *Further functional changes occur after birth as blood pressure increases and renal* vascular resistance decreases during the first postnatal weeks.[93,114] In term infants, GFR increases significantly during the first week of life[6,79,95,195] and continues to rise over the first two years of life.[4,209] The distal nephron is able to produce a dilute urine even in early gestation.[133] The limiting step to exclude excess water in the fetal or premature kidney is low GFR, not impaired distal nephron function.[133,183,184,209]

Immaturity of the distal nephron leads to reduced concentrating ability due to an anatomically shortened Loop of Henle[66,68,208] and a distal tubule and collecting system epithelium that is less responsive to arginine vasopressin (AVP).[66,115,182,184] Further, the interstitial urea concentration is low.[66-69]

Note: Compared to adults, term and preterm infants have to control a larger water volume per kg body weight with an immature renal excretion mechanism. Because of reduced ability of the immature kidney to concentrate urine, a higher water volume is needed to excrete the daily waste. Therefore there is need to supplement water, and adjust it to the actual requirements of neonates in a more precise way compared to adults.

2. Cardiovascular factors: Cardiac flow is proportional to ventricular filling. Therefore, if intravascular volume increases, cardiac output rises. The increased blood flow then increases renal perfusion and urine formation. However, blood pressure rather than flow is most directly correlated with increased urine production,[97,201] and blood pressure is also the prime stimulus to arterial mechanoreceptor afferents of the hormonal modulators in the ECF control system. The systemic vascular resistance, as maintained by the sympathetic nervous system and local metabolic needs, interacts with the direct effect of heart filling in the cardiovascular control of the ECF.[192,201] Term and preterm infants exhibit a blunted response to acute volume loading[23] due to an immature myocardium that has a high content of non-contractile tissue. The immature myocardium may limit the infants' adaptive response to acute loading of the ECF.

Note: Ability to enhance cardiovascular performance is limited in preterm and term newborns. Usually maximum contractility, and maximum endogenous stimulation by adrenergic substances are already achieved under normal physiological conditions

3. Hormonal factors:

Renin-Angiotensin-Aldosterone System (RAAS): The RAAS matures early in gestation. The limiting factor for the effectiveness of the system is immaturity of the kidney. The blunted response of renal tubules with only limited ability to concentrate urine leads to high plasma hormone concentrations in premature infants.[7,108] With kidney maturation, the physiologic stimuli for all components of the RAAS slowly decrease.[169,210]

Physiology: The RAAS regulates the volume of the extracellular compartment. Low sodium delivery to the distal nephron increases renin production by the kidney.[131,152,192] Renin cleaves angiotensinogen, forming angiotensin I. Angiotensin-converting enzyme (ACE), produced in the vascular endothelium, activates angiotensin I, which is then called angiotensin II. Angiotensin II raises blood pressure by vasoconstriction, which leads to a higher cardiac ejection fraction (Frank-Straub-Starling mechanism).[131] This leads to a higher GFR and higher sodium concentrations at the distal nephron, which decreases renin production

Arginine-Vasopressin (AVP, ADH): This antidiuretic hormone is secreted after 11 weeks of gestation: by the end of the second trimester, plasma concentrations in healthy fetuses or preterm infants are similar to those of term infants.[52,193,210] Besides the hyperosmolarity baroreceptor stimulation, there are different non-osmotic stimuli like low blood pressure, pain, hypoxia, and raised intracranial pressure.[52,98,134,175,180,185,224] In healthy term infants, plasma vasopressin concentrations rise in response to fluid hypertonicity if body weight loss exceeds 10%.[145] In preterm infants the immature kidney is the limiting factor of AVP efficiency with lower renal medullary solute concentration in term and premature infants.[66,69,126,208,215]

Physiology: AVP controls blood osmolality[180] by increasing water reabsorption in the collecting duct. This happens by increasing the cellular concentrations of cAMP, which increases water permeability of the collecting duct cells.[90]

Atrial Natriuretic Peptide (ANP): The principal action of ANP is to promote the renal excretion of water and sodium to reduce the extracellular fluid volume.[178,196] Only little is known about the maturity of the ANP-system after preterm delivery. High plasma

ANP concentrations are reported from Rozycki and Baumgart[187] in premature infants with respiratory distress syndrome (RDS). But there is no clear renal response measured, probably due to renal immaturity. During the first two days of life, a brisk diuresis of water and salt is observed in term neonates in combination with elevated ANP levels.[56]

Physiology: Plasma ANP concentrations rise if a high blood volume leads to mechanical distortion of the heart atrial walls. The prohormone is activated by plasma enzymes. The duration of action of ANP is probably very short-lived (a few minutes).[5] ANP levels rise shortly after birth (46 pg/ml) with a peak on day 3 (175 pg/ml), and then progressively decrease during the next two months (62 pg/ml).[80]

Note: All hormonal regulatory mechanisms are already present even in preterm infants. The limiting step, however, is the functional immaturity of the kidney.

Regulation of IVF:EVF ratio: A closer look to the IVF:EVF ratio is of interest because a critical intravascular volume must be sustained in order to assure cardiovascular function.

Under normal conditions, ie, when the capillary border is intact, the IVF:EVF ratio is mainly determined by blood pressure and by oncotic-hydrostatic pressure as well as by the overall permeability of the capillary wall. To explain the lower IVF:EVF ratio in preterm infants compared to term infants and adults,[83] it was theorized that the permeability of the capillary wall could be higher in preterm and term infants when compared to later life, but this theory was not confirmed in an animal study investigating the permeability of pulmonary capillaries in lambs. There was no difference in transmembranal protein turnover time between preterm and mature newborn sheep.[50] However, plasma oncotic pressure has been proven to be lower in term neonates and sometimes even lower in preterm infants compared to adults. This is especially the case in sick infants suffering from respiratory distress syndrome and may therefore explain the changes in IVF:EVF ratio.[30,31,70,123,206,231] Details about the mechanism of action of the hydrostatic-oncotic pressure are given in insert No. 2.

Under pathologic conditions like sepsis, the capillary walls tend to be "leaky".[118] Consequently fluid is shifted into the extravascular space, causing edema. Depending on the degree of capillary leakage, proteins may also migrate from intra- to extravascular fluid, thereby aggravating the loss of intravascular volume. Unfortunately, administration of albumin - which can help to raise oncotic pressure in the presence of intact capillary borders - may be deleterious in the presence of capillary leak because it rapidly distributes in equal parts between intra- and extravascular space, thereby affecting oncotic pressure on both sides in a parallel way. An alternative way to expand the intravascular fluid volume is to administer high-molecular substances like packed red cell transfusions. The application of HES (hydroxy ethyl starch) is under investigation.[105,119,132,233]

Note: In preterm and term neonates there is lower plasma oncotic pressure, combined with higher permeability of the capillary wall. Therefore the shift of water from intravascular to interstitial compartment is increased, and peripheral edema may develop more easily in these subjects.

Insert No. 2: Oncotic and Hydrostatic Pressure

A dynamic interaction of oncotic pressure and of hydrostatic pressure generated by the cardiovascular system[128] results in small, but important, differences between intravascular and extravascular volumes. These differences allow movement of water from the circulating blood into the surrounding tissues and back again.

Oncotic Pressure: Osmolality of body fluids is affected by the presence of large molecular weight plasma proteins (colloids) that do not pass freely through semipermeable membranes. These proteins are usually ionized at physiologic pH, so they have an associated electromotive force that causes an unequal distribution of the smaller diffusible ions (crystalloids) between body compartments (the Gibbs-Donnan equilibrium).[137,151,218,222] The increase in osmotic pressure of plasma water compared to the interstitial water due to the colloids (oncotic pressure) is approximately two-thirds directly related to the non-diffusible protein particles and one-third a result of the difference in diffusible particles. Plasma oncotic pressure is

25 to 28 mmHg in adults, 15 to 17 mmHg in term neonates, and sometimes lower (1-12 mmHg) in preterm infants with respiratory distress.[30,123,206]

Hydrostatic Pressure (Starling Relationship): *Water movement across an idealized capillary wall was described qualitatively by Starling in 1896*[211], *and the formal mathematical treatment of the component forces was presented 40 years ago by Landis and Pappenheimer.*[166,211,222]

The normal balance of these forces results in a small amount of water leaving the intravascular space at the arterial end of the capillary bed, while much of it re-enters at the venous end due to the fall in capillary hydrostatic pressure.[151,166] *The small amount of fluid that remains in the interstitium is then removed by lymphatic drainage. Disruption of the usual balance of forces within a tissue capillary bed may favor increased movement of fluid volume into the interstitium. The disruption may be caused by: 1) conditions of high plasma hydrostatic pressure; 2) increased vascular permeability; or 3) low plasma oncotic pressure. In these conditions the lymphatic drainage must increase or tissue edema will occur.*[151] *Since the ability to increase lymphatic drainage varies among the different tissue beds, some organs are more or less prone to develop edema. Other factors affecting lymphatic drainage include: 1) body movement, where lymphatic flow depends in part on tissue movement; 2) lymphatic obstruction due to tissue injury; and 3) mechanical factors.*

Fetal Water and Electrolyte Metabolism

In order to assess the postnatal needs of a preterm infant, a closer look at the intrauterine conditions to which the fetus is exposed is needed.

The intrauterine development of the fetus is in large part dependent on the metabolic capacity of the mother. The placenta represents the materno-fetal "interface": it supplies the fetus with oxygen, water, and fuels (glucose, amino acids etc), and it excretes waste products from fetal metabolism (urea, acids, carbon dioxide etc.). Expressed in medico-technical terms, the fetus may be considered as a "subject" that is given "life support," using:

1. Extracorporal membrane oxygenation,

2. Total parenteral nutrition, and

3. Chronic hemodialysis.

This condition is dramatically altered after birth. A rapid transition to an autonomic control of intake/excretion and self-controlled water homeostasis occurs. The degree of immaturity and/or the presence or absence of underlying disease (hypoxia/asphyxia, infection etc.) determine the amount of support needed during this period, and may be coupled to disturbances of water homeostasis.

During fetal life there is a transplacental net transfer of water to the fetus. Sodium and other electrolytes are actively transported:

1. Na^+/H^+-exchange via the NHE-1 transporter.[44,203]

2. Co-transport with inorganic ions and organic solutes, and

3. Na^+ conductance[229], such that an equilibrium between mother and fetus is established. The exchange is not rate-limited under normal conditions. Maternal plasma electrolyte concentrations determine fetal levels.

The *in utero* supply of the fetus with fluid and electrolytes may be compared to a continuous infusion with normotonic saline via the maternal circulation. The fetal mechanisms of water homeostasis react in this condition through high urinary output of fluid and electrolytes. In animals and humans, mean production of fetal urine increases during fetal life. Urine production first starts at five weeks of gestation.[153] At 20 and 32 weeks of gestation, 4.5 and 6 ml/kg/h are produced, respectively. At term (39 weeks), urinary production is up to 8 - 15 ml/kg/hour and up to 8 mmol sodium/kg/d, which is considerably higher than during postnatal life after completed adaptation.[107,153] Consequently, fetal urine osmolarity is low and usually does not exceed iso-osmotic concentrations; ie, fractional urinary Na excretion of the human fetus is high (ie, 8-18%) compared with postnatal life (<1%).[107] Normal fetal urine production, clinically most often reflected by normal amniotic fluid volumes, has been shown to be an indicator of fetal well-being.[107] Because of the excessive maternal donation of fluid and electrolytes, the fetal kidneys are not forced and/or able to produce

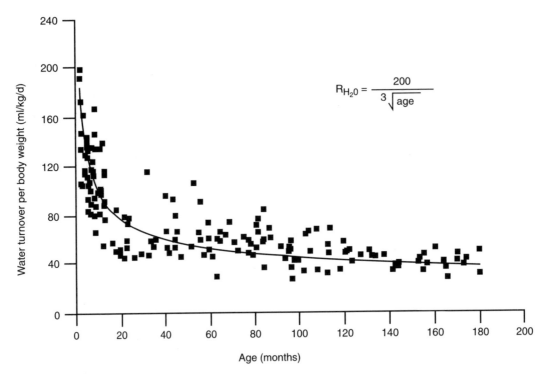

$$R_{H_2O} = \frac{200}{\sqrt[3]{age}}$$

Figure 7: Age-dependent changes of water turnover: normal values (per body weight) as measured by stable isotope elimination from early infancy to adolescence.[85]

concentrated urine of high osmolarity, a phenomenon that is also accompanied by the anatomic and physiologic immaturity of fetal kidneys (see insert No. 1, paragraph 1 and Figure 6). To assure fetal wellbeing, the placenta serves as the remote "backup" regulator of fetal fluid and electrolyte metabolism.

Water Turnover

Daily water turnover of healthy children decreases significantly during the first years of life (Figure 7). These remarkable changes are caused by age-dependent differences of body weight:surface ratio and by renal maturation mechanisms. Recommendations for fluid intake were calculated using a couple of assumptions on everyday *ad libitum* eating and drinking (protein intake, maximum renal molar clearance, maximum urine osmolarity to be achieved, etc.).

Most of the turnover data have been calculated from balance studies. There is only one study investigating the whole pediatric age range using the technique of stable

isotope dilution with subsequent elimination (Figure 7). Considerable differences between recommended intake and measured values were found, regardless of which technique used to assess spontaneous fluid intake.[85]

Physiology: The initial very high water turnover in preterm and term infants after birth is explained by the immaturity, or alternatively efficient physiological adaptation processes, of different organ functions.

Note: The regulation of the body water pool in preterm or term babies is more difficult compared to adults because there is more water per Kg body weight to be regulated and because water turnover is up to five-fold higher when compared to later life.

Factors Influencing Water Input

To understand how data on fluid requirements are obtained and on which assumptions they are based, the different factors that contribute to fluid intake and output in preterm infants will be discussed in the following paragraph.

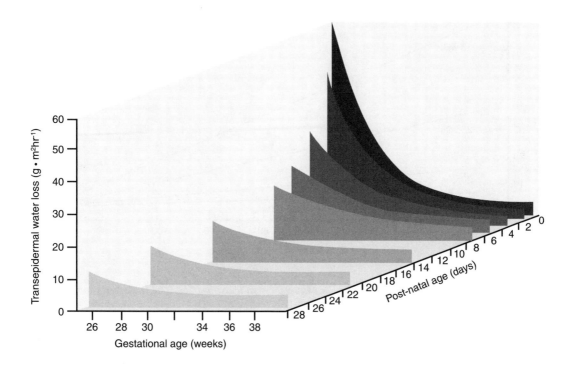

Figure 8: Transepidermal water loss of AGA infants in relation to gestational age and ambient relative humidity.[57]

Intake via Inspired Air. With each inspiration, water enters the respiratory tract: assuming 6 ml/kg body weight of tidal volume, respiratory rate of 40 min[-1], 85% of relative humidity and a maximum water content of 49 mg/l air at 37° C (pH$_2$O of 6.3 kPa), 14.4 ml of water per kg body weight per day enter the body via the lungs. Assuming that expired air is at 37° C and is fully saturated (100%) with water, a net loss of 2.5 ml/kg/d occurs.

Intake via Skin. Humidity water of ambient air is absorbed via the neonatal and premature skin, but there are no published data. However, under conditions met in daily routine, water output by insensible perspiration is usually considerably greater than hypothetical skin intake. This results in a net loss of water via skin and is discussed below.

Metabolic Water Production. When all metabolic pathways are correctly working, and the subject is under steady-state conditions, water is generated by oxidation of carbohydrates (0.6 ml H$_2$O per gm of carbohydrates) and fat (1.0 ml H$_2$O per gm of fat).

When proteins are also oxidized – which should occur only in small amounts because proteins normally should be used to establish lean mass and not to generate caloric equivalents – 0.4ml H$_2$O are produced per gram protein oxidized.[147]

Overall, this will result in daily production of metabolic water in the range of 5 to 15 ml/kg body weight, provided that the infant is adequately nourished and supplied with calories. Moreover, acceleration of metabolic rate due to environmental stress or disease may accelerate the production of metabolic water up to 20 ml/kg/d.[127,223]

However, these are all calculated data and currently there are no published data that have addressed the amount of metabolic water production in children and neonates. This issue may be answered by assessing the difference of registered water intake (by dietary nursery records) and water turnover measured by stable isotopes (oral intake plus metabolic water production).

Oral and Parenteral Intake. In fully autonomic subjects, this part is usually regulated by hunger and

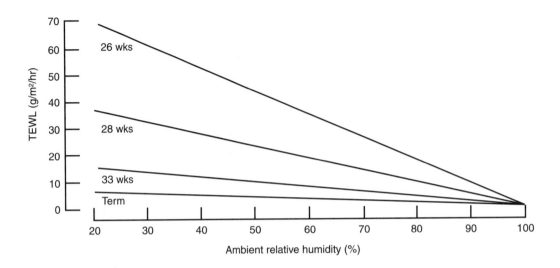

Figure 9: The effect of ambient relative humidity on transepidermal water loss (TEWL) (modified from the data of [99]).

thirst and/or intake regulated by social factors. These control mechanisms, however, are not effective in premature and term infants. The oral and parenteral intake is therefore completely under the control of the environment (e.g. nurses, doctors, parents).

Factors Influencing Water Output:
Insensible Water Loss via the Immature Skin.
Transcutaneous evaporation is a process with unpredictable amounts of water loss. From the exposed moist and immature epidermis, free water may be lost in vast quantities. In premature infants, the amount of insensible water loss mainly determines the need for exogeneous fluid administration during the first postnatal days. It decreases as skin matures and cornifies.

ELBW neonates below 1000 g birth weight especially experience disproportional high water losses[18,20,225]: in these infants the immature epidermis is only little cornified, and represents little barrier to passive evaporation. This effect is multiplied by the VLBW infant's ratio of surface area to body mass.[21,26,46,100,111,227,230] The sweat glands secrete little water, since apocrine function and thermal sensory-neural integration are immature before 34 weeks gestation.[45,46] Hammerlund et al.[100] and Sedin et al.[194]

measured a higher transdermal water loss in preterm babies compared with term-born infants. A loss of 10-15% of body weight in the first day occurs in preterm infants.[22] Figure 8 shows transepidermal water loss in relation to gestational age at birth at different postnatal ages in AGA infants.[57]

The often cited relationship between infant metabolic rate and transepidermal insensible water loss[202,228] cannot serve to guide replacement water volumes in preterm and term neonates.

Insert No. 3: Measures to Reduce Water Loss in Preterm Infants (An Overview of Measures– Proven and Unproven – To Reduce Transepidermal Water Losses).
The ratio of a large surface area and a low body mass combined with a weak epidermal barrier compounds a high evaporation rate in VLBW neonates. Different measures are proven to reduce significantly the insensible fluid loss:

1. Incubator treatment/humidity (Figure 9): Water diffuses through skin down a gradient of water vapor pressure. Under normal conditions water vapor pressure is high in tissues and low in surrounding air. The gradient of water pressure is high since the epidermal barrier offers little resistance to diffusion. The insensible water loss can be reduced if the water vapor pressure gradient is lowered by increasing the environmental humidity.[123a] The use of double wall incubators with controlled humidity and heat is "state of the art" in neonatology today concerning care of VLBW neonates. The theoretical disadvantage of an increase of infection rate due to moist conditions was not proven in controlled studies.[88a] Modern commercially available incubator systems are designed to minimize that risk and allow observation of the premature infant under environmental barrier conditions.

2. Double wall incubator treatment reduces insensible water loss in VLBW neonates by about 30% when a humidity of 90% is used at thermoneutral temperature. With maturation of the epidermal barrier, it is possible to reduce ambient humidity step by step, usually after the first 5 days of life.[100,100a]

3. Radiant warmers: Use of radiant warmers or single wall incubators for VLBW care may increase water loss and impair thermoregulation (i.e. thermoneutral conditions are less easily achieved). Such devices, however, are still in use in some hospitals because of lower costs, ease of access to the child, and supposed – but not proven – smaller risk of infection. There is a recent randomized study by Meyer et al comparing radiant warmers vs. incubators for use in VLBW infants (n=60). In the radiant warmer group, a higher initial weight loss was observed, which could be easily compensated for by adjusting fluid intake. However, adverse outcome (major morbidity: death, CLD, NEC, IVH > 2°, PVL, ROP > °2) was considerably lower in the radiant warmer-treated group (OR of 0.1, p < 0.05).[150] The findings of this study should induce more research in this area.

Little is known to accelerate the maturation process of the skin in premature infants. However, the skin barrier can be artificially increased by application of waterproof coverings, semipermeable membranes or emollient ointments:

4. The use of waterproof coverings (such as plastic films, plastic blankets, bubble blankets) in addition to treatment in an double wall incubator leads to further reduction of insensible water loss by 30-60%.[19]

5. A further increase in skin barrier is possible by the use of emollient ointments. There are emollients with different compositions currently in use. Little or no effect on fluid or thermal balance was shown by Nopper et al,[158a] but a reduction of systemic infections was reported in the group treated with a paraffin/lanolin mixture. In two studies published by Rutter et al. and by Lane et al, a decrease of insensible water loss of up to 50% was reported.[129,189]

6. Medical treatment influencing water turnover as side-effect; Ventilation: Endotracheal intubation and mechanical ventilation using warmed and humidified air significantly reduces insensible respiratory water loss. The amount of reduction is influenced by clinical status, respiratory frequency and humidity of breathing air during spontaneous ventilation. A reduction of up to 30% was reported by Sosulski et al.[207]

7. Phototherapy increases transdermal water loss significantly. Different investigators report an increase of 40-100% which is influenced by gestational age, postnatal age and ambient humidity.[230,234]

Breathing. Evaporation of water from upper respiratory passages accounts for approximately one third of net insensible water loss.[214,228] Because respiratory frequencies are higher in low-birth-weight premature infants, evaporative losses from the upper respiratory tract are larger (0.8-0.9 ml/kg/h[202,214]) when compared with water loss of term neonates (0.5 ml/kg/h) at room temperature in moderate relative humidity.[202] Diseases that lead to high ventilatory minute volumes may further enhance evaporation to more than 2.0 ml/kg/h (= 50 ml/kg/d) when dry oxygen-enriched gases are used.[57] The net water losses can be considerably reduced (near zero) when humidified (85 - 100% relative humidity) and warmed (37° C) air is applied.

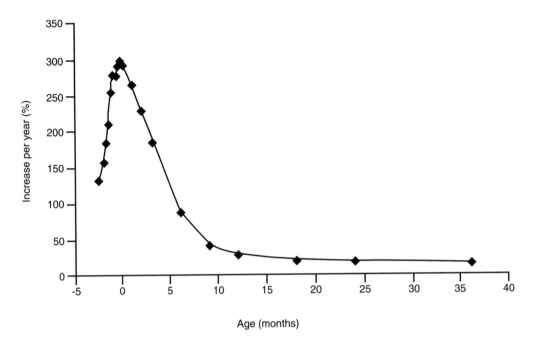

Figure 10: Gain of body weight during fetal and early postnatal period: weight gain velocity is highest during the last trimester of pregnancy and during the first few months, then sharply approaches a constant rate.

Urinary output. Water excretion via the renal system is necessary to remove waste products from the body (ie, urea and fixed acids). The minimum urinary fluid volume may be calculated from the potential renal solute load of the nutrition used, as well as from the capability of the newborn to produce concentrated urine. Due to the immature kidney, this ability is dependent on gestational and postnatal age (see Figure 6). A review of published data shows that in preterm infants with a birth weight of 2000 g, maximum water diuresis may be as high as 6.0 ml/kg/h of free water in the presence of a total urine production of 9.8 ml/kg/h.[134] Maximum urinary concentration up to 700 mosm/l can be achieved by term infants compared with 550 mosm/l in preterm newborns and 1200 mosm/l in adults.[53,174] Less mature infants may not be able to achieve these concentrations: Rees[174] reported maximum urine osmolarities of < 500 mosm/l in hypernatremic infants weighing 800 - 950 g. Svenningsen and Aronson[215] published average values of 360 - 520 mosm/l in 1- to

6-weeks old premature infants given an intranasal desmopressin test.

Figure 6 shows the postnatal maturation of renal function.[47] The premature infant may be placed at risk for volume depletion when a mismatch between renal solute load and ability to produce concentrated urine occurs. This has to be taken in account if sodium- containing nutrients or medications are given to neonates (eg, betalactam antibiotics with high sodium content).

Potential renal solute load (PRSL). The renal solute load is the sum of soluble waste products that must be excreted by the kidney. Because excretion of these solutes requires water, and because the capacity of the neonatal kidney to concentrate solutes is limited, the renal solute load exerts a major effect on water balance.[235] PRSL refers to solutes of dietary origin that would need to be excreted in the urine if none was diverted into formation of new tissue and none was lost through non-renal routes. The PSRL of a feeding assumes, therefore, full conversion

Variable	Effect	Reference
Increased activity	+20%	(230, 100)
Increased temperature	+20%	(230, 120)
Phototherapy	+40-100%	(230, 227)
Tachypnea	+20-30%	(56)
Intubation	-20-30%	(207)

Note: Plastic blankets/skin coverings have only little effect in incubator care (humidity 90%).

Table 2: Clinical conditions (variables) affecting water loss.

of protein to urea and is calculated as follows:

$$PRSL\ [mosm] = N/28\ [mg] + Na^+[mmol] + Cl[mmol] + K^+[mmol] + K^+[mmol]$$

where N is dietary nitrogen in milligrams, and electrolytes in mmol.[236] In preterm and term neonates, the apparent renal solute load is reduced by the amount of nitrogen that is stored in newly-formed body cell mass (see Chapter 3).

Fecal losses. Stool water loss is negligible in early life prior to establishing enteral feeding in premature infants.[117] When full enteral feeding is achieved, fecal losses (5 - 10 ml/kg/d[51]) are usually assumed to balance metabolic water production.

The combined effect of negligible stool loss, reduced respiratory water loss due to humidified inspired gases, and increased metabolic water may result in a bias towards free water retention in critically ill premature infants.

Growth (Figure 10). The formation of new cells and cell growth is only possible with an adequate water supply. The fetal/neonatal needs for water (in terms of net accretion) are determined by formation of new tissue during fetal/neonatal growth. A mean growth rate of 15 g/kg body weight/day results in a net storage of about 12 ml water and of about 1.0 -1.5 mmol Na$^+$ per kg body weight per day.

Note: The high growth rate which is preferentially seen in preterm and term babies leads to a need for a significant extra amount of stored water which has to be taken in account if water supplementation need is calculated.

Summary. Figures 11a and b and Table 2 give an overview about the different factors that determine water turnover at different gestational and postnatal ages.

Metabolism of Na$^+$, K$^+$ and Cl

Output

Urinary losses. Among the various ways by which electrolytes leave the body (fecal, sweat, urine, other), urinary output is the only one being actively regulated. Urinary excretion depends on intake: however, there are physiologic limits of preterm excretory function. As mentioned, urinary capacity to produce concentrated urine is dependent on gestational and postnatal age (see Figure 6). In VLBW infants, typical urinary electrolyte concentrations during states of normohydration are 20 - 40 mmol/l for Na$^+$ and 10 - 30 mmol/l for K$^+$ (Data calculated from Al-Dahhan et al[1] and Rees et al[176]).

Under normal physiologic conditions, there is an inverse correlation in healthy subjects between urinary volume and urinary electrolyte concentration; ie, in states of high normal hydration, large volumes of dilute urine are produced, whereas less urine but with high electrolyte concentration is produced when hydration status is in the low normal range. In other words, total amount of urinary electrolyte excretion is more or less constant, indicating that water and electrolytes are regulated independently; within physiological conditions.

However, under special circumstances, urinary volume may be high and may contain considerable amounts of electrolytes: the application of diuretics like furosemide may lead to urinary Na$^+$ concentrations up to 70 mmol/l (data recalculated using[176,177]). This may cause considerable sodium losses with subsequent hyponatremia accompanied by arterial hypotension.

Such losses may also occur when a subject recovers from renal failure with oliguria. During the following polyuric period, the regulation of electrolyte excretion in the distal/proximal tubule is impaired and can lead to massive electrolyte losses.

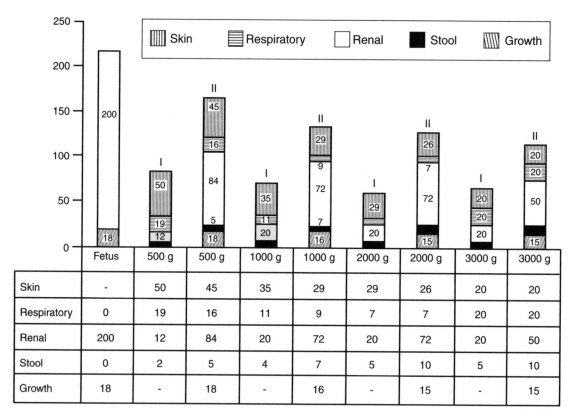

	Fetus	500 g	500 g	1000 g	1000 g	2000 g	2000 g	3000 g	3000 g
Skin	-	50	45	35	29	29	26	20	20
Respiratory	0	19	16	11	9	7	7	20	20
Renal	200	12	84	20	72	20	72	20	50
Stool	0	2	5	4	7	5	10	5	10
Growth	18	-	18	-	16	-	15	-	15

Figure 11a: Contributions to water turnover [ml/kg/day] as related to birth weight and postnatal age (I: day 1 of life, II: stable growth).

Comments: 1) For birth weights below 2000g, thermoneutral incubator treatment at 80-90% relative humidity was assumed, 2) Figures for AGA term infants are measured data (averaged from different studies (for references see text), corresponding figures for preterm infants are estimated (for references see text), 3) Figures for fetal period reflect last trimester conditions.

Losses by sweat. The authors are not aware of any published studies on electrolyte content of neonatal sweat or insensible perspiration.

Fecal losses. In term and preterm infants, fecal losses were found to be dependent on gestational age: immature infants (30 gestational weeks) lose more sodium (0.1 mmol/kg body weight/day) than mature infants (0.02 mmol/kg body weight/d). With increasing postnatal age, stool losses diminish to 30% of initial values. There is a clear correlation with postnatal age. Fecal potassium losses are about twice as high as sodium losses, but show no relation with gestational age.[2]

Other losses. Other electrolyte losses may occur under more pathological conditions: bowel obstruction due to congenital intestinal malformation, ileostoma due to necrotizing enterocolitis (NEC) surgery, pleural effusions due to chylothorax, peritoneal drainage for massive ascites due to hydrops fetalis, and external CSF drainage due to posthemorrhagic hydrocephalus. In these cases, the electrolyte content of lost fluids cannot be predicted precisely, though most of the fluid will be serum transudates with plasma-like levels of electrolytes. In clinical routine it is good advice to measure at least once the Na+ concentrations of such fluid losses in order to replace them.

Extra needs used for accretion of body mass during growth periods. The accretion of new body mass is

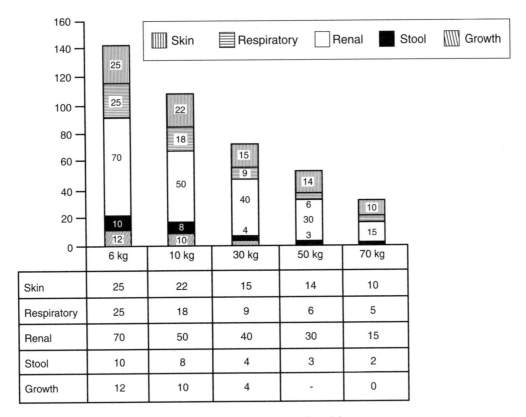

	6 kg	10 kg	30 kg	50 kg	70 kg
Skin	25	22	15	14	10
Respiratory	25	18	9	6	5
Renal	70	50	40	30	15
Stool	10	8	4	3	2
Growth	12	10	4	-	0

Figure 11b: Contributions to water turnover (mg/kg/day) during later life.

only possible with an adequate supply of electrolytes. Fetal and neonatal needs for electrolytes (in terms of net accretion) are determined by formation of new tissue during fetal and neonatal growth. A mean growth rate of 15 g/kg body weight/day results in a net storage of about 1.0 - 1.5 mmol Na^+ per kg body weight per day. It has been shown that restricted administration of sodium impairs longitudinal growth and weight gain in otherwise healthy preterm infants.[36,106] Though not separately investigated, it is reasonable to assume corresponding figures for K^+ and Cl^- to ensure optimal postnatal growth.

Intake

Oral and parenteral intake. There are no sources of endogenous production or any release of electrolytes into the human body. Therefore the human body is completely dependent on exogenous supply, either via oral ingestion or via parenteral administration. The enteral absorption is actively regulated, however, within certain limits. Because electrolyte homeostasis is one of the major components of overall body homeostasis, effective regulatory mechanisms for intake exist. In children, adolescents and adults, salt depletion results in specific "hunger for salty nutrients." In neonatal subjects, however, intake is almost completely controlled by others, and is dependent on the preparation of the nutrition used.

In neonatal care it should be taken into account that some drugs may contain considerable amounts of cations because they are prepared as the sodium or potassium salt of the drug (like aminopenicillin, fosfomycin etc).

Note: The high growth rate which is preferentially seen in preterm and term babies leads to need for significant extra amount of stored electrolytes, which has to be taken in account if electrolyte supplementation is calculated.

Postnatal Adaptation of Fluid and Electrolyte Homeostasis in VLBW Infants

General Aspects

With the delivery of the fetus a number of physiologic changes and adaptive processes occur that affect many organ systems. Some of these changes affect the metabolism of water and electrolytes and are given as follows:

- Changes with immediate impact on water and electrolyte metabolism
    1. Discontinuation of placental supply of fluids, electrolytes and nutrients.
    2. Discontinuation of placental clearance.
    3. Onset of considerable insensible water loss.
    4. Onset of infant thermoregulation.
- Changes with delayed impact on water and electrolyte metabolism
    5. Onset of autonomic renal regulation of fluids and electrolytes.
    6. Onset of oral intake of fluids and other nutrients.

The sudden discontinuation of placental supply, and of placental clearance, and the onset of insensible water loss, immediately start to compromise metabolism of water and electrolytes in different aspects. The compensatory regulative processes (like renal adaptation, oral intake, etc.), however, need time to counteract these effects on body water pools. Characteristic postnatal change of body water, like the well-known postnatal weight loss, occurs during this period of regulatory "mismatch." The time course of adaptational processes may be divided into three major phases:

- Period of transition (Phase I)
- Intermediate period (Phase II)
- Period of stable growth with regular gain of body weight (Phase III)

Besides the postnatal regulation of water balance, further adaptive processes occur simultaneously also in other organs (eg, respiratory or metabolic adaptation etc).

Postnatal Adaptation Phase I: The Early Stage - Rearrangement of Body Fluid Compartments

The immediate postnatal phase is characterized by a fall in urinary output that is due to a fall in GFR. The first urine formed postnatally is hypertonic to plasma, with increased concentration of urea, potassium and phosphate, but not of sodium and chloride.[153] The change in urine volume thus appears to be brought about by a decrease in free water clearance, which may be mediated by increased plasma concentrations of arginine vasopressine (AVP) present in the neonate around delivery.[136] This relative oliguria may last for a variable period (hours to days) that is mainly determined by the presence of underlying conditions and diseases like respiratory distress syndrome. This oliguria is then followed by a diuretic phase, during which body fluid compartments are rearranged by isotonic or hypertonic (ie, hypernatremic and hyperchloremic) contraction of extracellular fluid volume during the first postnatal days: these changes are caused by considerable evaporative water loss via the immature skin as well as by continuing natriuresis (as present during fetal life).[156] Both processes adapt to extrauterine conditions with different speed: the epidermal layer of the skin matures and cornifies during the first days of life, while the kidneys increase GFR and the ability to concentrate the urine over five to ten days (see Figure 6). It is unknown whether this continuing natriuresis reflects a delayed adaptation of renal regulation after birth or if it occurs as part of an active regulation of ICF contraction until a certain signal is received that ICF has sufficiently contracted.

The end of this transitional period is usually characterized by 1) urine volume < 2.0 ml/kg/hour, 2) urine osmolarity > serum osmolarity, 3) FE_{Na} diminishing from >3% to ≤1%, and 4) urine-specific gravity above >1.012.

In healthy preterm infants, the transitional period is usually completed after 3 to 5 days. In VLBW infants, the length of Phase I seems to be additionally modulated by the degree of respiratory insufficiency and may take up to 4 to 8 days.[1,13,14,16,17,102,103,143,155,176,197,200]

In clinical terms, Phase I starts at birth and ends

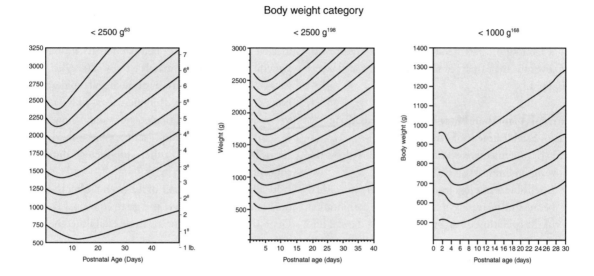

Figure 12: Normal values and time course of postnatal weight loss.[63,198,168]

usually when maximum weight loss is achieved.

Figure 12 summarizes the findings of three different studies in which the amount of postnatal weight loss was assessed in preterm infants with a birth weight of <2500 and <1000 gms, respectively. Postnatal weight loss expressed as percent of body weight seems to be inversely related to birth weight: infants <1000 g BW lose more fluids than infants with a birth weight between 1000 - 1500 g, or 1500 - 2000 g.[198] It has been shown in different studies that most of the weight loss of AGA infants is due to a loss of water, mainly of ECF, with only little change in ICF or body solids.[1,13,14,16,197-199]

Whether SGA infants behave differently from AGA infants in terms of initial postnatal hydration and subsequent adaptation is not fully elucidated: average weight loss of SGA infants is reported to be smaller than that of corresponding AGA infants (3.5 vs. 8-10%, respectively).[15,110,198,221] This finding may be in theory due to reduced water content of lean mass in SGA infants, indicating reduced content of ECF present already at birth. The nature of postnatal weight loss (ie, water or solids) could not be determined clearly in both studies. A recent study by Hartnoll et al using stable isotopes and bromide to measure TBW and ECF could show no difference of lean body tissue

hydration between SGA and AGA infants.[101]

The goals for fluid and electrolyte administration during this period are:

1. To allow contraction of ECF space without compromising intravascular fluid volume (IVF) and cardiovascular function,
2. To allow a negative net balance for sodium of 2 - 5 mmol/kg/d for the first postnatal days,
3. To maintain normal serum electrolyte concentrations
4. To allow sufficient urinary output to excrete waste products (like urea, acid equivalents, etc.) safely; and to avoid oliguria (<0.5 - 1.0 ml/kg/h) for longer than 12 hours,
5. To ensure regulation of body temperature by providing enough fluid for transepidermal evaporation,
6. To give enough caloric supply to meet energy maintenance needs during this period (equal to non-growth energy expenditure, approximately 40 - 60 kcal/kg/d).

Route of administration: Nowadays, "early oral feeding" is widely accepted in preterm infants. However, the volumes that can be fed are often too small to meet the needs of VLBW or ELBW infants during the first period. Therefore, parenteral administration (up to 100% of total needs) is usually started soon after birth. Even if oral feedings can be introduced without problems (ie, typical increments of 12 - 15 ml/kg/d), parenteral fluid administration will still cover the major part of total fluid needs at the end of Phase I.

Postnatal Adaptation Phase II: The Intermediate Phase - Establishment of Oral Feeding

Phase II (intermediate phase) is characterized by the following findings:

- Insensible water loss from the skin has diminished because of increasing maturation and cornification of the epidermis during the first 10-14 days of life.
- A fall in urine volume to less than 1-2 ml/kg/h and a low sodium excretion is effected through high plasma aldosterone concentrations. If no electrolyte supplementation is established, low serum electrolyte concentrations will develop due to continuing physiologic renal electrolyte and water losses.
- Intestinal ability to digest oral feedings is continuously increasing.

The goals for fluid and electrolyte administration during this period are:

1. To replete the body for electrolyte losses that may have inadvertently occurred during the first phase of ECF contraction (Phase I),
2. To replace actual water and electrolyte losses in order to maintain water and electrolyte homeostasis,
3. To try to augment oral feedings until sufficient calorie, protein and fluid intake is established.

Route of administration: During this Phase II, oral feedings can usually be augmented and subsequently the amount of parenteral fluid can be reduced. Total fluid intake is now related to ingested calories, protein and potential renal solute load. Due to this relation, which is more or less fixed in breast milk and commercially available formulas, total fluid intake generally amounts to 140 - 200 ml/kg/d.

Postnatal Adaptation Phase III: Stable Growth Phase

The subsequent Phase III (phase of stable growth) is then dominated by continuous weight gain, indicating now a positive net balance for sodium as well as the accretion of newly formed body tissue mass: ideally at a rate that is comparable to intrauterine growth rates (approximately 15 - 20 g/kg body weight/day). Cornification of neonatal epidermis is now complete, kidney function has fully adapted to extrauterine conditions, and may now react to different hydration states and fluid and electrolyte loads, by either producing dilute or concentrated urine.

Ideally, almost all intake of fluids and other nutrients may now be achieved via the gastrointestinal tract. In Phase III, equilibrium needs to be established between different needs such as:

1. Optimum calorie and protein supply (to optimize growth),
2. Optimum potential renal solute load (to assure safe excretion of waste products),
3. Total fluid volume (to respect limited intravascular capacity of VLBW preterm infants due to conditions like open ductus arteriosus) and,
4. Renal concentrating ability.

The goals of clinical strategies for fluid and electrolyte administration during this period are:

1. To replace losses of water and electrolytes in order to maintain water and electrolyte homeostasis,
2. To provide enough extra water and electrolytes to build up new tissue (80 g water and 8 mmol Na^+ and K^+ per 100 g weight gain) in order to allow tissue accumulation at intrauterine growth rates.

Route of administration: During Phase III usually the goal has been reached that most fluid, calorie and protein intake is achieved by oral feedings. Intravenous lines will only rarely be used, eg, to administer drugs still needed during this period (antibiotics, theophylline, etc.).

Duration of Phase I, II and III

In clinical routine, the end of Phase I and beginning of Phase III usually can be easily recognized. The duration of oliguria in Phase I and the time to achieve sufficient caloric intake during Phase II, however, are of varying clinical expression, and depend on gestational age and the presence of underlying diseases (RDS, sepsis, NEC etc): in clinical experience, Phase II seems to be of shorter duration in the more mature VLBW infants (ie, 30 - 34 gestational weeks) than in the very immature ones (ie, 23 - 26 gestational weeks). In other words: in a newborn infant of 32 gestational weeks, postnatal weight loss may be immediately followed by constant weight gain; in an infant of 25 gestational weeks, it may take an extra 10 to 20 days after completion of transitional period until stable weight gain is achieved. The time needed to achieve positive sodium balance seems to be considerably shorter in preterm infants of 30 - 34 weeks (2 to 5 days) when compared with infants of 26 - 28 weeks (7 - 10 days).[1] Another reason why Phase II is shorter in less immature infants may be that the length of this period is mainly defined by the time needed to achieve sufficient caloric intake. This period is usually short (7 to 10 days) in more mature VLBW infants because oral intake is less compromised. In the very tiny ELBW infants, however – despite early introduction of oral feeding– other compromising factors (sepsis, NEC etc.) may intervene and it can take several weeks until sufficient caloric intake is achieved enterally.

In a study by Heimler et al in preterm infants, weight changes and fluid compartments during the first week of life were related to calorie intake during that period as well as to the physiologic stability index (PSI).[110] It is likely that calorie intake and the degree of disease as indicated by PSI are highly correlated with each other.

Insert No. 4: The Teleological Meaning of Postnatal ECF Contraction: A Hypothesis
In newborn infants it seems reasonable that oral feedings are postnatally stepwise increased: during fetal life, the intestine has never been used to digest milk volumes of up to one-sixth of body weight. It may therefore be speculated that the delayed postnatal onset of lactation and its subsequent stepwise increase may therefore fit into the concept of intestinal adaptation. In term newborns,

full enteral feeding is usually achieved not before day 5 of life. Cumulated fluid deficit due to water loss by postnatally relevant insensible perspiration (60 ml/kg/d), and de facto achieved milk intake (25-100 ml/kg/d) may amount to more than 100 ml/kg for the first postnatal days. In order to assure and maintain minimum urinary flow during this period, water may be mobilized by contracting the ECF. The teleological meaning of "pumping up" the fetal ECF may be understood as generating a one-time store for body water in order to compensate for the delayed postnatal production of breast milk.

Data from Clinical Trials

Data from clinical trials may be used to generate recommendations for daily routine. Data from randomized and double-blinded studies are usually considered to be the gold standard, an approach that sometimes should be taken with care. In such trials outcome measures (primary and secondary) of two or more treatment regimens are usually compared by statistical means in order to find out the better treatment regimen. The outcome measures chosen in such studies, however, are often not standardized, and sometimes focus only on selected aspects (eg, percentage of babies being intubated, maximum oxygen concentration, days on ventilatory support etc.). Proven beneficial effects (eg, on selected items indicating short-term major morbidity or mortality) may be linked with less advantageous results when other outcome measures are tested (eg, frequency of patent ductus arteriosus or necrotising enterocolitis, length of stay, weight gain, neurological outcome). Results from clinical trials should therefore only be transferred into clinical guidelines recognizing the outcome measures assessed.

Transitional Phase (Phase I)
Transition without major problems/complications.
Unfortunately, a major question of physiology has not yet been answered: what is the normal weight loss that should be achieved after birth? What is the optimal weight loss for minimum overall morbidity?

Goals:

1. Expect weight loss during first 3-5 days of life
2. Maintain normal serum electrolyte concentrations:
   Sodium   135-145 mmol/L
   Potassium   3.5-5.0 mmol/L
   Chloride   98-108 mmol/L
3. Avoid oliguria   < 0.5 mL/kg/h for 8-12 hours

Phase 1 - Transition*: During the first 3-5 days of life is characterized by: 1) large transcutaneous water evaporation, and 2) renal diuresis of a large surfeit of extracellular salt and water.

Birthweight (grams)	Expected Weight Loss (%)	Water Intake+ (mL/kg/day)	Sodium Intake (mmol/kg/day)	Chloride Intake (mmol/kg/day)	Potassium Intake (mmol/kg/day)
< 1,000	15-20	90-140+++	0.0-1.0†	0.0-1.0	0.0-2.0§
1,000-1,500	10-15	80-120	0.0-1.0	0.0-1.0	0.0-2.0

Phase 2 - Stabilization: Contraction of ECF is completed, kidneys are able to concentrate urine. Enteral feeding is started but not sufficient. Variable length of 5-14 days, completed when birth weight is regained; transcutaneous water evaporation diminishing as neonatal epidermis cornifies.

Birthweight (grams)	Expected Weight gain (g/kg/day)	Water Intake (mL/kg/day)	Sodium Intake° (mmol/kg/day)	Chloride Intake (mmol/kg/day)	Potassium Intake (mmol/kg/day)
< 1,000	0-10	120-180	2.0-3.0	2.0	1.0-2.0
1,000-1,500	0-15	100-160	2.0-3.0	2.0	1.0-2.0

Phase 3 - Established Growth: Full enteral feeding is tolerated; objective is to match intrauterine growth rate for all weight categories in past two weeks. Oral intake is eventually ad libitum.

Expected Weight gain (g/kg/day)	Parenteral Volume (mL/kg/day)	Enteral Volume (mL/kg/day)	Sodium Intake (mmol/kg/day)	Chloride Intake (mmol/kg/day)	Potassium Intake (mmol/kg/day)
15-20	140-60	150-200	3.0-5.0 (- 7.0)	3.0-5.0 (- 7.0)	2.0-5.0

* The end of transition is recognized by: 1) Urine volume < 1.0 ml/kg/h, and urine osmolality > serum osmolality; 2) Fractional excretion of sodium diminishes form > 3 % to < 1 %; and 3) Urine specific gravity above 1.012.

+ Water intake volume should be 10 – 20 % less, with humidified incubator or artificial plastic shielding placed over the infant to conserve insensible water evaporation.

° Often 0.5-1.5 mmol/kg/day sodium is administered to these infants inadvertently with transfusions, medications and line infusion.

+++ Start with lower range, increase and adjust according to weight loss, sodium and chloride level, and clinical status. Avoid cardiovascular compromise.

§ Start K+ administration, but not before onset of diuresis; adjust according to calculated need, serum K level and urinary losses.

† Total sodium restriction may increase risk for hyponatremia.

Table 3: Recommendations for daily intake of water and electrolytes in preterm infants.

According to the authors' extensive data base research, no randomized clinical trials were identified that assessed the needs for fluid and sodium in healthy VLBW infants without RDS.

Though modern perinatal care has reduced the incidence of RDS in VLBW infants, most of these infants still experience adaptational disturbances linked to pulmonary immaturity. This might help explain the lack of data in healthy children.

Transitional Phase (Phase I) Complicated by Respiratory Distress Syndrome (RDS).

Pathophysiology. In the immature infant with RDS, the physiologic postnatal contraction in extracellular fluid volume is delayed.[153,217] The reason for this observation is unclear, but may be possibly related to pulmonary edema.[32,33,43,76,116] The start of the contraction process of the extracellular compartment in RDS patients usually occurs together with respiratory stabilization. Different suggestions for this phenomenon were published in the past: in one study, improved oxygenation was shown not to be the initial step in respiratory stabilization.[55,74,95,109,130] Some authors concluded that diuresis precedes respiratory improvement.[58,74,109,130] Modi and Hutton[156] concluded however that the start of diuresis followed respiratory improvement, and changes in sodium handling closely followed changes in respiratory function. Prior to improvement in respiratory function, infants continued to exhibit a net stimulus to retain sodium. Modi and Hutton speculated that the postnatal fall in pulmonary vascular resistance and increased left atrial return will lead to release of atrial natriuretic peptide (ANP). After respiratory stabilization of RDS patients there is also a fall in pulmonary vascular resistance, which increases left atrial pressure. The increase stimulates ANP release, which results in responses markedly different from those *in utero*.

Conclusion: Improvement in RDS leads to secondary normalization of fluid status.

Clinical trials on fluid and sodium intake. Much published data indicate that the initial regimen of fluid and sodium administration during postnatal adaptation is closely linked to later outcome of infants with RDS, i.e., development of chronic lung disease (CLD, BPD), and patent ductus arteriosus (PDA).[24,27,28,106,108,154,156,200,213,219,220]

Fluids. On the basis of improved understanding of physiologic adaptive processes there is first evidence that preterm infants might benefit from a restrictive fluid regimen. Lorenz et al[140] and Kavvadia and coworkers[122] published no adverse effects in randomized trials on short-term outcome with standard fluid administration versus a restricted fluid regimen. Lorenz et al controlled fluid intake in 88 VLBW infants to produce either 5-7% or 10-12% weight loss.[140] No differences concerning ICH, PDA, BPD, necrotizing enterocolitis, dehydration, or metabolic disturbances were found. The trial by Kavvadia et al compared a fluid regimen starting at 60 ml/kg/d and a one-week stepwise increment to 150 ml/kg/d, with a regimen that supplied 20% less fluid (n = 168).[122] Besides higher urinary osmolarities in the restricted group, no significant differences of acute and short-term adverse effects like jaundice, hypotension, hypoglycemia, or hyponatremia were noted.

From these findings, these authors concluded that fluid input in VLBW infants can be handled flexibly to allow gradual loss of 5-15% of birth weight during the first week of life without short or long term effects. The incidence of CLD was found to be coupled to the amount of fluid given on day 2 of life. For each increment of 10 ml/kg/d, CLD risk was increased by 6% (p < 0.05).

A meta-analysis of the Cochrane Data Base reviewed four randomized clinical studies with different levels of fluid intake during the first week of life.[25] A clear benefit of fluid restriction for the outcome (PDA, necrotising enterocolitis, death) can be proven. Trends, but not statistically significant differences, were found for the risk of dehydration (fluid restriction) and CLD (liberal fluids).

Conclusion: There seems to be sufficient data to recommend a careful restriction of water intake so that physiological needs are met, potentially benefitting cardiovascular and intestinal function without significant dehydration.[25,102,103,122,140]

Sodium. The aforementioned difficulty to compare and interpret outcome measures of clinical trials correctly are similar for clinical trials assessing sodium needs in preterm infants.

Costarino and co-workers compared two regimens of sodium prescription in a randomized, blinded therapeutic trial on VLBW infants (n=17). The infants in the restriction group received no sodium during the first five days, whereas the daily maintenance group received 3 to 4 mmol Na$^+$/kg/day.[59] In the sodium-restricted group, serum osmolarity was more likely to be normal and incidence of BPD was significantly lower than in the maintenance group. A 25%-incidence of hyponatremia was observed in the restriction group, whereas in the maintenance group 25% of the infants developed hypernatremia.

A higher incidence of hyponatremia in unsupplemented infants (37.5% vs. 13.6% in supplemented) was also confirmed by a study (n=46) of Al-Dahhan et al.[1,3] These authors recommend Na$^+$ intake of 5 mmol/kg/day to infants < 30 weeks and of 4 mmol/kg/d for infants between 30 to 35 weeks gestational age. In this study however, outcome measures were only parameters of short-term fluid and sodium homeostasis, but not those indicating major morbidity like CLD.

Considering all published data, there seems to be sufficient evidence that sodium intake should be restricted in VLBW infants during the period of ECF contraction until a weight loss of approximately 6% has occurred.[25,59,102,103] The rate of infants needing supplemental oxygen and developing BPD was considerably lower in those with restricted intake. However, infants with sodium restriction seem to lose more body weight than infants supplemented during the early period (weight difference between both groups up to 5 %). This difference does not seem to be caused by differences in fluid intake.[102,103] There is also evidence that infants on sodium restriction have a higher risk to develop hyponatremia.

In a recent study Hartnoll et al pointed out that the time point of sodium supplementation after birth does not affect outcome, but that the onset of postnatal sodium supplementation should be individually tailored and delayed until the onset of postnatal ECF contraction or marked clinical weight loss.[104]

Conclusion: Administration of fluids and sodium must be regarded as an integrative system. Both nutrients cannot be considered separately. Sodium and fluids must be in a relationship to each other that meets the current physiologic needs of the preterm organism during postnatal adaptation. To assure this process during daily clinical routine, a precise understanding of the underlying adaptive mechanisms is crucial.

However, it must be stated that we are often missing the target of normal electrolytes in these babies. With simple clinical means we are often not able to guess too little versus too much water when amounts of evaporation are so high and so variable from baby to baby.

Diuretics. Concerning the use of diuretics there are no recent data available. Furosemide, on one side, may reduce body water load, thus promoting closure of ductus arteriosus, but, on the other hand, interferes with prostaglandin metabolism and action and may therefore keep the ductus open. Therefore the routine use of furosemide must be weighed against the risk of developing a symptomatic patent ductus arteriosus.[41] Published investigations were all done before the era of prenatal steroids, surfactant and indomethacin.[146,191,232] In these studies, no benefit of furosemide administration on the clinical course of RDS and its outcome could be found. Elective administration of diuretics should be carefully weighed against the risk of precipitating hypovolemia and electrolyte imbalances. A recent Cochrane Data Base meta-analysis reviewing six studies did not prove any benefit of routine diuretic administration.

Capillary leak (sepsis, infection, shock). Physiology: Inflammatory mediators have the potential to lead to a structural instability of capillaries. This increases the loss of high molecular substances from the intravascular to the extravascular compartment, with the effect of lowering intravascular oncotic pressure and the occurrence of fluid shift from intra- to extracellular compartment. This clinical state presents clinically as edema or free fluid in the third space.

Conclusion: The treatment of the "capillary leak syndrome" is treatment of the underlying cause (eg, infection, allergic or toxic reaction). Symptomatic treatment of capillary leak can be achieved by administration of high molecular substances like erythrocyte concentrates. Erythrocytes have a molecular size which is bigger than capillary leaks. Because of the disadvantages of erythrocyte transfusion (potential risk of infection), high molecular substances like hydroxyethyl starch (HES) are potentially useful for symptomatic treatment of the capillary leak syndrome.[105,119,132,190,233] The intravenous use of protein solutions like human albumin with a low or medium molecular weight will lead only to a short-term positive effect. Due to the leaky capillary walls, protein molecules will leave the intravascular space and increase oncotic pressure in the extravascular space, thus worsening the situation.

Insert No. 5: Early Volume Expansion or Not? Inotropes?

Early volume expansion to improve morbidity and mortality of VLBW infants was investigated in different trials. In a study by Greenough and coworkers, ten sick but normotensive premature infants (mean gestational age of 29 weeks, range 24 - 36 weeks, mean birthweight of 1390 g, range 560 - 3315 g) with hypoalbuminemia (ie < 30 g/l) on ventilatory support were treated at the age of 1.7 days (range 24 hrs to 5 days) with 5 ml 20% salt poor albumin infusion. Mean pre- and post-infusion urinary output increased from 11.5 (range 1.3 - 23) to 21.1 (0.7 to 37) ml during the following 6-hr period.[91] However, the accompanying editorial comment criticized this study as lacking a control group.[188]

There is no evidence from randomized trials to support the routine use of early volume expansion in preterm infants without cardiovascular compromise. There is insufficient evidence to determine whether infants with cardiovascular compromise would benefit from volume expansion. There were no significant differences between the different types of volume expanders like 0.9% saline, albumin infusion or blood products.[163,205]

A second Cochrane review showed that dopamine was more successful than albumin at correcting low blood pressure in hypotensive preterm infants, many of whom had already received volume. However, neither intervention (early volume vs. inotrope) has been shown to be superior at improving blood flow, or improving mortality and morbidity.[164]

Asphyxia and cerebral edema. The authors are not aware of any published randomized trials investigating fluid and electrolyte regimens that improve outcome of preterm infants suffering from intrauterine asphyxia.

Intermediate and Stabilization Phase (Phase II and III)
General Aspects

In this period, renal and cardiovascular conditions are stabilized, and parenteral fluid administration is stepwise replaced by oral feeding. To the best knowledge of the authors there are no randomized, controlled clinical studies investigating appropriate fluid and electrolyte regimens during this dual period of enteral/parenteral fluid supply.

Therefore, in the following paragraphs, estimations of normal fluid and electrolyte requirements shall be derived on the basis of physiologic studies, observations and case reports.

Water. Coulthard and Hay have shown that healthy preterm infants (29 - 34 weeks) were able to cope with water intakes ranging from 96 to 200 ml/kg/day from the third day of life.[60] These figures may reflect the range of fluid load neonates can deal with, and they may serve as lower and upper limits for reasonable daily allowances.

Sodium Chloride. Based on metabolic balance studies, Ziegler and Fomon[236] determined that term breast-fed infants needed as little as only 0.35 to 0.7 mmol/kg/day of NaCl during the first 4 months of life to achieve adequate growth. The authors recommend 1.0 to 2.0 mmol/kg/day NaCl as a safe daily intake to cover incidental losses from skin or gastrointestinal tract.

Factors that link NaCl and water retention. Beside fluid intake, sodium balance is further positively influenced by protein intake and accretion of lean mass.[121] Sodium deficit is linked with impaired growth.

The greater weight gain in infants with excess sodium intake is caused by higher water retention in the ECF compared to those with a negative Na^+ balance.

The overall growth in terms of weight gain was shown to be greater in infants fed with more calories and was attributed to more fat deposition and higher Cl^- and K^+ retention.

Fluid and NaCl requirement. Because of insufficient data, the optimal fluid and NaCl requirement is only roughly definable (see above). Further, it is not known which initial weight loss is acceptable in term and preterm VLBW and ELBW neonates during the first week of extrauterine life. The published data show a slightly better outcome and a lower incidence for complications with a low initial NaCl (1 mmol/kg body weight/d) and fluid administration.

The individual variability of newborns with different birth weights, disease, losses and requirements makes an adaptation of fluid and electrolyte administration to the individual patient necessary. Assessment of individual requirements is roughly possible by the above mentioned methods to monitor the fluid status and laboratory measurements of plasma electrolytes (see above).

Potassium. Data on K+ supplementation to neonates are rare. Controversy about providing potassium to infants is often a matter of anxiety rather than related to data from controlled trials. The general concern about potassium supplementation was provoked by reports about cardiac arrhythmias due to high plasma potassium concentrations.

However, most episodes of hyperkalemia in the neonate have no observable consequences. In fact, the range of normal values for plasma K+ concentration given in standard references exceeds the upper limit for all other ages. Whether this is due to frequent occurrence of hemolysed blood specimens, blood sampling in a hypoperfused extremity, or a greater tolerance to extracellular K+ is uncertain.

Also, the reasons for the non-oliguric hyperkalemia which is seen in VLBW and ELBW preterm infants are not understood. Engle et al found urinary K+ excretion to be correlated with renal aldosterone excretion.[73] It could be that a rise in plasma K+ concentration following birth stimulates the renin-angiotensin-aldosterone axis in neonates, just as K+ loading does in rats.[157] Prevention of hyperkalemia should be directed more at keeping K+ within cells than providing the daily requirement recommended for stable and growing infants. Also, administration of protein solutions are under consideration to lower the

elevated plasma potassium concentration. If those measures fail, urinary K+ excretion can be increased by furosemide treatment due to 10 fold increase in PGE2 synthesis. This was shown in one neonate by Engle and Arant.[73]

Hyperkalemia varies (inversely) with urinary output, but not with K+ intake, arterial blood pH, asphyxia, respiratory distress, gestational age, or birthweight.[135] It is common practice to start potassium supplementation if plasma K+ concentration remains or returns to within the range of normal. Balance studies of different investigators[2,3,9,49,134] show that thriving preterm infants retain K+ at about 1.0 to 1.5 mmol/kg/d, which is about the same as fetal accretion. The amount of potassium usually recommended is similar to the amount provided in human milk, about 2 to 3 mmol/kg/d.[92] Milk formulas were studied which contained more K+ without any untoward effects on the infant, unless renal function is impaired or mineralocorticoid deficiency is present.

Enteral versus parenteral electrolyte intake. Recommendations usually do not differentiate between enteral or parenteral electrolyte intake. This is possible because electrolytes are almost completely absorbed from the intestine under healthy conditions. There are no data available about electrolyte absorption in preterm neonates or newborn infants.

Different investigators showed a correlation between fluid intake and sodium requirements. The following paragraph divides representative studies into three groups on the basis of fluid intake per kg body weight and day.

Phase II and III: Stabilization Without Problems

Daily fluid intake >170 ml/kg/d. Different authors show that sodium excretion increases with daily fluid intake. If daily fluid intake is as high as 170 ml/kg body weight or above, urinary Na+ excretion is high and sodium balance is usually negative in neonates. Even a Na+ intake as high as 10 mmol/kg body weight/d did not compensate for renal losses, and in half of the investigated infants hyponatremia developed.[72] When fluid therapy exceeds 200 ml/kg/d most ELBW infants will not be able to maintain NaCl-balance, regardless of the amount of NaCl provided.

Daily fluid intake 140-170 ml/kg/d. In different investigations, Bramhall[12], Raiha[172], Polberger[170] and day et al[64] provided infants with different sodium intake (between 1.1 or 3.0 mmol/kg/d) and a fluid intake between 140-170 ml/kg/d. Physiological Na+ concentrations were found in the investigated neonates. In all studies the growth rate was not related to sodium intake.

Daily Fluid intake <140 ml/kg/d. Different investigators reported that with a moderate volume of fluid (<140 ml/kg/d), a minimum NaCl intake of about 1 mmol/kg/d is adequate to maintain NaCl balance also in ELBW neonates.[10,59,71,75,125,140,200] There was no increase in morbidity among infants given less Na+ and less fluid. Even ELBW infants did well on a daily Na+ intake < 2 mmol/kg/d. Although not statistically significant, there was a tendency to higher incidences of patent ductus arteriosus and bronchopulmonary dysplasia in infants given more Na+ and a higher fluid intake.[28,43,59] If more fluid is administered, even to replace higher insensible water loss, additional NaCl must be prescribed.

Phase II and III: Stabilization with Problems (BPD/CLD eg)

General aspects. Bronchopulmonary dysplasia (BPD) is characterized by prolonged need for supplemental oxygen or even ventilator treatment. BPD per se is a problem during the phase of stable growth. PDA, on the other hand, may already be present during Phase I, and when major cardiovascular complication occurs, will usually be closed either using drugs or surgery. During the phase of stable growth, therefore, only PDA's with milder clinical signs are observed. In the following paragraph, treatments for both BPD/CLD and PDA are discussed that have an impact on fluid and sodium metabolism.

BPD: Effect of fluid restriction on water and electrolytes. During the phase of stable postnatal growth, fluid restriction is a common clinical first-line treatment for BPD because it is thought to diminish pulmonary edema. Though the clinical impression may be that this approach is sometimes effective, a close review of published data indicates that the benefit of fluid restriction has never been proven in clinical trials. Also, there are very limited data assessing the mechanism of action and other effects of fluid restriction to treat BPD/CLD during the phase of stable growth.[216]

Milder forms of BPD may be regarded as a self-limiting disease and may disappear during later postnatal growth because lung development is not completed before the age of two years. The achievement of appropriate postnatal growth must therefore be the main goal during this period because it is the only causal treatment of BPD/CLD. Fluid restriction using standard preterm formulas, however, bears the risk of insufficient calorie intake and may impair appropriate postnatal growth of the preemies. Puangco and Schanler report on a recent randomized trial in preterm infants with CLD who were fed a standard versus concentrated preterm ready-to-feed formula containing 30 kcal/oz. The authors found that the enriched formula enhanced postnatal growth pattern comparable to that of intrauterine growth.[171]

BPD: Effect of diuretics on water and electrolytes. Bronchopulmonary dysplasia (BPD) in preterm infants is often complicated by lung edema. Therefore diuretics are often prescribed on a regular basis in some hospitals. Brion and Primhak reviewed the published literature for the use of diuretics (enteral loop, distal loop or aerosolized).[38-40,42] Only concerning furosemide are there sufficient published data to perform a systematic review. Infants >3 weeks of age with chronic lung disease showed improved lung compliance and oxygenation under long term use of furosemide. There was no clear benefit for adding either spironolactone or metalazone.[112] In view of lack of data from randomized trials concerning long-term clinical outcomes, the use of diuretics, including furosemide, was not recommended by the reviewers.

BPD: Effect of postnatal steroids on water and electrolyte metabolism. Though steroids are frequently given in clinical routine to treat infants with prolonged need for supplemental oxygen, little has been studied about the impact of postnatally applied steroids on water and electrolyte homeostasis.

A well known clinical side effect is the increase of blood pressure.[61,65,120,149] The rise in blood pressure possibly is a consequence of increased renal sodium retention.[37] The increased blood pressure itself leads to a higher glomerular filtration rate (GFR) and therefore increases diuresis which then may affect body weight and electrolyte metabolism.

This indeed has also been found in preterm infants in two different recent studies.[35,89] Application of steroids at the age of 9 to 27 days of life led to pressure diuresis, weight loss and increase of osmolar load to the kidney. There are no published data available about sodium losses or balances after steroid treatment.

Conclusion: Starting treatment with steroids for BPD may have an impact on water/electrolyte metabolism and must therefore be monitored very carefully.

BPD: Effect of xanthines on water and electrolytes. Methylxanthines are sometimes used to treat infants with BPD because of their bronchodilatatory effect. Besides central stimulating effects, xanthines are known to increase diuresis and urinary volume and sodium output. There are many studies of xanthines in premature infants that show: 1) an inhibitory effect of solute reabsorption, 2) marked diuresis, and 3) increase of fractional sodium and potassium excretion. The effects were transient and disappeared after 24 hours despite continuing xanthine maintenance therapy.[148]

Special Cases
Changes of Fluid Balance Due to Prenatal Steroid Treatment.
Prenatal steroid treatment to prevent respiratory distress syndrome in preterm infants is suspected to enhance epithelial cell maturation, and improve skin barrier function.[11,160] Further it is thought that the maturation of the lung Na^+/K^+-ATPase activity leads to earlier postnatal reabsorption of fetal lung fluid.[161] Omar et al.[161] measured lower insensible water loss, a decreased incidence of hyponatremia, and an earlier diuresis and natriuresis in extremely low-birth-weight neonates.

In a randomized animal study in newborn lambs,

prenatal betamethasone leads to increased 2 hr-postnatal blood pressure, and urine flow and urinary Na^+ excretion as measured 17 hrs after corticoid administration.[204] This difference was further increased during a subsequent volume challenge of 2.5% saline infusion per kg body weight. This was accompanied by increased GFR and lower levels of renal hormones (plasma renin activity, angiotensin II, aldosterone, epinephrine and norepinephrine) when compared to the control group indicating a more mature renal and cardiovascular system in prenatally-treated animals.

Conclusion: Treatment with prenatal steroids affects fluid balance of the treated neonates via maturational processes of skin, renal and cardiovascular system. These effects stabilize fluid and electrolyte balance during the adaptational phase after birth.[29,77,78,161,204] There are no adverse or harmful effects on fluid balance reported.

Conditions of Excess and Deficiency of Water and/or Electrolytes
There are different reasons which relate to electrolyte derangements in neonates. The most usual ones concerning sodium, potassium, chloride, and water are discussed below.

Hypernatremia ($Na^+ > 145$ mmol/l)
Inadequate replacement of insensible water loss is the most often-noticed cause for plasma sodium concentrations above 145 mmol/l in neonates. Also, provision of a high sodium intake can cause hypernatremia. What is considered a "high" sodium intake in neonates is not a fixed number, because it is dependent on the renal ability to excrete Na^+. Therefore VLBW neonates are at increased risk for hypernatremia.

Moreover, hypernatremia has been reported in breast fed infants who received breast milk with a high sodium content.[138,167]

Diagnostic measures. In order to differentiate the causes which present with hypernatremia, the following should be checked: clinical investigation (signs of dehydration), change of body weight in the last few days, urine specific weight or gravity, acid base status, and hematocrit (see insert No. 7).

Pathophysiology. The excess Na⁺ in the ECF osmotically draws water from the intracellular space and leads to intracellular dehydration. Hypernatremia does not indicate total body sodium content, which can be high, low or normal depending on the cause of the hypernatremia and body water content. Hypernatremia can cause acute CNS dysfunction and even leave permanent CNS sequelae. Acute symptomatology was reported in children with plasma sodium concentrations above 158 mmol/l.[165]

Treatment. If dehydration is severe and shock is present, regardless of plasma sodium concentration, plasma volume should be repleted first by normal saline solution. Once perfusion is re-established, fluid containing Na⁺ 75-80 mmol/l should be given until urine is excreted. When urine output is established, hypotonic fluids are used to perform a slow correction of hypernatremia. There is time needed for the fluid exchange between different compartments (ECF/ICF). The slow correction of the hypernatremic state is needed to avoid intracellular edema, which can cause severe intracerebral complications (see above). A rate of reduction of plasma sodium concentration of 10 to 15 mmol/l per day is recommended. The degree of hypotonicity of the fluids is less important than the rate of correction. If other measures fail, the administration of a loop diuretic such as furosemide increases urinary Na⁺Cl⁻ losses.

Hyponatremia (Sodium <135 mmol/l)

Causes. Inadequate high fluid administration can cause low plasma sodium concentrations (relative hyponatremia). Longterm low sodium intake or gastrointestinal losses lead to absolute hyponatremia. Hyponatremia is often a secondary manifestation of other primary disease.

In preterm infants, the most common cause is relative hyponatremia, excess body water relative to a normal body Na⁺ content. Most often, inappropiate arginin-vasopression (AVP) secretion triggered by intrathoracic pressure that alters cardiac output is the underlying cause.[8,176]

Caveat. Hyponatremia can be an early sign of systemic infection.

Diagnostic measures. In order to differentiate the causes that present with hyponatremia, the following should be checked: clinical investigation (signs of infection/fluid status); change of body weight of the last few days; urine amount, specific weight or gravity; acid base status; hematocrit; and gastrointestinal losses (see insert No. 7).

Pathophysiology. Absolute Na⁺ deficiency is always related to volume loss of the extracellular compartment. This alters cardiovascular hemodynamics and organ perfusion, unless total body water has been maintained. In addition, the osmolarity of the extracellular space decreases and may increase the content of intracellular water (intracellular edema). This state can slow nerve conduction, reduce neuroexcitation of muscle tissue, and cause seizures. Also, the occurrence of neonatal apnea was found to be associated with hyponatremia.[62] If hyponatremia persists, there is potential risk for central pontine demyelinolysis.[48]

The mechanisms that lead to hyponatremia associated with systemic infection are not completely understood. The increase of plasma protein, fat and glucose concentrations reduce the relative water content of plasma. If this is not corrected, a lower plasma sodium content is measured.

Treatment. When absolute hyponatremia (ie, loss of total body sodium) is diagnosed, and even when the exact etiology of hyponatremia cannot be determined, sodium should be administered as a first line measure. If possible, sodium should be given orally, in order to correct a deficit over 24 hours or longer. If parenteral supplementation must be given, plasma osmolarity should not rise too fast. Therefore the sodium concentration in plasma should not increase by more than 2.5 mmol/l per day to prevent a reduction in brain water.[81] In case of seizures associated with hyponatremia, sodium administration may need to exceed this guideline. In symptomatic patients, hypertonic saline should be used to rapidly (within hours) correct the Na⁺ to 125 mmol/l.

If inappropriate AVP secretion is suspected as the underlying cause (eg, reduced urinary output despite adequate hydration), restriction of water intake is the method of choice until the plasma Na+ concentration is within normal range.

Late Hyponatremia in VLBW Infants

"Late" hyponatremia is defined when occurring beyond two weeks of life in otherwise healthy premature infants.[123b,186a,214a] Currently, there is no classical theory about the pathophysiology of this state: hypotheses include increased sodium requirements of VLBW infants; insufficient sodium intake; impaired ability to conserve sodium because of the immaturity of the renal function; increase in arginine-vasopressin resulting in enhanced renal water reabsorption; and hypoalbuminemia.

It is still a matter of debate whether late hyponatremia reflects a state of disease or is a transient, but otherwise normal state during VLBW growth. There are no accepted and approved guidelines for treatment of late hyponatremia. We suggest that the first line treatment should not be to increase sodium intake too much, but to try to supply sodium around maintenence doses and to carefully watch and monitor sodium levels. If growth rates are appropriate we would suggest not to increase daily sodium intake. We recommend to keep long-term serum sodium levels below 130 mmol/l. We would like to emphasize that this approach is suggested based on our clinical experience but has never been proven in randomized, controlled trials.

The administration of drugs leading to excessive sodium losses with hyponatremia (like caffeine or loop diuretics), however, might require another treatment (ie, sodium supplementation) in order to avoid decreased sodium stores, which might impair growth.

Hyperkalemia (K+ >5.5 mmol/l)

Causes. In preterm infants, hyperkalemia is often seen in the first 48 hours of life. It is possible to distinguish between oliguric and non-oliguric hyperkalemia. Further, cellular injury (hematoma, asphyxia, hypoxia), excess K+ administration, certain drugs, acidosis, or hypoglycemia can provoke hyperkalemia.

Diagnostic measures. Every VLBW infant should be monitored at regular intervals during the first 48 hours after birth to detect elevated plasma K+ concentrations. In order to differentiate the causes that present with hyperkalemia the following should be checked: clinical investigation (hematoma), acid base status, blood glucose concentration, urinary output (see insert No. 7).

Pathophysiology. States that lead to cellular injury increase the plasma K+ concentration by shifting intracellular K+ into the plasma due to injured cellular integrity. Metabolic imbalances like hypoglycemia or acidosis lead to shift of intracellular K+ to extracellular compartments. In case of oliguric hyperkalemia, the renal excretion of K+ is reduced. The mechanisms of the non-oliguric hyperkalemia are not fully understood. Electrocardiographic changes associated with increased K+ concentrations develop due to impaired membrane potential.

Treatment. In the event of symptomatic hyperkalemia (cardiac arrhythmia), additional glucose with insulin should be administered in order to drive K+ out of ECF into the intracellular space. Furosemide increases urinary K+ excretion. Calcium gluconate can be given intravenously in an emergency to treat arrhythmia, while other treatments are prepared. As a secondary measure, exchange resin may be given by enema. If K+ concentrations are increasing, yet the neonate is still asymptomatic, intravenous supplementation of aminoacid solution increases the renal microcirculation and leads to lower K+ levels by mechanisms which are not completely investigated. Salbutamol, a betamimetic agent, is under investigation.

Insert No. 6: Non-oliguric Hyperkalemia of the Very Immature Infant

VLBW, especially ELBW, infants may present with a currently unexplained non-oliguric hyperkalemia. These infants are typically very low gestational age and have no obvious clinical reason that could explain the potassium levels exceeding the normal range.[54,135,141] Besides the known mechanisms that are involved in the regulation of plasma potassium level (potassium intake, endogenous potassium loading due to cell breakdown; intra-/extracellular distribution; renal and fecal excretion; influences due to *pH; insulin:glucose ratio and glucagons; and adrenergic sympathetic tone), there must be further factors that lead to non-oliguric hyperkalemia. Clinical investigations identified no specific factor for the hyperkalemia in non-oliguric neonates.[113,141] One speculation is the combination of a high endogenous potassium shift due to cell breakdown (e.g., erythrocytes) in combination with other factors that increase plasma potassium levels (like impaired activity of the Na^+/K^+-ATPase) that could contribute to development of hyperkalemia in nonoliguric neonates. Another explanation could be hypernatremia per se, driving sodium ions into the intracellular space, defeating the membrane's pump, then causing leakage of potassium to the extracellular space. The incidence may be lowered by prenatal application of steroids.[162] Treatment is symptomatic (see section on hyperkalemia above). A prospective investigation of potassium balance in neonates with nonoliguric hyperkalemia is needed for better understanding of potassium metabolism and regulation in preterm neonates with very low gestational age.*

Hypokalemia (K <3.5 mmol/l)

Causes. Diuretic therapy or an inadequate (too low) potassium supplementation are common causes that lead to hypokalemia in neonates. Gastrointerstinal losses and alkalosis can provoke hypokalemia.

Diagnostic measures. Check for diuretic therapy, low K^+ supplementation, gastrointestinal losses and alkalosis.

Pathophysiology. An impaired membrane potential due to low plasma K^+ concentrations can provoke different clinical manifestations like ileus, lethargy, muscular weakness, or electrocardiographic changes like bradycardia and arrhythmia. Further, the renal concentrating ability is impaired due to low potassium state. Pseudo AVP resistance develops. Increased PGE^2 production, renin release, and increased angiotensin and aldosterone secretion worsens the potassium deficiency. If uncorrected, this leads to polyuria, dehydration, and hypernatremia.

Treatment. Slow correction of K^+ deficiency, preferably from oral administration, is indicated. Even with symptomatic hypokalemia, it is not appropriate to perform bolus injection of potassium solutions.

Grades of Dehydration	Loss of body weight	Clinical signs
I	<5% little	Dry mouth, reduced skin turgor
II	<10% moderate	I + Sunken fontanelle
III	>10% severe	I + II + Low blood pressure, increased heart rate, oliguria

Table 4: Clinical signs of dehydration.

Dehydration

Causes. Inadequate fluid administration, and high renal, insensible, or gastrointestinal losses are common causes in neonates.

Diagnostic measures. In order to diagnose dehydration, the following should be regularly checked: clinical investigation (signs of dehydration), change of body weight during the last few days, urine-specific weight or gravity, acid base status, plasma sodium concentration, plasma chloride concentration, and hematocrit (see insert No. 7). The amount of dehydration can be estimated by clinical signs (see Table 4). A good clinical marker for the state of hydration is the plasma chloride level (if chloride administration is adequate).

Pathophysiology. VLBW infants have increased insensible water loss in combination with reduced renal concentrating capacity (see above). These factors lead to a high vulnerability to develop dehydration.

Treatment. Before treatment is started, dehydration has to be further characterized. Differentiation among hypotonic (Na^+ <135 mmol/l), normotonic (Na^+ 135-155 mmol/l), or hypertonic dehydration (Na^+ >145 mmol/l) is indicated.

If severe normotonic dehydration is diagnosed (>10% of body weight, Na^+ 135-155 mmol/l), rehydration should take 48 - 72 hours. 50% of the estimated volume loss can be administered during the first 24 hours. The use of isotonic electrolyte solution like saline, Ringer's lactate or glucose electrolyte solution is adequate. Mild (<5%) or moderate (<10%) dehydration can be corrected within 24 hours.[48] If the dehydration is combined with derangement of electrolytes (hypo- or hypertonic dehydration), it is appropriate to follow the guidelines as described in the "treatment" paragraphs of the specific electrolyte disturbances (see above).

Caveat. CNS edema with the risk of subsequent seizures or brain damage may occur when treatment of hypertonic dehydration is done too quickly (guideline: first, correct severe dehydration with isotonic solutions, then start the specific treatment of the electrolyte imbalance.

Hyperhydration and Edema

Causes. Excess fluid administration, low renal fluid excretion, low protein status, capillary leakage.

Diagnostic measures. In order to diagnose hyperhydration or causes that lead to edema, the following should be checked: clinical investigation (edema), change of body weight during the last few days, urine-specific weight or gravity, acid base status, hematocrit, plasma chloride concentration, total plasma protein content (see insert No. 7).

Pathophysiology. Preterm and term neonates are prone to develop peripheral edema because of the immature vascular endothelium in combination with lower plasma proteins. Different clinical situations can contribute to the development of central or peripheral edema.

Treatment. There is no general treatment for hyperhydration or edema. The treatment has to be adapted to the underlying cause.

Insert No. 7: Monitoring Fluid Status in Neonates
In preterm infants, it is good clinical practice to monitor the fluid status. However, no consensus is established concerning time schedule and monitoring measures used. There are different ways to assess the hydration status which are divided into different categories:

1. Prophylactic monitoring measures
  Definition: Measures that have the potential to provide warning of fluid imbalances before they occur.
     - Calculation of future total fluid intake per time interval.
     - Monitoring of total fluid losses
     - Calculation of water balance per time interval

2. Early sign monitoring measures
  Definition: Measures that indicate minor changes of hydration.
     - Clinical evaluation of the patient (skin)
     - Measurement of body weight
     - Measurement of specific gravity of the urine
     - Measurements of electrolytes and acid base status (chloride)
     - Fractional excretion of sodium and of free water
     - Measurement of serum osmolality
     - Measurement of hematocrit.
     - Measurement of bioelectrical impedance (experimental).

3. Late sign monitoring measures
  Definition: Measures that indicate major changes of hydration (compromise of cardiovascular function).
     - Clinical evaluation of the patient (eyes, fontanelle, mucosal moistness)
     - Measurement of blood pressure.
     - Measurement of heart rate.
     - Measurement acid base status (presence of lactic acidosis)

4. Measures which are used for research: Tracers
  Stable isotope dilution (^2H_2O, $H_2^{18}O$), bromide space, Evans blue, sucrose

5. Recommendations for a clinical fluid monitoring
  There are no data available that give a scientific proof about the quality of different monitoring procedures. It is common practice to choose the monitoring measures and schedule the control intervals depending on the clinical status of the patient, on expected changes according to underlying pathophysiology and on the applied treatment. Usually several of the above mentioned measures are combined for optimal monitoring.

References

1. Al-Dahhan J, Haycock GB, Chantler C, Stimmler L. Sodium homeostasis in term and preterm neonates. I. Renal aspects. *Arch Dis Child* 1983a; 58:335-342.

2. Al-Dahhan J, Haycock GB, Chantler C, Stimmler L. Sodium homeostasis in term and preterm neonates. II. Gastrointestinal aspects. *Arch Dis Child* 1983b;58:343-345.

3. Al-Dahhan J, Haycock GB, Nichol B, Chantler C, Stimmler L. Sodium homeostasis in term and preterm neonates. III. Effect of salt supplementation. *Arch Dis Child* 1984;59:945-950.

4. Andersson B. Regulation of body fluids. *Annu Rev Physiol* 1977;39185-200:-200

5. Andersson S, Tikkanen I, Pesonen E, Meretoja O, Hynynen M, Fyhrquist F. Atrial natriuretic peptide in patent ductus arteriosus. *Pediatr Res* 1987;21:396-398.

6. Aperia A, Broberger O, Elinder G, Herin P, Zetterstrom R. Postnatal development of renal function in pre-term and full-term infants. *Acta Paediatr Scand* 1981;70:183-187.

7. Aperia A, Broberger O, Herin P, Zetterstrom R. Sodium excretion in relation to sodium intake and aldosterone excretion in newborn pre-term and full-term infants. *Acta Paediatr Scand* 1979;68:813-817.

8. Arant BS. Neonatal adjustments to extrauterine life. In: Edelmann CM, Bernstein J, Meadow R, Spitzer A, Trvis L, eds. Pediatric kidney disease. Boston: Little Brown, 1992:1015-1042.

9. Arant BS, Seikaly MG. Intrarenal angiotensin II may regulate developmental changes in renal blood flow. *Pediatr Nephrol* 1989;3:C142

10. Asano H, Taki M, Igarashi Y. Sodium homeostasis in premature infants during the early postnatal period: results of relative low volume of fluid and sodium intake. *Pediatr Nephrol* 1987;1:C38

11. Aszterbaum M, Feingold KR, Menon GK, Williams ML. Glucocorticoids accelerate fetal maturation of the epidermal permeability barrier in the rat. *J Clin Invest* 1993;91:2703-2708.

12. Babson SG, Bramhall JL. Diet and growth in the premature infant. The effect of different dietary intakes of ash-electrolyte and protein on weight gain and linear growth. *J Pediatr* 1969;74:890-900.

13. Bauer K, Bovermann G, Roithmaier A, Gotz M, Proiss A, Versmold HT. Body composition, nutrition, and fluid balance during the first two weeks of life in preterm neonates weighing less than 1500 grams. *J Pediatr* 1991;118:615-620.

14. Bauer K, Buschkamp S, Marcinkowski M, Kossel H, Thome U, Versmold HT. Postnatal changes of extracellular volume, atrial natriuretic factor, and diuresis in a randomized controlled trial of high-frequency oscillatory ventilation versus intermittent positive-pressure ventilation in premature infants <30 weeks gestation. *Crit Care Med* 2000;28:2064-2068.

15. Bauer K, Cowett RM, Howard GM, vanEpp J, Oh W. Effect of intrauterine growth retardation on postnatal weight change in preterm infants. *J Pediatr* 1993;123:301-306.

16. Bauer K, Versmold H. Postnatal weight loss in preterm neonates less than 1,500 g is due to isotonic dehydration of the extracellular volume. *Acta Paediatr Scand Suppl* 1989;36037-42:-42

17. Bauer K, Versmold H, Prolss A, De-Graaf SS, Meeuwsen-Van-der-Roest WP, Zijlstra WG. Estimation of extracellular volume in preterm infants less than 1500 g, children, and adults by sucrose dilution. *Pediatr Res* 1990;27:256-259.

18. Baumgart S. Radiant energy and insensible water loss in the premature newborn infant nursed under a radiant warmer. *Clin Perinatol* 1982;9:483-503.

19. Baumgart S. Reduction of oxygen consumption, insensible water loss, and radiant heat demand with use of a plastic blanket for low-birth-weight infants under radiant warmers. *Pediatrics* 1984;74: 1022-1028.

20. Baumgart S. Partitioning of heat losses and gains in premature newborn infants under radiant warmers. *Pediatrics* 1985;75:89-99.

21. Baumgart S, Engle WD, Fox WW, Polin RA. Radiant warmer power and body size as determinants of insensible water loss in the critically ill neonate. *Pediatr Res* 1981;15:1495-1499.

22. Baumgart S, Langman CB, Sosulski R, Fox WW, Polin RA. Fluid, electrolyte, and glucose maintenance in the very low birth weight infant. *Clin Pediatr* (Phila) 1982;21:199-206.

23. Baylen BG, Ogata H, Ikegami M, Jacobs H, Jobe A, Emmanouilides GC. Left ventricular performance and contractility before and after volume infusion: a comparative study of preterm and full-term newborn lambs. *Circulation* 1986;73:1042-1049.

24. Bell EF. Fluid therapie. In: Sinclair JC, Bracken M,

eds. Effective care of the newborn. Oxford: Oxford University Press, 1992:59-71.

25. Bell EF, Acarregui MJ. Restricted versus liberal water intake for preventing morbidity and mortality in preterm infants. Cochrane Database Syst Rev 2000;CD000503.

26. Bell EF, Neidich GA, Cashore WJ, Oh W. Combined effect of radiant warmer and phototherapy on insensible water loss in low-birth-weight infants. *J Pediatr* 1979;94:810-813.

27. Bell EF, Warburton D, Stonestreet BS, Oh W. High-volume fluid intake predisposes premature infants to necrotising enterocolitis. *Lancet* 1979;2:90

28. Bell EF, Warburton D, Stonestreet BS, Oh W. Effect of fluid administration on the development of symptomatic patent ductus arteriosus and congestive heart failure in premature infants. *N Engl J Med* 1980;302:598-604.

29. Berry LM, Polk DH, Ikegami M, Jobe AH, Padbury JF, Ervin MG. Preterm newborn lamb renal and cardiovascular responses after fetal or maternal antenatal betamethasone. *Am J Physiol* 1997;272:R1972-R1979.

30. Bhat R, Javed S, Malalis L, Vidyasagar D. Colloid osmotic pressure in healthy and sick neonates. *Crit Care Med* 1981;9:563-567.

31. Bhat R, Malalis L, Shukla A, Vidyasagar D. Colloid osmotic pressure in infants with hyaline membrane disease. *Chest* 1983;83 :776-779.

32. Bland RD. Edema formation in the newborn lung. *Clin Perinatol* 1982;9:593-611.

33. Bland RD. Edema formation in the lungs and its relationship to neonatal respiratory distress. *Acta Paediatr Scand Suppl* 1983;30592-9:-9

34. Boehles H. Ernaehrungsstoerungen im Kindesalter. Stuttgart: Wissenschaftliche Verlagsgesellschaft, 1991:26

35. Bos AF, van-Asselt WA, Okken A. Dexamethasone treatment and fluid balance in preterm infants at risk for chronic lung disease. *Acta Paediatr* 2000;89: 562-565.

36. Bower TR, Pringle KC, Soper RT. Sodium deficit causing decreased weight gain and metabolic acidosis in infants with ileostomy. *J Pediatr Surg* 1988;23: 567-572.

37. Brem AS. Insights Into Glucocorticoid-Associated Hypertension. *Am J Kidney Dis* 2001;37:1-10.

38. Brion LP, Primhak RA. Intravenous or enteral loop diuretics for preterm infants with (or developing) chronic lung disease. Cochrane Database Syst Rev 2000;CD001453.

39. Brion LP, Primhak RA, Ambrosio-Perez I. Diuretics acting on the distal renal tubule for preterm infants with (or developing) chronic lung disease. Cochrane Database Syst Rev 2000;CD001817.

40. Brion LP, Primhak RA, Yong W. Aerosolized diuretics for preterm infants with (or developing) chronic lung disease. Cochrane Database Syst Rev 2000; CD001694.

41. Brion LP, Soll RF. Diuretics for respiratory distress syndrome in preterm infants (Cochrane Review). Cochrane Database Syst Rev 2000;2:CD001454.

42. Brion LP, Yong SC, Perez IA, Primhak R. Diuretics and chronic lung disease of prematurity. *J Perinatol* 2001;21:269-271.

43. Brown ER, Stark A, Sosenko I, Lawson EE, Avery ME. Bronchopulmonary dysplasia: possible relationship to pulmonary edema. *J Pediatr* 1978;92: 982-984.

44. Brunette MG, Leclerc, Claveau D. Na+ transport by human placental brush border membranes: are there several mechanisms? *J Cell Physiol* 1996;167:72-80.

45. Brück K. Heat production and temperature regulation. In: Stave U, ed. Perinatal physiology. New York: Plenum Medical Publishing 1987:455.

46. Brück K. Neonatal thermal regulation. In: Polin RA, Fox WW, eds. Fetal and neonatal physiology. Philadelphia: Saunders W.B. 1992:488-514.

47. Bueva A, Guignard JP. Renal function in preterm neonates. *Pediatr Res* 1994;36:572-577.

48. Burcar PJ, Norenberg MD, Yarnell PR. Hyponatremia and central pontine myelinolysis. *Neurology* 1977;27:223-226.

49. Butterfield J, Lubchenco L, Bergstedt J, O'Brien D. Patterns in electrolyte and nitrogen balance in the newborn premature infant. *Pediatrics* 1960;26: 777-791.

50. Carlton DP, Cummings JJ, Scheerer RG, Bland RD. Lung vascular protein permeability in preterm fetal and mature newborn sheep. *J Appl Physiol* 1994;77:782-788.

51. Catzeflis C, Schutz Y, Micheli JL, Welsch C, Arnaud MJ, Jequier E. Whole body protein synthesis and energy expenditure in very low birth weight infants. *Pediatr Res* 1985;19:679-687.

52. Chard T, Hudson CN, Edwards CR, Boyd NR. Release of oxytocin and vasopressin by the human foetus during labour. *Nature* 1971;234 :352-354.

53. Chevalier RL. Developmental renal physiology of the low birth weight pre-term newborn. *J Urol* 1996; 156:714-719.

54. Chevalier RL. What are normal potassium concentrations in the neonate? What is a reasonable approach to hyperkalemia in the newborn with normal renal function? *Semin Nephrol* 1998;18: 360-361.

55. Cort R. Renal function in the respiratory distress syndrome. *Acta Paediatr Scand* 1962;51:313-323.

56. Costarino A, Baumgart S. Modern fluid and electrolyte management of the critically ill premature infant. *Pediatr Clin North Am* 1986;33:153-178.

57. Costarino AT, Baumgart S. Neonatal water and electrolyte metabolism. In: Cowett R, ed. Priciples of perinatal-neonatal metabolism. 2 Ed. New York: Springer 1998:1045-1075.

58. Costarino AT, Baumgart S, Norman ME, Polin RA. Renal adaptation to extrauterine life in patients with respiratory distress syndrome. *Am J Dis Child* 1985;139:1060-1063.

59. Costarino AT, Gruskay JA, Corcoran L, Polin RA, Baumgart S. Sodium restriction versus daily maintenance replacement in very low birth weight premature neonates: a randomized, blind therapeutic trial. *J Pediatr* 1992;120:99-106.

60. Coulthard MG, Hey EN. Effect of varying water intake on renal function in healthy preterm babies. *Arch Dis Child* 1985;60:614-620.

61. Cummings JJ, D'Eugenio DB, Gross SJ. A controlled trial of dexamethasone in preterm infants at high risk for bronchopulmonary dysplasia. *N Engl J Med* 1989;320:1505-1510.

62. Daily WJ, Klaus M, Meyer HB. Apnea in premature infants: monitoring, incidence, heart rate changes, and an effect of environmental temperature. *Pediatrics* 1969;43:510-518.

63. Dancis. *J Pediatr* 1948;33:547

64. Day GM, Radde IC, Balfe JW, Chance GW. Electrolyte abnormalities in very low birthweight infants. *Pediatr Res* 1976;10:522-526.

65. Durand M, Sardesai S, McEvoy C. Effects of early dexamethasone therapy on pulmonary mechanics and chronic lung disease in very low birth weight infants: a randomized, controlled trial. *Pediatrics* 1995; 95:584-590.

66. Edelmann CM, Barnett HL. Role of Kidney in water metabolism in young infants. *J Pediatr* 1960;56: 154-179.

67. Edelmann CM, Barnett HL, Stark H. Effect of urea on concentration of urinary nonurea solute in premature infants. *J Appl Physiol* 1966;21:1021-1025.

68. Edelmann CM, Trompkom V, Barnett HL. Renal concentrating ability in newborn infants. *Fed Proc* 1959;18:49-54.

69. Edelmann CM, Wolfish N. Diatary influence on renal maturation in preterm infants. *Pediatr Res* 1968;2:421-426.

70. Ekblad H. Postnatal changes in colloid osmotic pressure in premature infants: in healthy infants, in infants with respiratory distress syndrome, and in infants born to mothers with premature rupture of membranes. *Gynecol Obstet Invest* 1987;24:95-100.

71. Ekblad H, Kero P, Takala J, Korvenranta H, Valimaki I. Water, sodium and acid-base balance in premature infants: therapeutical aspects. *Acta Paediatr Scand* 1987;76:47-53.

72. Engelke SC, Shah BL, Vasan U, Raye JR. Sodium balance in very low-birth-weight infants. *J Pediatr* 1978;93:837-841.

73. Engle WD, Arant BS. Urinary potassium excretion in the critically ill neonate. *Pediatrics* 1984;74:259-264.

74. Engle WD, Arant BS, Wiriyathian S, Rosenfeld CR. Diuresis and respiratory distress syndrome: physiologic mechanisms and therapeutic implications. *J Pediatr* 1983;102:912-917.

75. Engle WD, Magness R, Faucher DJ, Arant BS, Rosenfeld CR. Sodium balance in the growing preterm infant. *Infant Pediatr Res* 1985;19:376a

76. Ertl T, Sulyok E, Bodis J, Csaba IF. Plasma prolactin levels in full-term newborn infants with idiopathic

edema: response to furosemide. *Biol Neonate* 1986;49:15-20.

77. Ervin MG, Berry LM, Ikegami M, Jobe AH, Padbury JF, Polk DH. Single dose fetal betamethasone administration stabilizes postnatal glomerular filtration rate and alters endocrine function in premature lambs. *Pediatr Res* 1996;40:645-651.

78. Ervin MG, Seidner SR, Leland MM, Ikegami M, Jobe AH. Direct fetal glucocorticoid treatment alters postnatal adaptation in premature newborn baboons. *Am J Physiol* 1998;274:R1169-R1176

79. Fawer CL, Torrado A, Guignard JP. Maturation of renal function in full-term and premature neonates. *Helv Paediatr Acta* 1979;34:11-21.

80. Fede C, Frisina N, Caracciolo A, Buemi M , Caruso MG, Ricca M. Changes in plasma concentrations of atrial natriuretic peptide during the first ten days and the second month of life. *Child Nephrol Urol* 1988;9:144-146.

81. Finberg L. The relationship of intravenous infusions and intracranial hemorrhage--a commentary. *J Pediatr* 1977;91:777-778.

82. Fomon SJ, Haschke F, Ziegler EE, Nemeth M. Body composition of reference children from birth to age 10 years. *Am J Clin Nutr* 1982;35:1169-1175.

83. Friis-Hansen B. Body water compartments in children: changes during growth and related changes in body composition. *Pediatrics* 1961;28:169-174.

84. Friis-Hansen B. Water - the major Nutrient. *Acta Paediatr Scand Suppl* 1982;299:11-16.

85. Fusch C, Hungerland E, Scharrer B, Moeller H. Water turnover of healthy children measured by deuterated water elimination. *Eur J Pediatr* 1993;152:110-114.

86. Fusch C, Keisker A, Blum WF, Moessinger AC. Serum leptin concentrations and body fat in healthy premature and term infants. *Pediatr Res* 1999; 42:231A(Abstract)

87. Fusch C, Scharrer B, Hungerland E, Moeller H. Body water lean body and fat mass of healthy children as measured by deuterium oxide dilution. *Isotopenpraxis Environ Health Stud* 1993;29: 125-131.

88. Fusch C, Slotboom J, Fuehrer U, Schumacher R, Kreisker A, Zimmermann W, Moessinger AC,

Boesch C, Blum J. Neonatal body composition: dual-energy X-ray absorptiometry, magnetic resonance imaging, and three dimensional chemical shift imaging versus chemical analysis in piglets. *Pediatr Res* 1999;465-473.

88a. Gaylord MS, Wright K, Lorch K, Lorch V, Walker E. Improved fluid management utilizing humidified incubators in extremely low birth weight infants. *J Perinatol* 2001 21:438-43

89. Gladstone IM, Ehrenkranz RA, Jacobs HC. Pulmonary function tests and fluid balance in neonates with chronic lung disease during dexamethasone treatment. *Pediatrics* 1989;84: 1072-1076.

90. Grantham JJ, Burg MB. Effect of vasopressin and cyclic AMP on permeability of isolated collecting tubules. *Am J Physiol* 1966;211:255-259.

91. Greenough A, Greenall F, Gamsu HR. Immediate effects of albumin infusion in ill premature neonates. *Arch Dis Child* 1988;63:307-30

92. Gross SJ. Growth and biochemical response of preterm infants fed human milk or modified infant formula. *N Engl J Med* 1983;308:237-241.

92a. Gruskay J, Costarino AT, Polin RA, Baumgart S. Non-oliguric hyperkalemia in the premature infant less than 1000 grams. *J Pediatr* 1988; 113:381-386.

93. Gruskin AB, Edelmann CM, Yuan S. Maturational changes in renal blood flow in piglets. *Pediatr Res* 1970;4:7-13.

94. Gruwel ML, Alves C, Schrader J. Na(+)-K(+)-ATPase in endothelial cell energetics: 23Na nuclear magnetic resonance and calorimetry study. *Am J Physiol* 1995;268:H351-H358

95. Guignard JP, Torrado A, Mazouni SM, Gautier E. Renal function in respiratory distress syndrome. *J Pediatr* 1976;88:845-850.

96. Gutin B, Litaker M, Islam S, Manos T, Smith C, Treiber F. Body-composition measurement in 9-11-y-old children by dual-energy X-ray absorptiometry, skinfold-thickness measurements, and bioimpedance analysis. *Am J Clin Nutr* 1996;63:287-292.

97. Guyton A, Scanlon L, Armstrong G. Effects of pressoreceptor reflex and cushing reflex on urinary output. *Fed Proc* 1952;11:61-62.

98. Hadeed AJ, Leake RD, Weitzman RE, Fisher DA. Possible mechanisms of high blood levels of vasopressin during the neonatal period. *J Pediatr* 1979;94:805-808.

99. Hammarlund K, Sedin G. Transepidermal water loss in newborn infants. III. Relation to gestational age. *Acta Paediatr Scand* 1979;68:795-801.

100. Hammarlund K, Sedin G, Stromberg B. Transepidermal water loss in newborn infants. VIII. Relation to gestational age and post-natal age in appropriate and small for gestational age infants. *Acta Paediatr Scand* 1983;72:721-728.

100a.Harpin VA, Rutter N. Humidification of incubators. *Arch Dis Child* 1985;60:219-224.

101. Hartnoll G, Betremieux P, Modi N. Body water content of extremely preterm infants at birth. *Arch Dis Child Fetal Neonatal Ed* 2000a;83:F56-F59

102. Hartnoll G, Betremieux P, Modi N. Randomised controlled trial of postnatal sodium supplementation on body composition in 25 to 30 week gestational age infants. *Arch Dis Child Fetal Neonatal Ed* 2000b;82:F24-F28

103. Hartnoll G, Betremieux P, Modi N. Randomised controlled trial of postnatal sodium supplementation on oxygen dependency and body weight in 25-30 week gestational age infants. *Arch Dis Child Fetal Neonatal Ed* 2000a;82:F19-F23

104. Hartnoll G, Betremieux P, Modi N. Randomised controlled trial of postnatal sodium supplementation in infants of 25-30 weeks gestational age: effects on cardiopulmonary adaptation. *Arch Dis Child Fetal Neonatal Ed* 2001b;85:F29-F32

105. Hausdorfer J, Hagemann H, Heine J. Vergleich der Volumenersatzmittel Humanalbumin 5% und Hydroxyathylstarke 6% (40.000/0,5) in der Kinderanasthesie. [Comparison of volume substitutes 5 percent human albumin and 6 percent hydroxyethyl starch (40,000/0.5) in pediatric anesthesia]. *Anasth Intensivther Notfallmed* 1986;21:137-142.

106. Haycock GB. The influence of sodium on growth in infancy. *Pediatr Nephrol* 1993;7:871-875.

107. Haycock GB. Development of glomerular filtration and tubular sodium reabsorption in the human fetus and newborn. *Br J Urol* 1998;81 Suppl 233-8:-8.

108. Haycock GB, Aperia A. Salt and the newborn kidney. *Pediatr Nephrol* 1991;5:65-70.

109. Heaf DP, Belik J, Spitzer AR, Gewitz MH , Fox WW. Changes in pulmonary function during the diuretic phase of respiratory distress syndrome. *J Pediatr* 1982;101:103-107.

110. Heimler R, Doumas BT, Jendrzejczak BM, Nemeth PB, Hoffman RG, Nelin LD. Relationship between nutrition, weight change, and fluid compartments in preterm infants during the first week of life. *J Pediatr* 1993;122:110-114.

111. Hey EN, Katz G. Evaporative water loss in the new-born baby. *J Physiol* 1969;200:605-619.

112. Hoffman DJ, Gerdes JS, Abbasi S. Pulmonary function and electrolyte balance following spironolactone treatment in preterm infants with chronic lung disease: a double-blind, placebo-controlled, randomized trial. *J Perinatol* 2000;20:41-45.

113. Hu PS, Su BH, Peng CT, Tsai CH. Glucose and insulin infusion versus kayexalate for the early treatment of non-oliguric hyperkalemia in very-low-birth-weight infants. *Acta Paediatr Taiwan* 1999;40:314-318.

114. Ichikawa I, Maddox DA, Brenner BM. Maturational development of glomerular ultrafiltration in the rat. *Am J Physiol* 1979;236:F465-F471

115. Imbert-Teboul M, Chabardes D, Clique A, Montegut M, Morel F. Ontogenesis of hormone-dependent adenylate cyclase in isolated rat nephron segments. *Am J Physiol* 1984;247: F316-F325.

116. Jefferies AL, Coates G, O'Brodovich H. Pulmonary epithelial permeability in hyaline-membrane disease. *N Engl J Med* 1984;311:1075-1080.

117. Jhaveri MK, Kumar SP. Passage of the first stool in very low birth weight infants. *Pediatrics* 1987;79:1005-1007.

118. Jobe A, Jacobs H, Ikegami M, Berry D. Lung protein leaks in ventilated lambs: effects of gestational age. *J Appl Physiol* 1985;58:1246-1251.

119. Kaplan SS, Park TS, Gonzales ER, Gidday JM. Hydroxyethyl starch reduces leukocyte adherence and vascular injury in the newborn pig cerebral circulation after asphyxia. *Stroke* 2000;31:2218-2223.

120. Kari MA, Heinonen K, Ikonen RS, Koivisto M, Raivio KO. Dexamethasone treatment in preterm infants at risk for bronchopulmonary dysplasia. *Arch Dis Child* 1993;68:566-569.

121. Kashyap S, Forsyth M, Zucker C, Ramakrishnan R, Dell RB, Heird WC. Effects of varying protein and energy intakes on growth and metabolic response in low birth weight infants. *J Pediatr* 1986;108:955-963.

122. Kavvadia V, Greenough A, Dimitriou G, Forsling ML. Randomized trial of two levels of fluid input in the perinatal period—effect on fluid balance, electrolyte and metabolic disturbances in ventilated VLBW infants. *Acta Paediatr* 2000;89:237-241.

123. Kero P, Korvenranta H, Alamaakala P, Selanne P, Kiilholma P, Valimaki I. Colloid osmotic pressure of cord blood in relation to neonatal outcome and mode of delivery. *Acta Paediatr Scand Suppl* 1983;30588-91:-91

123a. Kjartansson S, Arsan S, Hammarlund K, Sjors G, Sedin G. Water loss from the skin of term and preterm infants nursed under a radiant heater. *Pediatr Res* 1995;37:233-8

123b. Kloiber LL, Winn NJ, Shaffer SG, Hassanein RS. Late hyponatremia in very low birth weight infants: incidence and associated risk factors. *J Am Diet Assoc* 1996;96:880-884

124. Knutson DW, Chieu F, Bennett CM, Glassock RJ. Estimation of relative glomerular capillary surface area in normal and hypertrophic rat kidneys. *Kidney Int* 1978;14:437-443.

125. Kojima T, Fukuda Y, Hirata Y, Matsuzaki S, Kobayashi Y. Effects of aldosterone and atrial natriuretic peptide on water and electrolyte homeostasis of sick neonates. *Pediatr Res* 1989;25:591-594.

126. Kovacs L, Sulyok E, Lichardus B, Mihajlovskij N, Bircak J. Renal response to arginine vasopressin in premature infants with late hyponatraemia. *Arch Dis Child* 1986;61:1030-1032.

127. Kurzner SI, Garg M, Bautista DB, Sargent CW, Bowman CM, Keens TG. Growth failure in bronchopulmonary dysplasia: elevated metabolic rates and pulmonary mechanics. *J Pediatr* 1988;112:73-80.

128. Landis E, Pappenheimer J. Exchange of substances through the capillary walls. In: AnonymousHandbook

of Physiology. 2 Ed. Washington DC: American Physiologic Society, 1963:961-1034.

129. Lane AT, Drost SS. Effects of repeated application of emollient cream to premature neonates' skin. *Pediatrics* 1993;92:415-419.

130. Langman CB, Engle WD, Baumgart S, Fox WW, Polin RA. The diuretic phase of respiratory distress syndrome and its relationship to oxygenation. *J Pediatr* 1981;98:462-466.

131. Laragh JH, Seaman SL. The renin-angiotenson-aldosterone hormonal systemof sodium, potassium and blood pressure-electrolyte homeostasis. In: Orloff J, Berliner R, eds. Handbook of Physiology. Washington DC: American Physiological Society, 1973:831-908.

132. Laubenthal H. Einsatzstrategien fur Albumin. [Strategies for using albumin]. *Beitr Infusionsther* 1989;24102-11:-11

133. Leake RD, Zakauddin S, Trygstad CW, Fu P, Oh W. The effects of large volume intravenous fluid infusion on neonatal renal function. *J Pediatr* 1976a;89: 968-972.

134. Leake RD, Zakauddin S, Trygstad CW, Fu P, Oh W. The effects of large volume intravenous fluid infusion on neonatal renal function. *J Pediatr* 1976b;89: 968-972.

135. Leslie GI, Carman G, Arnold JD. Early neonatal hyperkalaemia in the extremely premature newborn infant. *J Paediatr Child Health* 1990;26:58-61.

136. Leung AK, McArthur RG, McMillan DD, Ko D, Deacon JS, Parboosingh JT, Lederis KP. Circulating antidiuretic hormone during labour and in the newborn. *Acta Paediatr Scand* 1980;69:505-510.

137. Linshaw MA. Selected aspects of cell volume control in renal cortical and medullary tissue. *Pediatr Nephrol* 1991;5:653-665.

138. Livingstone VH, Willis CE, Abdel-Wareth LO, Thiessen P, Lockitch G. Neonatal hypernatremic dehydration associated with breast-feeding malnutrition: a retrospective survey. *CMAJ* 2000;162:647-652.

139. Lorenz JM. The outcome of extreme prematurity. *Semin Perinatol* 2001;25:348-359.

140. Lorenz JM, Kleinman LI, Kotagal UR, Reller MD.

Water balance in very low-birth-weight infants: relationship to water and sodium intake and effect on outcome. *J Pediatr* 1982;101:423-432.

141. Lorenz JM, Kleinman LI, Markarian K. Potassium metabolism in extremely low birth weight infants in the first week of life. *J Pediatr* 1997;131:81-86.

142. Macknight AD, Leaf A. Regulation of cellular volume. *Physiol Rev* 1977;57:510-573.

143. Maclaurin JC. Changes in body water distribution during the first two weeks of life. *Arch Dis Child* 1966;41:286-291.

144. Mann JF, Johnson AK, Ganten D, Ritz E. Thirst and the renin-angiotensin system. *Kidney Int Suppl* 1987;21S27-34:-34

145. Marchini G, Stock S. Thirst and vasopressin secretion counteract dehydration in newborn infants. *J Pediatr* 1997;130:736-739.

146. Marks KH, Berman W, Friedman Z, Whiteman V, Lee C, Maisels MJ. Furosemide in hyaline membrane disease. *Pediatrics* 1978;62:785-788.

147. Martin D. Wasser und anorganische Elemente. In: Harpner H, Martin D, Mayes P, Rodwell V, eds. Medizinische Biochemie. 19 Ed. Berlin: Springer-Verlag, 1983:657-671.

148. Mazkereth R, Laufer J, Jordan S, Pomerance JJ, Boichis H, Reichman B. Effects of theophylline on renal function in premature infants. *Am J Perinatol* 1997;14:45-49.

149. Merritt TA, Hallman M, Berry C, Pohjavuori M, Edwards DK, Jaaskelainen J, Grafe MR, Vaucher Y, Wozniak P, Heldt G, et a. Randomized, placebo-controlled trial of human surfactant given at birth versus rescue administration in very low birth weight infants with lung immaturity. *J Pediatr* 1991;118:581-594.

150. Meyer MP, Payton MJ, Salmon A, Hutchinson C, de-Klerk A. A clinical comparison of radiant warmer and incubator care for preterm infants from birth to 1800 grams. *Pediatrics* 2001;108 :395-401.

151. Michel C. Fluid movements through capillary walls. In: AnonymousHandbook of physiology. 2 Ed. Bethesda: American Physiologic Society, 1984:

152. Mills IH. Renal regulation of sodium excretion. *Annu Rev Med* 1970;2175-98:-98

153. Modi N. Development of renal function. *Br Med Bull* 1988;44:935-956.

154. Modi N. Sodium intake and preterm babies. *Arch Dis Child* 1993;69:87-91.

155. Modi N. Adaptation to extrauterine life. *Br J Obstet Gynaecol* 1994;101:369-370.

156. Modi N, Hutton JL. The influence of postnatal respiratory adaptation on sodium handling in preterm neonates. *Early Hum Dev* 1990;21:11-20.

157. Nakamaru M, Misono KS, Naruse M, Workman RJ, Inagami T. A role for the adrenal renin-angiotensin system in the regulation of potassium-stimulated aldosterone production. *Endocrinology* 1985;117:1772-1778.

158. Nicholson J, Pesce M. Laboratory Testing and Reference Values in Infants and children. In: Nelson W, Behrman R, Kliegman R, Arvin A, eds. Textbook of Pediatrics. 15 Ed. Philadelphia: Saunders WB, 2002:2031-2084.

158a. Nopper AJ, Horii KA, Sookdeo-Drost S, Wang TH, Marcini AJ, Lane AT. Topical ointment therapy benefits premature infants. *J Pediatr* 1996;128:660-669. Comment in *J Pediatr* 1997;130:330-332. Comment in *J Pediatr* 1997;130:333-334 bis gleich.

159. Offringa PJ, Boersma ER, Brunsting JR, Meeuwsen WP, Velvis H. Weight loss in full-term negroid infants: relationship to body water compartments at birth? *Early Hum Dev* 1990;21:73-81.

160. Okah FA, Pickens WL, Hoath SB. Effect of prenatal steroids on skin surface hydrophobicity in the premature rat. *Pediatr Res* 1995;37:402-408.

161. Omar SA, DeCristofaro JD, Agarwal BI, La-Gamma EF. Effects of prenatal steroids on water and sodium homeostasis in extremely low birth weight neonates. *Pediatrics* 1999;104:482-488.

162. Omar SA, DeCristofaro JD, Agarwal BI, LaGamma EF. Effect of prenatal steroids on potassium balance in extremely low birth weight neonates. *Pediatrics* 2000;106:561-567.

163. Osborn DA, Evans N. Early volume expansion for prevention of morbidity and mortality in very preterm infants (Cochrane Review). Cochrane Database Syst Rev 1902a;4:CD002055.

164. Osborn DA, Evans N. Early volume expansion versus inotrope for prevention of morbidity and mortality in very preterm infants (Cochrane Review). Cochrane Database Syst Rev 1902b;2:CD002056.

165. Paneth N. Hypernatremic dehydration of infancy: an epidemiologic review. *Am J Dis Child* 1980; 134:785-792.

166. Pappenheimer J, Soto-Rivera. Effective osmotic pressure of the plasma proteins and other quantities associated with capillary circulation in the hind limb of cats and dogs. *Am J Physiol* 1948;152:471-491.

167. Paul AC, Ranjini K, Muthulakshmi, Roy A, Kirubakaran C. Malnutrition and hypernatraemia in breastfed babies. *Ann Trop Paediatr* 2000;20:179-183.

168. Pauls J, Bauer K, Versmold H. Postnatal body weight curves for infants below 1000 g birth weight receiving early enteral and parenteral nutrition. *Eur J Pediatr* 1998;157:416-421.

169. Pipkin FB, Smales OR. A study of factors affecting blood pressure and angiotensin II in newborn infants. *J Pediatr* 1977;91:113-119.

170. Polberger SK, Axelsson IA, Raiha NC. Growth of very low birth weight infants on varying amounts of human milk protein. *Pediatr Res* 1989;25:414-419.

171. Puangco MA, Schanler RJ. Clinical experience in enteral nutrition support for premature infants with bronchopulmonary dysplasia. *J Perinatol* 2000;20: 87-91.

172. Raiha NC, Heinonen K, Rassin DK, Gaull GE. Milk protein quantity and quality in low-birthweight infants: I. Metabolic responses and effects on growth. *Pediatrics* 1976;57:659-684.

173. Raubenstine DA, Ballantine TV, Greecher CP, Webb SL. Neonatal serum protein levels as indicators of nutritional status: normal values and correlation with anthropometric data. *J Pediatr Gastroenterol Nutr* 1990;10:53-61.

174. Rees L, Brook CG, Shaw JC, Forsling ML. Hyponatraemia in the first week of life in preterm infants. Part I. Arginine vasopressin secretion. *Arch Dis Child* 1984;59:414-422.

175. Rees L, Forsling ML, Brook CG. Vasopressin concentrations in the neonatal period. *Clin Endocrinol (Oxf.)* 1980;12:357-362.

176. Rees L, Shaw JC, Brook CG, Forsling ML. Hyponatraemia in the first week of life in preterm infants. Part II. Sodium and water balance. *Arch Dis Child* 1984;59:423-429.

177. Reiter PD, Makhlouf R, Stiles AD. Comparison of 6-hour infusion versus bolus furosemide in premature infants. *Pharmacotherapy* 1998;18:63-68.

178. Richards AM, Nicholls MG, Ikram H, Webster MW, Yandle TG, Espiner EA . Renal, haemodynamic, and hormonal effects of human alpha atrial natriuretic peptide in healthy volunteers. *Lancet* 1985;1:545-549.

179. Ritz P. Body water spaces and cellular hydration during healthy aging. *Ann N.Y Acad Sci* 2000; 904474-83:-83

180. Robertson G, Berl T. Water Metabolism. In: Brenner BM, Rector F, eds. The Kidney. Philadelphia: Saunders,WB, 1986:385-431.

181. Robillard JE, Kulvinskas C, Sessions C, Burmeister L, Smith FG. Maturational changes in the fetal glomerular filtration rate. *Am J Obstet Gynecol* 1975;122:601-606.

182. Robillard JE, Matson JR, Sessions C, Smith FG. Developmental aspects of renal tubular reabsorption of water in the lamb fetus. *Pediatr Res* 1979;13: 1172-1176.

183. Robillard JE, Nakamura KT. Hormonal regulation of renal function during development. *Biol Neonate* 1988;53:201-211.

184. Robillard JE, Weitzman RE. Developmental aspects of the fetal renal response to exogenous arginine vasopressin. *Am J Physiol* 1980;238:F407-F414.

185. Robillard JE, Weitzman RE, Fisher DA, Smith FG. The dynamics of vasopressin release and blood volume regulation during fetal hemorrhage in the lamb fetus. *Pediatr Res* 1979;13:606-610.

186. Roithmaier A, Arlettaz R, Bauer K, Bucher HU, Krieger M, Duc G, Versmold HT. Randomized controlled trial of Ringer solution versus serum for partial exchange transfusion in neonatal polycythaemia. *Eur J Pediatr* 1995;154:53-56.

186a. Roy RN, Chance GW, Radde IC, Hill DE, Willis DM, Sheepers J. Late hyponatremia in very low birth weight infants. *Pediatr Res* 1976;10:526-531.

187. Rozycki HJ, Baumgart S. Atrial natriuretic factor and

postnatal diuresis in respiratory distress syndrome. *Arch Dis Child* 1991;66:43-47.

188. Rutter N. Commentary. *Arch Dis Child* 1988;63: 309-309.

189. Rutter N, Hull D. Reduction of skin water loss in the newborn. I. Effect of applying topical agents. *Arch Dis Child* 1981;56:669-672.

190. Salmon JB, Mythen MG. Pharmacology and physiology of colloids. *Blood Rev* 1993;7:114-120.

191. Savage MD, Wilkinson AR, Baum JD, Roberton NRC. Furosemide in respiratory distress syndrome. *Arch Dis Child* 1975;50:709-713

192. Schrier RW. Pathogenesis of sodium and water retention in high-output and low-output cardiac failure, nephrotic syndrome, cirrhosis, and pregnancy (2). *N Engl J Med* 1988;319:1127-1134.

193. Schubert F, George JM, Rao MB. Vasopressin and oxytocin content of human fetal brain at different stages of gestation. *Brain Res* 1981;213:111-117.

194. Sedin G, Hammarlund K, Nilsson GE, Stromberg B, Oberg PA. Measurements of transepidermal water loss in newborn infants. *Clin Perinatol* 1985;12:79-99.

195. Sertel H, Scopes J. Rates of creatinine clearance in babies less than one week of age. *Arch Dis Child* 1973;48:717-720.

196. Seymour AA, Blaine EH, Mazack EK, Smith SG, Stabilito II, Haley AB, Napier MA, Whinnery MA, Nutt RF. Renal and systemic effects of synthetic atrial natriuretic factor. *Life Sci* 1985;36:33-44.

197. Shaffer SG, Bradt SK, Hall RT. Postnatal changes in total body water and extracellular volume in the preterm infant with respiratory distress syndrome. *J Pediatr* 1986;109:509-514.

198. Shaffer SG, Bradt SK, Meade VM, Hall RT. Extracellular fluid volume changes in very low birth weight infants during first 2 postnatal months. *J Pediatr* 1987;111:124-128.

199. Shaffer SG, Ekblad H, Brans YW. Estimation of extracellular fluid volume by bromide dilution in infants less than 1000 grams birth weight. *Early Hum Dev* 1991;27:19-24.

200. Shaffer SG, Meade VM. Sodium balance and extracellular volume regulation in very low birth weight infants. *J Pediatr* 1989;115:285-290.

201. Shapiro MD, Nicholls KM, Groves BM, Kluge R, Chung HM, Bichet DG, Schrier RW. Interrelationship between cardiac output and vascular resistance as determinants of effective arterial blood volume in cirrhotic patients. *Kidney Int* 1985;28:206-211.

202. Sinclair JC. Metabolic rate and temperature control. In: Smith CA, Nelson N, eds. The physiology of the newborn infant. 4 Ed. Springfield: Charles Thomas, 1976:354-415.

203. Smith CH, Moe AJ, Ganapathy V. Nutrient transport pathways across the epithelium of the placenta. *Annu Rev Nutr* 1992;12183-206:-206

204. Smith LM, Ervin MG, Wada N, Ikegami M, Polk DH, Jobe AH. Antenatal glucocorticoids alter postnatal preterm lamb renal and cardiovascular responses to intravascular volume expansion. *Pediatr Res* 2000;47:622-627.

205. So KW, Fok TF, Ng PC, Wong WW, Cheung KL. Randomised controlled trial of colloid or crystalloid in hypotensive preterm infants. *Arch Dis Child Fetal Neonatal Ed* 1997;76:F43-F46.

206. Sola A, Gregory GA. Colloid osmotic pressure of normal newborns and premature infants. *Crit Care Med* 1981;9:568-572.

207. Sosulski R, Polin RA, Baumgart S. Respiratory water loss and heat balance in intubated infants receiving humidified air. *J Pediatr* 1983;103:307-310.

208. Speller AM, Moffat DB. Tubulo-vascular relationships in the developing kidney. *J Anat* 1977;123:487-500.

209. Spitzer A. Renal physiology and function development. In: Edelmann CM, ed. The kidney and urinary tract. Boston: Little Brown, 1978:25-128.

210. Spitzer A. The role of the kidney in sodium homeostasis during maturation. *Kidney Int* 1982;21:539-545.

211. Starling E. On the absorption of fluid from the connective tissue spaces. *J Physiol* 1896;19:312-326.

212. Steen B. Body composition and aging. *Nutr Rev* 1988;46:45-51.

213. Stevenson JG. Fluid administration in the association of patent ductus arteriosus complicating respiratory distress syndrome. *J Pediatr* 1977;90:257-261.

214. Sulyok E, Jequier E, Prod'hom LS. Respiratory contribution to the thermal balance of the newborn infant under various ambient conditions. *Pediatrics* 1973;51:641-650.

214a. Sulyok E, Kovacs L, Lichardus B, Michajlovskij N, Lehotska V, Nemethova V, Varga L, Ertl T. Late hyponatremia in premature infants: role of aldosterone and aginine vasopressine. *J Pediatr* 1985;106: 990-994

215. Svenningsen NW, Aronson AS. Postnatal development of renal concentration capacity as estimated by DDAVP-test in normal and asphyxiated neonates. *Biol Neonate* 1974;25:230-241.

216. Tammela OK. Appropriate fluid regimens to prevent bronchopulmonary dysplasia. *Eur J Pediatr* 1995;154:S15-S18

217. Tang W, Ridout D, Modi N. Influence of respiratory distress syndrome on body composition after preterm birth. *Arch Dis Child Fetal Neonatal Ed* 1997; 77:F28-F31

218. Trachtman H. Cell volume regulation: a review of cerebral adaptive mechanisms and implications for clinical treatment of osmolal disturbances. I. *Pediatr Nephrol* 1991;5:743-750.

219. Van-Marter LJ, Allred EN, Leviton A, Pagano M, Parad R, Moore M. Antenatal glucocorticoid treatment does not reduce chronic lung disease among surviving preterm infants. *J Pediatr* 2001;138:198-204.

220. Van-Marter LJ, Leviton A, Allred EN, Pagano M, Kuban KC. Hydration during the first days of life and the risk of bronchopulmonary dysplasia in low birth weight infants. *J Pediatr* 1990;116:942-949.

221. vd-Wagen A, Okken A, Zweens J, Zijlstra WG. Composition of postnatal weight loss and subsequent weight gain in small for dates newborn infants. *Acta Paediatr Scand* 1985;74:57-61.

222. Webster HL. Colloid osmotic pressure: theoretical aspects and background. *Clin Perinatol* 1982;9: 505-521.

223. Weinstein MR, Oh W. Oxygen consumption in infants with bronchopulmonary dysplasia. *J Pediatr* 1981;99:958-961.

224. Weitzman RE, Fisher DA, Robillard J, Erenberg A, Kennedy R, Smith F. Arginine vasopressin response to an osmotic stimulus in the fetal sheep. *Pediatr Res* 1978;12:35-38.

225. Wheldon AE, Rutter N. The heat balance of small babies nursed in incubators and under radiant warmers. *Early Hum Dev* 1982;6:131-143.

226. Widdowson E. Changes of body composition during growth. In: Davis J, Dobbing J, eds. Scientific foundations of paediatrics. London: Heinemann, 1981:330-342.

227. Williams PR, Oh W. Effects of radiant warmer on insensible water loss in newborn infants. *Am J Dis Child* 1974;128:511-514.

228. Winters R. Maintenance Fluid therapy. In: Anonymous. The body fluids in pediatrics. Boston: Little Brown, 1973:113-133.

229. Wintour E. Water and electrolyte metabolism in the fetal-placental unit. In: Cowett R, ed. Priciples of perinatal-neonatal metabolism. 2 Ed. New York: Springer, 1998:511-534.

230. Wu PY, Hodgman JE. Insensible water loss in preterm infants: changes with postnatal development and non-ionizing radiant energy. *Pediatrics* 1974;54: 704-712.

231. Wu PY, Udani V, Chan L, Miller FC, Henneman CE. Colloid osmotic pressure: variations in normal pregnancy. *J Perinat Med* 1983;11:193-199.

232. Yeh TF, Shibli A, Leu ST, Ravel D, Pildes RD. Early furoesmide therapy in premature infants (2000g) with respiratory distress syndrome: a randomised controlled trial. *J Pediatr* 1984;105:603-609.

233. Yeh T, Parmar JM, Rebeyka IM, Lofland GK, Allen EL, Dignan RJ, Dyke CM, Wechsler AS. Limiting edema in neonatal cardiopulmonary bypass with narrow-range molecular weight hydroxyethyl starch. *J Thorac Cardiovasc Surg* 1992;104:659-665.

234. Yeh TF, Vidyasagar D, Pildes RS. Critical care problems of the newborn: insensible water loss in small premature infants. *Crit Care Med* 1975;3: 238-241.

235. Ziegler EE, Fomon SJ. Fluid intake, renal solute load, and water balance in infancy. *J Pediatr* 1971;78: 561-568.

236. Ziegler EE, Fomon SJ. Major minerals. In: Fomon SJ, ed. Infant Nutrition. 2 Ed. Philadelphia: Saunders,WB, 1974:267-297.

Calcium, Magnesium, Phosphorus and Vitamin D
Stephanie A. Atkinson, Ph.D. and Reginald Tsang, M.B.B.S.

Reviewed by Frank Pohlandt, M.D., Stephen Abrams, M.D., and Richard Cooke, M.D.

Key Messages
- *Parenteral nutrition – Intravenous delivery of Ca and P that is achievable in clinical practice will maintain a normal mineral biochemical status; but retention of mineral that parallels intrauterine accretion is rarely possible using inorganic salts. If organic phosphorus compounds like disodiumglycerophosphate are available, higher amounts of mineral may be delivered intravenously. In all instances, infants should be weaned to oral feedings as soon as medically possible in order to minimize complications of intravenous feeding and to support optimal early growth.*
- *Enteral feeding – Expressed or suckled breast milk should be encouraged for feeding to premature infants with the addition of Ca, P and Vitamin D as individual supplements or as part of a multinutrient human milk fortifier. This practice will ensure normophosphatemia and normal Vitamin D status, minimize hypercalciuria, and allow sufficient retention of mineral to meet intrauterine accretion of mineral and gain in bone mineral content. Similarly, formulas fed to premature infants in hospital should contain greater amounts of calcium, phosphorus, and magnesium than standard infant formulas.*

Physiology
Calcium (Ca), phosphorus (P), and magnesium (Mg) are essential for structural matrix of bone as well as function of soft tissues. The physiology and metabolism of these minerals are interrelated and modulated by other nutrients and hormones, including Vitamin D metabolites. Calcium and P form the major inorganic constituents of bone, with 99% of total body Ca and 80% of P being in the microcrystalline apatite $(Ca_5(PO_4)OH$, which forms in bone only when Ca and P are simultaneously available in optimal proportions. Magnesium is the second most common intracellular electrolyte (after potassium) in the body, and 60% of total body Mg is in bone mineral matrix. Calcium, P and Mg accrue linearly and in association with body weight gain in the fetus in the third trimester,[1,2] during which time about 80% of the mineral of the term infant is laid down.[3]

Estimates of calcium accretion for the period of 26 to 36 weeks of gestation are 2.3 to 3.2 mmol (90 - 120 mg) Ca/kg fetal body weight/d, although it might be slightly higher at 36 to 38 weeks of gestation, the time of peak fetal accretion of bone mineral.[4] Phosphorus accrues at about 1.9 to 2.5 mmol (60 - 75 mg)/kg/d during the third trimester, and Mg accretion is estimated at 0.1 to 0.14 mmol (2.5 - 3.4 mg)/kg/d.[4]

Using cross-sectional data on whole body bone mineral content (BMC) in infants of varying gestation at birth, and assuming that bone mineral contains 32.2% Ca, the total Ca that is accrued in utero to term is estimated to be 23.2 ± 35 g (mean ± SD).[5] The observation of a 5.5-fold increase in lumbar spine BMC as observed in a cross-sectional study of infants from 27 to 42 weeks and a 2.4-fold increase in the mid-humerus,[6] confirms the data on mineral accretion derived from cadavers that most bone deposition occurs from 24 weeks of gestation to term.[7] Longitudinal measures of whole body BMC from term date to one year of age demonstrated that both term-born[8] and prematurely born infants[9] experience

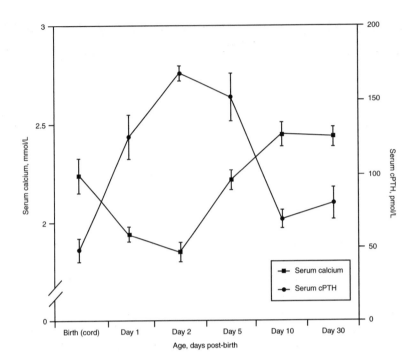

Figure 1: Early neonatal hypocalcemia in premature infants depicted as changes in total calcium (TCa) and carboxy-terminal parathyroid hormone (cPTH) concentrations in cord serum and at postnatal days 1,2,5,10 and 30. Data represent mean±SD for 15 preterm infants (mean birth weight of 1758 ± 78 g and gestational age 31.7 ± 0.5 weeks) as reported by Salle et al.[16] The mean values for TCa at days 1 and 2 and for cPTH at days 1,2 and 5 were significantly different from the values for cord serum (p<0.05).

an increase in BMC of 3.6- to 4.0-fold over the 12-month period.

Prematurely born infants may be at particular risk of having less-than-optimal normal bone mass since emerging evidence reveals that both genetics (measured as parental size at birth) and environmental factors, such as the diet and lifestyle habits of the mother, influence bone mineral accretion during fetal life. In a population-based cohort study, infants born at term whose mothers smoked during pregnancy had significantly lower (by 11%) whole body BMC than infants of non-smokers.[10] Maternal thinness as reflected in low triceps skinfold thickness and as well as more frequent and vigorous activity in late pregnancy were also associated with a lower BMC in the infants.[10] These maternal influences on newborn bone mass were independent of placental weight and thus not likely a result of reduced placental delivery of nutrients. It has

been hypothesized that variations in fetal skeletal development related to environmental influences via the mother occur as a result of perturbations in a fetal hormone regulatory pathway, such as the growth hormone/insulin-like growth factor axis.[11]

Maternal dietary intake of Ca also may be a factor in fetal bone mineral accretion. For women with low dietary Ca intakes (< 600 mg/day), a supplement of 2 grams of Ca from before 22 weeks of gestation resulted in higher BMC of the total body in infants born at term.[12] While the cited studies were conducted in term infants, large populations of mothers who deliver preterm infants are adolescents, a group known to have a high prevalence of smoking, thinness and low Ca intakes. In addition, birth weight is a predictor of bone mass in later life.[13,14]

When infants are born prematurely, there is a relatively urgent need to provide Ca either parenterally

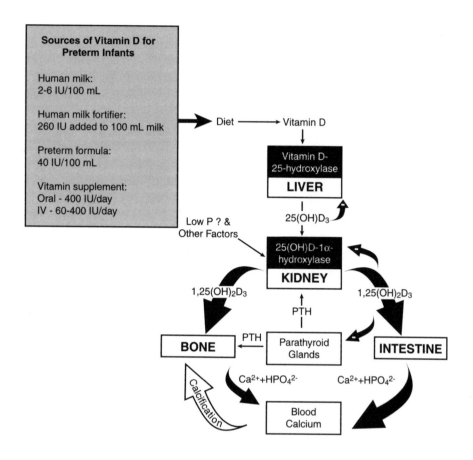

Figure 2: Vitamin D metabolism beginning with ingestion in the diet (from formula, human milk fortifier or vitamin supplement). Adapted from Holick MF.[162] Vitamin D: Photobiology, metabolism, mechanism of action and clinical application. In: Favus MJ, ed. Primer on the Metabolic Bone Diseases and Disorders of Mineral Metabolism, 3rd Edition, Philadelphia, PA: Lippincott-Raven; pp74-81; from Bone Primer by ASBMR.

or enterally to avoid early neonatal hypocalcemia (usually occurring within 12-24 hours and defined as total serum Ca < 1.75 mmol (70 mg)/L or serum ionized Ca < 1.1 mmol (44 mg)/L).[15] In some premature infants, a postnatal latency in the elaboration of parathyroid hormone (PTH) (for at least 48 hours postbirth) means that serum (plasma) Ca may not be hormonally regulated to protect against hypocalcemia.[16] However, other prematurely born infants may respond appropriately to hypocalcemia (Figure 1); serum PTH as well as serum 1,25-dihydroxyVitamin D may rise by 24-hours postnatally.[17,16] Early neonatal hypocalcemia can

be obviated with continuous infusion of intravenous Ca without blunting the PTH response,[17,18] but intravenous infusion of the active metabolite of Vitamin D (1,25-(OH)2D)[19] (except at pharmacological doses[20]) is not effective. It is usual that early hypocalcemia resolves within a few days after birth[21] and is not associated with any clinical symptoms in most premature infants. After serum Ca normalizes, infants should receive both Ca and P either by intravenous or oral feedings. The recommended amounts of Ca and P will be discussed in subsequent sections.

Vitamin D status in preterm infants at birth is

dependent on transplacental transfer from the mother. Transplacental transport of Vitamin D is mostly in the hydroxylated form 25-hydroxyVitamin D (25OHD). At birth, cord blood concentrations of this metabolite are about 20-30% lower than maternal circulating concentration, a relationship that appears similar in prematurely and term-born infants.[22]

Premature infants (at least those of > 28 weeks of gestation) appear to have the ability to absorb and hydroxylate Vitamin D to produce 25OHD and the active metabolite 1,25-dihydroxyVitamin D (1,25(OH)2D) from the first day of life[17,23] (Figure 1). Indeed, a sustained elevation in plasma 1,25(OH)2D up to three months postnatally[16,24] suggests an appropriate response to early neonatal hypocalcemia via stimulation of PTH. The physiological reason for the elevated 1,25 (OH)2D in preterm infants is not understood. In older infants and adults there is an absolute requirement for this active metabolite of Vitamin D to regulate transport of Ca and P across the intestinal mucosa and renal epithelium as depicted in Figure 2. Although Vitamin D stores may deplete rapidly postnatally, the demand for Vitamin D conversion to the active metabolite to facilitate absorption and retention of Ca and P in preterm infants is questionable, since there is evidence that these functions are independent of the availability of the active hormone at this stage of development.[25] At what postnatal age a dependency on Vitamin D-regulated transport of Ca and P begins is uncertain. The amount of Vitamin D required to support mineral absorption in prematurely born infants will be discussed below.

Magnesium has a strong inter-relationship with Ca in the body. Of total body Mg, 50-60% is found in bone or other cartilaginous tissues. Magnesium functions as a cofactor in many biological processes including the release of PTH, thus making it part of the calciotropic hormone axis. Neither plasma nor urine Mg is a sensitive marker of adequacy of dietary intake; nor is there a reasonable surrogate marker of Mg status at either the biochemical or functional level.[26] Thus, most studies on Mg status have relied on Mg balance and retention. Intestinal Mg

		mg	mmol
Calcium			
	Concentration (/L)	600	15
	Delivery (/kg/day)*	66	1.65
	Retention (% intake)**	92	92
	Apparent Retention (/kg/day)	61	1.5
	Intrauterine Accretion Rate (/kg/day)	90-120	2.3-3.2
Phosphorus			
	Concentration (/L)	465	15
	Delivery (/kg/day)*	51	1.65
	Retention (% intake)**	85	85
	Apparent Retention (/kg/day)	43	1.5
	Intrauterine Accretion Rate (/kg/day)	60-75	1.9-2.5
Magnesium			
	Concentration (/L)	72	3.0
	Delivery (/kg/day)*	7.9	0.3
	Retention (% intake)**	68	68
	Apparent Retention (/kg/day)	5.4	0.2
	Intrauterine Accretion Rate (/kg/day)	2.5-3.4	0.10-0.14

* Assumes fluid intake from amino acids of 110 ml/kg/d.
** % retention does not account for minimal fecal loss of mineral of about 2-4% of intake that can occur during parenteral nutrition feeding.[39]

Table 1: Projected net retention (balance) of Ca, P and Mg achievable from intravenous nutrition solutions containing 25 to 30 g amino acids/L compared to estimated intrauterine accretion of mineral.

absorption is not hormonally regulated. The efficiency of Mg absorption in preterm infants is generally greater from human milk than bovine-based formulas,[27,28] so lumenal factors may play a role in making this element more soluble and available for uptake across the brush border membrane.

Determination of Nutrient Requirements

Beyond the early neonatal period, the key criteria for assessment of the adequacy of intake of Ca, P and Mg are balance studies to determine accretion of nutrients, specific biochemical indices of endocrine or bone mineral status, and the measurement of bone mineral content as a functional outcome. Severe deficiency of these minerals in early life has also been associated with deformities of the skull,[29] a narrow palate, protruding eyeballs[30] and bone fractures.[31] While prevention of fractures in early life is important, a more physiologically relevant outcome is accretion of bone mass that is proportionate to linear growth as achieved by the fetus in utero, and subsequently the term-born infant over the first year of life.

Parenteral nutrition

Calcium and phosphorus: In the transition period, most very low birth weight (VLBW) infants will receive full or partial parenteral nutrition with the objective to maintain normal plasma status of Ca, P, Mg and Vitamin D. Early (first 24 to 72 hours of life) neonatal hypocalcemia is common and generally not associated with obvious clinical problems such as tetany. Calcium infusions of 1.25 - 1.88 mmol (50 - 75 mg)/kg/day will usually prevent or treat early neonatal hypocalcemia. The origin of the hypocalcemia likely relates to delayed elaboration of PTH in response to low blood Ca. As detailed previously, administration of the hormonal form of Vitamin D (1,25-(OH)2D) is not an effective treatment of early neonatal hypocalcemia.

After the first few postnatal days, prolonged total parenteral nutrition (TPN) in VLBW infants has been associated with hypocalcemia, hypophosphatemia, hypercalciuria[32-34], and mineral-deficient bone disease with or without fractures.[35-37] Such abnormalities are usually a direct result of inadequate amounts of Ca and P being added to the parenteral solutions. With intakes of minerals shown in Table 1, positive balance of Ca and P[38,39] and normal circulating Ca and P[39] can be achieved using available mineral salts. However, the retention of Ca and P will be lower than intrauterine accretion of these minerals (Table 1). Few studies have directly measured BMC as an outcome of intervention with varying parenteral intakes of Ca and P. In one study,[40] 35% higher intakes of Ca and P (with the higher intake at 1.7 Ca and 2.0 P mmol/kg/d) over 3 weeks produced a significantly higher rate of accretion and absolute radial BMC out to 8 weeks postnatally. The positive benefit to BMC occurred despite Ca retention being only 65% and P retention 85% of intrauterine accretion values.[40]

The lower limit of intake of Ca and P from TPN

that may contribute to a deficit in bone mineral accretion, eventual severe hypomineralization of bone, and risk of fracture has not been clearly defined. This lower limit is likely below 1.3 mmol/kg/d and perhaps below 1 mmol/kg/d but will be dependent on the duration of the TPN and the body weight of the baby. The smaller the baby, the more limited the body pool of P from soft tissue, and thus the more likely that demineralization of bone will occur. The target intake of parenteral Ca and P in order to achieve intrauterine accretion of mineral was calculated to be 3.0 mmol for Ca and 2.8 mmol for P /kg/d (or 23 mmol Ca/L and 21 mmol P/L).[38] In practice, such intakes are usually unachievable using the conventional injectable mineral salts available in North America but may be possible if organic phosphorus compounds are available, as currently occurs in Europe.

A realistic target for the optimal ratio of Ca:P in TPN would be the Ca:P of the whole body, which is 1:1 molar (1.60 w/w) or for the bone, which is 1.67 molar (2.15 w/w). Infusion of Ca:P in a molar ratio of 1:1 or slightly higher using Ca gluconate and potassium phosphate resulted in normal plasma biochemical indices of mineral status and was not associated with aberrant metabolic sequelae.[39,41] At a higher Ca:P molar ratio of 1.3:1 (1.7:1 mg:mg) using the same salts as the above study and providing intakes of 1.9 mmol Ca and 1.3 mmol P/kg/d, retention of Ca and P was superior compared to Ca:P infused at 1.55:1 or 1:1 molar.[42] While this study was a randomized trial, caution is required in interpreting these results. The balance period was short (24-hour), and the 48-hour adaptation period to TPN may not have provided adequate stabilization, given that there was no Ca and P intake for the 24 hours prior to the study, and that the protein intake changed daily over the study period.[42] An intake ratio as low as 0.8 - 0.85 mmol resulted in retention of Ca and P in a similar ratio, normal plasma biochemistry, and a gain in radial bone mineral content.[40] Thus, it appears that neonates tolerate and adjust to intake ratios of Ca:P over a range of 0.8 to 1.5 mmolar, which may in turn relate to variations in weight gain since

Feeding Group	n	Age, d	Weight, g	Al I	Al E (μg/kg/d)	Al R
Parenterally fed infants						
- PN + CaG+P	6	32 ± 10	1440 ± 138	30.4 ± 3.3	7.8 ± 1.6	22.2 ± 2.0
- PN + CaGly+P	12	26 ± 5	1428 ± 13	5.0 ± 0.9	3.1 ± 0.9	1.0 ± 1.0
Enterally fed infants						
- Mother's milk	5	26 ± 5	1492 ± 95	2.4 ± 0.4	1.7 ± 0.06	0.7 ± 0.5
- Premature formula	12	27 ± 8	1923 ± 141	64.1 ± 4.8	1.2 ± 0.2	62.9 ± 4.0

Table 2: Aluminum intake (I), excretion (E) and retention (R) in premature infants fed one of two parenteral nutrition (PN) solutions that differed only in the source of calcium and phosphorus added to the amino acid solution compared to infants fed mother's milk or preterm formula. CaG + P = calcium gluconate + potassium mono- and dibasic phosphate; CaGlyP = calcium glycerophosphate salt.[58]

mineral accretion is related to weight gain in utero[6] and postnatally.[43]

The major barrier to delivery of optimal amounts of Ca and P via TPN for neonates is the poor solubility of conventional mineral salts, especially in combination with moderate or low protein intakes. The degree of solubility of Ca and P in parenteral solutions varies with the pH, amino acid quantity and quality (sulphur amino acids increase Ca solubility), dextrose concentration, type of mineral salt used, and order of addition of Ca and P.[41] Greater solubilization of Ca and P may be achieved with higher concentrations of amino acids in TPN solutions;[41] however, the endogenous acid produced from the oxidation of excess sulphur amino acids may contribute to hypercalciuria.[44] By lowering the pH of the TPN solution with cysteine hydrochloride[40,41,45] or with acidic mineral salts,[46,47] delivery of soluble Ca and P may be improved. The lowered pH of the TPN solution may cause metabolic acidosis in very immature infants[47,48] but not be problematic for larger infants.[48] The risk of acidic and high sulfate solutions is that they may induce excessive renal Ca loss.[44] An acid load from use of cysteine hydrochloride as

an additive or the sulfate load from cysteine and Mg sulphate salt, may explain the hypercalciuria observed in infants provided with adequate amounts of Ca and P.[40]

Alternative sources of Ca and P have been investigated as a means of improving the amount of mineral delivered to infants receiving TPN. The conventional mineral salts used in neonatal parenteral solutions in North America are calcium gluconate and mono- and dibasic potassium phosphate, but they have limited solubility. The inorganic sodium and potassium phosphates such as sodium-glucose phosphate or –glycerophosphate,[49] fructose[1,6] di-phosphate[50] or glucose phosphate,[51] which are currently available in Europe, are quite soluble in water but the phosphate anion forms an insoluble precipitate when mixed with Ca ions. The key to this is to obtain alternative sources of P that do not precipitate with Ca 2+ ions. Calcium will maintain stability as an ion with salts such as the glycerophosphate-anion, glucosephosphate-anion or phosphoethanolamine. Although the salts are licensed for use in European countries, published clinical trials using such products are limited.

In-vitro testing of Ca glycerophosphate demonstrated good solubility in concentrations of 25 mmol/L of soluble Ca and P even at low amino acid concentration (8.3 gm/L) and a relatively alkaline pH of 6.3441. Similarly, Raupp et al[51] found the use of glycerophosphate as the sodium salt permitted the solubilization of 37.5 mmol/L Ca and 32.3 mmol/L P at amino acid concentrations of 12.5 - 25.5 gm/L, pH levels of 6.63 - 6.96, and a temperature of 37°C. In testing Ca glycerophosphate in TPN in a randomized clinical trial in small premature infants (mean birth weight of 1.4±0.1 kg and gestational age 30.6 ± 0.8 wk),[52] Ca and P intakes of about 2 mmol/kg/d, yielded a retention of Ca at 1.7 and of P at 1.6 mmol/kg/d representing 68% and 84% of the intrauterine accretion of Ca and P, respectively. The 72-hour balance studies were conducted after 5 days on the randomized intakes of Ca:P at ratios of 1.4:1.3, 2.0:2.1, or 2.5:1.1 mmol.[52] Normal serum ionized Ca, P, osteocalcin and urinary pH, titratable acidity, and net acid excretion were maintained.[51] At the highest Ca:P intake ratio, Ca was efficiently retained (89 - 93% intake) but hypophosphatemia and hypercalciuria occurred in the infants. The hypercalciuria was not associated with use of medications, such as diuretics or dexamethasone, or with Na intake or urinary Na and Ca.

A potential problem with higher parenteral Ca and P intakes is that the commercially available mineral salts for TPN are contaminated with aluminium. Aluminium overloading via parenteral nutrition solutions occurs because significant amounts of aluminium can be found in heparin, albumin and Ca and P salts,[53] or possibly leaching from glass vials (personal communication, F. Pohlandt, 2002). Excessive delivery of aluminium (reported to be 30 to 306 mg/L)[54] in TPN given to infants has been associated with greater retention of aluminium than from human milk or formula (Table 2);[55] accumulation of this element in infant tissues;[20] and reduced bone mineralization.[56,57] A unique feature of the calcium glycerophosphate salt is that the measured aluminium content was four- to five-fold lower than from Ca gluconate + P (Table 2). The lower parenteral

delivery of aluminium was reflected in a lower apparent retention of aluminium (Table 2).[58] Thus, the benefits Ca glycerophosphate in providing increased parenteral Ca and P for infants is also associated with a reduced risk of aluminium toxicity. As recognized by the FDA,[59] vigilance is needed as the aluminium content varies in different parenteral solutions.[20]

In summary, various regimens have been proposed for delivery of adequate Ca and P while circumventing the problem of Ca/P insolubility in parenteral solutions for small infants, but not all are practical for use in the clinical setting. Infusion of Ca-free and P-free solutions on alternate days or 12-hour periods does not improve retention,[60] reducing the pH of the solution puts the infant at risk of metabolic acidosis,[61] and the addition of sulphite compounds can actually exacerbate calciuria.[40, 44] Use of salts highly soluble in aqueous solutions such as calcium glycerophosphate or organic phosphate salts is a reasonable approach, but such products are currently only available in Europe. This limits the ability of pharmacists to prepare Ca and P from inorganic salts that will not precipitate out of solution.[62] Use of such salts would allow for delivery of Ca and P in amounts that will provide for retention of minerals similar to intrauterine accretion. However, we shall have to await universal availability of such products.

Magnesium: Intrauterine accretion of Mg is 0.10 - 0.14 mmol or 2.5 - 3.4 mg, per kg, per day. To achieve this rate, the predicted intake of Mg is 0.4 mmol (9.6 mg)/kg/d (3 mmol (72 mg) Mg/L).[38] However, in a clinical study[41] in which lower amounts (0.27 - 0.31 mmol/kg/day) of parenteral Mg were delivered intravenously, net retention (after correcting for fecal loss) was 0.16-0.19 mmol/kg/d, which meets the estimated intrauterine rate. The predicted adequate intake for Mg using regression analysis from Schanler's data[38] may have been an overestimate since they studied intakes of Mg close to 0.6 mmol/kg/d and urine losses were 0.2-0.3 mmol/kg/d or 2-3 times that in the study by Hanning et al.[41] Table 1 provides achievable intakes and estimated retention of Mg in parenterally fed preterm infants. Based on balance

	Preterm Human Milk + Ca/P supplement mmol	Preterm Human Milk + Fortifier mmol	Preterm Formula at 81 kcal/100cc mmol
Calcium			
(mg/kg•d)	200-250	84-168	160-240
(mmol/kg•d)	5-6.1	2-4	4-6
Phosphorus			
(mg/kg•d)	110-125	60-104	78-118
(mmol/kg•d)	3.6-4.1	2-3.3	3.3-4
Magnesium			
(mg/kg•d)	--	7.2-14.4	4.8-9.6
(mmol/kg•d)	--	0.3-0.6	0.2-0.4
Vitamin D			
(mg/kg•d)	400	800-1600	400
(mmol/kg•d)	10	20-40	10

Table 3: Comparison of recommendations for enteral nutrient intakes of low birth weight infants in the stable and growing period.

studies, varying the intake of infused Ca and P does not alter the utilization or renal excretion of Mg, and intrauterine accretion of Mg can be achieved.[41]

Vitamin D: For Vitamin D, parenteral nutrition bypasses the major role of 1,25-dihydroxyVitamin D to facilitate intestinal Ca uptake. Thus, only minimal amounts are required and principally only with extended use of TPN. Only the parent compound of Vitamin D need be infused as preterm infants have the capacity to hydroxylate to produce the active hormone. Infusion in amino acid/dextrose solution of about 30 IU Vitamin D/kg/d up to a maximum intake of 400 IU/day is appropriate.[39,42,63,64] If the Vitamin D is delivered in a lipid emulsion, 160 IU/kg/d up to a maximum of 400 IU/day is adequate to maintain normal Vitamin D status for infants requiring parenteral nutrition.[65] In extremely LBW infants (< 1000 g), infusion of 160 IU Vitamin D/kg/d resulted in plasma 25-hydroxyVitamin D in the low normal range.[40] Thus, the special population of extremely small infants may require higher intakes as their stores of Vitamin D from transplacental transport are likely minimal or none.

Enteral Nutrition

Current estimates of requirements for Ca, P, Mg and Vitamin D in premature infants vary between international sources of recommendations (Table 3). These recommendations represent the goals for the stable growing period when a reasonable target for oral intake of Ca, P and Mg is to achieve retention of mineral that is similar to intrauterine accretion.

Calcium and phosphorus: For the transitional period when infants are fed intravenously and being weaned to oral feeding, a practical clinical goal is to provide sufficient Ca and P to maintain normal plasma P and avoid hypercalciuria. Serum Ca is neither a specific nor sensitive marker of adequacy of Ca intake (see discussion under section on Monitoring). As noted above, it is possible to infuse sufficient Ca and P to maintain normal serum biochemistry without meeting the estimated requirements for whole body accretion of mineral that parallels intrauterine accretion. The latter is an achievable goal once the greater proportion of intake is from enteral feeds. However, to attain maximal retention of mineral, selection must be made of appropriate amounts of supplements or multi-nutrient fortifier to add to human milk, or a selection of a nutrient-enriched formula designed specifically for preterm infants.

Evaluation of the nutritional value of a wide variety of feedings for preterm infants has been conducted through clinical studies, some of which are rigorously designed randomized double-blind trials, but many of which are limited in interpretation by lack of randomization and inadequate power to achieve statistically significant results. The outcome criteria for nutritional adequacy used in clinical investigations vary but have included: one or a combination of plasma and urinary biomarkers of mineral homeostasis and bone turnover; growth in weight and length; BMC of the radius, spine or whole body; and nutrient balance. In the following discussion of enteral needs of Ca, P, Mg and Vitamin D, each of these outcome variables will be addressed, beginning with a focus on feeding of mother's milk for preterm infants.

Unfortified mother's milk provides only about 6.4 mmol (256 mg) Ca/L and 4.5 mmol (140 mg) P/L and thus intakes of mineral could not exceed 1 mmol Ca and 0.77 mmol P/kg/d. The Canadian recommendations for nutrient intake of preterm infants[66] stipulated that to meet predicted Ca and P needs, infants would have to consume a volume of mother's milk in excess of 200 ml/kg/d, generally an unachievable goal. Clinical studies have proven that preterm infants fed unfortified mother's milk in early life develop hypophosphatemia, with/without hypercalcemia[27,31,67] and hypercalciuria where the urinary loss of Ca represented about 10% of the measured Ca intake.[68]

While the fortification of mother's milk with Ca and P for growing LBW infants is now a universally accepted practice, there is no consensus as to the amount or form of mineral salt that is optimal. Some centers have used single supplements of Ca and/or P while others use a multi-nutrient fortifier, most commonly one of the commercially available bovine-based human milk fortifiers. Worldwide, there are at least seven such fortifiers available in a powdered form. The mineral content of the fortifiers per recommended daily dose ranges from 0.95 - 2.9 mmol (38 - 117 mg) for Ca, and 0.84 - 2.2 mmol (26 - 67 mg) for P. The fortifiers with lower mineral content also tend to have lower protein content (see chapter by Schanler and Atkinson[69] for details of nutrient composition of the fortifiers).

Normophosphatemia (defined as 1.8 – 2.6 mmol (5.6-8.1 mg)/L) and normocalciuria (defined as urinary Ca excretion of 0.1-0.5 mmol (4-20 mg)/kg/d) can be achieved by supplementing as little as 0.7 mmol (21 mg) P/kg/d to mother's milk.[70,71] When Ca alone was supplemented for a total intake of about 2.5 mmol (100 mg)/kg/d, hypercalciuria was exacerbated and fecal Ca also increased significantly in LBW infants compared to those fed mother's milk alone.[68] Fractional P excretion will escalate if absolute P intake is excessive[72,73] or if intake of absorbable Ca is inadequate.[38] By providing Ca and P in combination as supplements to human milk, normal plasma mineral biochemistry is usually achieved, although there are reports of small infants who develop hypercalcemia.[74,75]

Two published systematic reviews are relevant to the discussion of Ca and P needs of preterm infants fed mother's milk. In the recently updated review by Kuschel and Harding,[76] the objective was to determine if addition of Ca and P supplements to human milk improves growth and bone metabolism in preterm infants without significant adverse effects. Unfortunately, they found no randomized controlled trials on this topic on which to base practice recommendations.

Another systematic review[77] evaluated the effectiveness of multi-component fortification of human milk on the promotion of growth and bone mineralization in preterm infants. Ten trials (total of 596 infants) were included in the analysis, which represented random or quasi-random allocation to supplementation of human milk with multiple nutrients or no supplementation within a nursery setting. The trials varied considerably in the total amount of Ca and P provided in the fortifier, the volume of milk prescribed, the amount of Vitamin D provided, the duration of use of the fortifier, the timing of the outcome measures, and whether BMC (either radial or whole body bone) was measured or only biochemical markers of bone metabolism assessed.

The main results of the review were that fortification of mother's milk with multiple nutrients (including protein, Ca and P) is beneficial to short-term growth in weight, length and head circumference. While there was no effect of the fortification on biochemical markers of bone such as alkaline phosphatase, BMC did appear to be increased by the fortification. However, it is worthwhile to examine the specific studies that were analyzed in this review. Of the 5 studies in which BMC was measured, there were no statistical differences between control and treatment groups in 4 studies. A meta analysis of these 5 studies in which one study contributed 59 of a total of 79 infants, showed that there was a positive effect on BMC of fortification of mother's milk with a human milk fortifier (weighted mean difference [WMD] 8.3 mg/cm, 95% confidence interval [CI] 3.8 to 12.8 mg/cm). The incidence of hypercalcemia was similar between treatment groups when assessed, although both treatment groups were supplemented with minerals.[74,75] Plasma alkaline phosphatase was not different between treatment groups (see discussion of alkaline phosphatase under section on Clinical Monitoring).

Since the Cochrane review on multinutrient fortification of human milk,[77] additional trials (although not always of a randomized design) have examined the response of preterm infants to a variety of human milk fortifiers.[78-81] The design of the studies differed, either comparing "head to head" two different commercially available fortifiers, or fortified compared to non-fortified mother's milk or to preterm formula. Unfortunately, none of the studies reported BMC as an outcome. In all studies, mean values for plasma alkaline phosphatase, used as surrogate marker

of bone metabolism, were consistently within the normal range. In one study,[81] infants fed mother's milk plus fortifier had lower mean alkaline phosphatase than infants fed mother's milk alone, but had similar values to infants fed a preterm formula. In a study comparing two commercially available fortifiers,[79] a higher alkaline phosphatase was observed in the group with greater linear and weight growth rates.

Whole body BMC measured using dual energy x-ray absorptiometry (DXA) technology, has been evaluated in recent studies although mostly in infants after hospital discharge. Of relevance to outcomes related to in-hospital nutrition are measures of BMC at term-adjusted age. In two studies[75,82] of infants (gestational age of about 30 weeks and birth weight of about 1200-1400 g) fed fortified mother's milk, BMC was similar to infants fed preterm formula in hospital. In both studies, mean BMC of infants fed the fortified mother's milk was lower than the value observed in the respective studies for term infants at term-corrected age, but within – 1SD from the mean value for the term infants. Similarly, in a recent randomized blinded study of infants of < 32-weeks gestation (mean birth weight of diet groups was 1114 - 1308 g) from Denmark,[83] no differences in whole body BMC were observed at term-adjusted age between infants fed in hospital on mother's milk supplemented with added P (n=40) or a multi-nutrient fortifier (n=36) or those fed preterm formula (n=51). A sub-analysis of dietary groups found that infants fed mother's milk had significantly lower BMC than infants fed preterm formula (n=16) but the difference disappeared when the BMC was corrected for body size.[83] It is unfortunate that absolute intake of nutrients was not reported. Interpretation of the data in the latter study is further confounded since the group fed preterm formula also received variable amounts of mother's milk (since it was the feeding of choice in the study site).

In contrast to the findings of the three latter studies,[75,82,83] a recent study from Belgium in somewhat larger preterm infants (<1750 g birth weight, mean gestational age 31 weeks)[84] found that

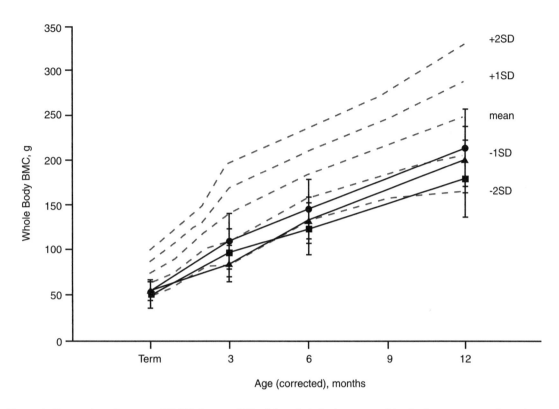

Figure 3: Bone mineral content (BMC) (mean±SD) of the whole body measured by dual energy x-ray absorptiometry in preterm infants at term-, 3-, 6- and 12-months-corrected age (adjusted for prematurity). The infant groups shown are as follows: ♦-------♦ infants (birth weight = 1154±239 g (mean ± SD); gestational age =30±3 wk; n=24) fed fortified breast milk in hospital and breast-feeding with only Vitamin D and iron supplementation after hospital discharge; ▲------▲ infants of extremely low birth weight (birth weight = 866±169 g ; gestational age = 26±1.5 wk; n=18); and ●------● infants of very low birth weight (birth weight = 1029±371 g; gestational age = 29±3 wk; n= 22), both latter groups fed preterm formula in hospital and standard term formula after hospital discharge. ------- represents reference values for mean ± 1 and ± 2 SD values for infants born at term and fed standard infant formula from birth to 1-year corrected age (data from S.A. Atkinson, McMaster University, Hamilton, Canada).

gain in whole body BMC was greater in infants fed premature formula   (n=34) than fortified mother's milk (n=20) (mother's own with/without added banked milk). Unfortunately, the difference in intake and absorption of minerals between diet groups was not reported for this study. An explanation for the discrepant findings in BMC between the studies of Faerk et al[83] and Pieltain et al[84] would be facilitated by more information regarding the intakes and absorption of minerals in the infant feeding groups. Since mixed feeding (a combination of fortified

human milk and formula) occurred in these studies,[83,84] it may be that the magnitude of the difference in absolute intakes of minerals was sufficiently variable between studies to influence a diet effect on bone mineral content at the age of approximately 36-37 weeks of gestation.

Some of the observed differences in BMC at term age between reported studies may relate to differences in birth size, particularly if the population studied included infants of extremely low birth weight or small for gestational age. As pointed out by Atkinson and

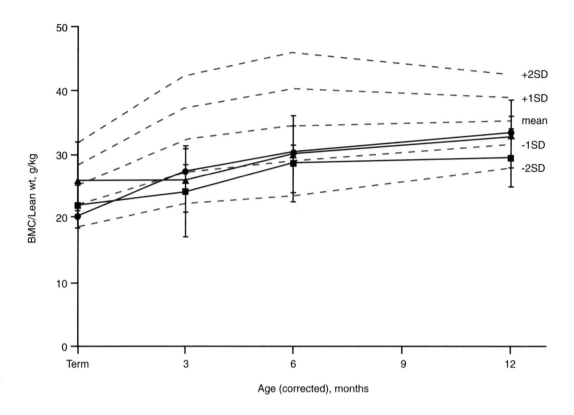

Figure 4: Bone mineral content (BMC) (mean±SD) of the whole body as a function of lean mass weight (BMC/Lean Wt) in preterm infants at term-, 3-, 6- and 12-months-corrected age as described in legend under Figure 3 (data from S.A. Atkinson, McMaster University, Hamilton, Canada). The infant groups shown are as follows: ◆-------◆ infants fed fortified breast milk in hospital and breast-feeding with only Vitamin D and iron supplementation after hospital discharge; ▲------▲ infants of extremely low birth weight; and ●------● infants of very low birth weight with both latter groups fed preterm formula in hospital and standard term formula after hospital discharge. ------- represents reference values for mean ± 1 and ± 2 SD values for infants born at term and fed standard infant formula from birth to 1-year-corrected age (data from S.A. Atkinson, McMaster University, Hamilton, Canada).

Wauben,[85] whole body BMC of preterm infants measured by DXA is best expressed as a function of lean mass since composition of fat and lean tissue varies with birth size and diet. Mean absolute BMC for preterm infants at term corrected age who were AGA was 16-30% lower, and for those who were small for gestational age (SGA) was 36% lower than BMC in term-born infants.[86] However, LBW infants were on average shorter and lighter at 40-weeks-adjusted age than term-born infants. When values for absolute BMC (Figure 3) are compared to values for BMC/lean mass (Figure 4) at term age, the latter deviate to a lesser

degree than absolute BMC from mean values for term-born infants.

Measurements of nutrient balance when conducted with adequate care and precautions[87] offer information on the amount of mineral intake required to achieve a net retention that is similar to estimates of intrauterine accretion of nutrients. If one accepts the hypothesis that achievement of intrauterine nutrient accretion and growth is an appropriate goal for nutritional management of LBW infants, then metabolic balance studies provide useful information on both the quantity and quality of growth. Such balance studies

	Preterm Human Milk + Ca/P supplement mmol	Preterm Human Milk + Fortifier mmol	Preterm Formula at 81 kcal/100cc mmol
Calcium			
Concentration (/L)*	NA	16-34	16-37
Delivery (/kg/day)	2.25-3.0	2.5-4.9	2.6-4.8
Retention (% intake)	73-79	50-82	40-72
Apparent Retention (/kg/day)	1.4-3.6	1.7-2.5	1.8-3.4
Intrauterine Accretion Rate (/kg/day)	2.3-3.2	2.3-3.2	2.3-3.2
	(90-120 mg)	(90-120 mg)	(90-120 mg)
Phosphorus			
Concentration (/L)	NA	16-21	14-26
Delivery (/kg/day)	2.0-4.0	2.3-2.8	2.5-3.9
Retention (% intake)	93	70-90	60-92
Apparent Retention (/kg/day)	1.7-2.5	1.9-2.8	1.5-2.5
Intrauterine Accretion Rate (/kg/day)	1.9-2.5	1.9-2.5	1.9-2.5
	(60-75 mg)	(60-75 mg)	(60-75 mg)
Magnesium			
Concentration (/L)	1.0-1.4	1.9-2.6	2.1-2.5
	(from breast milk)		
Delivery (/kg/day)	0.15-0.21	0.28-0.38	0.3-0.6
Retention (% intake)	84	73	40-60
Apparent Retention (/kg/day)	0.1-0.12	0.1-0.15	0.13-0.25
Intrauterine Accretion Rate (/kg/day)	0.1-0.14	0.1-0.14	0.1-0.14
	(2.5-3.4 mg)	(2.5-3.4 mg)	(2.5-3.4 mg)

Table 4: Projected net retention (balance) of Ca, P and Mg from preterm human milk with supplements of Ca and P alone, preterm human milk with added multi-nutrient fortifier and preterm infant formula compared to estimated intrauterine accretion rate. Concentration of nutrients represents published values for preterm milk at a mature stage of lactation without addition of Ca/P from supplement; preterm milk with commercially available powdered fortifier added in dose recommended by manufacturers; and bovine-based preterm formula of high Ca content. The infants represented in the cited balance studies were usually at a postnatal age of 3 weeks or more. The absorption and excretion of minerals might vary in infants of lesser postnatal ages. The range of values represent those available from published studies in which data were provided in tabular form.[55,68,75,82,87,88,89,92,93,97]

also allow an assessment of the efficiency of absorption of varying amounts and sources of mineral salts that are added as fortifiers to human milk or to preterm formulas. Unfortunately, due to the difficulty in properly performing metabolic balance studies and the associated high costs, especially if stable isotope tracers are used, there are few recent reports of nutrient balance in preterm infants fed currently marketed human milk fortifiers or preterm formulas. A summary of the available studies is provided in Table 4 for feedings of human milk with added Ca and P salts only, or with multi-nutrient fortifier, or preterm formulas.

Absorption of Ca from human milk (when

expressed as % of intake absorbed), with Ca and P salts added (73-79%), is usually somewhat greater than from human milk fortified with a multi-nutrient supplement (50-82%) and from preterm formula (40-72%) (Table 4). However, such observations are not consistent because of the variety of factors that confound absorption of Ca and P. For example, the efficiency of Ca absorption depends not only on the quantity and source of mineral salt fed, but on the amount and quality of fat, protein and phosphorus in the diet (reviewed in[88,89]), and whether the infants are being prescribed the steroid drug dexamethasone.[90] Phosphorus is absorbed very efficiently by preterm infants, usually at least 90% of intake, and does not vary greatly between types of feedings (Table 4). One exception is the observed lower availability of P from Ca triphosphate (only about 60% of intake) when it is the predominant mineral salt added to a preterm formula.[89] In some neonatal centers in Europe[43,91] the dose of supplemental Ca and P is prescribed individually and monitored by measuring urinary excretion of the minerals.

While normal serum and urinary biochemistry can be attained on Ca intakes as low as 2.5 mmol (107 mg)/kg/d and has high as 5.5 mmol (220 mg) /kg/d,[92] intrauterine accretion of Ca will only be achieved at the higher intakes. In one study using a powdered fortifier added to mother's milk,[93] a mean Ca intake of 5 mmol (196 mg)/kg/d resulted in apparent retention of Ca that just reached intrauterine accretion since the efficiency of Ca absorption was only about 50%. Phosphorus retention from an intake of 3.8 mmol (118 mg)/kg/d exceeded intrauterine retention as absorption of P was greater than 90%.[93] The data in Table 4 represent the range of values reported for intake, % absorption, and retention of Ca and P. This information serves as a guide to the expected retention of minerals in relation to intrauterine accretion depending on the type of feeding being provided to the infants.

The optimal ratio of dietary Ca:P of milk feedings for preterm infants has often been debated. The Ca:P of human milk is 1.6 molar (2.0 mg:mg). Most preterm formulas currently marketed have a Ca:P

ratio of 1.4-1.6 molar (1.8-2.0 mg:mg). The Ca:P of available human milk fortifiers ranges from 1.2 - 1.6 molar. The key factor in determining the ratio of Ca:P in fortifiers or formula is the availability of the Ca. If absorbed Ca is limiting, then the Ca:P ratio of the formula will have to be higher than the theoretical value derived from the ratio in bone apatite (1.7 molar) or the whole body (1.3 molar). It has been suggested that a Ca:P molar ratio of 2.2 or more is required to achieve a desirable retention of both minerals.[43] Few studies have experimentally addressed the issue of Ca:P ratio of feeds in relation to a specific outcome measure. In one study[94] in which three ratios of Ca:P were provided in high Ca containing formulas (24 mmol (948 mg)/L), a Ca:P of 1.1 molar (1.4 mg:mg) did not support radial bone mineral accretion to the same extent as the formulas with a Ca:P of 1.4-1.6 molar (1.7-2.0 mg:mg).

Magnesium: As for Ca and P, intakes and net retention of Mg vary with the type of feeding (Table 4). The Mg provided by mother's milk without supplemental Mg is marginally adequate to meet intrauterine accretion.[68,88] Magnesium absorption measured in classical balance studies is reported to be about 60-88%[68,93] from human milk but only 40-60% from preterm formula.[87,93] In studies in which human milk was intrinsically[95] or extrinsically[96] labeled with a stable isotope of Mg, fractional absorption was about 84-89% of intake. Whether Mg absorption is reduced by addition to mother's milk of other mineral salts or multi-nutrient fortifiers is controversial. Using classical balance studies, Lapillone et al[82] measured Mg absorption from human milk fortified with Ca (total intake of 2.5 mmol (101 mg)/kg/d) and P (intake of 2.5 mmol (78 mg)/kg/d) to be only 40%, and from preterm formula with similar Ca and P intakes to be 47%. This is a considerably lower efficiency of absorption than the approximately 60% from fortified mother's milk observed by Schanler et al.[93] Evidence of an interactive effect of Ca/P on Mg absorption was directly observed by Giles et al,[97] who found that high Ca and P intakes (5.5 mmol (220 mg) and 4 mmol (124) mg/kg/d, respectively) from formula with a Mg content of 2.25 mmol (54 mg)/L reduced Mg absorption so that retention of Mg was negative. While in most reports of Mg balance in preterm infants the net retention of Mg is positive; it is not always of an amount equal to maximum intrauterine retention of Mg (Table 4). Based on the data available, optimal Mg intake for preterm infants should be derived with recognition of the potential for negative influences of high dietary Ca and P on the availability of Mg for absorption in the intestine.

Vitamin D: Human milk is low in Vitamin D activity averaging about 80 IU/L in preterm milk, thus providing the preterm infants with only about 12-16 IU Vitamin D/kg/day.[98] At birth, preterm infants have normal cord blood or circulating 25-OH D that correlates with maternal Vitamin D status, albeit at concentrations about 20-30% lower in the infants.[22,99] Maternal Vitamin D deficiency will reduce the transplacental transfer to the fetus of 25-OHD, resulting in lower stores in the infant at birth.[22] In preterm infants born of Vitamin D replete mothers, a shortened gestation and low fat stores would limit the amount of Vitamin D stores considerably below that of term-born infants. Additionally, prolonged hospitalization prevents cutaneous synthesis as a source of Vitamin D. Thus, preterm infants require exogenous Vitamin D (Figure 2) but the recommended intake varies considerably across the world (Table 3). In preterm infants born in south central Canada with normal Vitamin D status (birth weight = 1350 ± 70 g, gestational age 30 ± 0.5 weeks) and given 800 IU Vitamin D daily from 3 to 7 weeks of age, plasma 25-OHD (34 ± 2 to 38 ± 2, ng/ml) was maintained (normal range 10-50 ng/mL).[99] In the United Kingdom, Vitamin D status was maintained in preterm infants in hospital when they received 400 IU/day of Vitamin D.[100]

In North America and Australia, supplementation with a single daily dose of Vitamin D of 400 IU/d is standard practice. The key study to support this recommendation is the randomized trial in infants of birth weight of 1200 g in which daily Vitamin D intakes of 200 IU (90 IU/kg), 400 (180 IU/kg) or 800 IU (360 IU/kg) given from 16 days of age for one

month, maintained normal Vitamin D status.[101] In addition, no radiological differences were observed between groups, all of whom were being fed high mineral containing formulas. A recent study substantiates the adequacy of Vitamin D intakes in the range of 200-400 IU/d. Intakes of Vitamin D from fortified human milk of about 325 to 374 IU/d, resulted in plasma 25-hydroxyVitamin D concentrations of 44 to 50 ng/mL representing the high normal range (normal range 10-50 ng/mL).[78] Plasma 25-OHD actually rose over two or more weeks from baseline values and concentrations of the active metabolite of 1,25-dihydroxyVitamin D were also in the normal range (48±4 to 47±5 pg/m; normal range 21-85 pg/ml).[78] Since absorption of Ca and P in preterm infants appears to be independent of Vitamin D,[25] there is little reason to believe that higher intakes of Vitamin D would serve a physiological function.

There are continental differences in recommendations for Vitamin D intake of preterm infants in that the Nutrition Committee for the European Society of Pediatric Gastroenterology, Hepatology and Nutrition[102] recommends a Vitamin D intake up to 1000 IU/d (Table 3). The rationale for the higher intake of Vitamin D for preterm infants is the risk of sub-clinical Vitamin D deficiency in women in Europe (and thus their newborn infants) owing to the lack of fortification of commercial cow milk with Vitamin D. However, in a clinical trial comparing 2000 vs 400 IU Vitamin D/d given to preterm infants fed human milk or standard term formula (both of which are relatively deficient in Ca and P relative to the recommended intakes for preterm infants), no differences in metabolic bone disease as assessed radiologically were observed.[103] Vitamin D status as measured by plasma 25-hydroxyVitamin D was within the normal range for both infant groups and at the upper limit of the normal range for those infants who received 2000 IU/d.[103]

Post-hospital discharge: For the postdischarge period, the key factors that influence bone mass accretion during the first year of life have not been delineated. In earlier studies that measured radial bone

	Calcium Intake, mmol/day				
Age, corrected	Term	3 mo	6 mo	12 mo	PRNI[66]
Breast-fed	5.6 ± 3.7	7.8 ± 3.8	13.3 ± 4.8	24.8 ± 7.7	6.3 ± 9.4
Formula-fed ELBW	5.3 ± 1.5	8.0 ± 3.0	13.0 ± 4.6	23.0 ± 9.0	6.3 ± 9.4
Formula-fed VLBW	7.0 ± 0.5	9.2 ± 3.0	15.2 ± 4.1	15.6 ± 4.9	6.3 ± 9.4

	Phosphorus Intake, mmol/day				
Age, corrected	Term	3 mo	6 mo	12 mo	PRNI
Breast-fed	3.8 ± 3.0	6.1 ± 3.8	12.7 ± 5.7	29.4 ± 9.0	3.4
Formula-fed ELBW	4.8 ± 1.5	7.0 ± 3.0	14.0 ± 6.0	27.0 ± 10.0	3.4
Formula-fed VLBW	5.9 ± 0.6	9.2 ± 3.0	15.6 ± 4.3	19.5 ± 4.9	3.4

Table 5: Calcium and phosphorus intakes at term-, 3-, 6-, and 12-months for preterm infants who were breast-fed (> 50% of fluid intake as breast milk) to 6-months-corrected age (BF); and extremely low birth weight (ELBW) infants and very low birth weight (VLBW) infants who were fed preterm formula in hospital, and standard term formula from hospital discharge to 1-year corrected age. A detailed description of infant groups is found under Figure 3. Nutrient intakes reflect the sum of intakes from measured volumes of breast milk and/or formula plus solid foods as recorded for 5 days at the time of each assessment. After 6 months of age, breast-fed infants were weaned either to formula or whole cow milk according to parental choice. Solid foods were introduced at the parents' discretion some time after 4-months-corrected age. ELBW infants were weaned to cow milk (at parenteral discretion) after 9 months of age. The Premature-Recommended Nutrient Intakes[66] (P-RNI) for infants after hospital discharge to 1 year of age are presented in the right-hand column for comparison.

mass using single photon absorptiometry, LBW infants fed either human milk or a standard term formula continued to have a lower radial BMC than infants fed a fortified formula up to one year of age.[104-106] However, the lower radial BMC observed in former LBW infants who were breast-fed until at least two months after hospital discharge (n=10) compared to those fed formula (n=11) up to 1 year of age, was no longer evident by 2 years of age.[107] In more recent studies in which BMC of the whole body was measured using DXA, supplemental dietary Ca and P after hospital discharge had a positive immediate benefit to BMC when the intervention was continued to 3-[108] or 9-[109] months-corrected age. However, such a

positive effect of early nutrition on BMC is not always sustained.[110,111]

Based on recent clinical trials from Atkinson's laboratory, whole body BMC of preterm infants to one-year-corrected age increases four-fold but still lags behind that of term-born infants (Figure 3). At term age, mean BMC of preterm infants falls close to −2 SD below the mean for term-born infants (Figure 3). No apparent difference was observed in BMC at term age between VLBW infants fed fortified breast milk in hospital followed by breast-feeding after hospital discharge and VLBW or extremely low birth weight (ELBW) infants who were fed preterm formula in hospital and standard term formula after discharge

(Figure 3). The infants originally breast-fed and the ELBW infants originally fed formula had cow milk introduced into their diet (at parental discretion) some time after 9-months-corrected age. By 12-months-corrected age some "catch-up" in BMC was observed, particularly for the VLBW infants fed formula but the mean value still fell below that for term-born infants. The poorest achievement in catch-up in BMC was observed in the breast-fed infants whose mean BMC remained lower than −1.5 SD at 12-months-corrected age. The reference values shown in Figure 3 are based on term infants fed standard term formula. No data yet exist on whole body BMC in term infants who were breast-fed to one year of age that could serve as appropriate reference data for preterm breast-fed infants.

Could the failure of preterm infants to achieve full "catch-up" in bone mineral content in the first year be due to mineral deficient diets? Mean Ca and P intakes (based on 5-day diet records) of the infants represented in Figure 3 are shown in Table 5 and compared to current recommended intakes for the first year of life of preterm infants. At term, mean Ca intakes are lower than the recommendations, but otherwise both Ca and P intakes to one year of age were at or above the current recommended intakes. In fact, due to the introduction of solid foods and cow milk for infants who had been weaned from breast milk or formula (the ELBW group), the intakes at 12 months were well in excess of recommendations.

In the 4th Edition of the *Pediatric Nutrition Handbook* by the American Academy of Pediatrics,[112] it is recommended that premature infants should attain growth and body composition similar to that of term-born infants. While this is theoretically a reasonable goal, it appears that, particularly in ELBW infants, even with enteral intakes of Ca in the range of 2.5-5 mmol (100-200 mg)/kg/d, P of 3-5 mmol (100-150 mg)/kg/d and Vitamin D of 400 IU/day or more given during hospitalization, whole body BMC is in the lower range of normal for term-born infants. The ELBW infant population is particularly disadvantaged as extended periods of TPN, especially when optimal delivery of Ca and P cannot be attained,

in addition to delayed weaning to enteral feeds containing sufficiently high enough amounts of Ca and P in early life, would not allow infants to achieve intrauterine accretion of bone minerals. It remains undetermined when and how to achieve the goal of whole body BMC in preterm infants similar to term infants. Follow-up of prematurely born infants at 8 to 10 years of age, demonstrated that BMC was significantly lower than for children of similar age born at term.[113] However, the preterm infants were also shorter and lighter so that their BMC was appropriate for body mass when compared with children born at term. An emerging hypothesis is that lower intakes of Ca and P in early life may be important in the programming of subsequent regulation of bone mineralization, but this has not been proven. In a secondary analysis of a longitudinal study,[104] the feeding of mother's milk to preterm infants in early life was associated with a greater bone mineral content at five years of age compared to infants who had been fed formula with higher mineral content. Physical activity is also a variable that impacts on bone mass accretion even in preterm infants in early neonatal life as measured using single photon absorptiometry[114] or DXA.[115] Using quantitative ultrasound of the tibia, early (about 2-weeks postnatal) intervention with brief daily passive range of motion exercise reduced the observed postnatal decline in tibial speed of sound (SOS) measures (see details of method under section on Clinical Monitoring).[116,117]

In summary, the multitude of factors that influence bone mass accretion in LBW infants during the first year or two of life has not been well delineated. There is evidence that higher amounts of minerals and protein provided in infant formulas support greater gains in BMC than in infants fed standard formulas designed for term infants. Somewhat disappointingly, this benefit to BMC is not always sustained after the dietary intervention period. Long-term follow-up of preterm infants on varying dietary intakes that includes measurement of activity will be required in order to determine whether a specific nutritional prescription, as yet not defined, is required to support skeletal mineralization parallel to that of infants born at term out to the age of adolescence (and peak bone mass). Clearly much more research is required into the multitude of factors controlling skeletal development in LBW infants.

Influence of Drugs on Requirements of Ca, P, Mg and Vitamin D

Dexamethasone: The potent exogenous steroid dexamethasone has been used widely in neonates to induce pulmonary compliance and earlier weaning from the ventilator.[118,119] Unfortunately, steroid therapy compromises nutritional status and growth in several ways. Exogenous steroid interferes with Ca and Vitamin D metabolism and alters bone formation and resorption resulting in a negative impact on skeletal development. Interference with the growth hormone-insulin-like growth factor axis[89,120] and promotion of protein catabolism[120,121] lead to somatic growth restriction. In addition, long-term follow-up of infants treated with dexamethasone in early life, show negative effects particularly on linear growth.[90]

When dexamethasone is used, infants may develop hypercalciuria and hyperphosphaturia, increased protein catabolism (elevated blood urea), and reduced circulating 25-OH Vitamin D. These biochemical measures will normalize following discontinuation of the drug, although it is unclear as to the long-term impact of early dexamethasone on length growth and bone mass accretion. Supplemental nutrition after hospital discharge to promote linear growth and bone mineral accretion has proven advantageous in very small infants with bronchopulmonary dysplasia who received dexamethasone in early life[108] but the amount and duration of need for a nutrient-enhanced diet requires more research.

Diuretics: Diuretic therapy for treatment of pulmonary congestion or edema in preterm infants with chronic lung disease, particularly with loop diuretics such as furosemide, induces excessive renal loss of Ca. Calcium loss occurs since sodium and Ca re-absorption in the distal tubule are blocked.[70,122,123] Use of thiazide diuretics with or without spironolactone also can induce renal loss of Ca.[122] If the definition of hypercalciuria in preterm infants is a 24-hour urinary Ca excretion >4-6 mg

(0.1 - 0.5 mmol)/kg/day as for term infants, then a hypercalciuric state may occur quite frequently when infants are prescribed furosemide. If these diuretic drugs are used chronically, secondary effects such as interstitial calcification of the kidney, nephrocalcinosis and renal Ca stones can occur.[122,124,125] Restricting Ca intake does not prevent diuretic-induced calciuria, since a daily Ca intake of only 100 mg (2.5 mmol)/kg/d in combination with prolonged furosemide administration may lead to hypercalciuria. However, other factors such as high sodium or Vitamin D intakes or low P intake may also contribute to calciuria.[122] Excessive renal loss of Ca in the presence of diuretic or supplemental sodium therapy may reflect excessive renal sodium loss since these minerals are co-transported in the proximal and distal kidney tubule.[122] In infants with hypercalciuria over extended periods during the hospitalized period, bone mineral accretion may be compromised.[126,127] Catch-up bone mineralization might be possible after diuretic therapy is concluded, but this may require close attention to providing extra Ca and P in the diet.

Special clinical populations

Infants of extremely low birth weight (ELBW) are particularly medically compromised due to extreme immaturity of their organ systems, dependence on assisted ventilation in early life (thus usually being maintained on parenteral nutrition for extended periods), and longer hospital stays than infants of larger birth weight. Many such infants develop chronic lung disease or bronchopulmonary dysplasia (BPD). Restricted volumes of fluid intake, especially as TPN, human milk or standard infant formula, may limit nutrient intakes below current recommendations for Ca, P and protein,[128] unless clinicians aggressively prescribe for optimal nutrition by fortifying human milk or providing nutrient-enriched preterm formulas in such situations. If Ca and P needs are not met in early life, whole body BMC of BPD infants will likely only reach the lower end of the reference range for term infants (ELBW group in Figures 3 and 4). The lack of catch-up in whole body bone mass up to one-year-corrected age,[111] parallels the observation of a previous study on radial bone mass in BPD infants.[127] Higher enteral intakes of Ca (3.8 ± 0.9 mmol (152 ± 36 mg) vs 1.7 ± 0.5 mmol (68 ± 20 mg)/kg/d) and P (3.0 ± 0.7 mmol (93 ± 22 mg) vs 1.6 ± 0.5 mmol (50 ± 15 mg)/kg/d) resulted in higher BMC (statistically significant only in males) after four months (at about 3-months-corrected age) of diet intervention.[108] However, once infants were changed to standard infant formula represented by the lower intakes above, the early benefit of higher mineral intakes to bone mass was not maintained.[111]

Deficiency

A deficiency of Ca and/or P for extended periods, especially in early life may be associated with deformities of the skull,[29] a narrow palate, protruding eyeballs[30] and metabolic bone disease, often referred to as osteopenia of prematurity, which when severe can cause rickets, with fracture (reviewed in).[31] In term-born infants, Vitamin D deficiency is the primary cause of rickets, but this is rarely the case in prematurely born infants. Deficiency of Ca/P and/or excess of aluminum delivered in parenteral nutrition solutions are the main causative factors of bone abnormalities in premature infants.[54,129]

Inadequate intakes of P can be identified by hypophosphatemia and non-detectable phosphate in the urine.[91] Aside from early neonatal hypocalcemia that occurs in the first 48-72 hours of life, serum Ca is not a sensitive indicator of inadequate calcium intakes, which may often occur in both parenterally and enterally fed infants (such as with unfortified mother's milk). Hypercalciuria will occur with phosphate depletion,[72] but collection of a representative urine sample is challenging in tiny infants in intensive care units. Trotter et al[43] suggests that a urine sample taken at any time of the day is adequate to monitor for hypercalciuria as there is no circadian rhythm for Ca/P excretion in urine. Specific clinical signs are unlikely to occur. Tetany is not a clinical sign except when it is secondary to hypoparathyroidism and severe hypocalcemia.

Before the 1990s, a high percent of infants, especially those of birth weight <1000 g, developed osteopenia and fractures.[130] Although not well documented, it is likely that severe osteopenia and fractures are less common in the last decade due to improved delivery of Ca/P intravenously (and shorter durations of parenteral nutrition which is deficient in Ca and/or P), and more global use of human milk fortifiers and preterm formulas that contain adequate amounts of absorbable Ca and P.

Vitamin D deficiency will only be found in infants who are born with low Vitamin D stores due to sub-clinical deficiency in the mothers and who do not receive Vitamin D via formula or as a supplement in the neonatal period. Preterm infants are born with plasma concentrations of 25-hydroxyVitamin D (the major circulating metabolite of Vitamin D) that are 20-30% lower than their mother's plasma 25-OHD.[22] Despite the efficient transplacental transport of 25-OHD that occurs in utero, the amount that has accumulated in stores of a preterm infant will be limited by the low amount of adipose stores in which it is usually deposited. Thus, to build up stores (as they would have had the preterm infant remained in utero) and to provide for needs for Vitamin D in early life, it is essential to provide Vitamin D as a supplement or as contained in a human milk fortifier or formula.

Toxicity

Toxicity associated with Ca, P and Mg is usually only associated with indiscriminant delivery of mineral via the parenteral route. Excessive infusion of calcium can cause tissue infiltration at the entry site. Excessive or unbalanced Ca and P in intravenous solutions may precipitate within the infusion line, especially at the warm temperatures of a neonatal unit.[126] Hypermagnesemia will occur if parenteral Mg is infused in too high amounts.

With parenteral or enteral feeding, hypercalciuria secondary to diuretic therapy (discussed above) can lead to nephrolithiasis and renal stones.[125,131] Supplementation of mother's milk with fortifiers containing Ca/P salts and high Vitamin D has been associated with anecdotal reports of hypercalcemia. Ca/P beozoars have been associated with Ca/P fortification of human milk to a total high

	Ca	P	Mg	Vit D[1]
Parenteral				
mmol/kg/d	1.5-2.0	1.5-2.0	0.18-0.3	1.5-10 µg/d
mg/kg/d	60-80	48-60	4.3-7.2	60-400 IU/d
Enteral				
mmol/kg/d	3.0-5.0*	2.0-3.5	0.3-0.4	5-25 µg/d
mg/kg/d	120-200*	70-120	7.2-9.6	200-1000 IU/d

[1]The recommended amounts of vitamin D represent the total daily intake. On a body
weight basis the minimum recommended oral intake is 2.25 µg (90 IU)/kg/day.
*For enteral nutrition the ratio of Ca:P should be maintained between 1.4-1.6 molar
(1.7-2.0 mg).

Table 6: Recommended reasonable range of intakes for parenteral and enteral nutrition for preterm infants during hospitalization.

intake of about 6.3 mmol (250 mg) Ca and 6.5 mmol (200 mg) P/kg/day.[132] Also, at very high intakes of Ca-supplemented formula (Ca of 40.6 (1840 mg) mmol/L formula or total intake of 5.9 mmol (235 mg) Ca/kg/day), three case reports of calcium-soap bezoars were published, two of which had ileal obstruction and intestinal perforation.[133] However, no controlled data are available to substantiate an increased risk for calcium-soap bezoars with high dietary Ca and P intakes. Hyperphosphatemia is rarely reported except when premature infants were fed evaporated or undiluted cow milk.[134]

Excessive chronic consumption of Vitamin D is well known to cause hypercalcemia and hypercalciuria and clinical symptoms such as anorexia, vomiting, failure to thrive, polyuria and ectopic calcification. This has usually been associated with very large intakes of >10,000 IU/kg/d or intermittent high-dose Vitamin D (600,000 IU every 2-3 months) for the prevention of rickets in older infants.[135] The recent report of the Dietary Reference Intakes set 1000 IU of Vitamin D as the tolerable upper limit for infants between birth and 12 months.[26] This would seem a safe upper limit for premature infants since there is one case of elevated serum 25-OHD and hypercalemia in a preterm infant (born at 816 g weight) who received about 1200 IU Vitamin D until about 16 months of age.[136] However, in parts of Europe, particularly in France, it has been general practice to provide up to 2000 IU Vitamin D

in hospital since most infants are born with low serum 25-OHD related to maternal sub-clinical Vitamin D deficiency.

Recommendations
Parenteral Nutrition

Infusion of 1.5[23] to 2.0[38,39] mmol Ca/kg/d, will support retentions of up to 1.8 mmol Ca and P /kg/d, and plasma Ca and P and urinary Ca excretion within a normal range can be maintained. Based on available studies a reasonable range for intake of Ca and P by parenteral nutrition is 1.5-2.0 mmol/kg/d (60-80 mg Ca and 45-60 mg P/kg/d) (Table 6), provided that amino acid intake is > 2-2.25 g/kg/d and the volume of infusate is > 100 ml/kg/d. Since solubility is a key issue, it is important to reduce the amount of Ca and P if the volume intake is restricted, otherwise the resultant high concentration of Ca and P leads to precipitates. With use of calcium glycerophosphate or disodium-glycerophosphate, which does not form precipitates with Ca-gluconate, greater amounts of Ca and P can be administered parenterally and retained. However, it is not possible to achieve amounts of retained mineral that are similar to that of intrauterine accretion when using currently available (in North America) injectable Ca and P salts.[38,39] In Europe, organic phosphorus compounds are licensed.

Enteral Nutrition

A range for Reasonable Recommended Intakes is provided in Table 6. For infants in transitional states or who have medical instability, intakes at the lower end of the range should support normal biochemical status but not necessarily intrauterine accretion of mineral. If the infant is stable and growing well, intakes at the upper range are recommended in order to potentiate retention of mineral that parallels intrauterine accretion. One possible approach is to adjust the supplemented amounts of Ca and P individually (and to monitor urinary excretion) in order to match the actual rate of growth and thus mineral needs.[43,91]

Calcium: The goal for net retention of Ca to match intrauterine accretion of Ca (about 120 mg (3 mmol)/kg/d[4]) and thereby optimize bone mineral

Biochemical Index	Range of Normal Values (mg/dl)
Phosphorus	1.8-2.6 mmol/L (5.6-8.1)
Blood ionized calcium	1.1-1.3 mmol/L (4.4-5.2)
Plasma total calcium if concerned about early neonatal hypocalcemia	2.2-2.5 mmol/L (8.8-10)
24-hour urinary calcium*	0.1-0.5 mmol/kg/d (4-20 mg/kg/d)
Alkaline phosphatase (bone isomer) (see discussion in text for limitations of interpretation of this measure)	150-400 units/L (depending on laboratory and assay used)
Measures of Bone Status X-ray of wrist for overt fractures or rickets	
Bone mineral content (to monitor accretion) by dual energy absorptiometry or quantitative ultrasound	Normative reference values not available as part of commercial software packages that come with the equipment

*Spot urine collections sampled over 4-hour periods may be adequate since excretion of Ca and P using this sampling method was reported to correlate well with that measured in 24-hour urine collections.[43]

Table 7: Clinical monitoring of calcium and phosphorus status during parenteral or enteral nutrition.

accretion during the hospital period will be dependent on a number of factors. First, during intravenous feeding, availability of organic phosphate salts is essential in order to infuse adequate amounts of Ca and P to meet intrauterine accretion. Second, the bioavailability of mineral from the oral feeds must be of the quality that allows for maximal intestinal absorption of Ca. It would be preferable that special formulas and human milk fortifiers are made available that contain adequate amounts and ratios of Ca and P. For cow-milk based formula this may require a Ca:P ratio in formula or human milk mixed with fortifier greater than 1.416 and up to 2.2 molar.[43] Also, the amount and type of the Ca salt should not impose any negative influences on absorption of other mineral elements such as magnesium, zinc or iron.

Minimum: 3.0 mmol (120 mg)/kg/d from human milk with added fortifier and 3.5 (140) mmol/kg/d from preterm formula.

Maximum: 5.0 mmol (200 mg)/kg/d from any feed with or without supplements.

Phosphorus: The minimum goal for P intake should be to maintain normophosphatemia and prevent excessive hypercalciuria. Intakes of 2.5 mmol (84 mg)/kg/d or greater will be required to achieve a retention of P of 1.9 - 2.5 mmol/kg/d, which represents intrauterine accretion.

Minimum: 2.0 mmol (62 mg)/kg/d for human milk with added fortifier or preterm formula.

Maximum: 3.5 mmol (109 mg)/kg/d from any feed with or without supplements.

Magnesium: The goal for Mg intake should be to achieve a retention of Mg of 0.1 to 0.14 mmol/kg/d, which represents intrauterine accretion of Mg. While Mg intake from human milk alone (0.2-0.25 mmol/kg/d) has proven to result in adequate retention, the addition of recommended amounts of Ca and P may reduce Mg absorption. Thus, a small amount of added Mg as part of a multi-nutrient fortifier is recommended. Higher intakes of Mg from formula are recommended because of the observed lower bioavailability of Mg from bovine-based formula.

Minimum: 0.3 mmol (7 mg)/kg/d from HMF or formula.

Maximum: 0.4 mmol (10 mg)/kg/d for HMF or formula.

Vitamin D: Based on the randomized trial of

Koo et al,[101] a minimum Vitamin D intake of 5 mg (200 IU)/day (or 90 IU/kg/d) would support a normal Vitamin D status. In Europe, Vitamin D in amounts from 500 up to 2000 IU per day is prescribed, but evidence is lacking for the physiologic need for the higher amount of vitamin. The upper level has thus been set at 1000 IU since this is the tolerable upper level established for term infants to 1 year of age by the Institute of Medicine report on Dietary Reference Intakes for Calcium, Phosphorus, Magnesium, Vitamin D and Fluoride.[26]

Minimum: total daily intake of 5 µg (200 IU).

Maximum: total daily intake of 25 µg (1000 IU).

Clinical Monitoring

The key clinical goal in prescribing Ca, P, Mg and Vitamin D for prematurely born infants is to maintain normocalcemia and normophosphatemia without excessive calciuria (see Table 7). In preterm infants fed unfortified human milk normophosphatemia cannot be maintained; although plasma Ca will be normal (after the first few days of life) (Atkinson et al, 1983) owing to the PTH-mediated regulation of circulating calcium. Infants fed human milk alone may develop moderate hypercalciuria, which is likely derived from loss of both tissue and dietary Ca (Abrams et al, 1994). In situations of inadequate intake of Ca and P, hypercalciuria may occur as a consequence of limited phosphorus intake (since the concentration of the two minerals in the blood is inadequate for deposition in the mineral of bone). Phosphaturia (defined as urinary P concentration >1 mmol/L) will occur primarily in very immature infants since renal phosphate threshold changes with advancing postmenstrual age.[138]

In general, normal plasma P and urinary Ca are maintained when infants are fed mineral-fortified human milk or nutrient-enriched preterm formulas.[28,82] When Ca and P were supplemented in amounts up to 10.2 and 5.3 mmol/kg/d, respectively, using inorganic salts on an individually adjusted basis, urinary Ca reached 1.4 - 5.8 mmol/kg/d and P reached 0.2 - 1.4 mmol/kg/d.[43] If this practice is adopted, careful monitoring for nephrocalcinosis is warranted,

especially if infants also receive diuretic therapy such as furosemide. Excessive delivery of Vitamin D or 1,25-dihydroxyVitamin D may also lead to hypercalciuria.

Suggested measures for clinical monitoring of mineral and Vitamin D status and ranges of normal values are provided in Table 7. Serum P is the most responsive to dietary intake. Hypophosphatemia (< 1.8 mmol/L)is certainly suggestive of inadequate P intake unless there is reason to suspect a renal leak of P owing to immaturity of the renal reabsorptive mechanism. Urinary Ca and P loss may occur with use of the steroid dexamethasone or with diuretics. Serum Ca concentration is so well controlled via PTH and 1,25-dihydroxyVitamin D, even in very immature premature infants, that it is not a sensitive indicator of inadequate Ca intake. Urinary Ca excretion in excess of 0.1 mmol (4 mg)/kg/day may reflect: a) phosphorus deficiency; b) secondary effect of diuretic therapy; c) hyperabsorptive hypercalciuria; d) Ca intakes that exceed growth needs; or e) bone resorption.

Alkaline phosphatase (AP) is an enzyme often used as an indirect biochemical marker for bone formation based on a spillover of excess or spent enzyme from active osteoblasts and precursors of osteoblasts in bone. Alkaline phosphatase accumulates in activated osteoblasts, hence its use as a marker of bone formation. However, just how the enzyme functions in the mineralization process remains elusive.[139] Since AP is present in blood in three isoforms, bone, liver and intestinal AP, a measure of total AP (the most likely measure conducted by a hospital clinical biochemist) may be misleading, especially since the fetal intestinal AP may represent up to 50% of the circulating enzyme in early neonatal life.[140] Circulating AP is higher in preterm compared to term infants and increases postnatally.[141,142] In most studies neither total nor bone AP predicted the rate of growth (weight gain) or bone mass accretion[140,143,144] although Crofton et al[145] found that bone AP positively correlated with rate of bone mineral accretion. In one study,[146] plasma AP explained only 4-6% of the observed variation in radial BMC.

When used to screen for osteopenia of prematurity,

an abnormally high circulating AP in preterm infants is usually only observed at the time of overt radiological evidence of rickets or fracture.[147] In term infants, AP was not elevated in infants with biochemical Vitamin D deficiency (plasma 25-OHD <15 nmol/L), and the mean value was similar to that of infants with normal plasma (25-OHD of >30 nmol/L).[148] In preterm infants, raised AP may reflect slower linear growth.[149,150] High plasma alkaline phosphatase may also reflect liver or gastrointestinal disease if the bone isoenzyme form (which constitutes about 50% of total circulating alkaline phosphatase) is not measured separately from total circulating alkaline phosphatase. Based on the available information, plasma AP in LBW infants is neither specific nor accurate for indicating bone turnover or identifying the risk of bone mineral deficits.

The most quantitative measure of bone mineral available for infants is dual energy x-ray absorptiometry (DXA), usually of the whole body, although software also exists for measures of spinal bone mineral content. Bone scans using DXA methodology have good precision, and the radiation dose is relatively low compared to x-ray or older measures by single and dual photon absorptiometry. Measures of BMC using DXA for research purposes have been reported in many studies[8,9,75,82,84,86,108,120,144,151,152] (and see Figures 3 and 4). Unfortunately, it remains difficult to adopt DXA measures for clinical use since the DXA machine manufacturers do not provide normal reference data upon which any measure conducted on an infant can be interpreted. Special software for DXA measures of infant whole body[151,153] and spine BMC[7] can be purchased if a clinical center has the appropriate instrument. However, appropriate methods must be used to conduct the DXA measures,[151,153] and the radiologist would have to use normal reference values for an appropriate population from the literature to make an interpretation of the DXA scan for an individual infant, which may not be appropriate given the variability between DXA machines. Sequential DXA scans can be used to monitor therapeutic intervention, such as supplemental Ca and P, provided that a reasonable duration of time between scans is

allowed so that any gain in bone is outside of the inherent errors in the measurement.[151,153]

An emerging method for estimation of bone mineral is that of speed of sound (SOS), a form of quantitative ultrasound (QUS), or sound waves possessing high frequency.[154] An ultrasound bone sonometer (Sunlight Omnisense®, Israel) is a non-invasive device that quantitatively measures the velocity of ultrasound waves propagating along the distal one-third of the radius bone or mid-shaft tibia.[155,156] QUS measures not only a quantitative aspect of bone but also qualitative factors that contribute to bone strength including bone elasticity, microarchitecture and fatigue damage.[155,157] Mid-tibial measures have been performed in children[158] and in very small preterm infants.[116,117,159,160] In premature infants (n=29) of medium birth weight 1264g and gestational age 31 weeks, tibial SOS in preterm infants at a median postnatal age of 7.5 weeks was lower than in term infants.[160] Of note, tibial SOS remained significantly lower in the preterm infatnts at term-corrected-age compared to term infants even though the preterm infants had received fortified human milk or preterm formula.[160] The QUS technique was recently shown to detect prevention of postnatal decline in bone SOS by daily exercise using passive motion from about two weeks of life in VLBW infants.[116,117] To date, QUS measures in infants have not been evaluated against DXA measures of whole body or spinal BMC. Also, normal reference data for QUS measures in preterm or term infants beyond birth have not been published. Assessment of bone status by QUS has potential as a clinical tool to assess osteopenia in preterm infants. The advantages of the SOS method include: cost, which is about one quarter or less of that of a DXA; machine portability compared to DXA, so it could be used at the bedside in the neonatal unit; and good in vivo precision at least in adults (intraobserver CV = 0.2 - 0.3%). Importantly, QUS does not involve use of ionizing radiation, whereas DXA exposes an infant to low-dose (about 2 mREM) radiation.

Case History

A female infant with a birth weight of 680 g is born at 26-weeks gestation with a complicated postnatal course. She requires prolonged ventilator support, one course of dexamethasone, and multiple intermittent doses of furosemide. She is weaned from supplemental oxygen by 8 months of age. Chest percussion (using a rubber conductive face mask) and chest vibration (using a battery-operated vibrator) are prescribed as therapeutic and preventive measures for pulmonary atelectasis. Passive exercise is also prescribed "to minimize increased muscle tone" of the infant. The infant receives repeated courses of PN (containing 1000 IU of Vitamin D2 [ergocalciferol], 4.5 mmol [180 mg] of elemental calcium, and 6 mmol [186 mg] of phosphorus per liter of infusate) via the peripheral and central venous route. Consistently adequate enteral feeding with preterm infant formula (100 kcal/kg/day) is not achieved until 16 weeks postnatally. Incidental skeletal abnormalities, including severe demineralization and fracture of ribs, are noted on a chest roentgenogram at 15 weeks postnatally. Roentgenograms of forearms and hands obtained immediately afterwards show rickets and fractures of radius and ulna.

Question: What are the important risk factors in this infant for osteopenia, fracture, and rickets?

Answer: Extremely low birth weight; low Ca and P content of PN solution; inadequate intake of enteral feeding during the first 3 months after birth; steroid and diuretic therapy; and physical therapy.

Question: Should 1,25(OH)2D be added to the therapeutic regimen?

Answer: With adequate mineral intake, 400 IU/day of Vitamin D is sufficient to maintain normal Vitamin D status. There is no documented advantage to using 1,25(OH)2D or other Vitamin D metabolites.

Question: What is the treatment for this infant if she has been fed human milk?

Answer: Powder or liquid fortifier for human milk, and in certain circumstances, direct Ca and P supplementation.

Question: What could have been done differently in this infant to prevent the osteopenia and fractures?

Answer: We suspect that a much more aggressive approach to maximize both parenteral and enteral mineral intake early in the course might have helped to prevent this condition. We also need to be careful to handle such "fragile" infants with gentleness, since "trauma" even in the form of chest percussion and physical therapy can precipitate fractures in a vulnerable infant.

References

1. Kelly HJ, Sloan, RE et al. Accumulation of nitrogen and 6 minerals in the human fetus during gestation. *Hum Biol.* 1951;23:61-74

2. Widdowson, EM and Spray, CM. Chemical development in utero. *Arch Dis Child.* 1951;26: 205-213.

3. Widdowson EM, Southgate DA, Hey E. Fetal growth and body composition. In: Linblad BS, ed. *Perinatal Nutrition.* New York, NY: Academic Press, Inc.; 1988;3-14.

4. Zeigler EE, O'Donnell Am, Nelson SE, Fomon SJ. Body composition of the reference fetus. *Growth* 1976;40:329-341.

5. Koo WWK, Walters J, Bush AJ, Chesney RW, Carlson SE. Dual energy x-ray absorptiometry studies of bone mineral status in newborn infants. *J Bone Miner Res* 1996;11:997-1002.

6. Pohlandt F and Mathers N. Bone mineral content of appropriate and light for gestational age preterm and term newborn infants. *Acta Paediatr Scand* 1989; 78: 835-839.

7. Koo WWK, Hockman EM. Physiologic predictors of lumbar spine bone mass in neonates. *Pediatric Research* 2000b;48:485-489.

8. Koo WWK, Bush AJ, Walters J, Carlson SE. Postnatal development of bone mineral status during infancy. *J American College Nutr* 1998b;17:65-70.

9. Wauben IPM, Atkinson SA, Shah JK, Paes B. Growth and body composition of preterm infants: influence of nutrient fortification of mother's milk in hospital and breast feeding post-hospital discharge. *Acta Paediatr* 1998b;87:780-785.

10. Godfrey K, Walker-Bone K, Robinson S, Taylor P, Shore S, Wheeler T, Cooper C. Neonatal Bone Mass: Influence of parental birthweight, maternal smoking, body composition, and activity during pregnancy. *J Bone Min Res* 2001;16(9):1694-1703.

11. Fall C, Hindmarsh P, Dennison E, Kellingray S, Barker D, Cooper C. Programming of growth hormone secretion and bone mineral density in elderly men: A hypothesis. *J Clin Endocrinol Metab* 1998;83:135-139.

12. Koo WW, Walters JC, Esterlitz J, Levine RJ, Bush AJ, Sibai B. Maternal calcium supplementation and fetal bone mineralization. *Obstet Gynecol* 1999;94(4): 577-582.

13. Jones G, Dwyer T. Birth weight, birth length, and bone density in prepubertal children: Evidence for an association that may be mediated by genetic factors. *Calcif Tissue Int* 2000;67:304-308.

14. Gale CR, Martyn CN, Kellingray S, Eastell R, Cooper C. Intrauterine programming of adult body composition. *J Clin Endocrinol Metab* 2001;86: 267-272.

15. Mimouni F and Tsang RC. Pathophysiology of neonatal hypocalcemia. In: Polin R, Fox W (eds.), *Fetal and Neonatal Physiology*, 2nd edition. Philadelphia, PA: W.B. Saunders Company, 1998;2329-2335.

16. Salle BL, Delvin EE, Lapillone A, Bishop NJ, Glorieux FH. Perinatal metabolism of Vitamin D. *Am J Clin Nutr* 2000:71(suppl):1317S-1324S.

17. Salle BL, Senterre J, Glorieux FH, Delvin EE, Putet G. Vitamin D metabolism in preterm infants. *Biol Neonate* 1987;52:119-30.

18. David L, Salle BL, Putet G et al. Serum immunoreactive calcitonin in low birth weight infants. Description of early changes; effect of intravenous calcium infusion; relationships with early changes in serum calcium, phosphorus, magnesium, parathyroid hormone and gastrin levels. *Pediatr Res* 1981;15:803-809.

19. Venkataraman PS, Tsang RC, Steichen JJ, Grey I, Neylan M, Fleishman AR. Early neonatal hypocalcemia in extremely preterm infants. High incidence, early onset, and refractoriness to supraphysiologic doses of calcitriol. *Am J Dis Child* 1986;140:1004-1008

20. Koo WWK, Kaplan LA, Bendon R, et al. Response to aluminum parenteral nutrition during infancy. *J Pediatr* 1986;109:877-883.

21. Scott SM et al. Effect of calcium therapy in the sick premature infant with early neonatal hypocalcemia. *J Pediatr* 1984;104:747-751.

22. Delvin EE, Gorieux FH, Salle BL et al. Control of Vitamin D metabolism in preterm infants: feto-maternal relationships. *Arch Dis Child* 1982;57:754-757.

23. Koo WWK, Tsang RC. Mineral requirements of low birth weight infants. *J Am Coll Nutr* 1991;10:474.

24. Schilling R et al. High total and free 1,25-dihydroxy Vitamin D concentrations in serum of premature infants. *Acta Pediatr Scand* 1990;79:36-40.

25. Bronner F, Salle BL, Putet G, Rigo J, Senterre J. Net calcium absorption in premature infants: results of 103 metabolic balance studies. *Am J Clin Nutr* 1992;56:1037-1044. [published erratum appears in *Am J Clin Nutr* 1993.57(3):451]

26. Institute of Medicine, Food and Nutrition Board. Dietary Reference Intakes for Calcium, Phosphorus, Magnesium, Vitamin D, and Fluoride. Washington, D.C.: National Academy Press, 1997.

27. Atkinson SA, Radde IC, Anderson GH. Macromineral balances in premature infants fed their own mother's milk or formula. *J Pediatr* 1983;102:99-106.

28. Schanler RJ, Rifka M. Calcium, phosphorus and magnesium needs for the low birth weight infant. *Acta Pediatr Suppl* 1994b;405:111-116.

29. Pohlandt, F. Bone mineral deficiency as the main factor of dolichocephalic head flattening in very low birth weight infants. *Pediatr Res* 1994a;35:701-703

30. Pohlandt, F. Hypothesis: myopia of prematurity is caused by postnatal bone mineral deficiency. *Eur J Pediatr* 1994b;153: 234-236

31. Koo WWK, Steichen JJ. Osteopenia and rickets of prematurity., In: Polin RA, Fox WW (eds). *Fetal and Neonatal Physiology*. Philadelphia, PA: WB Saunders, 1998a;2335-2349.

32. Vileisis RA. Effect of phosphorus intake in total parenteral nutrition infusates in premature infants. *J Pediatr* 1987;220:586-590.

33. Brown DR, Steranka BH. Renal cation excretion in the hypocalcemic premature human neonate. *Pediatr Res* 1981;15:1100-1104.

34. Goldsmith MA, Bahatia SS, Kanto WP, Kutrer MH, Ruadman D. Gluconate calcium therapy and neonatal hypercalciuria. *Am J Dis Child* 1981;135:538-545.

35. Klein GL, Cockburn JW. Parenteral nutrition: Effect on bone and mineral homeostasis. *Annu Rev Nutr* 1991;11:93-119.

36. Dabezies EJ, Warren PD. Fractures in very low birth weight infants with rickets. *Clin Orthopaedics Related Res* 1997;335:233-239.

37. Smith SL, Kirchhoff KT. Metabolic bone disease in very low weight infants: Assessment, prevention, and treatment by neonatal nurse practitioners. *JOGNN* 1997;26:297-302.

38. Schanler RJ, Shulman RJ, Prestridge LL. Parenteral nutrient needs of very low birth weight infants. *J Pediatr* 1994a;125:961-968.

39. Hanning RM, Atkinson SA, Whyte RK. Efficacy of calcium glycerophosphate vs conventional mineral salts for total parenteral nutrition in low birth weight infants: a randomized clinical trial. *Am J Clin Nutr* 1991;54:903-908.

40. Prestridge LL, Schanler RJ, Shulman RJ, Burns PA, Laine LL. Effect of parenteral calcium and phosphorus therapy on mineral retention and bone mineral content in very low birth weight infants. *J Pediatr* 1993;122:761-768.

41. Hanning RM, Mitchell MK, Atkinson SA. In-vitro solubility of calcium glycerophosphate versus conventional mineral salts in pediatric parenteral nutrition solutions. *J Pediatr Gastroenterol Nutr* 1989;9:67-72.

42. Pelegano JF, Rowe JC, Carey DE et al. Effect of calcium/phosphorus ratio on mineral retention in parenterally fed premature infants. *J Pediatr Gastroenterol Nutr* 1991;12:351-355.

43. Trotter, A and Pohlandt, F. Calcium and phosphorus retention in extremely preterm infants supplemented individually. *Acta Paediatr* 2002 91:1-4

44. Cole DEC, Zlotkin SH. Increased sulfite as an etiological factor in the hypercalciuria associated with total parenteral nutrition. *Am J Clin Nutr* 1983;37:108-113.

45. Fitzgerald KA, MacKay MW. Calcium and phosphate solubility in neonatal parenteral nutrition solutions containing TrophAmine. *Am J Hosp Pharm* 1986;43:88-93.

46. MacMahon P, Mayne PD, Blair M, Pope C, Kovar IZ. Calcium and phosphorus solubility in neonatal intravenous feeding solutions. *Arch Dis Child* 1990a;65:352-353.

47. Chessex P, Pineault M, Brisson G, Delvin EE, Glorieux F. Role of the source of phosphate salt in improving the mineral balance of parenterally fed low birth weight infants. *J Pediatr* 1990;116:765-772.

48. MacMahon P, Mayne PD, Blair M, Pope C, Kovar IZ. Acid-base state of the preterm infant and the formulation of intravenous feeding solutions. *Arch Dis Child* 1990b;65:354-356.

49. Costello, I, Powell, C and Williams, AF. Sodium glycerophosphate in the treatment of neonatal hypophosphataemia. *Arch Dis Child Fetal Neonatal Ed* 1994a;73(1):F44-45.

50. Prinzivalli, M and Ceccarelli, S. Sodium d-fructose-1, 6-diphosphate vs. sodium monohydrogen phosphate in total parenteral nutrition: a comparative in vitro assessment of calcium phosphate compatibility. *JPEN J Parenter Enteral Nutr* 1999;23(6):326-332.

51. Raupp P, Kries RV, Pfahl H-G, Mantz F. Glycero-vs glucose-phosphate in parenteral nutrition of premature infants: a comparative in vitro evaluation of calcium/phosphorus compatibility. *JPEN* 1991;15:469-473.

52. Atkinson S, Hanning R, Whyte R, Moss L. Altered amounts and ratios of calcium and phosphorus in total parenteral nutrition (TPN) for premature infants. *Pediatr Res* 1991;29:4.

53. Sedman AB, Klein GL, Merritt RJ, et al. Evidence of aluminum loading in infants receiving intravenous therapy. *N Eng J Med* 1985;312:1337-1343.

54. Koo WWK. Parenteral nutrition-related bone disease. *J Parenter Enteral Nutr* 1992b;16:386-394.

55. Atkinson SA, Shah JK. Calcium and phosphorus fortification of preterm formulas: Drug-mineral and mineral-mineral interactions. In: Hillman L, ed. *Mineral requirements for the premature infant.* New York, NY: Exerpta Medica 1990a:58-75.

56. Klein GL, Cannon RA, Diament M, et al. Infantile Vitamin D-resistant rickets associated with total parenteral nutrition. *Am J Dis Child* 1982;136:74-76.

57. Sedman AB, Alfrey AC, Miller NL, Goodman WG. Tissue and cellular basis for impaired bone formation in aluminum-related osteomalacia in the pig. *J Clin Invest* 1987;79:86-92.

58. Atkinson SA, Bahrey AL, Hanning RM. Aluminum intake and excretion in premature infants on enteral or parenteral feeds. *Pediatr Res* 1990c;27:4:279A (Abst 1660).

59. Anonymous. Aluminum in large and small volume parenterals used in total parenteral nutrition-FDA Proposed Rule. *Fed Regist* 1998;63:2:176-185.

60. Hoehn GJ, Carey DE, Rowe JC, Horak E, Raye JR. Alternate day infusion of calcium and phosphate in very low birth weight infants: Wasting of the infused mineral. *J Pediatr Gastroenterol Nutr* 1987;6:652-757.

61. Laine L, Shulman RJ, Pitre D, Lifschitz CH, Adams J. Cysteine usage increases the need for acetate in neonates who receive total parenteral nutrition. *Am J Clin Nutr* 1991;54:565-567.

62. Hicks, W., and Hardy G. Phosphate supplementation for hypophosphataemia and parenteral nutrition. *Curr Opin Clin Nutr Metab Care* 2001;4(3):227-233.

63. Koo WWK, Tsang RC, Steichen JJ, et al. Vitamin D requirement in infants receiving parenteral nutrition. *J Parenter Enteral Nutr* 1987b;11:172-176.

64. Koo WW, Tsang RC, Succop P, et al. Minimal Vitamin D and high calcium and phosphorus needs of preterm infants receiving parenteral nutrition. *J Pediatr Gastroenterol Nutr* 1989;8:225-233.

65. Baeckert PA, Greene HL, Fritx I, Oelberg DG, Adcock EW. Vitamin concentrations in very low birth weight infants given vitamins intravenously in a lipid emulsion: measurement of vitamins A, D, and E and riboflavin. *J Pediatr* 1988;113:1057-1065.

66. Canadian Pediatric Society - Nutrition Committee. Nutrient needs and feeding of premature infants. *Can Med Assoc J* 1995;152:1765-1783.

67. Rowe J, Rowe D, Horak E et al. Hypophosphatemia and hypercalciuria in small premature infants fed human milk: evidence for inadequate dietary phosphorus. *J Pediatr* 1984;104:112-7.

68. Atkinson SA, Chappell JA, Clandinin MT. Calcium supplementation of mother's milk for low birth weight infants: Problems related to absorption and excretion. *Nutr Res* 1987c;7:813-823.

69. Schanler RJ, Atkinson SA. Human Milk. In: Tsang RC et al, eds. *Nutrient Needs of Preterm Infants*, 2002, Cincinnati, Ohio, Digital Educational Publishing, Inc.

70. Rowe JC, Carey DE, Goetz CA, et al. Effect of high calcium and phosphorus intake on mineral retention in very low birth weight infants chronically treated with furosemide. *J Pediatr Gastroenterol Nutr* 1989;9: 206-211.

71. Senterre J, Putet G, Salle B, Rigo J. Effects of Vitamin D and phosphorus supplementation on calcium retention in preterm infants fed banked human milk. *J Pediatr* 1983;103:305-307.

72. Carey DE, Goetz CA, Horak E, Rowe JC. Phosphorus wasting during phosphorus supplementation of human milk feedings in preterm infants. *J Pediatr* 1985;107:790-794.

73. Giles MM, Fenton MH, Shaw B, Elton RA, Clarke M, Lang M, Hume R. Sequential calcium and phosphorus balance studies in preterm infants. *J Pediatr* 1987;110:591-598.

74. Lucas A, Fewtrell MS, Morley R, et al. Randomized outcome trial of human milk fortification and developmental outcome in preterm infants. *Am J Clin Nutr* 1996;64:142-151.

75. Wauben I, Atkinson SA, Grad TL, Shah JK, Paes B. Moderate nutrient supplementation to mother's milk for preterm infants supports adequate bone mass and short-term growth. A randomized controlled trial. *Am J Clin Nutr* 1998a;67:465-472.

76. Kuschel CA, Harding JE. Calcium and phosphorus supplementation of human milk for preterm infants. In: *The Cochrane Library*, Issue 4, 2001.

77. Kuschel CA, Harding JE. Multicomponent fortified human milk to promote growth in preterm infants (Cochrane Review). In: *The Cochrane Library*, Issue 2, 1999. Oxford, UK: Update Software.

78. Porcelli P, Schanler R, Greer F, et al. Growth in human milk-fed very low birth weight infants receiving a new human milk fortifier. *Ann Nutr Metab* 2000;44:2-10.

79. Reis BB, Hall RT, Schanler RJ, Berseth CL, Chan G, Ernst JA, Lemons J, Adamkin D, Baggs G, O'Connor D. Enhanced growth of preterm infants fed a new powdered human milk fortifier: A randomized, controlled trial. *Pediatrics* 2000;106:581-588.

80. Warner JT, Linton HR, Dunstan FD, Cartlidge PH. Growth and metabolic responses in preterm infants fed fortified human milk or a preterm formula. *Int. J Clin Pract* 1998;52:236-240.

81. Nicholl RM, Gamsu HR. Changes in growth and metabolism in very low birthweight infants fed with fortified breast milk. *Acta Paediatr* 1999;88: 1056-1061.

82. Lapillone AA, Glorieux FH, Salle B, et al. Mineral balance and whole body bone mineral content in very low birth weight infants. *Acta Pediatr Suppl* 1994;405:117-122.

83. Faerk J, Petersen S, Peitersen B, Fleischer Michaelsen K. Diet and bone mineral content at term in premature infants. *Pediatr Res* 2000;47:148-156.

84. Pieltain C, De Curtis M, Gerard P, Rigo J. Weight gain composition in preterm infants with dual energy x-ray absorptiometry. *Pediatr Res* 2001;49:120-124.

85. Atkinson SA and Wauben IPM. Reply to A Lapillone and BL Salle. *Am J Clin Nutr* 1999;69:154a-156.

86. Atkinson SA, Randall-Simpson J. Factors influencing body composition of premature infants at term-adjusted age. In: *Annals New York Academy of Sciences.* S. Yasumura (ed) 5th International Symposium on In-Vivo Body Composition Studies, New York, NY: 2000;904:393-400.

87. Cooke RJ, Perrin F, moore J, Paule C, Ruckman K. Methodology of nutrient balance in the preterm infant. J *Pediatr Gastroenterol Nutr* 1988;7:434-440.

88. Schanler RJ, Abrams SA. Postnatal attainment of intrauterine macromineral accretion rates in low birth weight infants fed fortified human milk. *J Pediatr* 1995;126:441-447.

89. Rigo J, De Curtis M, Pieltrain C, Picaud JC, Salle BL, Senterre J. Bone mineral metabolism in the micropremie. *Clin Perinatol* 2000;27(1):147-170.

90. Weiler HA, Paes B, Shah JK, Atkinson SA. Longitudinal assessment of growth and bone mineral accretion in prematurely born infants treated for chronic lung disease with dexamethasone. *J Early Hum Dev* 1997;47:271-286.

91. Pohlandt, F. Prevention of postnatal bone demineralization in very low birth weight infants by individually monitored supplementation with calcium and phosphorus. *Pediatr Res* 1994c;35:125-129

92. Mize CE, Uauy R, Waidelich D, Neylan MJ, Jacobs J. Effect of phosphorus supply on mineral balance at high calcium intakes in very low birth weight infants. *Am J Clin Nutr* 1995;62:385-391.

93. Schanler R J, Shulman R,J, Lau C. Feeding strategies for premature infants: beneficial outcomes of feeding fortified human milk versus preterm formula. *Pediatr* 1999;103:1150-1157.

94. Chan GM, Mileur L, Hansen JW. Calcium and phosphorus requirements in bone mineralization of preterm infants. *J Pediatr* 1988;113:225-229.

95. Liu Y-M, Neal P, Ernst J, et al. Absorption of calcium and magnesium from fortified human milk by very low birth weight infants. *Pediatr Res* 1989;25:496-502.

96. Wauben IPM, Paes B, Atkinson SA, Shah JK. Dietary bioavailability of Ca, Mg and Zn from supplemented mother's milk for preterm infants determined by stable isotope tracer and mass balance techniques. *Am Soc Clin Nutr* 1997;66:Abs.

97. Giles MM, Laing IA, Elton RA, Robins JB, Sanderson M, Hume R. Magnesium metabolism in preterm infants: effects of calcium, magnesium, and phosphorus, and of postnatal and gestational age. *J Pediatr* 1990;117:147-154.

98. Atkinson SA, Whyte RK, Gundberg C, Hollis BW. Vitamin D status and plasma osteocalcin in neonates fed supplemented mother's milk. *Fed Proc* 1987a;46(4):1015,A4072.

99. Atkinson SA, Reinhardt TA, Hollis BW. Vitamin D activity in maternal plasma and milk in relation to gestational stage at delivery. *Nutr Res* 1987b;7(10): 1005-1011.

100. Cooke R, Hollis B Conner C, Watson D, Werkman S, Chesney R. Vitamin D and mineral metabolism in the very low birth weight infant receiving 400 IU of Vitamin D. 1990;116:423-428.

101. Koo WWK, Krug-Wispe S, Neylan M, Succop P, Oestreich AE, Tsang RC. Effect of 3 levels of Vitamin D intake in preterm infants receiving high mineral-containing milk. *J Pediatr Gastroenterol Nutr* 1995b;21:182-189.

102. European Society for Pediatric Gastroenterology and Nutrition, Committee on Nutrition of the Preterm Infant, Nutrition and feeding of preterm infants. *Acta Paediatr Scand Suppl* 1987;336:1-14.

103. Evans JR, Allen AC, Stinson DA, et al. Effect of high-dose Vitamin D supplementation on radiographically detectable bone disease of very low birth weight infants. *J Pediatr* 1989;115:779-786.

104. Bishop J, Dahlenburg S, Fewtrell M, Morley R, Lucas A. Early diet of preterm infants and bone mineralization at age 5 years. *Acta Paediatr* 1996;85:230-236.

105. Chan GM. Growth and bone mineral status of discharged very low birth weight infants fed different formulas or human milk. *J Pediatr* 1993;123:439-443.

106. Abrams SA, Schanler RJ, Garza C. Bone mineralization in former very low birth weight infants fed either human milk or commercial formula. *J Pediatr* 1988;112:956-960.

107. Schanler RJ, Burns PA, Abrams SA, Garza C. Bone mineralization outcomes in human milk fed preterm infants. *Pediatr Res* 1992:31:583-586.

108. Brunton JA, Saigal S, Atkinson SA. Growth and body composition in infants with bronchopulmonary dysplasia up to 3 months corrected age: a randomized trial of a high-energy nutrient-enriched formula fed after hospital discharge. *J Pediatr* 1998;133:340-345.

109. Bishop NJ, King FJ, Lucas A. Increased bone mineral content of preterm babies fed with a nutrient enriched formula after discharge from hospital. *Arch Dis Child* 1993;68:573-578.

110. Rubinacci A, Sirtori P, Moro G, Galli L, Minoli I, Tessari L. Is there an impact of birth weight and early life nutrition on bone mineral content in preterm born infants and children? *Acta Pediatr* 1993;82:711-713.

111. Brunton JA, Saigal S, Atkinson S. Nutrient intake similar to recommended values does not result in catch-up growth by 12 months of age in very low birth weight infant (VLBW) with bronchopulmonary dysplasia (BPD). *Am J Clin Nutr* 1997b;55(i) Abst. 102.

112. American Academy of Pediatrics. Committee on Nutrition Nutritional needs of preterm infants. In: *Pediatric Handbook*, 4th ed. Kleinman, RE, ed. Elk Grove Village, IL:American Academy of Pediatrics; 1998:55-87.

113. Fewtrell MS, Prentice A, Jones SC, et al. Bone mineralization and turnover in preterm infants at 8-12 years of age: the effect of early diet. *J Bone Miner Res* 1999;14:810-820.

114. Moyer-Milleur L, Brunstetter V, McNaught TP, Gill G, Chan GM. Daily physical activity program increases bone mineralization and growth in preterm very low birth weight infants. *Pediatrics* 2000;106:1082-1092.

115. Moyer-Milleur L, Brunstetter V, McNaught TP, Gill G, Chan GM. Daily physical activity program increases bone mineralization and growth in preterm very low birth weight infants. *Pediatrics* 2000;106:1082-1092.

116. Nemet D, Dolfin T, Litmanovitz I, Shainkin-Kestenbaum R, Lis M, Eliakim A. Evidence for exercise-induced bone formation in premature infants. *Int J Sprots Med* 2002;23:1-4.

117. Litmanovtz I, Fridland O, Dolfin T, Arnon S, Regev R, Shainkin-Kestenbaum R, Lis M, Eliakim A. Early physical activity intervention prevents decrease of bone strength in very low birth weight premature infants. *Pediatrics* 2002; in press.

118. Halliday HL, Ehrenkranz RA. Early postnatal (<96 hours) corticosteroids for preventing chronic lung disease in preterm infants. (Cochrane Review). In: *The Cochrane Library*, Issue 1, 2001. Oxford: UpdateSoftware.

119. Halliday HL, Ehrenkranz RA. Delayed (>3 weeks) postnatal corticosteroids for chronic lung disease in preterm infants. (Cochrane Review). In: *The Cochrane Library*, Issue 2, 2001. Oxford: Update Software.

120. Ward WE, Atkinson SA , Donovan S, Paes B. Bone metabolism and circulating IGF-1 and IGFBPs in dexamethasone-treated preterm infants. *Early Human Develop* 1999;56:127-141.

121. Van Goudoever JB, Wattimena JDL, Camlelli PV, et al. Effect of dexamethasone on protein metabolism in infants with bronchopulmonary dysplasia. *J Pediatr* 1994;124:112.

122. Atkinson SA, Shah J, McGee C, Steele BT. Mineral excretion and bone mineral density in premature infants receiving various diuretic therapies. *J Pediatr* 1988;113:540-545.

123. Jacinto JS, Modanlou HD, Crade M, et al. Renal calcification incidence in very low birth weight infants. *Pediatrics* 1988;82:31-35.

124. Glasier CM, Stoddard RA, Ackerman NB Jr, et al. Nephrolithiasis in infants: Association with chronic furosemide therapy. *AJR* 1983;140:107-108.

125. Gilsanz V, Fernal W, Reid BS, et al. Nephrolithiasis in premature infants. *Radiology* 1985;154:107-110.

126. Venkataraman PS, Brissie EO, Tsang RC. Stability of calcium and phosphorus in neonatal parenteral nutrition solutions. *J Pediatr Gastroenterol Nutr* 1983;2:640-643.

127. Greer FR, McCormick A. Bone growth with low bone mineral content in very low birth weight premature infants. *Pediatr Res* 1986;20:925-928.

128. Atkinson SA. Special nutritional needs of infants for prevention of and recovery from bronchopulmonary dysplasia. *J Nutr* 2001;131:9428-9465.

129. Koo WWK, Krug-Wispe SK, Succop P, Bendon R, Kaplan LA. Sequential serum aluminum and urine aluminum:creatinine ratio and tissue aluminum loading in infants with fractures and rickets. *Pediatrics* 1992a;89:877-881.

130. Koo WWK, Sherman R, Succop P et al. Sequential bone mineral content in very low birth weight infants with and without fractures and rickets. *J Bone Miner Res* 1988;3:193-197.

131. Ezzeden F, Adelman RD, Ahlfors CE. Renal calcification in preterm infants: pathophysiology and long-term sequelae. *J Pediatr* 1988;113:532-539.

132. Cleghorn GJ, Tudehope DI. Neonatal intestinal obstruction associated with oral calcium supplementation. *Aust Paediatr J* 1981;17:298-299.

133. Koletzko B, Tangermann R, von Kries R, et al. Intestinal milk-bolus obstruction in formula-fed premature infants given high doses of calcium. *J Pediatr Gastroenterol Nutr* 1988;7:548-553.

134. Barltrop D, Oppe TE. Dietary factors in neonatal calcium homeostasis. *Lancet* 1970;2:1333-1335.

135. Markestad T, Hesse V, Siebenhuner M, Jahreis G, Aksnes L, Plenert W, Aarskog D. Intermittent high-dose Vitamin D prophylaxis during infancy: effect on Vitamin D metabolites, calcium and phosphorus. *Am J Clin Nutr* 1987;46:652-658.

136. Nako Y, Fukushima N, Tomomasa T, Nagshima K, Kuroume T. Hypervitaminosis D after prolonged feeding with a premature formula. *Pediatrics* 1993;92:862-864.

137. Abrams SA, Yergey AL, Schanler RJ, Vieira NE, Welch TR. Hypercalciuria in premature infants receiving high mineral-containing diets. *J Pediatr Gastroenterol Nutr* 1994;18:20-24.

138. Mihatsch, WA, Muche R, et al. The renal phosphate threshold decreases with increasing postmenstrual age in very low birth weight infants. *Pediatr Res* 1996;40:300-303.

139. Akesson K. Biochemical markers of bone turnover. *Acta Orthop Scand* 1995;66:376-386.

140. Bhandari V, Fall P, Raisz L, Rowe J. Potential biochemical growth markers in premature infants. *Am J Perinatol* 1999;14:389-395.

141. Beyers N, Alheit B, Taljaard J, Hall J, Hough S. High turnover osteopenia in preterm babies. *Bone* 1994;15:5-13.

142. Shiff Y. Eliakim A, Shainkin-Kestenbaum R, Arnon S, et al. Measurements of bone turnover markers in premature infants. *J Pediatr Endocrinol Metab* 2001;14:389-95.

143. Pittard WB III, Geddes KM, Hulsey TC, Hollis BW. Osteocalcin, skeletal alkaline phosphatase and bone mineral content in very low birth weight infants: a longitudinal perspective. *Pediatr Res* 1992;31: 181-185.

144. Faerk B, Sadres E, Constantini N, Eliakim A, Zigel L, Foldes AJ. Quantitative ultrasound (QUS) of the Tibia: A sensitive tool for the detection of bone changes in growing boys. *J Pediatr Endocrinol Metab* 2000;13:1129-1135.

145. Crofton PM, Shrivastava A, Wade JC, Kelnar SR, Lyon AJ, McIntosh N. Bone and collagen markers in preterm infants: relationship with growth and bone mineral content over the first 10 weeks of life. *Pediatr Res* 1999;46:581-587.

146. Ryan SW, Truscott J, Simpson M, James J. Phosphate, alkaline phosphatase and bone mineralization in preterm neonates. *Acta Paediatr* 1993;82:518-521.

147. Glass EJ, Hume R, Hendry GMA, Strange RC, Forfar JO. Plasma alkaline phosphatase activity in

rickets of prematurity. *Arch Dis Child* 1982;57: 373-376.

148. Zeghoud F, Vervel C, Guillozo H, Walrant-Debray O, Boutignon H, Garabedian M. Sub-clinical Vitamin D deficiency in neonates: definition and response to Vitamin D supplements. *Am J Clin Nutr* 1997;65:771-778.

149. Lucas A, Brooke Ogm Baker BA, Bishop N, Morley R. High alkaline phosphatase activity and growth in preterm neonates. *Arch Dis Child* 1989;64:902-909.

150. James JA, Mayne PD, Barnes IC, Kovar IZ. Growth velocity and plasma alkaline phosphatase activity in the preterm infant. *Early Hum Dev* 1985;11:27-32.

151. Brunton JA, Weiler HA, Atkinson SA. Improvement in the accuracy of dual energy X-ray absorptiometry for whole body and regional analysis of body composition. Validation using piglets and methodological considerations in infants. *Pediatr Res* 1997a;41:1-7.

152. Koo WWK, Walters JC, Hockman EM. Body composition in human infants at birth and postnatally. *J Nutr* 2000a;130:2188-2194.

153. Koo WWK, Walters J, Bush AJ. Technical considerations of dual-energy x-ray absorptiometry-based bone mineral measurements for pediatric studies. *J Bone Miner Res* 1995a;10:1998-2004.

154. Barkmann R, Kantorovich E, Singal C, Hans D, Genant HK, Heller M, Gluer CC. A new method for quantitative ultrasound measurements at multiple skeletal sites. *J Clin Densitomm* 2000;3:1-7.

155. Prins SH, Jorgensen HL, Jorgensen LV, Hassager C. The role of quantitative ultrasound in the assessment of bone: a review. *Clin Physiol* 1998;18:3-17.

156. Falk B, Sadres E, Constantini N, Eliakim A, Zigel L, Foldes AJ. Quantitative ultrasound (QUS) of the Tibia: A sensitive tool for the detection of bone changes in growing boys. *J Pediatr Endocrinol Metab* 2000;13:1129-1135.

157. Foldes AJ, Rimon A, Keinan DD, Popovitzer MM. Quantitative ultrasound of the tibia: A novel approach for assessment of bone status. *Bone* 1995;17:363-377.

158. Jaworski M, Lebiedowski M, Lorenc RS, Trempe J. Ultrasound bone measurements in pediatric subjects.

Calcif Tissue Int 1995;56:368-371.

159. Wright LL, Glade MJ, Gopal J. The use of transmission ultrasonics to assess bone status in the human newborn. *Pediatr Res* 1987;22:541-544.

160. Nemet D, Dolfin T, Wolach B, Eliakim A. Quantitative ultrasound measurements of bone speed of sound in premature infants. *Eur J Pediatr* 2001;160:736-730.

161. American Academy of Pediatrics. Committee on Nutrition (1985a). Nutritional needs of low birth weight infants. *Pediatrics* 1985;75:976-983.

162. Holick MF. Vitamin D: Photobiology, metabolism, mechanism of action, and clinical applications. In: Favus, MJ ed. *Primer on the Metabolic Bone Diseases and Disorders of Mineral Metabolism.* Fourth Edition. 1999; Chapter 15, 92-98.

Microminerals
Raghavendra Rao, M.D. and Michael Georgieff, M.D.

Reviewed by Stanley Zlotkin, M.D., Ph.D., and James Friel, Ph.D.
Acknowledgement: Richard Ehrenkranz, M.D., RM Reifen, M.D.,
and Stan Zlotkin, M.D., Ph.D. from previous edition

Nine trace elements (or trace minerals) are nutritionally essential for the human: iron, zinc, copper, selenium, molybdenum, chromium, manganese, and iodine. This chapter reviews the major metabolic functions of these minerals, comments on the currently recommended intakes of these minerals, and gives specific recommendations, where appropriate, on the need for supplementation in the very low birth weight (VLBW) preterm infant and other survivors of preterm birth.

Although quantitatively, the trace elements make up a small fraction of the total mineral content of the human body, they play an important role in numerous metabolic pathways. Clinical deficiencies have been described for six of the elements. The infant born prematurely is at increased risk of developing trace mineral deficiencies. Premature birth is associated with low stores at birth, because accretion of trace minerals takes place during the last trimester of pregnancy. Rapid postnatal growth, unknown requirements, and variable intake of trace minerals also put the preterm infant at risk for deficiencies.

The content of trace minerals in human milk is the accepted "gold standard" for the full-term infant, provided that an adequate volume of milk is ingested. For the infant born prematurely, there is no gold standard for trace mineral intakes. There are, however, three acceptable objectives for trace mineral intakes: (1) intake of an amount that will prevent trace mineral deficiencies; (2) intake of an amount that will allow for accretion of stores that would have been deposited in the developing fetus had the infant stayed in the womb until term; and (3) avoidance of toxicity from excess intakes.

Key Message: The exact requirements for premature infants of most of the microminerals remain poorly defined because of a paucity of randomized controlled trials that assess efficacy and safety. Recent studies have better delineated the range of suggested micromineral delivery to this population.

Iron

Iron is a paradoxical nutrient. On the one hand, it is a critical component of many basic biological mechanisms including DNA replication, cellular energetics, and oxygen delivery.[1] Iron deficiency during development adversely affects erythropoiesis, neurodevelopment, cardiac and skeletal muscle function, and gastrointestinal function.[2-5] Conversely, iron is one of the most toxic elements to humans. In its free (non-protein bound) state, iron reacts with oxygen to create reactive oxidant species that disrupt cell membranes and result in cell death.[6-8] Iron overload syndromes cause brain dysfunction and hepatic and cardiac failure. Free iron has been implicated in the pathophysiology of reperfusion injuries in the brain, intestine, and heart following hypoxic-ischemic insults.[8] Because preterm infants have limited iron binding capacity, iron delivery to the body and trafficking within the body must be tightly regulated.[9-12] The therapeutic:toxic ratio for this element is more narrow than for most nutrients as the human does not tolerate iron overload or iron underload states for long periods.

The preterm infant requires iron for erythropoiesis, brain development, muscle function, and cardiac function. In order to determine the iron needs of the preterm infant, one must take into consideration the iron endowment of the preterm infant at birth (maternal-fetal transport), the distribution of iron in the newborn infant, the projected rate of utilization based on the infant's growth and expansion of the red cell volume, and the potential sources of iron loss from the infant, such as through phlebotomy. Each of these aspects of iron metabolism has been assessed in preterm infants. Clinical trials of iron supplementation of preterm infants have estimated the iron requirements of the infants and then assessed the impact of various levels of supplementation on mostly hematologic outcome parameters. The following sections review: the biochemical basis for the essentiality of iron; general principles of iron trafficking and prioritization among and within organs; the iron status of the newborn preterm infant; the effect of postnatal stressors on iron status; and ultimately, the range of intake expected to keep the preterm infant iron sufficient.

The Biochemical Basis for Iron

Every dividing cell needs iron both for replication and for cellular energetics. Iron is an integral component of ribonucleotide reductase, an enzyme critical for initiating DNA replication. Iron is also found in cytochromes that promote electron transfer during oxidative phosphorylation and the creation of ATP in the mitochondria. Iron deficiency results in decreased cell number and reductions in cellular metabolism and energy production.[2,3] Iron also serves a vital role in its porphyrin form as a component of hemoglobin and myoglobin and thus in tissue oxygen delivery. Iron deficiency results in a microcytic, hypochromic anemia characterized clinically by lethargy and lassitude, presumably on the basis of reduced tissue oxygenation.[1,13,14] Severe anemia has been associated with poorer growth rates in the preterm infant. In skeletal and cardiac muscle, iron deficiency reduces muscle contractility most likely through the combined negative effects on oxygen delivery (myoglobin) and cellular energetics (cytochromes).[2,3] Muscle oxygen delivery is dependent in part on the tissue concentration of myoglobin, the iron-containing protein of the porphyrin family. As

with the related compound hemoglobin, myoglobin synthesis is impaired by the lack of iron substrate. The lower muscle myoglobin concentration impairs oxygen delivery much in the same way that low hemoglobin concentrations do. Iron deficiency can similarly decrease tissue concentrations of cytochromes, which are another set of iron-containing hemoproteins. The resultant physiologic effect is impaired electron transport and ATP synthesis. Heart failure and fatigue are the accompanying clinical symptoms. Iron is also important in brain development, since it is an integral component of enzymes that affect brain growth (ribonucleotide reductase), myelination (delta-9 desaturase), energetics (cytochrome c oxidase), and dopamine metabolism (tyrosine hydroxylase). Iron deficiency in young infants and animal models results in both motor and cognitive developmental delays that are only partially reversible by iron repletion through supplementation.[15-18]

One of the intriguing aspects of iron metabolism is the ability of the body to prioritize available iron. A predictable pattern of prioritization occurs among organs and also within organs when iron supply does not meet iron demand in the fetus, neonate, or older infant. Among organ systems, typically hepatic iron stores are lost first, followed by lower priority tissues such as skeletal muscle and the intestine. With greater stress on the system, cardiac iron is compromised, followed by brain iron and finally red cell iron. Thus, in the developing human, rat and sheep, iron is prioritized to the red cells, even apparently at the expense of the heart and brain.[1,19] The liver iron stores, mostly in the form of ferritin, represent a buffer to protect vital organs from iron shortage. There is no known physiologic consequence of loss of storage iron other than a higher risk for subsequent iron deficiency. Once liver iron stores are depleted, the non-heme, non-storage tissues are at risk for iron deficiency and attendant dysfunction. The classic symptoms of iron deficiency are due primarily to loss of tissue-based iron and not simply the anemia.[1]

Intraorgan prioritization also occurs. In the perinatal rat brain, iron-dependent cytochrome oxidase activity is compromised to a greater extent in the hippocampus, a region that subserves recognition memory processing, than in the striatum, an area involved in procedural memory.[20] Similarly, myoglobin production is spared at the expense of cytochrome concentrations in the iron-deficient perinatal sheep heart.[19] The mechanisms of inter- and intra-organ prioritization are not currently known.

In summary, there is a clear biochemical need for iron throughout the body for normal growth and development in the perinatal and neonatal period. The symptoms of iron deficiency are due to tissue-level losses of iron containing enzymes and iron-sulfur proteins, not just to anemia. The body prioritizes iron to the red cells at the expense of non-heme tissues during periods of negative iron balance. Thus, screening for iron deficiency by assessing red cell indices appears to be a late indicator of tissue-level iron deficiency, making prevention a far better option than treatment.

Iron Status at Birth

The infant born any time during the third trimester or at term has a relatively constant total body iron content of approximately 75 mg/kg body weight.[9,21-24] This iron is distributed as 55 to 60 mg/kg in red cells, mostly as hemoglobin, 10 to 12 mg/kg in liver, mostly as ferritin, and 8 mg/kg as non-heme tissue enzymes, such as myoglobin and cytochromes.[24,25] The fetal rate of accretion during the third trimester is between 1.6 and 2.0 mg/kg/day and is regulated primarily by fetal need rather than maternal supply.[21-26] Nevertheless, severe maternal iron deficiency (maternal hemoglobin concentration <85 g/L) will compromise fetal and thus neonatal iron status.[27,28] Although severe maternal iron deficiency is relatively rare in the developed world, 30% to 50% of pregnancies in certain developing countries are complicated by this condition. Other gestational conditions that negatively affect newborn iron status include placental insufficiency with fetal growth restriction, maternal gestational or insulin-dependent diabetes mellitus, and fetal blood loss through fetal-maternal or twin-twin hemorrhage.[24,30-32] Iron overload can occur secondary to twin-twin transfusion or, more significantly, to

congenital hemochromatosis. In the latter condition, infants present with symptoms of hepatic and cardiac failure due to iron overload. The condition is often fatal and is not due to the same mutation of the HFE gene that is responsible for hereditary hemochromatosis.

Iron status at birth can also be affected by perinatal events. Early clamping of the umbilical cord, placenta previa or abruptio, and umbilical cord accidents can decrease the total body iron load; while late cord clamping, especially with the infant held below the level of the placenta, and stripping of the umbilical cord before clamping, can increase the iron endowment. The infant's hemoglobin concentration (once equilibrated after birth) and the cord serum ferritin concentration combine to give the best estimate of total body iron status. Normal hemoglobin concentrations at birth are a function of gestational age but generally range from 145 to 180 g/L.[24] The fifth percentile for cord serum ferritin concentration is between 55 and 60 µg/L at birth.[33,34]

In summary, the preterm and term newborn have similar iron loads on a per kilogram body weight basis. The 24-week-gestational-age infant weighing 500 grams only has an endowment of 37.5 mg, while a term 3-kg infant has closer to 225 mg. Thus, the most premature infant has less than 20% of the iron that will be needed by 40 weeks post-conceptional age, assuming extrauterine growth at the intrauterine rate.

Determining Postnatal Iron Requirements

The largest iron need for the preterm infant is for erythropoiesis (see below). The neonatal blood volume expands proportionally with growth. Since the rate of catch-up growth can be very high, the attendant increase in blood volume and hemoglobin requires relatively high rates of iron delivery. For each gram of hemoglobin synthesized, 3.47 mg of elemental iron are required. Preterm infants increase their total body iron content by approximately fivefold to achieve similar hematopoietic and iron status as their term counterparts during infancy.[35-37] In addition to having a higher baseline iron requirement for normal physiologic processes, the preterm infant also encounters stressors that promote negative iron balance that the typical term infant does not. Sick preterm infants face large phlebotomy losses, occasionally require exchange transfusions, and are treated with recombinant human erythropoietin, which, unlike blood transfusions, taps rather than restores total body iron.[38-40] In summary, the infant's birth weight, initial hemoglobin and ferritin concentration, rate of growth, and balance between blood withdrawn by phlebotomy and blood replaced by red cell transfusion will determine the postnatal iron requirements.

Oski has estimated that, in the absence of iron supplementation and blood loss, the VLBW preterm infant has enough iron stores to last two months, half as long as a term infant.[41] The average iron needs during the first year can be estimated based on the initial birth weight and subsequent growth rate. For example, an infant having a birth weight of 1 kg and an initial hemoglobin concentration of 17 g/dL will require about 280 mg of additional iron to become a 10-kg, 1-year-old with a hemoglobin concentration of 11 g/dL (assuming a blood volume of 75 ml/kg, 3.47 mg of iron/g of hemoglobin, and iron tissue needs of about 7 mg/kg).[41] This would require an iron accretion of 0.83 mg/day. Oski's estimates were published in 1985 when it was rarer for <1 kg birth weight infants to survive. The survival rates for infants between 500 and 1000 grams have risen steadily since the mid-1980s. Thus, it should be recognized that these extremely low birth weight infants have even lower total body iron loads, although their iron content per kilogram body weight is similar at 75 mg/kg.[21] The smaller the infant is at birth, the greater the amount of catch up, and the higher the dose of iron that is necessary.

Iron is not fully absorbed by the intestine at any age. Ehrenkranz et al used stable isotope techniques to demonstrate a 30% to 40% rate of iron uptake from the preterm infant intestine.[42] Their data confirmed more simple non-isotopic balance studies performed previously by Shaw, Dauncey et al, and Salvioli et al.[43-45] Using an absorption rate of 40%, the daily enteral iron need in the non-phlebotomized 1-kg, preterm infant is 2 mg/kg/day. This figure becomes substantially higher when adjusted for non-compensated phlebotomy losses and the number of days when the infant does not receive iron because of feeding intolerance or illness.

The Role of Postnatal Erythropoiesis in Determining Iron Requirements

Postnatal erythropoiesis has been divided into three stages.[22,41,46] In the first stage, which begins immediately after birth and lasts during the first 6 to 8 weeks of life in a term infant, there is an abrupt decrease in erythropoiesis. This decrease reflects the increased postnatal delivery of oxygen to tissues and is manifested by a decrease in marrow erythroid precursors, a fall in the reticulocyte count, and a fall in the hemoglobin concentration. The rate of decline in hemoglobin concentration is largely related to the shorter life span of fetal RBCs, about two-thirds that of normal adult RBC. Because erythropoiesis is depressed, reticuloendothelial iron stores become augmented and serum ferritin concentrations increase. This "physiological anemia" apparently cannot be prevented in the term infant by the provision of iron; rather, it appears that the term infant stores the excess iron or excretes it in the stool. The preterm infant exhibits a similar early anemia, but the hemoglobin concentration at the nadir is 2 to 3 g/dL lower than in the term infant for, as yet, undetermined reasons.[22,41,46] Supplementation of preterm infants with iron may reduce the degree of anemia. For example, the magnitude of the erythropoietic response in the preterm infant to recombinant human erythropoietin (rh-Epo) administration is directly related to the amount of iron provided, suggesting that iron primes the response.[47,48] This priming response does however appear to have an upper limit. For example, an enteral iron dose of 16 mg/kg/day does not result in a more efficacious erythropoietic response than a dose of 8/mkg/day.[49] The finding that the erythropoietic response of therapeutic rh-Epo is primed by iron suggests that iron supplementation might be expected to prevent or diminish the degree of anemia in preterm infants.

An equally interesting and unknown issue

revolves around whether "anemia of prematurity" is a physiologic or pathologic condition. The latter is supported by the findings that the anemia is more profound in preterm infants who have lower iron stores and is modified by rh-Epo and iron therapy. Of greater importance is whether non-heme, non-storage tissues such as the brain are compromised during this anemia by either the degree of anemia or a component of iron deficiency. No studies have assessed this issue in the human to date.

The second stage in term infants occurs between postnatal months 2 and 4 and is characterized by active erythropoiesis in response to mild tissue hypoxia associated with the preexisting physiologic anemia from stage one. Blood erythropoietin, erythroid precursors in the marrow, and reticulocyte count all increase.[22,41,46] Although the total body hemoglobin increases (and thus requires a proportionate amount of iron delivery), the concentration of hemoglobin in the blood may not rise substantially because of dilution of the red cell mass by the expanded plasma volume that results with increased body weight. During this period of active erythropoiesis, iron demands are increased; the sources of iron include liberation of ferrous iron from ferritin and increased iron absorption from the intestine. Serum transferrin receptor concentrations increase and ferritin concentrations decrease.[13,38,50-52] This second stage begins proportionately earlier in preterm infants since they reach their "physiologic nadir" by 6 to 8 weeks of age.[22,41,46] Extremely premature infants will still be in the hospital at this point. Their iron requirements to support stage two erythropoiesis are likely higher (on a per kilogram body weight basis) than term infants because their absolute total body iron content is lower, their rate of postnatal weight is greater, and they likely have experienced non-compensated phlebotomy.

The third stage of postnatal erythropoiesis begins after the fourth month of life in term infants and is characterized by its dependence on dietary iron.[22,41,46] Infants who receive sufficient dietary iron to maintain body iron stores are able to support the increased erythropoiesis started in the second stage and will maintain a relatively constant hemoglobin concentration

during the remainder of the first year. However, if the decreased iron stores are not replenished by provision and absorption of sufficient dietary iron, that increased erythropoiesis will not be maintained and iron-deficiency anemia will develop. The third stage of erythropoiesis is even more dependent on dietary iron in the preterm infant and begins at an earlier post-conceptional age. Essentially, this dietary iron-dependent stage begins when the infant can no longer rely on the iron stores accreted in utero. The dose of dietary iron required to sustain adequate erythropoiesis will be directly related to the rate of growth, which is greater in the preterm infant, and inversely related to the fetal iron stores, which are lower in the preterm infant. In summary, the preterm infant will require higher iron dosing to maintain effective erythropoiesis and prevent iron-deficiency anemia in the first postnatal year when compared to a term infant.

Key Message: The need for erythropoiesis drives iron needs to a large extent in the premature infant. Ineffective erythropoiesis will occur if the there is not a readily available source of iron.

Mechanisms of Iron Absorption in Preterm Infants

Great strides have been made in our understanding of intestinal iron absorption in the past five years with the discovery of two new iron transporters, divalent metal transporter-1 (DMT-1) and ferroportin-1 (FPN-1).[53-55] Their discovery helped determine the primary form (ferrous) in which iron is absorbed and excreted by the duodenal epithelial cell, and helped clarify why no transferrin receptors are found on the apical surface of these cells. Prior to their discovery, the only known iron transport receptor was the transferrin receptor found in abundance on red cells, neurons, and hepatocytes. This receptor binds diferric transferrin and the cell endocytoses the entire complex, after which the elemental iron is released by an unknown mechanism for utilization by the cell. The lack of transferrin receptors on the apical surface of the intestinal absorptive cell implies that iron is not absorbed from the gut bound to transferrin, and thus another transporter is involved. The cloning of DMT-1, also known as Nramp2 and DCT-1, in 1997 resulted in the identification of copious amounts of this ferrous iron transporter in the duodenal epithelium.[53,55] This transporter has affinity for all divalent cations including zinc, copper and lead, but the affinity is highest for iron. Like transferrin receptor, DMT-1 expression increases with iron deficiency as the body attempts to upregulate iron transport to correct the deficiency. It remains unclear whether this membrane protein endocytoses with iron or remains membrane bound and simply shuttles iron from the lumen. This transporter relies on conversion of dietary ferric iron to its ferrous state by ascorbic acid or by a ferroreductase located on the brush border membrane. Thus, it has been postulated that a suboptimal Vitamin C status, as is seen in the first two weeks after preterm birth, may hinder iron absorption.[56] Ferrous iron is not the only form of iron found in the intestine; iron can be absorbed as dietary ferritin or as hemoproteins. The latter, found in meats, are thought to be absorbed intact and are particularly bioavailable. Yet, the transporters for ferritin and hemoprotein-derived iron remain unknown.

The fate of ferrous iron after absorption across the brush border membrane remains unclear. Ultimately, it is transported across the basolateral membrane to the serum, but only recently have the transporters that are involved been elucidated. The leading candidate for basolateral transport is ferroportin, also known as MTP-1 or IREG-1.[53] All studies investigating these transporters have been performed in the adult animal model so that the developmental expression remains unknown. Thus, whether the preterm infant has a fully regulated intestinal iron absorptive system remains hotly debated but unknown. Isotope and balance studies in response to varying iron status have yielded mixed results.[42,57-60] The issue of unregulated iron absorption is not a trivial one, since lack of regulation would imply that the preterm infant would be "at the mercy" of dietary iron status. The infant could potentially become iron overloaded when presented with an enteral iron dose if unable to down-regulate iron transporters. Conversely, the inability to up-regulate

iron transporters during low dietary iron delivery would place the infant at higher risk for iron deficiency.

Absorption and Bioavailability of Iron in Preterm Infants

Neonatal iron absorption rates and the preterm neonate's response to iron treatment have been extensively studied.[36,39,42-45,57,61-64]

Iron is primarily absorbed in the duodenum. The intestinal iron absorption rate of preterm infants ranges from as low as 0.3% to as high as 74%, depending on the iron status of the infant, the form of iron given, and the age of the preterm infant.[61-64] Stable isotope studies have measured the rate at between 34% and 42%, standing in stark contrast to the 7% to 12% rate registered in term infants.[42,57,58] Using simple non-isotopic balance studies, Shaw, Dauncey et al and Salvioli et al confirmed the need for supplemental iron to avoid negative iron balance and continued accretion at intrauterine rates.[43-45] Factors that enhance absorption in preterm infants include postnatal age, relative iron deficiency, dosing between meals, human milk feedings, and normal Vitamin C status.[58,62,63,65,66] Factors that suppress intestinal iron absorption include formula feeding and recent erythrocyte transfusions.[44] Interestingly, gestational age, postconceptional age, and rh-Epo therapy have been shown to have only a minimal effect on iron absorption.[58,62]

Unlike adults, where 90% of enterally absorbed iron is incorporated into red cell hemoglobin, preterm infants incorporate only 4.7% to 12%.[58,67] The rest is presumably taken up by liver iron stores as ferritin since it is not immediately excreted in the stool, but definitive proof of the fate of this absorbed iron is lacking. Widness et al reported a second late phase (after 3 weeks) of isotope appearance in red cells, suggesting that the initial dose had been sequestered elsewhere.[58]

Response to Iron Treatment

Preterm infants with birth weights between 1000 and 2000 grams receiving human milk or low-iron formulas deplete their iron stores by 3 months of age and become anemic before liver stores are completely depleted.[36] Simple dose response studies and balance studies have generated a range of iron doses between 2 and 5 mg/kg/day to maintain normal iron status, defined as prevention of iron deficiency (low ferritin concentration) or matching of intrauterine accretion rates. Most of these studies suffer from low power and having been performed in healthy preterm infants in the non-modern era. Nevertheless, they established a baseline expectation that a dose of 1 mg/kg/day of iron as given to term infants is insufficient to maintain iron status in the preterm infant, resulting in an iron deficiency anemia rate of 37% at one year of age.[45,60,68-71] Anemia could be prevented with an additional supplement of 2 mg/kg/day for the first five months of life. Lundstrom et al demonstrated that 2 mg/kg/day of ferrous sulfate prevented iron deficiency at six months of age.[36] Dauncey et al found that an intake of 5 to 6 mg/kg/day resulted in iron accretion rates similar to intrauterine rates.[44]

A meta-analysis of studies published prior to 1992 demonstrated that iron supplementation reduces the incidence of iron deficiency in premature infants.[72] The two studies most relevant to current neonatal management are randomized, double-blind trials in premature infants by Hall et al[61] and by Friel et al.[73] In the former, three groups of infants less than 1800-grams birth weight were studied. They received either 3 or 15 mg/L of iron in preterm formula, or fortified breastmilk supplemented to an iron content of 1.7 mg/L.[61] Assuming a consumption of 150 cc/kg/day, the respective iron doses would prorate to 0.45 and 2.25 mg/kg/day. Hall et al found a 70% rate of anemia and a 79% rate of low ferritin concentrations at hospital discharge in the low-iron formula group compared with a 26% rate of anemia and 67% rate of low ferritin concentrations in the high-iron group. At two months after hospital discharge, the prevalence of iron deficiency remained higher, and the mean MCV was lower in the low-iron group despite receiving a standard infant formula with 12 mg/L of iron after discharge. This study was performed in the pre-rh-Epo era, but suggests that iron delivery of 2.25 mg/kg/day marginally maintains iron status in

relatively healthy preterm infants. Subsequently, Friel et al randomly assigned 58 infants near or at the time of discharge to receive an infant formula containing either 13.4 mg/L or 20.7 mg/L of iron until one year of age.[73] The mean weight at study entry was approximately 2300 grams. The effective iron doses of these formulas when fed at the standard 150cc/kg/day were 2.0 and 3.1 mg/kg/day, respectively. The group fed the higher iron content formula had a trend toward higher hemoglobin concentrations at 3 months of age (123 versus 118 g/L; p=0.07), but this trend completely disappeared by 6-months. No infants in either group had iron-deficiency anemia, and the rate of iron-deficiency without anemia was low and comparable in both groups. The infants receiving the higher dose of iron had a trend toward lower zinc and copper levels suggesting some competition among these divalent cations in the intestine. Although there was little evidence for increased oxidant stress in the higher iron group, there were more respiratory infections in the first year in the higher iron group. No developmental advantage was conferred by the higher iron dose. Overall, this study supports the notion that iron doses between 2 and 3 mg/kg/day in the post-discharge period maintain relative iron sufficiency in relatively large preterm infants (birth weights averaging 1400 grams).

The effect of rh-Epo treatment on iron requirements must be considered. The effectiveness of rh-Epo treatment depends on available iron. Since the intent of this treatment is to reduce the number of transfusions (and hence the exogenous iron load), the preterm infant will be dependent on endogenous iron stores to support the erythropoietic response.[38,58] Serum ferritin concentrations decline rapidly by 14 days after initiation of rh-Epo and occurs in spite of intravenous iron supplementation of up to 3 mg/kg/day.[47,74] Based on data from the national collaborative trial on rh-Epo administration, the American Academy of Pediatrics (AAP) recommends giving 6 mg/kg/day of enteral iron to preterm infants treated with rh-Epo.[65,75] Others have supplemented these infants with 2 mg/kg/day of intravenous iron to provide immediate support for erythropoiesis, and

	Preterm Human Milk*	Preterm Infant Formula at 81 Kcal/100cc**	Preterm Post-Discharge Formula at 74 Kcal/100cc**
Iron			
Concentration (mg/L)	0.3	14.52	13.48
Delivery (mg/kg/day)‡	0.045	2.20	2.02
Typical Percent Absorption	50%	33%	12%
Projected Retention (mg/kd/day)	0.023	0.73	0.24
Intrauterine Accretion Rate (mg/kg/day)†	1.8	1.8	--
Zinc			
Concentration (mg/L)‡	2.2	12.1	9.18
Delivery (mg/kg/day)‡	0.33	1.82	1.38
Typical Percent Absorption	60%	30%	30%
Projected Retention (mg/kd/day)	0.20	0.55	0.41
Intrauterine Accretion Rate (mg/kg/day)†	0.85	0.85	--
Copper			
Concentration (mcg/L)	508	1512 (1008-2016)	899
Delivery (mcg/kg/day)‡	76	227 (151-300)	135
Typical Percent Absorption	60%	15%	15%
Projected Retention (mcg/kd/day)	46	34 (23-45)	20
Intrauterine Accretion Rate (mcg/kg/day)†	50	50	--
Selenium			
Concentration (mcg/L)	17.4	14.5	17.2
Delivery (mcg/kg/day)‡	2.6	2.2	2.6
Typical Percent Absorption	80%	80%	80%
Projected Retention (mcg/kd/day)	2.1	1.8	2.1
Intrauterine Accretion Rate (mcg/kg/day)†	1	1	--
Chromium			
Concentration (mcg/L)	0.3	15	15
Delivery (mcg/kg/day)‡	0.05	2.25	2.25
Typical Percent Absorption	n/a	n/a	n/a
Projected Retention (mcg/kd/day)	n/a	n/a	n/a
Intrauterine Accretion Rate (mcg/kg/day)†	n/a	n/a	--
Molybdenum			
Concentration (mcg/L)	2.0	133	n/a
Delivery (mcg/kg/day)‡	0.3	20	n/a
Typical Percent Absorption	>80%	>80%	n/a
Projected Retention (mcg/kd/day)	0.24	16	n/a
Intrauterine Accretion Rate (mcg/kg/day)†	1	1	--
Manganese			
Concentration (mcg/L)	7.5	74 (51-97)	94 (75-113)
Delivery (mcg/kg/day)‡	1.1	11.1 (7.7-14.6)	14.1
Typical Percent Absorption	8%	2%	2%
Projected Retention (mcg/kd/day)†	0.09	0.22 (0.15-0.29)	0.28
Intrauterine Accretion Rate (mcg/kg/day)†	9	9	--
Iodine			
Concentration (mcg/L)	160§,Δ	125 (48-202)	112
Delivery (mcg/kg/day)‡	24	18.8 (7.2-30.3)	16.8
Typical Percent Absorption	50%§	50%§	50%§
Projected Retention (mcg/kd/day)	12	9.4 (3.6-15.2)	8.4
Intrauterine Accretion Rate (mcg/kg/day)†	1	1	--

* Values for iron, zinc, copper, selenium, chromium, and manganese are based on published average values of mature preterm mother's milk at 21-30 days lactation.[84-86]
 The values for the remaining micronutrients are based on data from term human milk.
** Formula contents are averages of available products and thus do not represent any single product. Where a discrepancy of >50% in a nutrient content between two products exists, the mean and range are given.

‡ Delivery is based on average daily intake of 150 cc/kg body weight

† Average third trimester rate of fetal nutrient accretion

§ Term data (preterm value unknown)

Δ Value from lactating women in United States

n/a- figures not available or unknown

Table 1: Micronutrient content of enteral foods fed to premature infants.

9 mg/kg/day of oral iron to meet phlebotomy losses and support iron requirements for growth.[74] A recent trial, however, demonstrated that doubling the enteral iron supplementation from 8 mg/kg/day to 16 mg/kg/day did not further enhance erythropoeisis or preserve iron stores.[49]

An additional issue raised by the latter study is the optimal time and route of iron administration to preterm infants. The main considerations are safety and efficacy. For example, Lundstrom et al addressed the issue of efficacy in 1977 and demonstrated that initiating oral iron therapy at a dose of 2 mg/kg/day was more effective in preventing later anemia than waiting to initiate therapy after 2 months of age.[36] Franz et al performed a prospective randomized trial of early versus late enteral iron supplementation in VLBW infants who were on conservative transfusion protocols and did not receive rh-Epo.[76] The infants were randomized to early treatment of either 2 or 6 mg/kg/day of iron starting on a median of 15 days of age, or late iron treatment starting on median day 32. Overall, the early treated group had a lower incidence of iron deficiency and had received fewer red blood cell transfusions by 61 days of age. No increase in putative oxidative diseases (eg, BPD, necrotizing enterocolitis) was seen in the early treatment or the high dose treatment groups. Hall et al also used relatively early supplementation (ie, the time of tolerating enteral feeds) to demonstrate the effect of 2.25 mg/kg/day on the prevention of subsequent anemia but did not specifically test early versus late iron supplementation.[61] Winzerling and Kling demonstrated that 1200-gram birth weight infants with a postnatal age of 6 weeks and a mean hematocrit of 32.4% at hospital discharge have a significant component of iron-deficient erythropoiesis as documented by an elevated blood zinc protoporphyrin/heme ratio.[77] Their findings suggest that the routine "anemia of prematurity" seen in preterm infants may indeed have a component of iron-deficiency anemia. Whether the etiology of the iron-deficient erythropoiesis is nutritional (eg, low iron delivery) or functional (eg, decreased iron availability) remains to be determined and will in turn affect iron supplementation recommendations. These

studies appear to support the concept that anemia of prematurity has an iron deficiency component to it, and that early iron therapy is efficacious and low risk in modulating the course of anemia in preterm infants.

Conversely, there are safety and efficacy considerations that suggest later rather than earlier therapy is indicated. There is also concern that the Vitamin C status of the infant needs to be intact for adequate absorption to occur in the gut and for adequate quenching of free oxygen radicals.[56,78] Berger et al have suggested that this does not occur until at least 2 weeks of age.[56] Furthermore, incorporation of iron is better when administered at the time of erythropoiesis, suggesting that early iron supplementation when the infant is in phase one of postnatal erythropoiesis (see above) will be ineffective. Thus, iron supplementation appears unnecessary before 2 weeks of age and may carry a significant risk of oxidative injury. Iron supplementation between 2 and 8 weeks of age may be ineffective if the infant has no endogenous or exogenous (ie, rh-Epo) erythropoietic drive, but nevertheless appears to be safe when delivered enterally (see below). After that age, iron supplementation is necessary to ensure adequate substrate for erythropoiesis and growth.

An increasing number of preterm infants are receiving human milk for the putative intellectual, feeding tolerance, and immunologic benefits. As with term milk, preterm milk has a low iron content ranging from 0.3 to 1.1 mg/L (Table 1).[74-86] Although absorption rates may be as high as 50% to 75%, the low iron content of the milk prevents adequate iron accretion for growth and erythropoiesis, even if the absorption rate were 100%.[87] Greater than 80% of preterm infants fed unsupplemented human milk are iron deficient by 6 months of age.[87] Supplementation with 2 to 4 mg/kg/day reduces the incidence of iron deficiency and iron-deficiency anemia.[45] In response to the documented iron needs of these infants, human milk fortifiers now contain iron and will deliver between 0.5 and 2.2 mg/kg/day when mixed to create a 24 kcal/oz diet fed at 150 cc/kg/day.

Since preterm infants frequently receive the majority of their nutrition parenterally, the issue of parenteral iron dosing has arisen. Parenteral iron administration has been studied during rh-Epo administration.[64,74,88,89] A dose of 1 mg/kg/day appears to be effective in achieving positive iron balance.[64] A greater percentage of intravenous iron is incorporated into red cells, consistent with the fact that there is no need to take a rate of enteral absorption into account. Thus, a dose of 1 mg/kg/day of intravenous iron appears to be equivalent to an enteral dose of 3 mg/kg/day. The concern with intravenous iron administration is the potential for exceeding the total iron binding capacity, which is lower in the preterm infant compared with the term infant, placing the infant at risk for oxidant injury.[10-12] Indeed, malondialdehyde levels, an indicator of reactive oxidant species, are elevated following intravenous iron infusion, although it is unclear whether actual oxidant injury occurs.[74]

At this time, the risk/benefit ratio does not favor giving parenteral iron during transition for the following reasons: (1) the infant is not growing during transition thus there is little pressure to expand the iron pool (the major need for iron is to match the expanding red cell mass that in turn is dependent on the rate of somatic growth); and (2) there is an as yet unresolved issue of a potential risk of iron toxicity with IV iron. This is supported by Berger's data suggesting a major anti-oxidant system (Vitamin C) is not fully mature until about 2 weeks of age.[78] On the other hand, once iron is started during the stable growth phase, the highest parenteral dose tested that did not cause any signs of toxicity is 250 µg/kg/d, although it still left infants in negative iron balance.[64] Further studies of toxicity will need to determine whether doses between 250 µg/kg/day[64] and 2 mg/kg/day[74] are safe and whether the chemical form of parenteral iron modifies the effectiveness and toxicity.

Key Message: Most studies suggest that 2 mg/kg/day of enteral iron marginally supports erythropoiesis in the growing preterm infant.

Iron Toxicity and Nutrient Interactions

Iron is a potentially very toxic element.[8] Normally, it never circulates freely in the serum because of the risk of its ability to react with oxygen. This reaction generates oxygen species that peroxidate lipid membranes, causing cell death. Instead, it is normally bound predominantly to transferrin, a molecule that, by its three-dimensional structure, can effectively shield the iron. Iron is taken up into cells by the transferrin receptor via binding and endocytosis of transferrin.

The premature infant is theoretically at higher risk for iron-induced oxidant injury because of a lower total iron binding capacity and less mature antioxidant systems.[8,10,90,91] Researchers have been concerned that bronchopulmonary dysplasia and retinopathy of prematurity (ROP) may be caused by oxygen-derived free radicals, which in turn may be produced by iron overload. Little direct evidence implicates enteral iron intake in the pathogenesis of these two diseases. Most studies have assessed the relationship between the number of red cell transfusions and the prevalence of these diseases, and have found that infants with these diseases had more transfusions and higher serum ferritin levels. Cooke et al studied red cell storage and free-iron status, along with free-radical reacting substances, such as thiobarbituric acid reacting substances, in the first month of life in 73 preterm infants.[92] They found that infants with bronchopulmonary dysplasia (BPD) had more transfusions and higher ferritin and free-iron concentrations, but no evidence of increased 2-thiobarbituric acid reaction products (an index of oxidative products). They concluded that the higher ferritin levels were not surprising since the transfusions were essentially dosing the infants with iron, but that in absence of free radical formation, blood transfusion and the iron from it does not contribute to the risk of BPD. The obvious confounding variable is that sicker infants are likely to get more transfusions and are also more likely to be ventilated longer, increasing their risk of BPD. The two may not be pathophysiologically related.

Two similar studies have assessed the risk of transfusions, iron load and ROP. Hesse et al found a significant relationship between the amount of transfused blood and the incidence of ROP in VLBW

	Transitional Period (0-14 days)		Stable/Postdischarge Periods	
	Enteral (μg/kg/day)	Parenteral (μg/kg/day)	Enteral (μg/kg/day)	Parenteral (μg/kg/day)
Fe	0	0	2000-4000	250-670
Zn	500-800	150	1,000-2000*	400
Cu	120	0, = 20[†]	120-150	20[†]
Se	1.3	0, = 1.3	1.3-4.5	1.5-4.5
Cr	0.5	0, = 0.05	0.1-2.25	0.05-0.3
Mo	0.3	0	0.3-4.0	0.25-1.0[‡]
Mn	0.75	0, = 0.75[†]	0.75-7.5	1.0[†]
Iodine	11-27	0, = 1.0	10-60	1.0

*Postdischarge supplement of 0.5 mg/kg/day for infants fed human milk.

[†]Should be withheld when hepatic cholestasis is present.

[‡]For long-term TPN only.

Table 2: Recommended micromineral intakes for preterm infants.

infants, but could find no relationship between the infants' iron status and the disease.[93] They concluded that VLBW infants transfused with more than 15 cc/kg (one standard transfusion of packed red blood cells) are six times more likely to get ROP than those receiving less blood, but that the relationship, "was not mediated via an increased iron load." Perhaps most importantly, no study has demonstrated a relationship between enteral iron intake and so-called "oxidant stress" diseases such as BPD and ROP. This may be related to the ability of preterm infants to load iron into ferritin effectively if the iron is dosed slowly; ie, by the enteral route.[42] It should be noted, however, that there probably is a threshold level of iron intake beyond which reactive oxidant species will appear. Melhorn and Gross demonstrated that 8 to 10 mg/kg/day of enteral iron in Vitamin E deficient premature infants results in lower hemoglobin levels, which they interpreted as being due to hemolysis.[94] The threshold in Vitamin E sufficient infants remains to be determined.

Iron can compete with other divalent cations, such as zinc and copper, for binding sites on transporters. Although each divalent cation has its own set of species-specific transporters for which it has the highest affinity, competition will occur when the designated cation is in short supply. Thus, lead will bind to transferrin and be transported by transferrin receptor when iron is absent (iron deficiency). Friel et al have demonstrated that a zinc:iron ratio as high as 4:1 does not interfere with red cell iron incorporation.[95] Manipulating the zinc:iron ratio may affect either zinc or iron status of the infant. For example, the improved growth and zinc nutriture observed by Walraens and Hambidge in infants fed a zinc-fortified (5.8 mg/L), iron-fortified (12 mg/L) formula compared with the growth in infants fed a non-zinc-fortified (1.8 mg/L), iron-fortified formula has been attributed to increased zinc bioavailability due to the change in the iron:zinc ratio from 6.7:1 to 2.1:1.[96] Salvioli et al showed that a supplemental dose of iron in the 2 mg/kg/day range does not affect zinc status.[45] Yip et al and Haschke et al failed to demonstrate significant iron-zinc or iron-copper interactions with the currently recommended levels of iron supplementation or iron fortification of formulas.[97,98] Similarly, the AAP Committee on Nutrition stated that, given the levels of zinc and copper in infant formulas, iron fortification of the formulas does not impair the absorption of those minerals to a nutritionally important degree.[99] The zinc and copper contents of preterm formulas as currently constituted do not present a risk for nutrient interactions.

Key Message: No study has demonstrated oxidative toxicity from enteral iron given at conventional doses in preterm infants.

Conclusions and Recommendations

In summary, preterm infants need supplemental iron starting after 2 weeks of age. The enteral route appears safest. Iron can be supplied by preterm formula, human milk fortifier, or medicinal iron drops. The enteral dose for the preterm infant not receiving rh-EPO ranges from 2 to 4 mg/kg/day (Table 2), depending on the degree of prematurity and the amount of uncompensated phlebotomy. Recent studies using stable isotopes and randomized controlled trials of varying iron doses confirm Siimes' estimate over 20 years ago with respect to the dose range. The recent introduction of rh-Epo puts a greater stress on iron balance, forcing the infant to mobilize endogenous iron stores at a faster rate. For infants receiving this medication, an enteral dose of 6 mg/kg/day is recommended. Supplemental iron is not usually required during total parenteral nutrition unless it is the sole source of nutrition for over two months or if iron deficiency develops. However, if these conditions exist, parenteral iron, 0.1 to 0.2 mg/kg/day, can be delivered with parenteral alimentation. The optimal form for parenteral iron (iron dextran, saccharated iron) has not been determined. Studies are currently addressing the need for iron after discharge in preterm infants. Their iron needs will likely remain greater than that of term infants because of their more rapid relative rate of growth, and therefore, blood volume expansion. Recommendations regarding when to follow iron status will be forthcoming. In the meantime, given their lower endogenous iron stores, it would be prudent to screen these infants earlier (eg, two months postdischarge) than term infants.

Recommended Enteral Iron Intake (Table 2)

Transition period: 0 µg/kg/day

Stable and postdischarge periods: 2000-4000 µg/kg/day

Recommended Parenteral Iron Intake

Transitional period: 0 µg/kg/day

Stable and postdischarge periods: 250-670 µg/kg/day

Zinc

Zinc is a ubiquitous trace metal essential for subcellular metabolism and plays a catalytic, co-catalytic or synthetic role.[100] At least one zinc-containing enzyme is present in each of the six classes of enzyme systems that participate in carbohydrate and protein metabolism, nucleic acid synthesis, heme synthesis, and other vital functions.[101] Carbonic anhydrase, alkaline phosphatase, and DNA and RNA polymerase are some of the over 300 zinc-containing enzymes that have been discovered. Zinc is required for cellular division and differentiation. In addition to DNA synthesis, zinc regulates gene expression of transcription factors and nuclear hormonal receptors through its role in determining the configuration of the zinc finger motif.[100,102] Growth-stimulating hormones, such as insulin and insulin-like growth factors, need zinc for their activity.[103] Zinc is also involved in regulation of apoptosis.[104]

Zinc homeostasis is maintained over a wide range through regulation of fractional absorption and endogenous excretion in the gastrointestinal tract. Fecal excretion correlates with the amount of zinc ingested. Full-term infants and preterm infants of gestational ages 32 weeks and higher are capable of intestinal conservation of endogenous zinc at an early postnatal stage.[105,106] Urinary losses are the major route of excretion of parenteral zinc supplementation, but do not participate in homeostasis of enterally administered zinc.[107] Integumental zinc losses have not been determined in preterm infants but are unlikely to play a significant role in zinc homeostasis.

Zinc Status at Birth

Zinc is essential during embryogenesis, but the most significant fetal accretion occurs during the third trimester of pregnancy. The average daily accretion between 24 and 34 weeks is 850 µg/kg.[108] Cord blood

Factors Enhancing Fractional Absorption
Smaller dose Body zinc deficiency state Administration with human milk Amino acids: histidine, cysteine, methionine Lactose Citrate, Vitamin C
Factors Decreasing Fractional Absorption
Large dose Body zinc sufficiency state Casein in bovine milk Phytates and fibers Alkaline pH Other cations: calcium, iron, cadmium Human milk fortification Dexamethasone

Table 3: Factors affecting fractional absorption of enterally administered zinc.

plasma zinc levels[109] as well as brain, heart and kidney zinc contents are similar in full-term and preterm infants.[110] The skeletal muscle zinc content increases from 110 µg/g to 160 µg/g between 20 and 40 weeks and accounts for 40% of the total body zinc at term.[110] Hepatic metallothionein, the major zinc-binding protein in the liver, is considered the major source of zinc stores in the fetus and may protect the infant from developing zinc deficiency during the immediate postnatal period. Metallothionein levels in preterm infants are comparable to those seen in full-term infants. However, due to the small size of their livers, the total zinc stores of preterm infants are lower when compared with full-term infants.[111] Hepatic metallothionein levels decrease soon after birth and reach those seen in older children by 4 months of age. Plasma zinc levels also decrease soon after birth and reach a nadir between 6 and 12 weeks before starting to rise again.[110]

Zinc Absorption

Intestinal absorption and retention of zinc is incompletely understood, but likely involves specific zinc transporter proteins and divalent metal transporter-1 (DMT-1).[112] Intestinal metallothionein levels may also have a regulatory role in zinc absorption and retention. Dietary zinc is absorbed mostly in the distal duodenum and proximal jejunum.[113] However, the colon may participate in zinc absorption, especially following small-bowel disease or resection.[114] Following cellular uptake, zinc is actively secreted into the portal circulation. Two-thirds of zinc in plasma is bound to albumin, one-third to α_2-macroglobulin, and a small fraction to amino acids.

Absorption and retention of zinc is affected by several factors: (1) the amount of zinc administered; (2) the presence of promoting or inhibiting dietary factors in the intestinal lumen; and (3) the status of body zinc sufficiency (Table 3).[113] Generally, the fractional rate of zinc absorption is inversely related to the amount of zinc present in the lumen of the intestine. However, even though the fractional rate of absorption is lower with larger amounts of supplementation, the absolute amount of zinc absorbed and retained is proportionally higher. Zinc administered with human milk is better absorbed than that given with bovine milk;[115,116] over 60% of zinc given with preterm human milk is absorbed, compared with only 14% to 24% of that given with a formula.[117] Fortification of human milk appears to decrease fractional absorption rate. The lower rate of zinc absorption from bovine milk could be related to the high concentration of casein in bovine milk. Casein binds with zinc in the intestinal lumen and prevents its absorption. Using a casein hydrolysate formula and providing iron supplementation mixed with milk, rather than as a separate supplementation, are some of the measures that can be used to overcome the inhibitory effects of dietary factors on zinc absorption.[118,119]

The fractional absorption of zinc in preterm infants has been variously described to be between 0.22 and 0.42;[105,117,120,121] a value of 0.30 appears to be representative. VLBW infants of = 29 weeks gestational age appear to have lower fractional absorption rates.[120] More than 50% of parenterally administered zinc is retained by preterm and full-term infants.[107]

Sources of Zinc in the Diet

The concentration of zinc in colostrum is high (5.4 mg/L).[84-86,103] Zinc concentration of transitional preterm human milk is 4.8 mg/L,[84-86,122] decreasing to 2.2 mg/L at 1 month and to 1.1 mg/L at 3 months (Table 1).[84-86] Due to the higher fractional absorption, this concentration would provide approximately 1000-1500 μg of zinc per day to a full-term infant during the first three months of life and meet the demands of growth. Unfortified human milk is unlikely to provide the daily needs of zinc to preterm infants. Currently available human milk fortifiers in the United States provide an additional 7 to 10 mg of zinc per liter. The zinc concentration of commonly available preterm formulas varies between 8 and 12 mg/L. Full-term formulas contain 5-7 mg/L.[65]

Zinc Deficiency

The effects of severe zinc deficiency in older children and adults are protean and include growth failure, diminished food intake, skin lesions, poor wound healing, hair loss, decreased protein synthesis, and depressed host defense. In severe deficiency states, distinctive skin lesions, diarrhea, growth failure, and behavioral changes are seen.[102] While such florid zinc deficiency states as acrodermatitis and enteropathica have been described in preterm infants,[122,123] they are fortunately uncommon.

The true incidence of subclinical zinc deficiency is unknown because of the extreme difficulty of accurate diagnosis. Plasma or serum zinc concentration may be normal or modestly lower and lack sufficient sensitivity. Failure to grow while receiving adequate calories may suggest zinc deficiency. Other markers of body zinc status, such as hair zinc levels, have not been well defined. As zinc retention positively correlates with onset of catch-up growth, demonstration of an increase in growth velocity following dietary zinc supplementation has been considered evidence of preexisting zinc deficiency.[102] The fact that any number of other conditions, including repletion of other nutrients such as protein and energy, stimulate catch-up growth demonstrates the weakness of this method of diagnosing subclinical zinc deficiency.

The following groups of infants appear to be at highest risk of zinc deficiency: extremely low birth weight (ELBW) infants receiving total parenteral nutrition with inadequate zinc content;[124] preterm SGA infants;[109] and growing preterm infants fed unfortified human milk. In developing countries, maternal zinc supplementation during pregnancy may improve the zinc endowment of the fetus and prevent early zinc deficiency.[125] There is no evidence that maternal zinc supplementation is beneficial in the developed world.

Response to Zinc Supplementation

Several randomized controlled trials have assessed the response of the preterm infant to zinc supplementation in the hospital and after discharge. Obladen et al found that more than 50% (14/26) of rapidly growing VLBW infants in Germany developed subclinical zinc deficiency as indexed by serum zinc concentrations <7.6 mcg/L at the time of hospital discharge.[126] These surprisingly low serum values occurred despite a calculated range of zinc intake from 600 to 2000 mcg/kg/day. The levels were low whether the infants received primarily fortified human milk or preterm infant formula. Their data contrast with those of Wauben et al, who demonstrated that preterm infants remain zinc sufficient through 6 months corrected age when they are fed zinc fortified mother's milk during hospitalization and mother's milk after discharge.[127] The apparent zinc dose in the latter study was similar to that in Obladen et al. Rajaram et al also documented zinc sufficiency in preterm infants fed a discharge infant formula supplying 1800 μg/Kg/day of zinc.[128] Friel et al used a randomized control trial to demonstrate that zinc supplementation after hospital discharge increases plasma zinc concentrations, linear growth velocity and scores for motor development.[129]

Recommended Enteral Zinc Intake (Table 2)
Transition period: 500 to 800 μg/kg/day
Stable and postdischarge periods: 1000-2000 μg/kg/day

Acute zinc deficiency cases have not been reported in ELBW infants during the first weeks of life.[101] In spite of greater fractional absorption of zinc from human milk,[117] unsupplemented human milk will not meet the daily zinc needs of growing preterm infants. One-third to one-half of preterm infants receiving suboptimal zinc supplementation develop marginal body zinc status during infancy.[122,126,130] The AAP recommends zinc supplementation of >500 µg/day until six months of age to growing preterm infants receiving human milk.[64] However, more recent studies suggest that doses up to 1800 µg/kg/day are safe and promote better growth in the postdischarge period.[128] ELBW infants and infants with excessive gastrointestinal (diarrhea and ileostomy losses) or urinary zinc (high output renal failure) losses, and preterm infants with BPD, may need additional zinc supplementation.[101,131]

Recommended Parenteral Zinc Intake
Transitional period: 150 µg/kg/day
Stable and postdischarge periods: 400 µg/kg/day

VLBW preterm infants who receive inadequate amounts of zinc in TPN are at risk for developing zinc deficiency.[124] A parenteral intake of 150 µg/day during the transition period and 400 µg/day during the stable and postdischarge periods has been recommended. While these doses may not achieve zinc retention to the same degree as intrauterine accretion rates, they maintain serum zinc levels and meet the demands of growth.[102,132] As 87% of unretained parenterally administered zinc is excreted in the urine, the dose may have to be adjusted in acute and chronic renal conditions.[107]

Key Message: Zinc sufficiency is critical for adequate growth and development. Because zinc deficiency is difficult to diagnose accurately, it is better to err on the side of early zinc supplementation.

Copper
Copper is essential because of its presence in a number of proteins displaying redox activity.[123] The copper-containing enzyme, cytochrome c oxidase, is the terminal enzyme involved in oxidative phosphorylation. The most abundant group of copper-containing enzymes, superoxide dismutases, help protect cell membranes from oxidative damage. Dopamine ß-hydroxylase, catechol oxidase, and lysyl oxidase are some of the other copper-containing enzymes that play essential roles in the body. Ceruloplasmin, which functions as a copper transporter in the plasma, also has ferroxidase activity and is necessary for release of iron from hepatic stores and for its binding with transferrin. In addition, copper-dependent transcription factors participate in gene expression.[133]

Copper Status at Birth
The fetus is dependent on maternal copper status during pregnancy. The intrauterine accretion rate is approximately 50 µg/kg/day and principally occurs during the second half of pregnancy.[134] Fifty percent to 60% of copper is stored in the fetal liver as metallothionein. The copper content of the liver increases from 3 mg at 26 weeks gestation to approximately 10 to 12 mg at full term.[110] Eighty percent of hepatic copper can be considered as its storage form. After birth, hepatic copper decreases steadily to meet the demands of growth and to offset fecal copper losses associated with an increase in biliary secretion. In full-term infants, plasma copper and ceruloplasmin levels begin to rise 6 to 12 weeks after birth and reach adult values by six months of age. Plasma copper levels in preterm infants tend to be lower and reach the values present in full-term infants at birth only at around four months of age.[135] Depending upon the gestational age, mean serum copper levels in preterm infants range from 20 to 50 µg/dL and ceruloplasmin levels from 20 to 30 µg/dL when measured at 1 week of postnatal age.[133,135] Ceruloplasmin synthesis begins earlier in gestationally mature infants.

Copper Absorption
Copper is primarily absorbed from the upper small intestine. The mechanisms involved in intestinal copper absorption are incompletely understood. Similar to zinc, preterm infants fed human milk are capable of absorbing over 60% of copper, while those receiving bovine milk absorb only 16%.[117] Copper absorption from soy-based formulas is even lower.[136]

Twenty percent to 25% of copper in breast milk is bound to ceruloplasmin. Animal studies have demonstrated that ceruloplasmin-bound copper has better absorbability.[137] Preterm infants on human milk can achieve copper retention rates that approach intrauterine accretion rates.[133] Fructose, other refined sugars, cysteine, ascorbic acid, and high zinc and iron levels decrease copper absorption.[98,138] The fractional absorption of copper is halved when presented in a formula containing 10.2 mg/L of iron when compared with the one containing 2.5 mg/L.[98] With increasing amounts of copper in the intestinal lumen, the fractional absorption rate decreases while fecal copper losses increase. Fecal copper losses are also higher in conditions of fat malabsorption. Only small amounts of copper are normally lost in urine. Homeostasis is achieved by regulating biliary excretion.

After absorption from the intestine, copper is transported to the liver and the kidney bound to plasma proteins, albumin, and transcuprein. In the liver, it is incorporated into ceruloplasmin and metalloenzymes or is excreted via the biliary tract. The metallothionein-bound copper in the liver provides a source of copper soon after birth when dietary intakes are likely to be minimal. In addition, the liver plays a central role in copper metabolism through synthesis of ceruloplasmin, the principal copper transporter in the plasma. The second phase of copper transport, from the liver to other body tissues, is mediated through ceruloplasmin.[137] After birth, concentrations of copper in the liver remain constant throughout life, except in states of copper deficiency.

Sources of Dietary Copper

The mean concentration of copper in human milk is approximately 508 mcg/L (Table 1).[79,84-86] Preterm human milk contains 800 mcg/L soon after birth, and decreases gradually to 500 mcg/L at 4 weeks of age.[82,84-86] Cow milk copper concentration is lower and is of poor bioavailability. Commonly available full-term and preterm formulas contain approximately 0.5 to 0.6 mg/L and 0.7 to 2.0 mg/L of copper, respectively.[65] The copper concentration of preterm discharge formulas is 0.9 mg/L while human milk fortifiers provide an additional 0.44 to 1.7 mg/L.

Copper Deficiency

Overt copper deficiency is rare. The mean age of presentation is 3 to 4 months, with a range of 4 weeks to 8 months.[110,133,139] Common clinical manifestations include failure to thrive, pallor, hypothermia, apneic episodes, hypotonia, and bone abnormalities.[110] Anemia may be associated with hypoferremia but will not respond to iron supplementation. Neutropenia is one of the earliest manifestation.[139] Bone changes may include osteoporosis, fractures of long bones and ribs, and delayed bone age.[133] Decreased pigmentation of the skin and hair, skin lesions akin to seborrheic dermatitis, edema and hypoproteinuria, diarrhea, and hepatosplenomegaly are other rare signs of copper deficiency. These symptoms have not been reported in the neonatal period in premature infants.

Copper deficiency occurs if insufficient amounts are provided or if the amount supplemented is poorly absorbed. Preterm infants <34 weeks are theoretically at risk for copper deficiency[139] because their hepatic copper stores are lower and their copper requirements for growth are higher than full-term infants. Infants fed bovine milk or those with diarrhea or gastrointestinal malabsorption disorders are particularly prone to copper deficiency. Inadequate copper supplementation during total parenteral nutrition can result in copper deficiency. High oral zinc and iron intakes can result in copper deficiency, probably by competing with its absorption.

Menkes disease, a rare X-linked genetic disorder, is associated with abnormalities in copper absorption. The genetic abnormality has been mapped to the gene ATP7A. The clinical features of this disorder are low copper levels in blood, liver and hair, hypothermia, defective keratinization of hair, prominence of superficial veins, metaphysial lesions, degenerative changes in aortic elastin, and progressive mental deterioration. The clinical condition is rarely manifest during the first month of life, with the typical age of onset being 2 to 3 months. Aggressive early copper supplementation has been tried, but the overall prognosis remains poor.[140,141] Wilson's disease (due to a mutation in gene ATP7B) and aceruloplasminemia are other genetic disorders of copper metabolism. Wilson's disease is characterized by excessive copper accumulation in the serum due to a defect in tissue copper exporter.[142] Clinical features of aceruloplasminemia are similar to those seen with hemochromatosis and are due to tissue deposition of excess iron. The lack of ceruloplasmin does not allow the conversion of ferrous to ferric iron to occur at the cell membrane, thereby inhibiting iron egress from the cell.[143]

Low serum copper and ceruloplasmin concentrations as indicators of copper deficiency lack specificity.[139] Low serum copper concentrations soon after birth in preterm infants could be due to decreased hepatic release and may not indicate a deficiency state. Similarly, low ceruloplasmin concentrations soon after birth could be due to poor hepatic production in these infants. Unlike in older infants and adults, these low ceruloplasmin concentrations do not respond to copper supplementation. Ceruloplasmin concentrations can be falsely elevated due to inflammation. Erythrocyte superoxide dismutase is a better indicator of copper status in the preterm infant compared with plasma levels.[144] A therapeutic response (reticulocytosis and resolution of anemia, neutrophilia, onset of catch-up growth, and reversal of bone abnormalities) to a copper dose of 2 to 5 µg/kg/day has been considered diagnostic of preexisting copper deficiency.[110,139]

Copper Toxicity

Acute copper toxicity is rare. Chronic excessive intake or reduced biliary excretion can result in hepatic cirrhosis.

Recommended Enteral Copper Intake (Table 2)

Transitional period: 120 µg/kg/day
Stable and postdischarge periods: 120 to 150 µg/kg/day

The Committee on Nutrition of the AAP recommends a daily copper intake of 90 µg/100 kcal.[134] Based on a caloric intake of 120 to 140 kcal/day, this amounts to 108 to 120 µg/kg/day. Since the hepatic stores meet the minimal needs of

copper during the initial 1 to 2 weeks of life, copper supplementation is not necessary soon after birth. Both human milk and preterm infant formulas meet the daily requirement when consumed at 150 ml/kg/day. Additional copper supplementation is not necessary except in rare instances where bovine milk or soy milk are used for prolonged periods. Early copper supplementation is undertaken in Menkes disease but does not appear to improve the outcome.

Recommended Parenteral Copper Intake (Table 2)

Transitional period: May be omitted, if given = 20 µg/kg/d
Stable and postdischarge periods: 20 µg/kg/d
Note: Copper should be withheld when hepatic cholestasis is present.

Copper needs of preterm infants are minimal during the transitional period. There is no requirement for growth, and biliary excretion is minimal in an infant who is yet to be enterally fed. The low serum copper levels seen in these infants is essentially due to poor hepatic mobilization and can be considered physiological. Hence, the Committee on Nutrition of the AAP recommends that copper may be omitted from total parenteral nutrition that is limited to 1 to 2 weeks in preterm infants. If copper supplementation is considered necessary, a daily supplementation of 16 µg/kg/day meets the daily needs and prevents copper deficiency.[107] For long-term parenteral nutrition, an intake of 20 µg/kg/day is recommended. Copper should be omitted in the presence of obstructive jaundice.[65] Lockitch et al demonstrated normal serum copper levels with parenteral intake between 19 and 38 µg/kg/day.[132]

Key Message: Like zinc, copper deficiency is difficult to diagnose reliably in preterm infants and is probably quite rare. Supplying an adequate source of parenteral and enteral copper is not difficult or toxic and thus can be started immediately after birth.

Selenium

Although selenium deficiency has been described infrequently in the infant, selenium is recognized as a nutritionally essential trace element.[145] The role of selenium in perinatal nutrition has recently been reviewed.[110] Its established enzymatic functions include four glutathione peroxidases and the iodothyronine deiodinases. The glutathione peroxidases are involved in protecting cell membranes from peroxidase damage through detoxification of peroxides and free radicals. Selenium plays a role in thyroid metabolism by regulating the expression of the deiodinases, leading to activation of T_3. Selenium may play an important role in brain development; indeed, it is one of a handful of nutrients (including iron, zinc, iodine, protein, energy and Vitamin A) that have an impact on cognitive development, affecting brain thyroid concentration and expression of thyroid responsive genes, myelination, and neurotransmitter synthesis.[146-149]

Selenium deficiency is one of the etiologic factors responsible for Keshan disease, an often fatal cardiomyopathy primarily affecting children and young women in more than a dozen provinces within the belt of endemic selenium deficiency in China.[150,151] Cases of cardiac and skeletal myopathy resembling Keshan disease have been reported in patients with depressed selenium status in the United States. Two of these patients were on long-term total parenteral nutrition (TPN) and had little or no selenium in their parenteral formulations.[152] Loss of hair pigment and macrocytosis, apparently attributable to selenium deficiency, have also been reported in intravenously fed children.[153] Clinical selenium deficiency has not been described in preterm infants, although biochemical evidence of selenium deficiency (low serum concentrations and decreased glutathione peroxidase activity) has been cited. The preterm infant is at risk because of low stores at birth and use of selenium-free TPN.[154]

One of the main issues with respect to maintaining adequate selenium status in VLBW premature infants relates to their high risk of oxidative diseases. In theory, adequate anti-oxidant status, including nutrients such as selenium and Vitamin E, may have a protective effect. Sluis et al suggested that selenium deficiency is a risk factor for BPD.[155] Infants with BPD have lower selenium levels at 28 days than infants without BPD, although infants with BPD are generally more malnourished in the first month; thus, the role of selenium per se is difficult to isolate.[156,157] Two recent prospective trials addressed whether selenium supplementation reduces the prevalence of BPD in high-risk infants born in selenium-deficient endemic areas.[157,158] Darlow et al supplemented 268 infants with 7 µg/kg/day of parenteral or 5 µg/kg/day of enteral selenium (versus placebo for the control group) and found no difference in the prevalence of ROP or BPD. Interestingly, however, they did find that infants born to mothers with low selenium concentrations had a higher risk of BPD.[158]

All soluble selenium compounds, including selenite, selenomethionine, and selenocysteine are absorbed in the duodenum. Ehrenkranz et al, using stable isotopes of selenium in a study of 20 premature infants, demonstrated absorption of 60% to 80% of dietary selenium in formula.[159] Selenium absorption and retention were not found to correlate with gestational age, post-conceptional age, or weight gain. Although selenium is generally thought to be lost from the body via the urine following metabolism, about twice as much selenium is excreted in stool as in urine.[159] Human milk, bovine milk, and infant formulas all provide biologically available sources of dietary selenium (Table 1). Colostrum contains twice as much selenium as mature human milk. The selenium content of mature human milk falls from 17.4 µg/L at 1 month postpartum to 15 µg/L at 3 and 6 months postpartum.[84-86] The selenium content of infant formulas varies according to the amounts of intrinsic selenium in the ingredients. Dietary selenium is normally associated with proteins. The content of selenium in formula, therefore, depends mainly on the amount, source, and type of protein in the formulation. A usual range is 7 to 14 µg/L.

Infants born prematurely have decreased hepatic selenium stores compared to full-term infants.[154] Intrauterine accretion of selenium during the third trimester of gestation is estimated to be 1 µg/kg/day.[110,160] This estimate is likely an underestimate of gestational accretion, since it was based on tissues obtained from fetuses in New Zealand, where tissue selenium contents are known to be low. Ehrenkranz and colleagues, using a stable isotope methodology, showed that preterm infants who were enterally fed selenium at a rate of 3 µg/kg/day were able to absorb and retain dietary selenium at a rate that exceeded this rate of intrauterine selenium accretion.[159] Nevertheless, Friel et al showed that selenium dependent glutathione peroxidase activity declines during the first six postnatal months in VLBW infants, suggesting that earlier supplies of selenium were inadequate.[161] A randomized trial of parenteral selenium supplementation showed that 3 µg/kg/day of selenous acid maintained selenium status.[162] Since 60% to 80% of enteral zinc is absorbed, minimal if any dose adjustments need to be considered between enteral and parenteral dosing. An enteral dose of 1 µg/kg/day appears to be sufficient to maintain normal serum selenium levels for six weeks, although plasma glutathione peroxidase activity declines.[163] Smith et al demonstrated that premature infants fed either preterm human milk (selenium content 24 µg/L), standard premature formula (7.8 µg/L), or premature formula supplemented with 30 µg/L of selenium, had similar plasma and red blood cell selenium and glutathione peroxidase levels.[164] Tyrala et al used a randomized controlled study design to show that infants fed a formula fortified with 28.4 µg/L (average daily dose of 4.5 µg/kg/day) had higher red cell and plasma selenium levels, but similar growth, to age-matched preterm infants fed a formula with 10 µg/L (average daily dose of 1.5 µg/kg/day).[165] The glutathione activity remained similar in the infants until three months, at which time the supplemented infants had greater values.

The relationship between serum selenium concentrations and plasma glutathione activity, which serves as a biological marker of selenium activity, is complex. Whole blood selenium concentrations below 100 µg/L have a linear relationship with glutathione activity.[110,160] However, glutathione activity can be affected by steroid exposure and oxygen exposure, disassociating its relationship from selenium intake. Clinical symptoms of selenium deficiency, such as increased red cell hemolysis, are seen at serum concentrations less than 40 µg/L, with myopathies evident at about one-quarter of that level.[110,160]

Previous recommendations of selenium intake were 1.3 to 3 µg/kg/day enterally and 1.5 to 2.0 µg/kg/day parenterally. Agget suggests 1.3 to 2 µg/kg/day for both parenteral and enteral usage.[110] The Institute of Medicine recommended an adequate intake of 2.1 µg/kg for infants up to six months of age.[166] More recent data suggest that slightly higher deliveries (eg, up to 4.5 µg/kg/day) are well tolerated and result in higher serum selenium concentrations, and ultimately, more glutathione activity.[110,158,165] Thus, the recommended enteral selenium intake can range from 1.5 to 4.5 µg/kg/day.

Recommended Enteral Selenium Intake (Table 2)

Transitional period: Equivalent to human milk (1.3 µg/kg/day)
Stable and postdischarge periods: 1.3 to 4.5 µg/kg/day

Recommended Parenteral Selenium Intake (Table 2)

Early transitional period: may be omitted; if given, = 1.3 µg/kg/day
Stable and postdischarge periods: 1.5 to 4.5 µg/kg/day
Note: Because selenium is excreted primarily by the kidneys, the dosage should be lowered in the presence of decreased renal output.

Key Message: Since 1993, a great deal more has become known about the importance of maintaining selenium status. Not only is it a potent anti-oxidant, but its role in the developing brain is now being elucidated.

Chromium

Chromium is involved in the prevention of glucose intolerance by an unknown mechanism. Early work suggested that chromium is part of, or necessary for, a glucose tolerance factor described as being a water-soluble component of liver, blood, plasma, and other biologic cells.[167] Yamamoto et al[168] reported the isolation from liver and milk of an amino acid component containing chromium that had biologic activity, stimulated adipocytes to take up glucose, and potentiated insulin action. The role of chromium in glucose homeostasis continues to be investigated in human adults. Two studies have addressed its status in infants with glucose homeostasis abnormalities.[169,170] Serum chromium levels were similar in hypoglycemic preterm and term infants when compared to normoglycemic infants matched for birth weight and gestational age.[169] Only intrauterine growth-retarded infants had lower chromium levels when compared to gestational age-matched controls.[169] No other biological role outside of glucose homeostasis appears to exist for the mineral. Chromium is found in human milk.

Adults absorb less than 2% of a chromium load and excrete chromium in the urine in an amount proportional to dietary intake.[171] Chromium deficiency, characterized by weight loss, peripheral neuropathy, hyperglycemia, and insulin resistance in adults, has not been described in children or infants.[172,173] It is unclear whether this is because the syndrome does not exist in infants or whether infants on long-term TPN have not had their chromium status assessed.

Chromium is ubiquitous, making trace amounts in blood or urine extremely difficult to detect from background contamination.

The concentration of chromium in bovine milk and formula based on bovine milk (15 μg/L) is considerably higher than the concentration in human milk (Table 1). The chromium content of human milk is 0.3 to 0.5 μg/L.[84,174,175]

Data are insufficient to recommend a specific chromium intake for the infant born prematurely. Plasma chromium levels are not different in premature versus control infants at birth or in the first postnatal month.[176] Because infants fed their own mother's milk have not become obviously chromium deficient, this intake is likely adequate for the preterm infant. Furthermore, because infants fed formula with a significantly higher amount of chromium have not developed overt toxicity, there is likely a wide safe range of intake.

Since deficiency has not been documented in preterm infants receiving their own mother's milk, a safe enteral dose of chromium would appear to be 0.05 μg/kg/day. The lack of toxicity in formula-fed infants suggests a dose up to 2.25 μg/kg/day is safe.

Infants on long-term TPN can likely be given the dose used to prevent chromium deficiency in adults (0.3 μg/kg/day).

Recommended Enteral Chromium Intake (Table 2)

Transitional period: Equivalent to human milk (0.05 μg/kg/day)
Stable and postdischarge periods: 0.1 to 2.25 μg/kg/day

Recommended Parenteral Chromium Intake (Table 2)

Early transitional period: May be omitted; if given, = 0.05 μg/kg/day
Stable and postdischarge periods: 0.05 to 0.3 μg/kg/day
Note: Because chromium is excreted primarily via the kidneys, the dosage should be lowered in the presence of decreased renal output.

The Committee on Clinical Practice Issues of the American Society of Clinical Nutrition recommended parenteral intakes of chromium at 0.2 μg/kg/day for the preterm infant. This recommendation was based on the dose known to prevent chromium deficiency in adults on long-term TPN (0.3 μg/kg/day). No adverse effects have been reported in infants receiving this amount of chromium. There are no data to justify an intake higher than that received by the breastfed infant.

Molybdenum

Molybdenum is necessary in very small amounts for the function of three mammalian enzymes: xanthine, aldehyde, and sulfite oxidases. Xanthine oxidase is necessary for the terminal oxidation of purines to allow their excretion as uric acid. Sulfite oxidase is necessary for the disposal and excretion of sulfur.

Reports of molybdenum toxicity are exceedingly rare.[177] As with several other nutrients discussed in this chapter, deficiency occurs when adult patients are on very-long-term TPN not supplemented with a particular nutrient. Molybdenum deficiency in adults results in cardiac and neurologic symptoms including tachycardia and coma. An associated rise in uric acid levels has been noted. The diagnosis is made by monitoring the response to provision of molybdenum, which in this case was given at a dose of 2.5 µg/kg/day. Neither toxicity nor deficiency states have been described in preterm infants on long-term TPN. Molybdenum is readily absorbed from the intestine, and excretion is via the urine.

Only one study has examined the fetal accretion of molybdenum. Abumrad has estimated the intrauterine accretion rate to be 1 µg/kg/day,[178] although that may be an overestimate. Mature preterm human milk contains 2 µg/L, ensuring an effective dose of 0.3 µg/kg/day when consumed at 150 cc/kg/day (Table 1).[84-86] The bioavailability of molybdenum from preterm and term human milk appears to be high. Although human milk contains only 4% of the molybdenum of term infant formula and 1.5% of preterm formula, infants fed human milk have higher serum molybdenum concentrations and a higher associated uric acid excretion (implying that dietary molybdenum has been actively metabolized) than formula-fed infants.[179] The molybdenum content of term and preterm human milk decreases over time.[85]

There have been no randomized controlled trials of molybdenum administration, either enterally or parenterally, in preterm infants. Sievers et al performed the only molybdenum balance study in premature infants and found they excreted more than 60% of either a high or low dose in the urine.[180] These 34-week-gestational-age infants were studied at a postconceptional age of 37+ weeks. During the low-dose studies, they received 0.024 micromol/kg/day and excreted 0.02 micromol/kg/day. The high-intake studies delivered over 10 times that amount (0.284 micromol/kg/day), yet the infants excreted 0.243 micromol/kg/day. Retention ranged from -0.03 to 0.378 micromol/kg/day. Friel et al performed a balance study that demonstrated VLBW infants require 1µg/kg/d of intravenous molybdenum and 4 to 6 µg/kg/day of enteral molybdenum.[181]

Based on these minimal data, the enteral intake of molybdenum could range up to 4 µg/kg/day.

Recommended Enteral Molybdenum Intake (Table 2)

Transitional period: Equivalent to human milk (0.3 µg/kg/day)

Stable and postdischarge periods: 0.3-4.0 µg/kg/day

Recommended Parenteral Molybdenum Intake (Table 2)

Early transitional period: 0

Stable and postdischarge periods: 0.25-1.0 µg/kg/day

The Committee on Clinical Practice Issues of the American Society of Clinical Nutrition recommended parenteral intakes of molybdenum at 0.25 µg/kg/day for the preterm infant. This intake is probably in the appropriate range. However, because molybdenum deficiency has not been described in the pediatric population, intravenous molybdenum is recommended only for those infants needing long-term TPN.

Manganese

Manganese is known to function in three main areas of metabolism: (1) it acts as an activator of the gluconeogenic enzymes pyruvate carboxylase and isocitrate dehydroxygenase; (2) it is involved in protecting mitochondrial membranes through superoxide dismutase, a manganese-containing enzyme; and (3) it activates glycosyl transferase, which is involved in mucopolysaccharide synthesis.

Manganese deficiency has not been conclusively demonstrated in humans. Manganese deficiency in animals, however, has a significant effect on the production of hyaluronic acid, chondroitin sulfate, heparin, and other mucopolysaccharides that are important for growth and maintenance of connective tissue, cartilage, and bone. The subsequent clinical symptoms include growth retardation, impaired collagen formation, glucose intolerance, and abnormal lipid metabolism. Although manganese is involved as a cofactor in numerous enzyme systems, manganese deficiency does not appear to have broad effects other than on mucopolysaccharides and lipopolysaccharide formation. This is probably because magnesium can be substituted for manganese in many of its enzyme-related functions. Its role in pulmonary superoxide dismutase has been recently studied in the baboon model of BPD.[182] Mn superoxide dismutase mRNA and protein levels increase in lungs with BPD or with chronic infection, suggesting a role for the micronutrient in responses to oxidative injuries. The effect of Mn deficiency on these responses to mechanical ventilation and pulmonary infection was not studied.

Whereas manganese deficiency has not been reported in humans, manganese toxicity has been well described. Miners of manganese in India and Peru, for example, develop a toxicity syndrome that consists of extrapyramidal signs similar to those seen in Parkinson's disease.[183] Apparently, manganese crosses the blood-brain barrier and displaces catecholamines from storage sites in the central nervous system, resulting in a central catecholamine depletion state.[184] The signs of manganese toxicity respond quickly to treatment with levodopa, thus confirming the depletion of brain catecholamines.

Adult populations are protected from manganese toxicity by three barriers: the intestinal barrier; the blood-brain barrier; and the liver. Newborn premature infants, especially those receiving manganese-supplemented TPN, may be at increased risk of toxicity because manganese homeostasis is poorly developed in the premature infant. In addition, absorptive control (in the intestine) is bypassed by TPN, and because little or no stool is passed, excretion is minimal.[185] Intravenous infusions likely result in altered tissue distribution.[186] Finally, the blood-brain barrier of the preterm infant is immature, and therefore, more permeable. Zlotkin and Buchanan[187] looked for manganese toxicity in parenterally fed preterm infants by measuring the urinary excretion of catecholamine metabolites. Despite high manganese intakes in the infants studied (48 µg/kg/day), no evidence of manganese toxicity was detected. Unfortunately, there are no readily usable laboratory assays to assess manganese status adequately.

Manganese absorption in humans is low. In adults, 2% of the manganese from bovine milk was absorbed, 8% from human milk, and <1% from soy formula.[188] Studies in animals show that absorption varies inversely with the level of manganese.[189] In the plasma, manganese is bound to transferrin. More than 90% of manganese is excreted through the bile, with only a small portion excreted through the kidneys.[190] Manganese is rapidly cleared from the blood, with only 1.5% of an ingested adult dose being retained 10 days later.[191]

The manganese content of human milk is about 7.5 µg/L.[85] With a milk intake of 150 mL/kg/day, the intake of manganese would be 1.1 µg/kg/day (Table 1). Formulas contain variable amounts of manganese, ranging from undetectable amounts to 340 µg/L. Isotope studies in rat pups indicate that manganese absorption and retention from human milk or infant formula exceed 83%.[192] Formula-fed infants may receive between 5 and 37.5 µg/kg/day, depending on the formula provided. Soy protein-based formulas deliver the highest manganese dose, while preterm infant formulas supply between 6.5 and 14.5 µg/kg/day (Table 1). There is no evidence that the low intake of manganese in breast-fed infants, even premature infants, is associated with manganese deficiency, nor is there any indication that higher intake with the use of formulas is associated with toxicity. We therefore conclude that the safe and adequate range for manganese intake is 0.75 to 7.5 µg/kg/day. Based on data reported by Casey and Robinson,[193] a 1-kg infant would accumulate manganese at a rate of 9 µg/kg/day during the last trimester of pregnancy. Although the above recommendation would not duplicate intrauterine accretion rates, the absence of deficiency signs in infants receiving these lower intakes, combined with the potential for toxicity in the small preterm infant, leads to recommendation of the lower amounts.

Recommended Enteral Manganese Intake (Table 2)
Transitional period: Equivalent to human milk (0.75 µg/kg/day)
Stable and postdischarge periods: 0.7 to 7.5 µg/kg/day

Recommended Parenteral Manganese Intake (Table 2)
Transitional period: May be omitted; if given, = 0.75 µg/kg/day
Stable and postdischarge periods: 1.0 µg/kg/day
Note: Manganese supplements should be withheld when hepatic cholestasis is present.

Parenteral solutions contain variable quantities

of manganese contaminants.[194] For example, Zlotkin and Buchanan[187] found levels of 7 ± 1 µg/L in apparently manganese-free TPN formulations. Little manganese is secreted into the gut during TPN; thus, retention of intravenously infused manganese is close to 100%.[187] The majority of premature infants on TPN will be in positive manganese balance with intakes of 1.0 µg/kg/day. Quantities 10 times that high have been used without evidence of toxicity, although serum manganese levels are elevated above normal. The addition of 5 µg/L has been associated with normal concentrations of serum manganese except in cholestatic liver disease.[195]

The Committee on Clinical Practice Issues of the American Society of Clinical Nutrition deemed parenteral intakes of manganese at 1.0 µg/kg/day to be in the appropriate range for the preterm infant.

Iodine

The only known role of iodine is in thyroid function, where it is part of triiodothyronine (T_3) and tetraiodothyronine (T_4) (60% iodine by weight). However, since the effects of hypothyroidism are protean and include abnormal neurodevelopment, maintaining iodine sufficiency is of paramount importance. The physiologic response to iodine deficiency in humans is increased secretion of thyroid-stimulating hormone, thyroid hyperplasia and hypertrophy, increased thyroid iodine uptake, and increased ratio of secretion of T_3 relative to T_4. Iodine deficiency depresses the production of thyroid hormones, especially T_4. Endemic goiter occurs in specific geographic areas throughout the world when dietary iodine intake is <15 µg/day.

In the intestinal tract, iodine is converted to I- prior to absorption. Iodine is stored in the thyroid gland, and after peroxidation it becomes attached to the tyrosine residues of thyroglobulin.

The major concern regarding iodine nutrition in infants is endemic cretinism due to maternal iodide deficiency. Indeed, maternal and fetal iodine status is mainly a reflection of maternal dietary iodine intake. Overt cretinism is said to occur in 5% to 15% of cases of endemic neonatal goiter. Milder degrees of iodine deficiency, both in utero and after birth, may have detrimental effects on growth and intellectual performance.

Excess iodine intake can also cause hypothyroidism, especially in the 4% of the population who are sensitive to excess iodine. Even in a patient who receives no iodine by mouth or parenterally, iodine intake may be excessive from skin absorption of iodine in topical disinfectants, detergents, and other sources.

In infants born prematurely, mechanisms to deal with iodine excess and deficiency are immature. When the diet is deficient in iodine, the premature infant is not able to compensate by retaining more iodine; thus, a higher iodine intake is needed to maintain a euthyroid state. Iodine excess can also be deleterious to young infants.[196,197] If premature infants (<34 weeks gestation) are exposed to high iodine intakes (>100 µg/day) via cutaneous administration of providone-iodine and alcohol-iodine solutions, decreased T_4 and increased serum thyroid-stimulating hormone may result.[198,199]

Because of the variability in iodine status in the preterm infant and the association of low-circulating thyroid hormone with poor neurodevelopmental outcome, Roghan et al performed a randomized trial of standard (10.2 µg/kg/day) versus high (40.8 µg/kg/day) iodine intake in a total of 121 preterm infants.[200] No differences were seen in thyroid status between the two groups at 41 weeks postconceptional age. The study was performed in an area where iodine deficiency is not endemic (Liverpool, UK). Long-term neurodevelopmental status was not assessed. The study, however, clearly shows that a dose of 10.2 µg/kg/day will maintain iodine sufficiency (as indexed by thyroid status) in preterm infants born to presumably iodine-sufficient mothers. In contrast, premature infants born in countries with endemic low iodine intake may develop transient hypothyroidism on iodine intakes of 10 to 30 µg/kg/day.[196,197] These infants are at increased risk because of low iodine stores at birth and the low iodine content of their mother's milk.

The content of iodine in human milk is variable, depending on the dietary intake of the mother.

The average iodine content of mature human milk in European mothers is 70 to 90 µg/L; in the United States, the iodine content is higher, 140 to 180 µg/L (Table 1). An American infant ingesting 150 mL/kg/day will receive iodine at about 24 µg/kg/day. The average iodine content of bovine milk, also quite variable, is about three times higher than that of human milk (average 415 µg/L). Formulas based on bovine milk contain between 41 and 101 µg/L iodine, while special premature formulas contain between 41 and 202 µg/L. The concentrations of iodine in formula are well below the advised upper safety limit of 333 µg/L recommended at a symposium on upper limits in infant formulas,[201] and 233 µg/L by Raiten et al.[202]

Delange has suggested a daily iodine requirement of >30 µg/kg/day for the preterm infant (personal communication). Some premature infants may be in negative iodine balance on intakes of <30 µg/kg/day.[203] Based on the average iodine content of human milk, human milk from European mothers would definitely not be an adequate iodine source for the preterm infant, while human milk from mothers in the United States would be only slightly below this recommended intake.

Recommended Enteral Iodine Intake (Table 2)

Transitional period: Equivalent to human milk (11 to 27 µg/kg/day)
Stable and postdischarge periods: 10 to 42 µg/kg/day

Recommended Parenteral Iodine Intake (Table 2)

Transitional period: May be omitted; if given, = 1.0 µg/kg/day
Stable and postdischarge periods: 1.0 µg/kg/day

Most infants receiving TPN will have iodine-containing disinfectants or detergents used on their skin. Thus, one may assume a significant amount of iodine absorption through the skin. Based on this assumption, the Committee on Clinical Practice Issues of the American Society of Clinical Nutrition recommended parenteral intakes of iodine at 1.0 µg/kg/day for the preterm infant. In patients on long-term TPN, 1 µg/kg/day will avoid any risk of iodine deficiency, and yet does not add significantly to the risk of toxicity from topical iodine absorption.

Key Message: The dose of iodine for the preterm infant is highly dependent on whether the infant resides in an area of the world that is endemic for low iodine intake. Infants born in low iodine areas will have higher needs to maintain adequate thyroid status.

Case Study

A 7-month-old, former 28-week-gestation female infant is brought to the NICU follow-up clinic for routine assessment of growth and neurodevelopment. Her parents state that she has been in good health and has been growing adequately. She is achieving appropriate developmental milestones. Her history is remarkable for her birth at 28-weeks gestation because of maternal hypertension. She weighed 700 grams and her parents recall that the neonatologists had remarked that she was "small for her dates." She had a benign neonatal course not requiring mechanical ventilation. They could not recall her requiring blood transfusions, and they stated that other than routine laboratories each week, blood drawing was minimal. Her initial hemoglobin was 143 g/L. She had mild hyperbilirubinemia (peak serum bilirubin concentration of 10.3 with no direct component) and her blood type was A-positive, the same as her mother. No hemolysis was noted on her initial blood smear. She began trophic feedings of her mother's milk within 3 days of birth, and except for some brief stoppages of feeding due to "NEC scares," she worked up to full enteral feedings of her mother's milk within two weeks of birth. The feedings were fortified with a human milk fortifier (without iron) to a caloric density of 80 kcal/100 cc. She did not receive recombinant human erythropoietin, nor did she receive iron supplementation in the nursery. At the time of discharge, her hemoglobin was 8.1 which her attending physician ascribed to anemia of prematurity. Since discharge she has been exclusively breastfed with no supplemental foods.

On physical examination in clinic, she was well developed and nourished, although her growth remains at the 10th percentile for weight and height and at the 25th percentile for head circumference on the IHDP growth curves for VLBW premature girls. She was developmentally appropriate for her corrected age. Her lungs were clear and she showed no signs of chronic disease. She is pale.

Because of her pallor, a complete blood count was obtained that demonstrated a hemoglobin concentration of 51 g/L with a mean corpuscular volume (MCV) of 61. Additional blood work was obtained that showed a serum ferritin concentration of 1 ng/ml, a total iron binding capacity of 512 mg/dl and percent TIBC saturation <10%. The reticulocyte count was 1.2%.

A diagnosis of iron-deficiency anemia was made and the infant was started on supplemental iron sulfate therapy at a dose of 6 mg/kg/day. A repeat analysis at 8-months corrected age demonstrated a hemoglobin concentration of 11.1 g/L with a ferritin concentration of 15 ng/ml.

Commentary

This infant has iron-deficiency anemia and demonstrates many of the risk factors for this disease in premature infants. First, the infant was quite premature at 28-weeks gestation. Since iron is accreted by the fetus during the last trimester, this infant effectively missed out on most of her transplacental load of iron. At 700 grams birth weight, she only had about 50 mg of total body iron, compared with the expected 225 mg of a term infant. Second, she was small for gestational age, which up to 30% of premature infants are. Up to 50% of small for gestational infants have decreased hepatic iron stores, most likely due to poor maternal-fetal iron transport during placental insufficiency due to maternal hypertension. Her low hemoglobin concentration at birth also suggests low total body iron status. Third, like many small-for-dates preterm infants, she had minimal lung disease and was generally quite mature for her gestational age. Thus, although she had minimal blood drawing, she also had no red blood cell transfusions that would have been a postnatal source of iron. Fourth, she did not receive an iron source during her NICU stay because she was fed human milk. Until very recently, human milk fortifiers did not contain adequate (or in some cases any) iron. Many physicians

are reluctant to supplement human milk with iron because of concerns that it binds the lactoferrin, thereby reducing the latter's anti-infective capacity. There is no evidence for this concern in the preterm infant. Fifth, although she was noted to have a low hemoglobin concentration at hospital discharge, this was ascribed to physiologic anemia of prematurity. There are now data to suggest that anemia of prematurity has a component of iron deficiency (see above and reference 77). Sixth, she grew relatively well for an SGA infant in the follow-up period. A rapid rate of postdischarge growth implies a rapid expansion of the blood volume that requires a high rate of iron delivery of at least 2 mg/kg/day. Unsupplemented human milk does not provide that amount of iron.

Management changes that could have been made in this case would have included measuring a ferritin concentration at birth. A value less than 50 ng/ml at birth is consistent with abnormally low hepatic iron stores. Iron supplements should have started after feedings were established (approximately 2 weeks of age). A dose of 2 mg/kg/day as medicinal iron drops would have been appropriate. Alternatively, a human milk fortifier that delivers that effective dose would suffice. It is useful to know these infants' iron status (hemoglobin, MCV, reticulocyte count) at hospital discharge so that the primary care physician has a baseline value from which to work. Iron supplementation should continue after hospital discharge at a dose of 2 mg/kg/day. Earlier screening for iron deficiency is indicated in preterm and SGA infants. The AAP suggests screening at 6 months instead of 9 months. This infant's rapid recovery of iron sufficiency is typical of adequate treatment.

References

1. Dallman PR. Biochemical basis for the manifestations of iron deficiency. *Ann Rev Nutr.*1986; 6:13-40.
2. Mackler B, Grace R, Finch CA. Iron deficiency in the rat: effects on oxidative metabolism in distinct types of skeletal muscle. *Pediatr Res* 1984; 18:499-500.
3. Blayney L, Bailey-Wood R, Jacobs A, Henderson A, Muir J. The effects of iron deficiency on the respiratory function and cytochrome content of rat heart

mitochondria. 1976; 39:744-748.

4. Ercan O, Ulukutlu L, Ozbay G, Arda O. Intestinal effects of iron deficiency anemia in children. *Turk J Pediatr* 1991; 33:85-98.

5. Berant M, Khourie M, Menzies IS. Effect of iron deficiency on small intestinal permeability in infants and young children. *J Pediatr Gastroenterol Nutr* 1992; 14:17-20.

6. Inder TE, Clemett RS, Austin NC, Graham P, Darlow BA. High iron status in VLBW infants is associated with an increased risk of retinopathy of prematurity. *J Pediatr* 1997; 131:541-544.

7. Lackmann GM, Hesse L, Tollner U. Reduced iron-associated anti-oxidants in premature newborns suffering intracerebral hemorrhage. *Free Radic Biol Med* 1996; 20:407-409.

8. Jansson LT. Iron, oxygen stress, and the preterm infant. In: Lonnerdal B, ed. *Iron Metabolism in Infants.* Boca Raton, FL: CRC Press; 1990: 73-85.

9. Gulbis B, Jauniaux E, Decuyper J, Thiry P, Jurkovic D, Campbell S. Distribution of iron and iron-binding proteins in first-trimester human pregnancies. *Obstet Gynecol* 1994; 84:289-293.

10. Scott PH, Berger HM, Kenward C, Scott P, Wharton BA. Effect of gestational age and intrauterine nutrition on plasma transferrin and iron in the newborn. *Arch Dis Child* 1975; 50:796-798.

11. Lackmann GM, Schnieder C, Bohner J. Gestational age-dependent reference values for iron and selected proteins of iron metabolism in serum of premature human neonates. *Biol Neonate* 1998; 74:208-213.

12. Chockalingam U, Murphy E, Ophoven JC, Georgieff MK. The influence of gestational age, size for dates, and prenatal steroids on cord transferrin levels in newborn infants. *J Ped Gastroenterol Nutr* 1987; 6:276-280.

13. Josephs HW. Iron metabolism and the hypochromic anaemia of infancy. *Medicine* 1953; 32:125-157.

14. Dallman PR, Siimes MA, Stekel A. Iron deficiency in infancy and childhood. *Am J Clin Nutr* 1980; 33: 86-118.

15. Lozoff B. Perinatal iron deficiency and the developing brain [In Process Citation]. *Pediatr Res* 2000; 48: 137-139.

16. Lozoff B, Klein NK, Nelson EC, McClish DK, Manuel M, Chacon ME. Behavior of infants with iron-deficiency anemia. *Child Dev* 1998 69:24-36.

17. Walter T. Effect of iron-deficiency anaemia on cognitive skills in infancy and childhood [Review]. Baillieres *Clinical Haematology* 1994; 7:815-827.

18. Felt BT, Lozoff B. Brain iron and behavior of rats are not normalized by treatment of iron deficiency anemia during early development. *J Nutr* 1996; 126:693-701.

19. Guiang SF, III, Georgieff MK, Lambert DJ, Schmidt RL, Widness JA. Intravenous iron supplementation effect on tissue iron and hemoproteins in chronically phlebotomized lambs. *Am J Physiol* 1997; 273:R2124-2131.

20. deUngria M, et al. Perinatal iron deficiency decreases cytochrome c oxidase activity in selected regions of neonatal rat brain. *Pediatr Res* 2000; 48:169-176.

21. Widdowson EM, Spray CM. Chemical development in utero. *Arch Dis Child* 1951; 26:205-214.

22. Dallman PR, Siimes MA. *Iron deficiency in infancy and childhood: a report for the international nutritional anemia consultative group.* Washington, DC: The Nutrition Foundation, 1979.

23. Shaw JCL. Parenteral nutrition in the management of sick low birth weight infants. *Pediatr Clin N Am* 1973; 20:333-358.

24. Oski FA, Naiman JL. The hematologic aspects of the maternal-fetal relationship. In: Oski FA, Naiman JL, eds. *Hematologic Problems in the Newborn. 3rd ed.* Philadelphia, PA; WB Saunders; 1982:32-55.

25. Singla PN, Gupta VK, Agarwal KN. Storage iron in human foetal organs. *Acta Paediatr Scand* 1985; 74:701-706.

26. Petry C, et al. Placental transferrin receptor in diabetic pregnancies with increased iron demand. *Am J Physiol* 1994; 121:109-114.

27. Stekel A. Iron requirements in infancy and childhood. In: *Iron Nutrition in Infancy and Childhood.* New York, NY: Raven Press; 1984:1-10.

28. Dallman PR. Review of iron metabolism. In: Filer LJ, ed. *Dietary Iron: Birth to Two Years.* New York, NY: Raven Press; 1989:1-18.

29. Kilbride J, Baker TG, Parapia LA, Khoury SA. Incidence of iron-deficiency anaemia in infants in a prospective study in Jordan. *Eur J Haematol* 2000;

64:231-236.

30. Chockalingam U, Murphy E, Ophoven JC, Weisdorf SA, Georgieff MK. Cord transferrin and ferritin levels in newborn infants at risk for prenatal uteroplacental insufficiency and chronic hypoxia. *J Pediatr* 1987; 111:283-286.

31. Georgieff M, et al. Abnormal iron distribution in infants of diabetic mothers: Spectrum and maternal antecedents. *J Pediatr* 1990; 117:455-461.

32. Petry C, et al. Iron deficiency of liver, heart, and brain in newborn infants of diabetic mothers. *J Pediatr* 1992; 121:109-114.

33. Saarinen UM, Siimes MA. Serum ferritin in assessment of iron nutrition in healthy infants. *Acta Paediatr Scand* 1978; 67:745-751.

34. Rios E, Lipschitz DA, Cook JD, Smith NJ. Relationship of maternal and infant iron stores as assessed by determination of plasma ferritin. *Pediatrics* 1975; 55:694-699.

35. Siimes MA, Koerper MA, Licko V, Dallman PR. Ferritin turnover in plasma: an opportunistic use of blood removed during exchange transfusion. *Pediatr Res* 1975; 9:127-129.

36. Lundstrom U, Siimes MA, Dallman PR. At what age does iron supplementation become necessary in low-birth weight infants? *J Pediatr* 1977; 91:878-883.

37. Halliday HL, Lappin TR, McClure G. Iron status of the preterm infant during the first year of life. *Biol Neonate* 1984; 45(5):228-35.

38. Strauss RG. Recombinant erythropoietin for the anemia of prematurity: Still a promise, not a panacea. *J Pediatr* 1997; 131:653-655.

39. Widness JA, Seward VJ, Kromer IJ, Burmeister LF, Bell EF, Strauss RG. Changing patterns of red blood cell transfusion in VLBW infants. *J Pediatr* 1996; 129:680-687.

40. Maier RF, Sonntag J, Walka MM, Liu G, Metze BC, Obladen M. Changing practices of red blood cell transfusions in infants with birth weight less than 1000 g. *J Pediatr* 2000; 136:220-224.

41. Oski FA. Iron requirements of the premature infant. In: Tsang RC, ed. *Vitamin and Mineral Requirements in Preterm Infants.* New York, NY: Marcel Dekker; 1985:9-21.

42. Ehrenkranz RA, Gettner PA, Nelli CM, Sherwonit EA, Williams JE, Pearson HA, et al. Iron absorption and incorporation into red blood cells by VLBW infants: studies with the stable isotope 58Fe. *J Pediatr Gastroenterol Nutr* 1992; 15:270-278.

43. Shaw JC. Iron absorption by the premature infant. The effect of transfusion and iron supplements on the serum ferritin levels. *Acta Paediatr Scand* 1982; 299: [Suppl] 83-89.

44. Dauncey MJ, Davies CG, Shaw JC, Urman J. The effect of iron supplements and blood transfusion on iron absorption by low birth weight infants fed pasteurized human breast milk. *Pediatr Res* 1978; 12:899-904.

45. Salvioli GP, Faldella G, Alessandroni R, Lanari M, Benfenati L. Plasma zinc concentrations in iron supplemented low birth weight infants. *Arch Dis Child* 1986; 61:346-348.

46. Dallman PR. Nutritional anemia of infancy: iron, folic acid, and vitamin B12. In: Tsang RD, Nichols BL, eds. *Nutrition During Infancy.* Philadelphia: Hanley and Belfus, 1988:216-235.

47. Carnielli VP, Da Riol R, Montini G. Iron supplementation enhances response to high doses of recombinant human erythropoietin in preterm infants. *Arch Dis Child Fetal Neonatal Ed* 1998; 79:F44-F48.

48. Bechensteen AG, Halvorsen S, Haga P, Cotes PM, Liestol K. Erythropoietin (Epo), protein and iron supplementation and the prevention of anaemia of prematurity: effects on serum immunoreactive Epo, growth, and protein and iron metabolism. *Acta Paediatr* 1996; 85:490-495.

49. Bader D, Kugelman A, Maor-Rogin N, Weinger-Abend M, Hershkowitz S, Tamir A, Lanir A, Attias D, Barak M. The role of high-dose oral iron supplementation during erythropoietin therapy for anemia of prematurity. *J Perinatology* 2001; 21: 215-220.

50. Kling PJ, Roberts RA, Widness JA. Plasma transferrin receptor levels and indices of erythropoiesis and iron status in healthy term infants. *J Pediatr Hematol Oncol* 1998; 20:309-314.

51. Abbas A, Snijders RJ, Sadullah S, Nicolaides KH. Fetal blood ferritin and cobalamin in normal pregnancy.

Fetal Diagn Ther 1994; 9:14-18.

52. Siimes MA. Hematopoiesis and storage iron in infants. In: Lonnerdal B, ed. *Iron Metabolism in Infants.* Boca Raton, FL: CRC Press; 1990:33-62.

53. Andrews NC. Disorders of iron metabolism. *N Engl J Med* 1999; 341:1986-1995.

54. Andrews NC. The iron transporter DMT1. *Int J Biochem Cell Biol* 1999; 31:991-994.

55. Gunshin H, Mackenzie B, Berger UV, Gunshin Y, Romero MF, Boron WF, et al. Cloning and characterization of a mammalian proton-coupled metal-ion transporter. *Nature* 1997; 388:482-488.

56. Berger TM, Polidori MC, Dabbagh A, Evans PJ, Halliwell B, Morrow JD, et al. Antioxidant activity of vitamin C in iron-overloaded human plasma. *J Biol Chem* 1997; 272:15656-15660.

57. Zlotkin SH, Lay DM, Kjarsgaard J, Longley T. Determination of iron absorption using erythrocyte iron incorporation of two stable isotopes of iron (57Fe and 58Fe) in VLBW premature infants. *J Pediatr Gastroenterol Nutr* 1995; 21:190-199.

58. Widness JA, Lombard KA, Ziegler EE, Serfass RE, Carlson SJ, Johnson KJ, et al. Erythrocyte incorporation and absorption of 58Fe in premature infants treated with erythropoietin. *Pediatr Res* 1997; 41:416-423.

59. Oettinger L, et al. Iron absorption in premature and full-term infants. *J Pediatr* 1954; 45:305-306.

60. Gorten MK, et al. Iron metabolism in premature infants, I: absorption and utilization of iron as measured by isotope studies. *J Pediatr* 1963; 63: 1063-1071.

61. Hall RT, Wheeler RE, Benson J, Harris G, Rippetoe L. Feeding iron-fortified premature formula during initial hospitalization to infants less than 1800 grams birth weight. *Pediatrics* 1993; 92:409-414.

62. Moody GJ, Schanler RJ, Abrams SA. Utilization of supplemental iron by premature infants fed fortified human milk. *Acta Pediatr* 1999;88:763-7.

63. McDonald MC, Abrams SA, Schanler RJ. Iron absorption and red blood cell incorporation in premature infants fed an iron-fortified infant formula. *Pediatr Res* 1998; 44:507-511.

64. Friel J, Andrews W, Hall M, et al. Intravenous iron administration to very low-birth weight newborns receiving total and partial parenteral nutrition. *J Parenteral Enteral Nutri* 1995; 19:114-118.

65. American Academy of Pediatrics Committee on Nutrition. Nutritional needs of preterm infants. In: Kleinman RE, ed. *Pediatric Nutrition Handbook.* Elk Grove Village, IL: American Academy of Pediatrics; 1998:55-87.

66. Fomon SJ, Nelson SE, Ziegler EE. Retention of iron by infants [In Process Citation]. *Ann Rev Nutr* 2000; 20:273-290.

67. Larsen L, Milman N. Normal iron absorption determined by means of whole body counting and red cell incorporation of 59Fe. *Acta Med Scand* 1975; 198:271-274.

68. Gorten MK, Cross ER. Iron metabolism in premature infants, II: prevention of iron deficiency. *J Pediatr* 1964; 64:509-520.

69. Doyle JJ, Zipursky A. Neonatal blood disorders. In: Sinclair JL, Bracken MB, eds. *Effective Care of the Newborn Infant.* Oxford, UK: Oxford University Press; 1992:426-453.

70. James JA, Combes M. Iron deficiency in the premature infant. Significance, and prevention by the intramuscular administration of iron-dextran. *Pediatrics* 1960; 26:368-374.

71. Hammond D, Murphy A. The influence of exogenous iron on formation of hemoglobin in the premature infant. *Pediatrics* 1960; 25:362-374.

72. Doyle JJ, Zypursky A. Neonatal blood disorders. In: Sinclair JC, Bracken MR, eds: *Effective care of the newborn infant.* Oxford, UK: Oxford University Press; 1992; 425-451.

73. Friel JK, Andrews WL, Aziz K, Kwa PG, Lepage G, L'Abbe MR. A randomized trail of two levels of iron supplementation and developmental outcome in low birth weight infants. *J Pediatr* 2001; 139:254-260.

74. Pollak A, Hayde M, Hayn M, Herkner K, Lombard KA, Lubec G, et al. Effect of intravenous iron supplementation on erythropoiesis in erythropoietin treated premature infants. *Pediatr* 2001; 107:78-85.

75. Shannon KM, Keith JF, 3rd, Mentzer WC, Ehrenkranz RA, Brown MS, Widness JA, et al. Recombinant human erythropoietin stimulates erythropoiesis and

reduces erythrocyte transfusions in VLBW preterm infants [see comments]. *Pediatrics* 1995; 95:1-8.

76. Franz AR, Mihatsch WA, Sander S, Kron M, Pohlandt F. Prospective randomized trial of early versus late enteral iron supplementation in infants with a birth weight of less than 1301 grams. *Pediatrics* 2000; 106:700-706.

77. Winzerling J, Kling P. Iron-deficient erythropoiesis in premature infants measured by blood zinc protoporphyrin/heme. *J Pediatr* 2001; 139:134-136.

78. Berger HM, Mumby S, Gutteridge JM. Ferrous ions detected in iron-overloaded cord blood plasma from preterm and term babies: implications for oxidative stress. *Free Radic Res* 1995; 22:555-559.

79. Dorea JG. Iron and copper in human milk. *Nutrition* 2000; 16:209-220.

80. Atinmo T, Omololu A. Trace element content of breastmilk from mothers of preterm infants in Nigeria. *Early Hum Dev* 1982; 6:309-313.

81. Lemons JA, Moye L, Hall D, Simmons M. Differences in the composition of preterm and term human milk during early lactation. *Pediatr Res* 1982; 16:113-117.

82. Mendelson RA, Anderson GH, Bryan MH. Zinc, copper and iron content of milk from mothers of preterm and full-term infants. *Early Hum Dev* 1982; 6:145-151.

83. Trugo NM, Donangelo CM, Koury JC, Silva MI, Freitas LA. Concentration and distribution pattern of selected micronutrients in preterm and term milk from urban Brazilian mothers during early lactation. *Eur J Clin Nutr* 1988; 42:497-507.

84. Aquilo E, Spagnoli R, Seri S, Bottone G, Spennati G. Trace element content of human milk during lactation of preterm newborns. *Biol Trace Elem Res* 1996; 52: 63-70.

85. Friel JK, Andrews WL, Jackson SE, et al. Elemental composition of human milk from mothers of premature and full-term infants during the first three months of lactation. *Biol Trace Elem Res* 1999; 67:225-247.

86. Perrone L, DiPalma L, DiToro R, Gialanella G, Moro R. Interaction of trace elements in a longitudinal study of human milk from full-term and preterm mothers. *Biol Trace Elem Res* 1994; 41:321-30.

87. Iwai Y, Takanashi T, Nakao Y, Mikawa H. Iron status in low birth weight infants on breast and formula feeding. *Eur J Pediatr* 1986; 145:63-65.

88. Bader D, Blondheim O, Jonas R, Admoni O, Abend-Winger M, Reich D, et al. Decreased ferritin levels, despite iron supplementation, during erythropoietin therapy in anaemia of prematurity. *Acta Paediatr* 1996; 85:496-501.

89. Ohls RK, Harcum J, Schibler KR, Christensen RD. The effect of erythropoietin on the transfusion requirements of preterm infants weighing 750 grams or less: a randomized, double-blind, placebo-controlled study [see comments]. *J Pediatr* 1997; 131:661-665.

90. Buonocore G, Zani S, Perrone S, Caciotti B, Bracci R. Intraerythrocyte nonprotein-bound iron and plasma malondialdehyde in the hypoxic newborn. *Free Radic Biol Med* 1998; 25:766-770.

91. Buonocore G, Zani S, Sargentini I, Gioia D, Signorini C, Bracci R. Hypoxia-induced free iron release in the red cells of newborn infants. *Acta Paediatr* 1998; 87:77-81.

92. Cooke RW, Drury JA, Yoxall CW, James C. Blood transfusion and chronic lung disease in preterm infants. *Eur J Pediatr* 1997; 156:47-50.

93. Hesse L, Eberl W, Schlaud M, Poets CF. Blood transfusion: Iron load and retinopathy of prematurity. *Eur J Pediatr* 1997; 156:465-470.

94. Melhorn DK, Gross S. Vitamin E-dependent anemia in the premature infant. I. Effects of large doses of medicinal iron. *J Pediatr* 1971; 79:569-580.

95. Friel JK, Serfass RE, Fennessey PV, Miller LV, Andrews WL, Simmons BS, et al. Elevated intakes of zinc in infant formulas does not interfere with iron absorption in premature infants. *J Pediatr Gastroenterol Nutr* 1998; 27:312-316.

96. Walraens PA, Hambidge KM. Growth of infants fed a zinc supplemented formula. *Am J Clin Nutr* 1976; 29:114-121.

97. Yip R, Reeves JD, Lonnerdal B, Keen CL, Dallman PR. Does iron supplementation compromise zinc nutrition in healthy infants? *Am J Clin Nutr* 1985; 42:683-687.

98. Haschke F, Ziegler EE, Edwards BB, Fomom SJ. Effect of iron fortification of infant formula on trace mineral absorption. *J Pediatr Gastroenterol Nutr* 1986; 5:768-773.

99. American Academy of Pediatrics Committee on Nutrition. Iron-fortified infant formulas. *Pediatrics* 1989; 84:114-115.

100. McCall KA, Huang C, Fierke CA. Function and mechanism of zinc metalloenzymes. *J Nutr* 2000; 130:1437S-14346S.

101. Zlotkin SH, Atkinson S, Lockitch G. Trace elements in nutrition for premature infants. *Clin Perinatol* 1995; 22:223-240.

102. Hambidge M. Human zinc deficiency. *J Nutr* 2000; 130:1344S-1249S.

103. Herrmann T, Krebs NF. Zinc nutrition in the fetus and preterm neonate. *Sem Neonatal Nutr Metabol* 2000; 7:5-7.

104. Zalewski PD, Forbes IJ, Seamark RF, et al. Flux of intracellular labile zinc during apoptosis (gene-directed cell death) revealed by a specific chemical probe, Zinquin. *Chem Biol* 1994; 1: 153-161.

105. Wastney ME, Angelus PA, Barnes RM, Subramanian KN. Zinc absorption, distribution, excretion, and retention by healthy preterm infants. *Pediatr Res* 1999; 45:191-196.

106. Krebs NF, Reidinger CJ, Miller LV, Hambidge KM. Zinc homeostasis in breast-fed infants. *Pediatr Res* 1999; 39:661-665.

107. Zlotkin SH, Buchanan BE. Meeting zinc and copper intake requirements in the parenterally fed preterm and full-term infant. *J Pediatr* 1983; 103:441-446.

108. Widdowson EM, Southgate DA, Hey E. Fetal growth and body composition. In: Lindblad BS, ed. *Perinatal Nutrition*. New York, NY: Academic Press, Inc; 1988:3-14.

109. Bahl L, Chaudhuri LS, Pathak RM. Study of serum zinc in neonates and their mothers in Shimla hills (Himachal Pradesh). *Indian J Pediatr* 1994; 61: 571-575.

110. Aggett PJ. Trace elements of the micropremie. *Clin Perinatol* 2000; 27:119-129.

111. Zlotkin SH, Cherian MG. Hepatic metallothionein as a source of zinc and cysteine during the first year of life. *Pediatr Res* 1988; 24: 326-329.

112. Cousins RJ, McMahon RJ. Integrative aspects of zinc transporters. *J Nutr* 2000; 130:1384S-1387S.

113. Krebs NF. Overview of zinc absorption and excretion in the human gastrointestinal tract. *J Nutr* 2000; 130:1374S-1377S.

114. Hara H, Konishi A, Kasai T. Contribution of the cecum and colon to zinc absorption in rats. *J Nut* 2000; 130:83-89.

115. Sandstrom B, Cederblad A, Lonnerdal B. Zinc absorption from human milk, cow's milk, and infant formulas. *Am J Dis Child* 1983; 137:726-729.

116. Solomons NW. Factors affecting the bioavailability of zinc. *J Am Diet Assoc* 1982; 80:115-121.

117. Ehrenkranz RA, Gettner PA, Nelli CM, et al. Zinc and copper nutritional studies in VLBW infants: comparison of stable isotopic extrinsic tag and chemical balance methods. *Pediatr Res* 1989; 26: 298-307.

118. Krebs NF, Reidinger CJ, Miller LV, Borschel MW. Zinc homeostasis in healthy infants fed a casein hydrolysate formula. *J Pediatr Gastroenterol Nutr* 2000; 30:29-33.

119. Lonnerdal B. Dietary factors influencing zinc absorption. *J Nutr* 2000; 130:1378S-1383S.

120. Friel JK, Andrews WL, Simmons BS, Miller LV, Longerich HP. Zinc absorption in premature infants: comparison of two isotopic methods. *Am J Clin Nutr* 1996; 63:342-347.

121. Wastney ME, Angelus P, Barnes R M, Subramanian KN. Zinc kinetics in preterm infants: a compartmental model based on stable isotope data. *Am J Physiol* 1996; 271:R1452-1459.

122. Atkinson SA, Whelan D, Whyte RK, Lonnerdal B. Abnormal zinc content in human milk. Risk for development of nutritional zinc deficiency in infants. *Am J Dis Child* 1989; 143:608-611.

123. Zimmerman AW, Hambidge KM, Lepow, Greenberg RD, Stover ML, Casey CE. Acrodermatitis in breast-fed premature infants: evidence for a defect of mammary zinc secretion. *Pediatrics* 1982; 69: 176-183.

124. Friel JK, Penney S, Reid DW, Andrews WL. Zinc, copper, manganese, and iron balance of parenterally fed VLBW preterm infants receiving a trace element supplement. *J Parenter Enteral Nutr* 1988; 12:382-386.

125. Caulfield LE, Zavaleta N, Figueroa A. Addition zinc

to prenatal iron and folate supplements improves maternal and neonatal zinc status in Peruvian population. *Am J Clin Nutr* 1999; 69:1257-1263.

126. Obladen M, Loui A, Kampmann W, Renz H. Zinc deficiency in rapidly growing preterm infants. *Acta Paediatr* 1998; 87:685-961.

127. Wauben I, Gibson R, Atkinson S. Premature infants fed mothers' milk to 6 months corrected age demonstrate adequate growth and zinc status in the first year. *Early Hum Dev* 1999; 54:181-194.

128. Rajaram S, Carlson SE, Koo WWK, et al. Plasma mineral concentrations in preterm infants fed a nutrient-enriched formula after hospital discharge. *J Pediatr* 1995; 126:791-796.

129. Friel JK, Andrews WL, Matthew JD, et al. Zinc supplementation in VLBW infants. *J Pediatr Gastroenterol Nutr* 1993; 17:97-104.

130. Friel JK, Gibson RS, Balassa R, Watts JL. A comparison of the zinc, copper and manganese status of VLBW preterm and full-term infants during the first twelve months. *Acta Paediatr Scand* 1984; 73:596-601.

131. Brunton JA, Saigal S, Atkinson SA. Growth and body composition in infants with bronchopulmonary dysplasia up to 3 months corrected age: a randomized trial of a high-energy nutrient-enriched formula fed after hospital discharge. *J Pediatr* 1998; 133: 340-345.

132. Lockitch G, Godolphin W, Pendray MR, Riddell D, Quigley G. Serum zinc, copper, retinol-binding protein, prealbumin, and ceruloplasmin concentrations in infants receiving intravenous zinc and copper supplementation. *J Pediatr* 1983; 102:304-348.

133. Uauy R, Olivares M, Gonzalez M. Essentiality of copper in humans. *Am J Clin Nutr* 1998; 67:952S-9S.

134. Widdowson EM. Trace elements in foetal and early postnatal development. *Proc Nutr Soc* 1974; 33: 275-84.

135. Beshgetoor D, Hambidge M. Clinical conditions altering copper metabolism in humans. *Am J Clin Nutr* 1998. 67: 1017S-21S.

136. Lonnerdal B, Bell JG, Keen CL. Copper absorption from human milk, cow's milk and infant formulas using a sucking rat model. *Am J Clin Nutr*

1985; 42: 836-44.

137. Linder MC, Wooten L, Cerveza P, Cotton S, Shulze R, Lomeli N. Copper transport. *Am J Clin Nutr* 1998; 67: 965S-71S.

138. Turnlund JR. Copper nutriture, bioavailability, and the influence of dietary factors. *J Am Diet Assoc* 1988; 88: 303-8.

139. Cordano A. Clinical manifestations of nutritional copper deficiency in infants and children. *Am J Clin Nutr* 1998; 67: 1012S-16S.

140. Kaler S.G. Diagnosis and therapy of Menkes syndrome, a genetic form of copper deficiency. *Am J Clin Nutr* 1998; 67: 1029S-34S.

141. Mercer F. Menkes syndrome and animal models. *Am J Clin Nutr* 1998; 67: 1022S-28S.

142. Brewer GJ. Wilson disease and canine copper toxicosis. *Am J Clin Nutr* 1998; 67: 1087S-90S.

143. Gitlin JD. Aceruloplasminemia. *Pediatric Research* 1998; 44: 271-6.

144. L'Abbe MR, Friel JK. Copper status of VLBW infants during the first 12 months of infancy. *Pediatr Res* 1992; 32:183-88.

145. Combs FR Jr, Combs SB. The role of selenium in nutrition. In: Walker WA, Watkins JB, eds. *Nutrition in Pediatrics: Science and Clinical Application.* Boston, MA: Little Brown, 1985; 17-45.

146. Gu J, et al. Selenium is required for normal upregulation of myelin genes in differentiating oligodendrocytes. *J Neurosci Res* 1997;47:626-635.

147. Castano A, Ayala A, Rodriquez-Gomez JA. Low selenium diet increases dopamine turnover in prefrontal cortex of the rat. *Neurochem Internat* 1997;30:549-555.

148. Watanabe C, Satoh H. Brain selenium status and behavioral development in selenium-deficient preweanling mice. *Physiol Behav* 1994;56:927-932.

149. Campos-Barros A, et al. Effects of selenium and iodine deficiency on thyroid hormone concentration in the central nervous system of the rat. *Eur J Endocrinol* 1997;136:316-323.

150. Chen X, et al. Studies on the relations of selenium and Keshan disease. *Biol Trace Elem Res* 1980;2: 91-107.

151. Sokoloff L. Kashin-Bech disease: current status.

Nutr Rec 1988;46:113-119.

152. Levander OA, Burk RF. Report on the 1986 ASPEN Research Workshop on Selenium in Clinical Nutrition. *JPEN* 1986;10:545-549.

153. Vinton NE, et al. Macrocytosis and pseudoalbinism: manifestations of selenium deficiency. *J Pediatr* 1987;111:711-717.

154. Bayliss PA, et al. Tissue selenium accretion in premature and full-term human infants and children. *Biol Trace Elem Res* 1985;7:755-761.

155. Sluis KB, et al. Selenium and glutathione peroxidase levels in premature infants in a low selenium community (Christchurch, New Zealand). *Pediatr Res* 1992;32:189-194.

156. Darlow BA, et al. The relationship of selenium status to respiratory outcome in the VLBW infant. *Pediatr* 1995;96:314-319.

157. Winterbourn CC, et al. Protein carbonyls and lipid peroxidation products as oxidation markers in preterm infant plasma: associations with chronic lung disease and retinopathy and effects of selenium supplementation. *Pediatr Res* 2000;48(1):84-90.

158. Darlow BA, et al. The effect of selenium supplementation on outcome in very low birth weight infants: a randomized controlled trial. The New Zealand Neonatal Study Group. *J Pediatr* 2000;136(4):473-480.

159. Ehrenkranz RA, et al. Selenium absorption and retention by very low birth weight infants: studies with the extrinsic stable isotope tag 74 Se. *J Pediatr Gastroentrol Nutr* 1991;13:125-133.

160. Abbas A, et al. Fetal blood ferritin and cobalamin in normal pregnancy. *Fetal Diagn Ther* 1994;9:4-18.

161. Friel JK, Andrews WL, Long DR, L'Abbe MR. Selenium status of VLBW infants. *Pediatr Res* 1993; 34: 293-296.

162. Daniels L, Gibson R, Simmer K. Randomised clinical trial of parenteral selenium supplementation in preterm infants. *Arch Dis Child Fetal Neonat ed* 1996;74:F158-164.

163. Rudolph N, et al. Hematologic and selenium status of low birth weight infants fed formulas with and without iron. *J Pediatr* 1981;9:57-62.

164. Smith AM, et al. Influence of feeding regimens on

selenium concentrations and gluthathione peroxidase activities in plasma on erythrocytes of infants. *J Trace Elem Exp Med* 1988;1:209-216.

165. Tyrala EE, Borschel MW, Jacobs JR. Selenate fortification of infant formulas improves the selenium status of preterm infants. *Am J Clin Nutr* 1996;64:860-865.

166. Institute of Medicine. Selenium. In: *Dietary Reference Intakes for Vitamin C, Vitamin E, Selenium, and Carotenoids. A Report of the Panel on Dietary Anti-oxidants and Related Compounds, Subcommittees on Upper Reference Levels of Nutrients and Interpretation and Uses of Dietary Reference Intakes and the Standing Committee on the Scientific Evaluation of Dietary Reference Intakes.* Washington, DC: National Academy Press; 2000: 284-324.

167. Mertz W. Chromium occurrence and function in biological systems. *Physiol Rev* 1969;49:163-239.

168. Yamamoto A, Waso O, Suzuki H. Purification and properties of biologically active chromium complex from bovine colostrum. *J Nutr* 1988;118:39-45.

169. Kitapci F, et al. Plasma chromium levels in hypoglycemic preterm, full-term and in intrauterine-growth retarded babies. *Biol Neonate* 1994;66(5):267-271.

170. Yurdakok M, et al. Plasma chromium levels in small-for-gestational-age newborn infants. *Turk J Pediatr* 1993; Jan-Mar;35(1):37-40.

171. Anderson RA, Kozlovsky AS. Chromium intake, absorption and excretion of subjects consuming self-selected diets. *Am J Clin Nutr* 1985;41: 1177-1183.

172. Jeejeebhoy DN, et al. Chromium deficiency, glucose intolerance, and neuropathy reversed by chromium supplementation, in a patient receiving long-term total parenteral nutrition. *Am J Clin Nutr* 1977;30:531-538.

173. Freund H, Atamian S, Fischer JE. Chromium deficiency during total parenteral nutrition. *JAMA* 1979;241:496-499.

174. Kumpulaninen J, Vuori E. Longitudinal study of chromium in human milk. *Am J Clin Nutr* 1980;33:2299-2302.

175. Casey CE, Hambidge KM. Chromium in human milk from American mothers. *Br J Nutr* 1984;52:73-77.

176. Bougle D, et al. Chromium status of full-term and preterm newborns. *Biol Trace Elem Res* 1992; Jan-Mar;32:47-51.

177. Johnson J, Wadman SK. Molybdenum cofactor deficiency. In: Scriver CR, Beaudet AL, Sly WS, Valle D, eds. *Metabolic Basis of Inherited Diseases.* 6th ed. New York, NY: McGraw Hill; 1989; 1463-1475.

178. Abumrad NN. Molybdenum—is it an essential trace metal? *Bull NY Acad Med* 1984;60:163-171.

179. Bougle D, et al. Molybdenum in the premature infant. *Biol Neonate* 1991;59(4):201-203.

180. Sievers E, et al. Molybdenum balance studies in premature male infants. *Euro J Pediatr* 2001;160(2):109-113.

181. Friel JK, MacDonald AC, Mercer CN, Belkhode SL, Downton G, Kwa PG, Aziz K, Andrews WL. Molybdenum requirements in low-birth weight infants receiving parenteral and enteral nutrition. *J Parenter Enteral Nutr* 1999; 23:155-159

182. Clerch JB, Wright AE, Coalson JJ. Lung manganese superoxide dismutase protein expression increases in the baboon model of bronchopulmonary dyslpasia and is regulated at a post-transcriptional leve. *Pediatr Res* 1996;39:253-258.

183. Cotzias GC, et al. Manganese and catecholamines. *Adv Neurol* 1974;5:235-243.

184. Mena I, et al. Modification of chronic manganese poisoning. *N Engl J Med* 1970;282:5-10.

185. Papavasiliou PS, Miller ST, Cotzias GC. Role of liver in regulation distribution and excretion of manganese. *Am J Physiol* 1966;211:211-216.

186. Cotzias GC, et al. Chronic manganese poisoning. *Neurology* 1968;18:376-382.

187. Zlotkin SH, Buchanan BE. Manganese intake in intravenously fed infants. *Biol Trace Elem Res* 1986;9:271-279.

188. Davidson L, et al. Manganese retention in man: a method for estimating manganese absorption in man. *Am J Clin Nutr* 1989;49:170-179.

189. Weigand E, Kirchgessner M. Radioisotope studies on true absorption of manganese. In: Mills CF,

Bremner I, Chesters JK, eds. *Trace Elements in Man and Animals.* Slough, UK: Commonwealth Agricultural Bureaux, 1985; 5:506-509.

190. Gan LS, Tan KT, Kwok SF. Biological threshold limit values for manganese dust exposure. *Sing Med J* 1988;29:105-109.

191. Mena I, et al. Chronic manganese poisoning: individual susceptibility and absorption of iron. *Neurology* 1964;19:1000.

192. Knudsen E, Sandstrom B, Andersen O. Zinc and manganese bioavailability from human milk and infant formula used for VLBW infants, evaluated in a rat pup model. *Biol Race Elem Res* 1995; Jul;49(1):53-65.

193. Casey CE, Robinson MF. Copper, manganese, zinc, nickel, cadmium and lead in human foetal tissue. *Br J Nutr* 1978;39:639-646.

194. Kurkus J, Alcock NW, Shiles ME. Manganese content of large volume parenteral solutions and of nutrient additives. *JPEN* 1984;8:254-257.

195. Hambidge KM, et al. Plasma manganese concentrations in infants and children receiving parenteral nutrition. *JPEN* 1989;13:168-171.

196. Delange F, et al. Increased risk of primary hypothyroidism in preterm infant. *J Pediatr* 1984;105:462-469.

197. Delange F, et al. Physiopathology of iodine nutrition during pregnancy, lactation, and early postnatal life. In: Berger H, ed. *Vitamins and Minerals in Pregnancy and Lactation. Nestle Nutrition Workshop Series, vol. 16.* New York, NY: Raven Press, Ltd., 1988; 205-214.

198. Castaing H, et al. Thyroide du ne et surcharge en iode apres la naissance. *Arch Rf Perinatal* 1979;36(4)365-368.

199. Linder N, et al. Topical iodine containing anitseptics and subclinical hypothyroidism in preterm infants. *J Pediatr* 1997;131:434-439.

200. Rogahn K, et al. Randomised trial of iodine intake and thyroid status in preterm infants. *Arch Dis Child Fetal Neonatal Ed* 2000; Sep;83(2):F86-90.

201. Fischer DA. Upper limit of iodine in infant formulas. *J Nutr* 1989;119:1865-1868.

202. Raiten DJ. Assessment of Nutrient Requirements for infant formulas. *J Nutrition* 1998; 128 (11S):

2167S-2169S.

203. Delange F, Bourdoux P, Senterre J. Evidence of a high requirement of iodine in preterm infants. *Pediatr Res* 1984;18:106.

Enteral Nutrition: Practical Aspects, Strategy and Management

Victor Y.H. Yu, M.D., M.Sc., FRACP, FRCP, FRCPCH and Karen Simmer, M.B.B.S., Ph.D., FRACP, FRCPCH

Reviewed by Sudha Kashyap, M.D.

Nutrition of the preterm infant has been a focus of research over the last decade with the increasing evidence from animal and human studies that early nutrition has a major impact on longterm health and intelligence. *In utero* growth retardation is associated with impaired neurodevelopment[1] and vascular disease.[2] Survival rates of infants born at the end of the second trimester and in the third trimester are high, but they often suffer extreme disturbances in nutrition. An association between poor growth and poor development has been reported in very low birth weight[3] and extremely low birth weight infants.[4] The mechanisms for this association remain uncertain. Disturbances in nutrition at different times of fetal and neonatal development, and adaptations to these disturbances, are likely to have varying effects. Attempts to enhance catch-up growth may not be beneficial.[5] Quantity and quality of nutrition in the preterm period is likely to impact the quality of the survival.

In this chapter, practical aspects and strategies of enteral nutrition in preterm infants and the management of common clinical problems are addressed in the light of information from physiological studies and randomized clinical trials (RCTs). Recommended intakes are discussed in other chapters. Intakes of preterm infants fed human milk are not necessarily the gold standards. *In utero* accretion rates, although difficult to achieve, may be a better standard, and the safety of high intakes of some nutrients must be evaluated.

Human Milk

The American Academy of Pediatrics has acknowledged the advantages of human milk feeding with the statement that it is the preferred feeding for all infants, including those born preterm.[6] Human milk protein is unique and considered to be of superior quality to cow milk, but the quantity of protein in human milk is less than that in formula, and this is associated with poor weight gain.[7] Human milk better meets the amino acid requirements of preterm infants, particularly with respect to taurine and cysteine. Human milk contains many nucleotides, hormones and growth factors, which are not in formula milk. Approximately 20% of the total nitrogen content of human milk is represented by non-protein nitrogen, and up to 20% of the latter consists of free nucleotides.[8] These are believed to be important in the growth and maturation of the gastrointestinal tract and in the development of neonatal immune function.[9] Dietary nucleotides have been found to favorably alter bowel microflora and to reduce the risk of diarrhea.[10,11] RCTs have enhanced mononuclear cell function and antibody responses in infants fed human milk.[12,13] The biological importance of human milk hormones and growth factors to the preterm infant remains uncertain.[14] Insulin-like growth factor-1, epidermal growth factor (EGF) and transforming growth factor alpha are believed to have trophic effects on the developing gastrointestinal tract.[15] Compared to formula-fed infants, those fed human milk have more rapid gastric emptying[16,17] and increased stool frequency.[18] Preterm infants fed human milk tolerate full enteral feeds more quickly and require less parenteral nutrition.[7]

There is epidemiological evidence that feeding human milk protects against the development of diabetes.[19,20] Formula milk with protein of bovine origin may interfere with the normal immune tolerance in genetically predisposed individuals, resulting in an autoimmune process preceding the onset of insulin-dependent diabetes (IDDM). A meta-analysis of twenty RCTs confirms that formula milk feeding is associated with the development of IDDM in childhood.[21] Breastfeeding or the use of formula with hydrolyzed protein has been associated with a reduced risk of wheeze, atopic disease, vomiting and diarrhea.[22] Possible mechanisms include: minimizing the dose of foreign protein; inducing earlier maturation of the natural mucosal barrier against entry of foreign protein; and/or providing passive protection against the entry of foreign protein (secretory IgA). In a RCT comparing preterm infants fed formula milk and banked human milk, the prevalence of allergic disease at eighteen months of age was unaffected,[23] but in the subgroup with a family history of allergy in first-degree relatives, formula-fed infants had more eczema, asthma and reactions to foods and drugs. Another study of preterm infants at eleven years of age has shown that symptoms of atopy were more frequent in those fed human milk.[24] Food allergens can pass into human milk and recommending a low allergen diet for the mother has been shown in RCT to reduce symptoms of colic.[25]

Preterm infants have reduced pancreatic and lingual lipase activities, and reduced bile acid pool. Human milk contains at least 60 enzymes, including lipase, which has been shown to enhance intestinal lipolysis and improve fat absorption.[26] Compared to formula milk, human milk has a higher content and unique pattern of longchain polyunsaturated fatty acids (LCPUFA) and gangliosides. LCPUFA are believed to be important for eicosanoid synthesis and cell membrane, cerebral and retinal function. Controversy remains over whether preterm infants are able to synthesize sufficient amounts of LCPUFA to satisfy the needs of their developing brain and retina.[6,27] Human milk gangliosides, which contain one or more sialic acid moieties, are also believed to have biological significance regarding neuronal development, as well as somatic growth and development of intestinal

immunity.[28,29] Clinical studies on ganglioside supplementation of formula milk have yet to be performed.

In addition to its nutritional advantages, human milk has anti-infective advantages when compared to formula milk. It contains live cells (macrophages, polymorphonuclear leukocytes, T and B lymphocytes) and a range of antimicrobial factors (secretory IgA, lactoferrin, lysozyme, B_{12} and folate-binding proteins, complement, fibronectin, mucin, and antiviral factors).[30] In developing countries, there is good RCT evidence in preterm infants that human milk feeding reduces the risk of infection.[31] This benefit remains when formula milk is used with fresh human milk,[32] but not if used with pasteurized human milk.[33] In developed countries, human milk feeding in preterm infants has also been shown to reduce the risk of infection (odds ratio [OR] = 0.43; 95% confidence interval [CI] 0.23, 0.81) and septicaemia/meningitis (OR = 0.47; 95% CI 0.23, 0.95).[34] Another study reported a significant reduction in the number of late-onset sepsis and the number of positive blood cultures.[35] The incidence of necrotizing enterocolitis (NEC) is reduced in preterm infants fed human milk.[36,37] Exclusively formula-fed preterm infants are reported to have a rate of NEC that is six times higher than those exclusively fed human milk, and three times higher than those fed human milk plus formula milk.[37]

Human milk cells and antimicrobial factors probably play a major role in conferring local immunological protection to the preterm gastrointestinal tract. The protection afforded by breastfeeding may also be partially explained by the regular nursery visits and skin-to-skin contact between mother and infant. The potential exists for the enteromammary immune system to function effectively in the preterm infant-mother dyad. The mother produces secretory IgA antibodies specific to the microorganisms she is exposed to when she visits the nursery and makes contact with her preterm infant. Ingestion of milk containing maternal antibodies against the nosocomial pathogens in the nursery environment and in her infant could potentially aid to promote the host defense of the infant. To this end, an open visiting policy, early skin-to-skin contact between mothers and their own infants, and human milk feeding are to be encouraged.

Preterm infants fed human milk, compared with those fed formula milk, have been shown to have improved cognitive performance at 18 months[38] and at 8 years of age.[39] An 8-point advantage in IQ (half a standard deviation) remained even after adjustment for mother's education and social class. Other studies comparing breastfed with formula-fed infants lose the association between breastfeeding and intelligence once confounding factors are considered; after multivariate analysis, only maternal IQ and environment/home score correlated with intelligence.[40] It is possible that genetic and/or environmental factors associated with the choice to breastfeed result in increased performance rather than the composition of human milk. The role that nutrients in human milk play in enhancing neurodevelopment remains an active research area as the majority of preterm infants receive more formula than human milk over the first year of life. Randomizing mothers to breastfeed or not is not possible. This fact and the complex confounding factors affecting the development of the sick preterm infant prevent concise studies. Follow-up of large numbers of preterm infants randomized to receive formula with varying compositions is feasible, but production of a formula that mimics the unique composition of human milk is unlikely.

Donor's Term Milk

The composition of human milk varies during the course of lactation and during a feed. With the exception of lactose, most nutritional components of human milk decline in concentration during the first few months of lactation, in particular protein, sodium, zinc and copper. Expressed donor milk obtained before an infant has had a breast feed (foremilk) has a lower fat and energy content, while that obtained after a breastfeed (hindmilk) has a higher fat and energy content. Drip breast milk collected from the contralateral breast during breast feeding has a lower protein, fat

and energy content (as low as 45 kcal/100ml).[41] Donors to human milk banks are likely to have given birth at term, and therefore well established for months into their lactation. RCTs comparing preterm infants fed banked term human milk with those fed formula milk have shown that the former had reduced growth rate, energy and nitrogen retention; lower serum phosphorus and higher alkaline phosphatase and higher bilirubin concentrations; lower scores on Brazelton neonatal behavioral assessment; and longer hospitalization.[42-47] Donor milk from mothers who have had a term delivery is nutritionally inadequate for preterm infants. For this reason and the fact that human immunodeficiency virus, human T-lymphotropic virus type 1, cytomegalovirus (CMV) and other viruses are excreted in breast milk,[28] the popularity of human milk banking declined.[48]

Mothers of preterm infants have varying success at expressing milk and breastfeeding, and some elect not to try. In 1980, the WHO and UNICEF jointly declared, "Where it is not possible for the biological mother to breastfeed, the first alternative, if available, should be the use of human milk from other sources. Human milk banks should be made available in appropriate situations."[49] The WHO/UNICEF Global Baby-Friendly Hospital Initiative[50] has since led to a revival of interest in milk banks. The few studies that compare fortified preterm milk with preterm formula suggest that the improved health (reduced incidence of NEC and sepsis) with human milk outweigh the slower weight gain. Larger RCTs comparing fortified pasteurized donor milk with preterm formula are required before consistent evidence-based recommendations can be made. At present, the Royal College of Paediatrics and Child Health in the United Kingdom[51] and the Human Milk Banking Association of North America[52] have both published guidelines for the establishment and operations of human milk banks. In 1991, the German Paediatric Society issued a position statement[53] in support of human milk banking. In 1995, the Canadian Paediatric Society issued a position statement[54] which did not support human milk banking. The Royal Australasian College of Physicians recommends the use of donor human milk only for preterm infants in clinical trials.[55]

Own Mother's Preterm Milk

Over 25 studies have been published to show that milk from mothers who have delivered before term has a different composition to milk from mothers who have delivered at term.[56] The former has a higher concentration of macrophages, secretory IgA and immune proteins, as well as protein, non-protein nitrogen, total lipid, LCPUFA, energy, sodium, chloride, calcium, magnesium, zinc, copper, iron, and vitamins such as retinol, tocopherol and D. The differences between preterm and term milk are particularly marked in early lactation (colostrum and transitional milk). However, there is considerable variation in the composition of preterm milk in late lactation, which might be even greater than the difference in mean composition between preterm and term milk. A RCT comparing feeding preterm milk with term milk has shown a shorter time to regain birthweight and an improvement in all growth parameters with preterm milk.[56] RCTs comparing unfortified preterm milk with both standard and preterm formula milk have shown that standard formula results in a similar growth rate as unfortified preterm milk, but preterm formula results in better growth and mineral status than unfortified preterm milk, although the size of the difference is less than that when preterm formula is compared with unfortified term milk.[57-59]

Feeding preterm infants with human milk from their own mothers has social and psychological benefits. Mothers become part of the team caring for the infants at a time when much of that care is delegated to others and suckling is impossible. Mothers of preterm infants need to be motivated to maintain their supply of express breast milk. They need to be given adequate emotional support and skilled assistance by sympathetic nursing staff. In an Australian study of preterm infants <1500g, 75% received preterm milk from their own mother and their breast-feeding rate was 44% at 3 months and 23% at 6 months.[60] This was similar to breastfeeding

rates in the community reported at the time of the survey. For optimal milk production, mothers need to express more than four times a day and cumulatively more than 100 minutes per day.[61,62] An electric breast pump is more effective than the hand pump or manual expression.[63] Oral metoclopramide, 10 mg eight hourly for one week, is effective in raising the basal serum prolactin level and in more than doubling milk production in mothers who have difficulty maintaining lactation after delivering preterm.[64] Another antidopaminergic agent, domperidone (10 mg eight hourly) also increases milk supply[65] and, unlike metaclopromide, is not excreted in human milk and does not cross the blood-brain barrier. Human growth hormone, 0.2 IU/kg/d given subcutaneously to a maximum of 16 IU/d for seven days, increases milk production by over 30% in mothers whose milk production is insufficient for their preterm infants' needs.[66] Mothers who are unable to maintain lactation during the period when their infants are too preterm or ill can be successfully induced to relactate after the immediate postpartum period.[67]

Collection, Storage and Processing

Human milk undergoes significant quantitative and qualitative changes through collection, storage, processing and refeeding. Manual expression of breast milk is associated with less bacterial contamination compared to the use of electric breast pumps.[68] Data are contradictory whether the practice of discarding the first few millilitres of expressed milk, which has a higher bacterial colony count than the remainder, is effective in reducing bacterial contamination.[69,70] Significant bacterial growth does not occur in human milk when stored in room temperature for up to 24 hours after expression for colostrum, and up to six hours for mature milk, because of bacteriostatic properties of human milk.[71] Heat treatment of human milk as a means to destroying microorganisms reduces nitrogen retention, fat absorption (enzymes including milk lipase are destroyed) and the concentration of water soluble vitamins.[72-74] Infants fed with raw preterm milk have been shown in an RCT to have greater weight gain than those fed with pasteurized preterm milk.[75] More than ten publications have shown that heat treatment also destroys or reduces antimicrobial factors such as viable leukocytes, immunoglobulins, lactoferrin, lysozyme, C3 complement, specific antibody to Escherichia coli, and vitamin B_{12} and folate binding proteins.[76] Only short low-temperature (56° C for 15 min)[77] or rapid high-temperature (72° C for 5-15 sec)[78] treatments reduce bacterial contamination without destroying most antimicrobial factors in human milk. However, equipment for such precise pasteurizing processes is not generally available.

Because heat treatment is either a detrimental or an expensive process, it is advisable for human milk to be refrigerated to retard bacterial growth if not used soon after expression. It has been shown that storage of human milk at 3-4° C maintains stability of nutrients (except Vitamin C) and preserves viability and function of leukocytes and concentration of antimicrobial proteins.[79,80] Paradoxically, there is a progressive decrease in the bacterial colony count and positive bacterial culture rate over a 5-day period, partly due to the refrigeration process itself and partly to the inhibitory effect of antimicrobial factors in human milk.[81] Since no study had extended beyond 5 days, human milk stored for a longer period should be frozen. Freezing destroys milk leukocytes, but most nutrients and antimicrobial proteins are preserved.[80,82,83] A microwave oven should not be used to thaw frozen human milk or to warm refrigerated human milk, as microwave destroys most of its antimicrobial factors.[84] No agreement has been reached on the need for bacteriological surveillance of expressed and stored human milk.[85] Such routine screening is not performed in most neonatal units. If surveillance is done, colony counts of greater than 10,000/ml are considered unacceptable contamination by most human milk banks. Although microorganisms arising from the skin and mammary ducts and bacterial pathogens do contaminate expressed human milk, serious morbidity is rare.[86] Of concern is the fact that CMV is transmitted to the infant via milk of a seropositive mother.[87] In preterm infants, this can cause significant disease.[88] Freezing the milk at -20° C will reduce the risk. This is not routinely done in most neonatal units, even though great effort is taken to eliminate the risk of CMV transmission via donor blood transfusions.

Fortified Preterm Milk

The initial growth rate and accretion rates of nitrogen, fat, sodium, potassium and chloride in preterm infants fed their own mother's milk approximate expected intrauterine rates.[89-92] However, as the nutrient concentration progressively drops with time, preterm milk collected after thirty days postpartum has a protein, sodium, calcium, phosphorus and magnesium content that is too low to meet the requirements of growing preterm infants. Feeding with expressed hindmilk results in improved weight gain as it has a higher fat content than foremilk.[93] Alternatively, through a process of human milk lacto-engineering, human milk can be fortified with skim and cream components derived from heat-treated, lyophilized mature donor human milk to produce a "human milk formula."[94-99] This method of fortification avoids cow's milk proteins, but it is impractical for most neonatal units, since it involves a complex process and requires a large supply of donor milk.

Preterm human milk fortified with protein of bovine origin has become the standard practice in most neonatal units. One study comparing a fortifier containing bovine-derived proteins with one derived from freeze-dried human milk, showed no difference in nitrogen balance, fat absorption and weight gain.[100] There are more than half a dozen commercially available "human milk fortifiers" which, when added to human milk, provide 2.5 g/kg/d protein and 120 kcal/kg/d energy. They vary in composition qualitatively and quantitatively but in general, they contain bovine whey-predominant protein (intact or hydrolyzed), carbohydrate which is mainly or exclusively glucose polymers or maltodextrins, and macronutrients such as sodium, calcium, phosphorus and magnesium. Some fortifiers contain fat and/or lactose. Some also contain micronutrients (zinc and copper) and vitamins, though RCTs comparing fortifiers with or without these components have revealed no differences in growth, plasma calcium, phosphorus and copper concentrations, and zinc status up to one year of age.[101,102]

Cochrane Reviews have concluded that protein supplementation or multicomponent fortification of human milk increases nitrogen retention, short-term weight gain, linear and head growth, and bone mineral content (BMC), but there is no such evidence to recommend fat supplementation.[103-105] The data are insufficient, however, to evaluate long-term growth and neurodevelopment. Developmental scores at eighteen months in one RCT were found to be higher in the fortified group, though the difference did not reach statistical significance.[106] Most RCTs show that preterm infants fed fortified preterm milk have a growth rate equivalent to that in infants fed preterm formula, while those fed unfortified preterm milk have a slower growth rate similar to that in infants fed standard formula. Short-term fortification of calcium and phosphorus supplementation for 5-6 weeks does not improve mineral status.[107-109] However, preterm infants fed at least 8-12 weeks of fortified preterm milk have been shown to have significant improvements in calcium and phosphorus balance, serum calcium, phosphorus and alkaline phosphatase, tubular reabsorption of phosphate and BMC compared with those fed unfortified milk.[110,111] One study, which measured BMC of the infant's whole body by dual energy X-ray absorptiometry, demonstrated that the BMC of infants fed fortified human milk was similar to that of those fed preterm formula at 3 months.[112] Their BMC were similar to that of term infants, having caught up regardless of diet by 6 months post-term. Recently, preterm infants who were randomized to receive donor human milk or preterm formula in the neonatal period were reported to have similar BMC measured by dual X-ray absorptiometry at 9-12 years of age despite large differences in early mineral intake.[113] In summary, there is little evidence that fortification of human milk has a long-term effect on BMC.

Routine analysis of human milk to guide fortification rarely occurs. However, considerable variation occurs in the composition of human milk during breast expression, depending on the stage of lactation and the mother, and the simple addition of a fixed proportion of fortifier could potentially lead to either inadequate or excessive nutrient intakes. It has been estimated that in general, an intake of 180 ml/kg/d of fortified preterm milk is required to achieve optimal nutrient intake, compared to about 160 ml/kg/d of preterm formula.[114] For preterm infants above 32 weeks gestation or over 1500 g birthweight, fortification is probably unnecessary if they are able to tolerate at least 180 ml/kg/d of preterm milk.[56] The use of a human milk fortifier is recommended for the more immature or smaller preterm infants, beginning from the time when they are able to tolerate 100 ml/kg/d of milk. The delay in commencing fortification is because of concerns that it might increase feed intolerance or the rate of sepsis and NEC. Conflicting results were obtained on the effect of fortification on the rate of gastric emptying, probably because of differences in the composition of the fortifier and the gestational and postnatal ages of the study infants.[115,116] Clinical observations, including one RCT, have not shown an association between the use of fortifiers and feed intolerance, as manifest by abdominal distension, increased gastric aspirate, vomiting or change in stool frequency.[106,117] Preterm infants receiving fortifiers were found in one RCT to have significantly more infections, but the incidence of NEC was not significantly increased.[106] Some anti-infective properties of human milk are affected by the addition of fortifier, (for example, lysozyme activity is reduced).[118] However, IgA concentration is not affected, and it has been found to be safe to store human milk for 24 hours after the addition of fortifier before it is used.[119]

Formula Milk
Term Formula

The composition of standard formula is modeled on that of mature term human milk. Protein, sodium, calcium, phosphorus and several micronutrients do not meet the needs of the preterm infant. It is therefore nutritionally inadequate as well as lacking in the non-nutritive factors present in human milk. Soy-based formulas in particular should not be used.

Soy protein is of low bioavailability and there is increased loss of macronutrients, micronutrients and vitamins, some of which are bound to phytate. Other problems reported include low plasma levels of methionine (growth impairment), chloride (hypochloraemic metabolic alkalosis) and iodine, and the composition of soy formula has been amended to avoid these deficiencies. Concerns have also been expressed over the high content of aluminium and phytoestrogen of soy formula.

Preterm Formula

If human milk from the preterm infant's own mother is not available for use with the addition of human milk fortifier, the next best choice is preterm formula. These are designed to meet the increased nutritional needs of preterm infants. Compared to unfortified human milk or term formula, preterm formula contains more protein, sodium, calcium, phosphorus, zinc, copper and vitamins, often in a form that is more easily absorbed and metabolized.[120] Most have an energy content of about 80 kcal/100 ml (24 kcal/oz). In spite of the higher carbohydrate and mineral content, the osmolality of preterm formulas remains low at around 250-320 mOsm/kg H_2O.

Preterm formulas contain at least 2 g/100 ml of protein so that the preterm infant will receive 3 g/kg/d of protein when fed at 150 ml/kg/d. During the stable growing period, a protein intake of 3.5-4.0 g/kg/d is recommended for preterm infants born <1000 g and 3.0-3.6 g/kg/d for those born >1000 g.[121] RCTs have shown that raising the protein intake from 2 to 4 g/kg/d improves weight gain, linear growth, nitrogen retention and serum albumin.[122-127] Increasing the protein intake further from 4 to 6 g/kg/d does not result in more weight gain[122] but is associated with fever and lethargy, and on follow-up, an increased incidence of strabismus and low developmental scores.[127] Since protein cannot be utilized efficiently when energy intake is low, 100 kilocalories should be provided for every 2-3 grams of protein intake. RCTs have shown that preterm infants tolerate whey-predominant protein better than casein-predominant protein with lower blood ammonia, phenylalanine and

tyrosine levels and higher taurine levels.[122,128] The whey-predominant preterm formulas, with their higher protein content, have been shown to be metabolically safe with normal plasma aminograms.[129,130] The use of protein hydrolysates in some preterm formulas is aimed to reduce the risk of atopy associated with exposure to intact cow milk protein.[131] However, these formulas have been reported to result in reduced nitrogen absorption and retention and phosphorus absorption when compared with formulas containing intact cow milk protein.[132]

The carbohydrate content in preterm formula is around 8-9 g/100 ml, but the lactose content is reduced to 40-80% of the total carbohydrate content to minimize the risk of lactose intolerance, while not eliminating the stimulus necessary for induction of intestinal lactase activity.[133] The balance of the carbohydrate content is provided by high molecular weight glucose polymers, which have a similar glycemic response, but with a lesser insulin response compared to lactose in preterm infants.[134] Reducing the lactose in preterm formulas is beneficial, as intestinal lactase activity remains low up to 25-weeks gestation when it rises slowly until 32 weeks, following which there is a rapid increase.[135]

Some preterm formulas are supplemented with LCPUFA. A Cochrane Review has concluded that LCPUFA supplementation confers no benefit in preterm infants, but there is evidence that their early rate of visual maturation is increased.[136] No studies to determine long-term effects have been performed. Improving the ratio of the precursor essential fatty acids, linoleic acid and alpha linolenic acid, to enhance the infant's ability to synthesize their own LCPUFA may be sufficient. A recently published large RCT of LCPUFA supplementation of preterm formula confirms the benefit on visual acuity reported by the Cochrane Review as well as demonstrates a significantly higher Bayley Motor Developmental Index at 12 months in infants below 1250 g birth weight.[137] Preterm infants have poor absorption of long-chain triglycerides, due mainly to a reduced pancreatic lipase activity and reduced bile acid pool size and secretion rate.[26] The digestion of medium-chain triglycerides (MCT) is independent of bile salts and, in some preterm formulas, MCT is 40% of the fat. However, RCTs have shown that MCT-enriched formulas may not result in improvement in fat absorption, energy storage, nitrogen retention or growth[138-142] (ie, MCT supplements reduce levels of circulating docosahexaenoic acid).[143] RCTs which compare preterm formulas with a high or low MCT content have shown that the former is associated with a higher incidence of adverse gastrointestinal effects including abdominal distension, increased gastric aspirate, vomiting, loose stools and NEC.[144,145]

Preterm infants fed preterm formula have been shown to grow at a rate that is at or above intrauterine growth rate.[144-151] Infants fed formula have a higher body fat content but whether this is a good adaptation to the extra-uterine environment or deleterious in the long-term, is not known. RCTs have reported significant benefits of preterm formula over term formula, with higher growth rate and developmental scores at eighteen months.[42,152] The gains with preterm formula are especially striking in small for gestational age infants and in males, both of whom are particularly at higher risk for developmental delay. The rate of NEC among infants fed preterm formula is similar to those fed term formula.[40] An RCT comparing the use of preterm formula versus donor human milk, used exclusively or as a supplement to preterm human milk, reports higher developmental scores at nine-months-corrected age with preterm formula,[153] though the differences at eighteen months do not remain statistically significant.[154]

Practical Aspects
Tube Feeding
Nasogastric or orogastric gavage feeding is the most common method of enteral feeding in preterm infants before 32-34 week's gestation who lack coordination of sucking, swallowing and breathing. A nasogastric tube is easier to fix in place than an orogastric tube, but it increases airway resistance and work of breathing and decreases minute ventilation.[155,156] An RCT has shown an increased incidence of periodic breathing and

central apnea when a nasogastric tube is used.[157] Removal of the gavage tube results in reduced apnea rates and improved oxygenation. Intermittent placement will overcome the problems of an indwelling tube, but correct placement is vital. The position can be checked by testing the gastric aspirate for acidity with litmus paper or by "syringing" into the tube several millilitres of air whilst listening with a stethoscope placed over the stomach.

Should the preterm infant, who as a fetus is fed continuously, be fed in the same manner or be fed intermittently? Oxygenation falls consistently after an intragastric bolus feed in preterm infants recovering from respiratory distress, even with a small volume of 5 ml/kg delivered slowly by the gravity method.[158-162] Higher feed volumes result in a significant decrease in tidal volume, minute ventilation, dynamic compliance, functional residual capacity and cerebral perfusion, and a significant increase in pulmonary resistance and oxygen consumption.[163-168] Energy expenditure has been found to be higher with intermittent feeding compared to continuous feeding.[169] However, continuous tube feeding is associated with increased bacterial contamination, and loss of nutrients which adhere to the internal wall of the infusion set. Nutrient losses are significantly greater than those with bolus feeding: 24% for energy, 34% for fat and 5% for protein.[170,171] Since fat tends to float to the top of the syringe, fat loss during continuous milk infusion can be reduced by using eccentric nozzle syringes with the nozzle in an uppermost position and set at an angle so that the nozzle end of the syringe is higher than its plunger end.[172] Losses also occur for macronutrients and micronutrients when human milk fortifier in the powder form is added to milk: 43% for calcium, 40% for phosphorus, 9% for magnesium, 26% for zinc and 12% for copper.[173] Such losses are less pronounced when a liquid fortifier is used. Significant increases in aerobic flora and coliforms have been documented in human milk from the syringe kept at ambient room temperature in the neonatal unit.[174] Although advocates of continuous intragastric feeding are adamant that there is "little reason for the routine use of bolus feeds in the small preterm infant,"[175] a

Cochrane Review has concluded that infants on continuous intragastric feeding take longer to reach full enteral feeds compared with those on intermittent bolus feeding (weighted mean difference 3 days, 95% CI 0.7, 5.2).[176] Bolus feeds will likely increase gastric capacity and stimulate the gastric-colic reflex without increasing the frequency of apneas, growth rate, length of hospital stay, or incidence of NEC. Most neonatal units routinely use intermittent intragastric feeding, but if difficulties with feed tolerance occur, continuous intragastric feeding might be worth trying.

A number of RCTs have examined the possible benefits of routine continuous nasoduodenal or nasojejunal feeding over intragastric feeding in preterm infants.[177-183] They show no difference in energy intake, growth rate or complications such as aspiration pneumonia, diarrhea and NEC. Absorption of nitrogen and fat decreases with transpyloric feeding; it bypasses the stomach, where gastric and lingual lipases normally hydrolyzes one-third of the ingested triglycerides. A meta-analysis of RCTs published over a decade ago has indicated that not only was there no benefit, there was an increase in mortality rate by about 15% with transpyloric feeding.[184] Transpyloric feeding might be useful in selected preterm infants with extremely poor gastric emptying and symptomatic gastro-esophageal reflux (GOR), but intragastric feeding should be resumed as soon as feasible. Gastrostomy feeds are not usually recommended for preterm infants. One RCT comparing gastrostomy with conventional feeding showed no difference in milk intake or growth rate and showed a higher mortality rate with gastrostomy feeding.[185]

Non-nutritive Sucking

Thirteen RCTs have examined the benefits of giving preterm infants the opportunity to suck on a pacifier before, during or after gavage feeding. The rationale is that non-nutritive sucking facilitates development of sucking behavior and transition to nipple feeding, as well as improves digestion by stimulating lingual lipase. A Cochrane Review has concluded that non-nutritive sucking shortens transition from tube to sucking feeds and the length of hospital stay.[186] No

consistent benefits are found with respect to heart rate, oxygen saturation, gastric emptying, intestinal transit, energy intake or weight gain. No negative effect on breastfeeding or on the incidence of later oral aversion has been reported, which is different to the situation in term infants where pacifier use is thought to inhibit the initiation of breastfeeding. Most preterm infants appear to learn to breast and bottle feed. A recent large RCT of pacifier and/or cup feeding in preterm infants found no effect of pacifier use and a marginal benefit of encouraging cup over bottle supplementation on the rate of breastfeeding at discharge.[187] Pacifiers may be useful for sedating infants in the neonatal unit, but prolonged use after discharge may be deleterious to development. One study of term infants reported an association between pacifier use and lower intelligence.[188]

Strategy

Trophic Feeding

It is often impossible to rely only on enteral feeding alone in preterm infants who are <1000 g or are critically ill. Although parenteral feeding is the main source of nutrition in such infants where nutritive enteral feeding is impossible, inadequate or hazardous, early introduction of nutritionally inconsequential amounts of enteral trophic feeding is vital. Colostrum should be used for the first feed, but if aspiration is a major concern, sterile water should be used, as glucose water elicits as much of an inflammatory reaction in the lung as milk.[189] Hourly feeds are generally used in infants <1000 g but subnutritional quantities of milk may be commenced at one millilitre every 2-4 hours. "Trophic feeding" is synonymous with "minimal enteral nutrition," "gut priming," and "early hypocaloric feeding." Gut atrophy develops rapidly in experimental animals and preterm infants maintained on total parenteral feeding. Plausible explanations include an absence of agents in milk that are trophic to the gastrointestinal tract,[15] lack of induction of gastrointestinal motor activity development,[190] lack of luminal nutrients, and failure to release trophic enteric hormones.[191]

A Cochrane Review reports that trophic feeding

reduces the number of days to full enteral feeding, total days that feeding has to be withheld, and length of hospital stay.[192] Another Cochrane Review compared early (mean or median age four days or less) and late (over four days) initiation of progressive enteral feeding, and reports that the former group has fewer days on parenteral nutrition and fewer infants have interruption of feeds, require percutaneous central venous catheters, or have sepsis evaluation.[193] One study reports that early enteral feeds increase the risk of NEC when formula milk is used but not when human milk is used.[37] Care needs be taken when adding medications to small volume feeds, as many medications have an osmolality of over 3000 mOsm/kg H_2O. An osmolality of over 600 mOsm/kg H_2O has been associated with NEC.[194] None of the RCTs has reported adverse effects of trophic feeding, in particular NEC.[195] Individually, some RCTs have reported enhanced whole gut motility and less indirect hyperbilirubinaemia, cholestatic jaundice and osteopenia of prematurity.[196-198] A recently published large RCT confirms the benefits reported by the Cochrane Reviews as well as demonstrates other benefits including greater energy intake and head growth, fewer days on oxygen therapy, and half as many episodes of infection.[199] The latter could be secondary to a decreased need for parenteral nutrition, but it might be explained by a reduction in the translocation of enteric pathogens into the circulation because of the decreased mucosal permeability secondary to enhanced gut maturation induced by the trophic effects of enteral feeds.[200]

Progression of Feeds

Preterm infants commenced on trophic feeding can have their feed volume progressively increased as their clinical condition stabilizes and feed tolerance improves over the ensuing days or weeks. In order to determine feed tolerance, the gavage tube should be aspirated regularly before a feed. Gastric aspirates are usually measured four hourly in the infants less than 32-weeks gestation. The aspirate is returned to reduce loss of enzymes and electrolytes. Repeated aspiration of volumes of over two-thirds of the previous feed usually

signifies feed intolerance, and feeds should be reduced or ceased. Conflicting results have been reported in RCTs assessing the benefits of full-strength versus half-strength formulas during the grading-up process.[201,202] Dilute feeds do not promote maturation of gut motility as well as full-strength feeds,[203] and there is little rationale behind the practice of diluting feeds. Studies using historical controls[204-206] and case-controlled studies[207-209] have suggested that rapid advancement of enteral feeds may increase the risk of NEC. However, a Cochrane Review has concluded that a more rapid rate of advancing feeds results in a shorter time to achieve full enteral feeds and shorter time to regain birth weight, with no effect on NEC (relative risk = 0.90, 95% CI 0.46, 1.77).[210] The ideal rate of advancement remains unclear, though daily increments in the range of 10-35 ml/kg appear to be safe. If abdominal distension, bile-stained aspirates or diarrhea develops, feeds should be reduced or ceased.

Healthy preterm infants who are >1500 g often do not require intravenous therapy after birth and should be commenced on gavage feeds as soon as feasible before 2 hours of age. A volume of 60-90 ml/kg/d is commonly employed on the first day, given 4-hourly for infants >2000 g, 3-hourly for 1500-2000 g, and 2-hourly for 1000-1500 g. The volume can generally be increased to 100-150 ml/kg/d by the end of the first week and 150-200 ml/kg/d by the end of the second week. Only one RCT compared demand feeding with scheduled feeding in preterm infants after they have established full enteral feeds on a 4-hourly regimen.[211] It shows that although demand-fed infants have similar daily milk intakes, they require fewer gavage feeds and are able to be discharged from hospital earlier. Some sucking feeds need be established before term to avoid the development of a feeding dyspraxia. Mother's own milk is the preferred feed, and stored milk is fed in the order that it was expressed. If this is unavailable, a preterm formula should be chosen. Vitamin and mineral supplementation will depend on the composition of the fortifier or formula chosen.[120]

Medium-chain triglyceride oil or glucose polymers are occasionally used as an energy supplement for preterm infants with chronic lung disease or heart disease. Studies have shown that, whereas glucose polymers will increase weight gain,[212] the metabolic cost of MCT oil negates any benefit.[213]

After discharge, growth may slow initially, especially if full breastfeeding is being established. The growth standard by tradition is based on formula-fed infants, and breastfeeding growth curves differ from formula-feeding growth curves partly due to the increased fat deposition in formula-fed infants. In one study, breastfeeding of SGA infants after discharge promoted faster growth than formula feeding.[214] Breastfeeding from predominantly one breast per feed is often recommended for term infants.[215] For preterm infants, especially those with chronic lung disease, breastfeeding from both breasts at each feed, before the infant tires, is likely to result in increased intake compared with feeding from predominantly one breast per feed, as most milk is consumed in the first five minutes of feeding from each breast. If growth failure occurs after discharge due to inadequate intake, fortification of expressed human milk or the use of a "follow-on" preterm formula will provide more nutrition than increasing the strength of term formula or adding standard formula to human milk.

Management
Gastrointestinal Dysmotility
Functional immaturity of gastrointestinal motility predisposes preterm infants to feed intolerance. Motilin is a gastrointestinal peptide that stimulates gastric emptying and propagative contractile activity in the proximal small intestine. Erythromycin, a macrolide antibiotic, is a motilin agonist with potent prokinetic properties. It has been used to improve gastrointestinal motility in selected preterm infants who fail to establish full enteral feeding at several weeks of age after an obstructive lesion of the gastrointestinal tract has been ruled out. Low oral doses (1-3 mg/kg/dose) enhance the phase 3 migrating motor complex at the antral level, whereas high doses (up to 12.5 mg/kg/dose) result in sustained antral contractile activity and improve antroduodenal coordination.[216] From earlier reports, erythromycin appears to be less effective in infants below 32-weeks

gestation, and a Cochrane Review based on two RCTs is inconclusive with regard to its effectiveness.[217] However, a recent RCT reports that oral erythromycin at a dose of 12.5 mg/kg/dose every six hours is effective in preterm infants <1500 g with moderately severe gastrointestinal dysmotility who tolerate less than half their daily intake by the enteral route by 14 days of age.[218] The median times taken to establish half or full enteral feeding in the placebo group are almost twice as long. Although oral erythromycin does not have the adverse cardiac effects of intravenous erythromycin and does not appear to promote the emergence of resistant organisms, it should not be used prophylactically in preterm infants.

Gastro-oesophageal Reflux
GOR is a commonly suspected problem in preterm infants, especially in those with chronic lung disease, although most GOR episodes are asymptomatic and there does not appear to be a clear association between GOR and apnea.[219] Although oesophageal pH studies over a 24-hour period provide useful information not available from other methods of investigating GOR, there is considerable variability in the pH pattern between "normal" infants[220] and between repeated studies on the same infant.[221] Positioning, feed thickening, antacids and cholinergics have not been shown to be effective in GOR. Formulas thickened by replacing some of the lactose with carob bean flour, rice starch or pregelatinized corn starch, are marketed for the treatment of GOR. There is little evidence that thickened formulas reduces GOR and some evidence that they actually delay gastric emptying and exacerbate symptoms of GOR.[222,223] Cisapride[224] and fundoplication[225] are being used in the treatment of GOR. However, RCTs have shown that cisapride does not decrease the time to establish enteral feeds; instead, it delays gastric emptying and whole gastrointestinal transit time.[226,227] Many neonatal units have stopped using cisapride because it predisposes to cardiac arrhythmia, especially when the QTc is over 450 msec and can potentially cause sudden infant death.[228]

Lactose Intolerance

The relatively high lactose content of human milk and term formula can be a problem for the preterm infant. Excessive lactose intake results in diarrhea and metabolic acidosis, and is one of the factors postulated in the pathogenesis of NEC. Undigested lactose, fermented by bacteria to lactate and hydrogen gas, accounts for the increase in fecal-reducing substances, urinary D-lactate excretion and breath hydrogen excretion found prior to or coincident with the onset of NEC. Excess carbohydrate in the small intestine is fermented by bacteria to organic acids, which combine with the undigested protein and results in the pathological changes of NEC in the preterm gut.[229] Excessive lactose can also reach the colon in preterm infants[230] where it increases bacterial proliferation and, together with bacterial antigens, exerts a local inflammatory effect on colonic mucosa.[231] Rarely, physiological lactose intolerance results in weight loss and requires treatment with a low lactose formula. Alternatively, lactose in human milk can be digested with lactase. This needs to be done prior to feeding as lactase is neutralized by gastric acid.[232] Caution needs to be taken when treating lactose intolerance in preterm infants, as the signs may be due to early NEC.

Conclusions

The statement has been made that the extremely preterm infant born under 1000 g presents a "nutritional emergency."[233] Even with the best efforts to commence parenteral nutrition from day one and to establish enteral feeds as early as possible, weight loss exceeds 10% and birth weight is not regained for two weeks[234,235] due to inadequate energy intake, especially in those with respiratory failure.[236] The deficit in the first postnatal weeks is of sufficient magnitude to make catch-up growth virtually impossible, even though by the fourth week, a growth rate at or above the intrauterine growth rate can be achieved.[234] Extrauterine growth retardation is a serious problem that results in a doubling of the number of infants below the third percentile for weight between birth and hospital discharge.[3,4,56] Although these studies have reported some catch-up growth after

weaning from milk feeding, the idea of "nutritional programming" has been suggested in which a stimulus or insult applied at a critical and sensitive period of the preterm infant's development could have a lifetime impact on the quality of survival. With increasing evidence that a suboptimal diet and early growth deficits have long-lasting effects including short stature, impaired health, and poor neurodevelopmental outcomes,[3,4] more definitive targeted RCTs designed to test both short and long-term safety and efficacy of specific nutritional management in preterm infants are encouraged. In spite of the fact that this chapter has listed over sixty RCTs and twelve meta-analyses of published RCTs, many of the presumptions used in making choices on enteral nutrition in preterm infants are yet to be evidence-based. Nonetheless, whatever practice is adopted within a given neonatal unit, it must be consistent enough that its outcome can be audited and correlated to the clinical approach that has been chosen.

Case Study

Baby C was born at 26-weeks gestation weighing 800 gms. Baby C was incubated and ventilated soon after birth for respiratory distress syndrome. He received artificial surfactant and was extubated to nasal CPAP on day 5 and to headbox oxygen on day 10. Baby C received intravenous caffeine prior to extubation.

Parenteral nutrition was commenced on day 2. Minimal enteral feeding with expressed breast milk (EBM) 1ml every 3 hours was commenced on day 3. This was increased to 1ml every 2 hours on day 4 and 1ml hourly on day 5. EBM was increased by 1ml every hour each day to 5mls per hour on day 9.

There was a large aspirate (6mls) on day 9 but this was not bile-stained and there was no abdominal distension or diarrhea. Feeds were held for 4 hours.

On day 10, the EBM was fortified with a human milk fortifier to 85 calories per 100mls. On day 11, the intravenous caffeine was changed to oral caffeine and feed volume increased to 180mls per kilo per day. Suck feeds occurred from week 5.

Baby C was discharged home at 10 weeks of age weighing 2.2kgs. The human milk fortifier was ceased prior to discharge. Baby C's weight gain was slow for the first two weeks at home. Mother was breastfeeding frequently (2-3 hourly during the day and 3-5 hourly over night). By week 3 Baby C was gaining weight at 150-200gms per week. Oral multi-vitamins and iron were commenced at week 4 and continued until 6 months of age.

References

1. Harvey D, Prince J, Bunton J, Parkinson C, Campbell S. Ability of children who were small for gestational age. *Pediatrics* 1982;69:296-300.

2. Barker DJP. Mothers, babies and health in later life. Edinburgh, Churchill Livingstone 1998.

3. Astbury J, Orgill AA, Bajuk B, Yu VYH. Sequelae of growth failure in appropriate for gestational age, very low-birthweight infants. *Dev Med Child Neurol* 1986;28:472-479.

4. Connors JM, O'Callaghan MJ, Burns YR, Gray PH, Tudehope DI, Mohay H, Rogers YM. The influence of growth on development outcome in extremely low birthweight infants at 2 years of age. *J Paediatr Child Health* 1999;35:37-41.

5. Eriksson JG, Forsen T, Tuomilehto J, Winter PD, Osmond C, Barker DJP. Catch-up growth in childhood and death from coronary heart disease: longitudinal study. *BMJ* 1999;318:427-431.

6. American Academy of Pediatrics. Work Group on Breastfeeding. Breastfeeding and the use of human milk. *Pediatrics* 1997;100:1035-1039.

7. Simmer K, Metcalf R, Daniels L. The use of breast milk in a neonatal unit and its relationship to protein and energy intake and growth. *J Paediatr Child Health* 1997;33:55-60.

8. Thorell L, Sjöberg L, Hernell O. Nucleotides in human milk: sources and metabolism by the newborn infant. *Pediatr Res* 1996;40:845-852.

9. Carver JD, Walker WA. The role of nucleotides in human nutrition. *J Nutr Biochem* 1995;6:58-72.

10. Balmer SE, Hanvery LS, Wharton BA. Diet and faecal flora in the newborn: nucleotides. *Arch Dis Child* 1994;70:F137-F140.

11. Brunser O, Espinoza J, Araya M, Cruchet S, Gil A. Effect of dietary nucleotide supplementation on diarrhoeal disease in infants. *Acta Paediatr* 1994;83:188-191.

12. Carver JD, Pimentel B, Cox WI, Barness LA. Dietary nucleotide effects upon immune function in infants. *Pediatrics* 1991;88:359-363.

13. Pickering LK, Granoff DM, Erickson JR, Reed J, Masor ML, Cordle CT, Schaller JP, Winship, TR, Raule CL, Hilty MD. Modulation of the immune system by human milk and infant formula containing nucleotides. *Pediatrics* 1998;101:242-249.

14. Hay WW Jr, Lucas A, Heird WC, Zieler E, Levin E, Grave GD, Catz C, Yaffe SJ. Workshop summary: nutrition of the extremely low birth weight infant. *Pediatrics* 1999;104:1360-1368.

15. Carver JD, Barness LA. Trophic factors for the gastrointestinal tract. *Clin Perinatol* 1996;23:265-285.

16. Cavell B. Gastric emptying in infants fed human milk or infant formula. *Acta Paediatr Scand* 1981;70:639-641.

17. Ewer AK, Durbin GM, Morgan MEI, Booth IW. Gastric emptying in preterm infants. *Arch Dis Child* 1994;71:F24-F27.

18. Weaver LT, Ewing G, Taylor LC. The bowel habit of milk-fed infants. *J Pediatr Gastroenterol Nutr* 1988;7:568-571.

19. Mayor EJ, Hainman RF, Gay EL, Lezott DS, Santz DA, Klingensmith GJ. Reduced risk of IDDM among breastfed infants. *Diabetes* 1988;87:1625-1632.

20. Virtanen SM, Rasanen L, Aro A, Lindstrom J, Sippola H, Lounamaa R, Toivanen L, Toumclenta J, Akersblom HR. Infant feeding in children <7 years of age with newly diagnosed IDDM. *Diabetes Care* 1991;14:415-417.

21. Gerstein HC. Cows' milk exposure and type 1 diabetes mellitus. *Diabetes Care* 1994;17:13-19.

22. Karjalainen J, Martin JM, Knip M, Ilonen J, Robinson BH, Savilanti E, Alcerblom HK, Dosch HM. A bovine albumin peptide as a possible trigger of insulin dependent diabetes. *N Engl J Med* 1992;327:302-307.

23. Lucas A, Brooke OG, Morley R, Cole TJ, Bamford MF. A randomised prospective study of early diet and later allergic or atopic disease. *BMJ* 1990;300:837-840.

24. Savilahti E, Tuomikoski-Jaakkola P, Jarvenpaa A, Virtanen M. Early feeding of preterm infants and

allergic symptoms during childhood. *Acta Paediatr* 1993;82:340-344.

25. Hill DJ, Hudson L, Sheffield LJ, Shelton MJ, Menaham S, Hosking CS. A low allergen diet is a significant intervention in infantile colic: results of a community-based study. *J Allergy Clin Immunol* 1995;96:886-892.

26. Rey J, Schuri ZJ, Amedee-Manesmo O. Fat absorption in low birthweight infants. *Acta Pediatr Scand* 1982;296(suppl):81-84.

27. Kurlak LO, Stephenson TJ. Plausible explanations for effects of long chain polyunsaturated fatty acids (LCPUFA) on neonates. *Arch Dis Child* 1999;80: F148-F154.

28. Rueda R, Maldonado J, Narbona E, Gil A. Neonatal dietary gangliosides. *Early Hum Dev* 1998;53(suppl):S135-S147.

29. Pan XL, Izumi T. Variation of the ganglioside compositions of human milk, cow's milk and infant formulas. *Early Hum Dev* 2000;57:25-31.

30. May JT. Antimicrobial factors and microbial contaminants in human milk: recent studies. *J Paediatr Child Health* 1994;30:470-475.

31. Narayanan I, Prakash K, Gujral VV. The value of human milk in the prevention of infection in the high-risk low birth weight infant. *J Pediatr* 1981;99:496-498.

32. Narayanan I, Prakash K, Bala S, Verma RK, Gujral VV. Partial supplementation with expressed breast milk for prevention of infection in the low birth weight infant. *Lancet* 1980;2:561-563.

33. Narayanan I, Prakash K, Murthy NS, Gujral VV. Randomised controlled trial of effect of raw and holder pasteurised human milk and of formula supplements on incidence of neonatal infection. *Lancet* 1984;2:1111-1113.

34. Hylander MA, Strobina DM, Dhanireddy R. Human milk feeding and infection among very low birthweight infants. *Pediatrics* 1998;102:630-635.

35. Schanler RJ, Shulman RJ, Lau C. Feeding strategies for premature infants: beneficial outcomes of feeding fortified human milk versus preterm formula. *Pediatrics* 1999;103:1150-1157.

36. Beeby PJ, Jeffery H. Risk factors for NEC: the influence of gestational age. *Arch Dis Child* 1992;67:432-435.

37. Lucas A, Cole TJ. Breast milk and neonatal necrotising enterocolitis. *Lancet* 1990;336:1519-1523.

38. Morley R, Cole TJ, Lucas PJ, Lucas A. Mothers' choice to provide breast milk and developmental outcome. *Arch Dis Child* 1988;63:1382-1385.

39. Lucas A, Morley R, Cole TJ, Lister G, Leeson-Payne C. Breast milk and subsequent intelligence quotient in children born preterm. *Lancet* 1992;339:261-264.

40. Jacobson SW, Chiodo LM, Jacobson JL. Breastfeeding effects on intelligence quotient in 4- and 11-year old children. *Paediatrics* 103(5):e71, 1999 May.

41. Gibbs JAH, Fisher C, Bhattacharya S, Goddard P, Baum JD. Drip breast milk: its composition, collection and pasteurization. *Early Hum Dev* 1978;1:227-245.

42. Lucas A, Brooke OG, Baker BA, Bishop N, Morley R. High alkaline phosphatase activity and growth in preterm neonates. *Arch Dis Child* 1989;64:902-909.

43. Davis DP. Adequacy of expressed breast milk for early growth of preterm infants. *Arch Dis Child* 1977;52: 296-301.

44. Tyson JE, Lasky RE, Mize CE, Richards CJ, Blair-Smith N, Whyte R, Beer AE. Growth, metabolic response, and development in very low birthweight infants fed banked human milk or enriched formula. I. Neonatal findings. *J Pediatr* 1983;13:95-104.

45. Gross SJ. Growth and biochemical response of preterm infants fed human milk or modified infant formula. *New Engl J Med* 1983;308:237-241.

46. Lucas A, Gore SM, Cole TJ, Bamford MF, Dossetor JF, Barr I, Dicarlo L, Cork S, Lucas PJ. Multicentre trial on feeding low birthweight infants: effects of diet on early growth. *Arch Dis Child* 1984;59:722-730.

47. Roberts SB, Lucas A. The effects of two extreme of dietary protein accretion in preterm infants. *Early Hum Dev* 1985;12:301-307.

48. Davies DP. Future of human milk banks. *BMJ* 1992;305:433-4.

49. WHO/UNICEF Joint Statement. Meeting in Infant and Young Child Feeding. *J of Nurse-Midwifery* 1980;25:31-38.

50. WHO/UNICEF Joint Statement. Protection, Promotion and Support of Breastfeeding: the Ten Steps to Successful Breastfeeding. 1999.

51. Guidelines for the establishment and operation of human milk banks in the United Kingdom. British Paediatric Association. 1994.

52. Guidelines for the establishment and operation of donor human milk banks. Human Milk Banking Association of North America: 8th ed. Tully MR (ed). Raleigh, NC. 1999.

53. Deutsche Gesellschaft for Kinderheilkunde. Hansesches Verlagskontor: Lukeck. *Jahresbericht* 1992:13.

54. Human Milk Banking and Storage. Canadian Paediatric Society (ref no N95-03). 1995.

55. Human Milk Banking. Royal Australasian College of Physicians (Paediatric Division). Position Statement. 2001.

56. Atkinson SA. Human milk feeding of the micropremie. *Clin Perinatol* 2000;27:235-247.

57. Svenningsen NW, Lindroth M, Lindquist B. Growth in relation to protein intake of low birth weight infants. *Early Hum Dev* 1982;6:47-58.

58. Bell A, Halliday H, McClure G, Reid M. Controlled trial of new formulae for feeding low birth weight infants. *Early Hum Dev* 1986;13:97-105.

59. Modanlou HD, Lim MO, Hansen JW, Sickles V. Growth, biochemical status, and mineral metabolism in very-low-birth-weight infants receiving fortified preterm human milk. *J Pediatr Gastroenterol Nutr* 1886;5: 762-767.

60. Yu VYH, Jamieson J, Bajuk B. Breast milk feeding in very low birthweight infants. *Aust Paediatr J* 1981;17:186-190.

61. Green D, Moye L, Schreiner RL, Lemons JA. The relative efficacy of four methods of human milk expression. *Early Hum Dev* 1982;6:153-159.

62. deCarvalho M, Anderson DM, Giangreco A, Pittard WB III. Frequency of milk expression and milk production by mothers of nonnursing premature neonates. *Am J Dis Child* 1985;139:483-85.

63. Hopkinson JM, Schanler RJ, Garza C. Milk production by mothers of premature infants. *Pediatrics* 1988;81:815-820.

64. Ehrenkranz RA, Ackerman BA. Metoclopramide effect on faltering milk production by mothers of premature infants. *Pediatrics* 1986;78:614-620.

65. Petraglia F, Deheo V, Sardelli S, Pieroni ML, D'antona N, Genazzani AR. Domperidone in defective and insufficient lactation. *Europ J Obstet Gynec Reprod Biol* 1985;19:281-287.

66. Gunn AJ, Gunn TR, Rabone DL, Breier BH, Blum WF, Gluckman PD. Growth hormone increases breast milk volumes in mothers of preterm infants. *Pediatrics* 1996;98:279-282.

67. Bose CL, D'Ercole J, Lester AG, Hunter RS, Barrett JR. Relactation by mothers of sick and premature infants. *Pediatrics* 1981;67:565-569.

68. Liebhaber M, Lewiston NJ, Asquith, Sunshine P. Comparison of bacterial contamination with two methods of human milk collection. *J Pediatr* 1978;92:236-237.

69. Asquith MT, Harrod JR. Reduction of bacterial contamination in banked human milk. *J Pediatr* 1979;95:993-994.

70. Carroll L, Osman M, Davies DP. Does discarding the first few millilitres of breast milk improve the bacteriological quality of bank breast milk? *Arch Dis Child* 1980;55:898-899.

71. Pittard WB III, Anderson DM, Cerutti ER, Boxerbaum B. Bacteriostatic qualities of human milk. *J Pediatr* 1985;107:240-243.

72. Williamson S, Finucane E, Ellis H, Gamsu HR. Effect of heat treatment of human milk on absorption of nitrogen, fat, sodium, calcium and phosphorus by preterm infants. *Arch Dis Child* 1978;53:555-563.

73. Putet G, Senterre J, Rigo J, Salle B. Nutrient balance, energy utilization, and composition of weight gain in very low birth weight infants fed pooled human milk or a preterm formula. *J Pediatr* 1984;105:79-85.

74. van Zoeren-Grobben D, Schrijver J, van den Berg H, Berger HM. Human milk vitamin content after pasteurisation, storage or tube feeding. *Arch Dis Child* 1987;62:161-165.

75. Stein H, Cohen D, Herman AAB, Rissik J, Ellis U, Bolton K, Pettifor J, MacDougall L. Pooled pasteurized breast milk and untreated own mother's milk in the feeding of very low birth weight babies: a randomized controlled trial. *J Pediatr Gastroenterol Nutr* 1986;5:242-247.

76. Yu VYH. Enteral feeding in the preterm infant. *Early Hum Dev* 1999;56:89-115.

77. Wills ME, Han VEM, Harris DA. Short time low temperature pasteurisation of human milk. *Early Hum Dev* 1982;7:71-80.

78. Goldblum RM, Dill CW, Albrecht TB, Alford ES, Garza C, Goldman AS. Rapid high-temperature treatment of human milk. *J Pediatr* 1984;104:380-385.

79. Paxson CL, Cress CC. Survival of human milk leukocytes. *J Pediatr* 1979;94:61-64.

80. Garza C, Johnson CA, Harrist R, Nichols BL. Effects of methods of collection and storage on nutrients in human milk. *Early Hum Dev* 1982;6:295-303.

81. Sosa R, Barness L. Bacterial growth in refrigerated human milk. *Am J Dis Child* 1987;141:111-112.

82. Liebhaber M, Lewiston NJ, Asquith MT, Olds-Arroyo L, Sunshine P. Alterations of lymphocytes and of antibody content of human milk after processing. *J Pediatr* 1977;91:897-900.

83. Evans TJ, Ryley HC, Neale LM, Dodge JA, Lewarne VM. Effect of storage and heat on antimicrobial proteins in human milk. *Arch Dis Child* 1978;53: 239-241.

84. Quan R, Yang C, Rubinstein S, Lewiston NJ, Sunshine P, Stevenson DK, Kerner JA Jr. Effects of microwave radiation on anti-infective factors in human milk. *Pediatrics* 1992;89:667-669.

85. Hodge D, Puntis JWL. The use of expressed breast milk for the premature newborn. *Clin Nutr* 2000;19:75-77.

86. Law BJ, Urias BA, Lertzman J, Robson D, Romance L. Is ingestion of milk-associated bacteria by premature infants fed raw human milk controlled by routine bacteriological screening? *J Clin Microbiol* 1989;27:1560-1566.

87. Wee J, Tang ZY, Wu YX, Li WR. Acquired CMV infection of breastmilk in infancy. *Clin Med J* 1989;102:124-128.

88. Dasorsky M, Yon M, Stajno S, Pass RF, Alford C. CMV infection of breastmilk and transmission in infancy. *Pediatrics* 1983;72:395-399.

89. Atkinson SA, Bryan MH, Anderson GH. Human milk feeding in premature infants: protein, fat and carbohydrate balances in the first two weeks of life. *J Pediatr* 1981;99:617-624.

90. Spencer SA, Hendrickse W, Roberton D, Hull D. Energy intake and weight gain of very low birthweight babies fed raw expressed breast milk. *BMJ* 1982; 285:924-926.

91. Atkinson SA, Radde IC, Anderson GH. Macromineral balances in premature infants fed their own mother's milk or formula. *J Pediatr* 1983;102:99-106.

92. Chessex P, Reichman B, Verellen G, Putet G, Smith JM, Heim T, Swyer PR. Quality of growth in premature infants fed their own mothers' milk. *J Pediatr* 1983;102:107-112.

93. Valentine C, Hurst N, Schanler R. Hindmilk improves weight gain in low birthweight infants fed human milk. *J Pediatr Gastroenterol Nutr* 1994;18:474-477.

94. Lucas A, Lucas PJ, Chavin SL, Lyster RLJ, Baum D. Human milk formula. *Early Hum Dev* 1980;4:15-21.

95. Hagelberg S, Lindblad BS, Lundsjo A, Carlsson B, Fonden R, Fujita H, Lassfolk G, Lindqvist B. The protein tolerance of very low birth weight infants fed human milk protein enriched mother's milk. *Acta Paediatr Scand* 1982;71:597-601.

96. Ronnholm KAR, Perheentupa J, Siimes MA. Supplementation with human milk protein improves growth of small premature infants fed human milk. *Pediatrics* 1986;77:649-653.

97. Voyer M, Senterre J, Rigo J, Charlas J, Satge P. Human milk lacto-engineering. Growth, nitrogen metabolism and energy balance in preterm infants. *Acta Paediatr Scand* 1984;73:302-306.

98. Schanler RJ, Garza C, Nichols BL. Fortified mothers' milk for very low birth weight infants: Results of growth and nutrient balance studies. *J Pediatr* 1985;107:437-445.

99. Polberger SKT, Axelsson IA, Raiha NCE. Growth of low birth weight infants on varying amounts of human milk protein. *Pediatr Res* 1989;25:414-419.

100. Boehm G, Muller DM, Senger H, Borte M, Moro G. Nitrogen and fat balances in very low birth weight infants fed human milk fortified with human milk or bovine milk protein. *Eur J Pediatr* 1993;152:236-239.

101. Metcalf R, Dilena B, Gibson R, Marshall P, Simmer K. How appropriate are commercially available human milk fortifiers? *J Paediatr Child Health* 1994;30:350-355.

102. Wauben I, Gibson R, Atkinson S. Premature infants fed mothers' milk to 6 months corrected age

demonstrate adequate growth and zinc status in the first year. *Early Hum Dev* 1999;54:181-194.

103. Kuschel CA, Harding JE. Protein supplementation of human milk for promoting growth in preterm infants (Cochrane Review). In: The Cochrane Library, 2, 2001. Oxford: Update Software.

104. Kuschel CA, Harding JE. Multicomponent fortified human milk for promoting growth in preterm infants (Cochrane Review). In: The Cochrane Library, 2, 2001. Oxford: Update Software.

105. Kuschel CA, Harding JE. Fat supplementation of human milk for promoting growth in preterm infants (Cochrane Review). In: The Cochrane Library, 2, 2001. Oxford: Update Software.

106. Lucas A, Fewtrell MS, Morley R, Lucas PJ, Baker BA, Lister G, Bishop NJ. Randomized outcome trial of human milk fortification and developmental outcome in preterm infants. *Am J Clin Nutr* 1996;64:142-151.

107. Gross SJ. Bone mineralization in preterm infants fed human milk with and without mineral supplementation. *J Pediatr* 1987;111:450-458.

108. Carey DE, Rowe JC, Goetz CA, Horak E, Clark RM, Goldberg B. Growth and phosphorus metabolism in premature infants fed human milk, fortified human milk, or special premature formula. *Am J Dis Child* 1987;141:511-515.

109. Greer FR, McCormick A. Improved bone mineralization and growth in premature infants fed fortified own mother's milk. *J Pediatr* 1988;112:961-969.

110. Kashyap S, Schilze KF, Forsyth M, Dell RB, Ramakrishnan R, Heird WC. Growth, nutrient retention, and metabolic response of low-birthweight infants fed supplemented and unsupplemented preterm human milk. *Am J Clin Nutr* 1990;52: 254-262.

111. Hayashi T, Takeuchi T, Itabashi K, Okuyama K. Nutrient balance, metabolic response, and bone growth in VLBW infants fed fortified human milk. *Early Hum Dev* 1994;39:27-36.

112. Lapillonne AA, Glorieux FH, Salle B, Braillon PM, Chambon M, Rigo J, Putet G, Senterre J. Mineral balance and whole body bone mineral content in very low-birthweight infants. *Acta Paediatr*

1994:405(Suppl):117-122.

113. Fewtrell MS, Prentice A, Jones SC, Bishop NJ, Stirling D, Buffenstein R, Lunt M, Cole TJ, Lucas A. Bone mineralisation and turnover in preterm infants at 8-12 years of age: the effect of early diet. *J Bone Min Res* 1999;14:810-820.

114. Schanler RJ. The role of human milk fortification for premature infants. *Clin Perinatol* 1998;25:645-657.

115. Ewer AK, Yu VYH. Gastric emptying in preterm infants: the effect of breast milk fortifier. *Acta Paediatr* 1996;85:1112-1115.

116. McClure RJ, Newell SJ. Effect of fortifying breast milk on gastric emptying. *Arch Dis Child* 1996;74: F60-F62.

117. Moody GJ, Schanler RJ, Lau C, Shulman RJ. Feeding tolerance in premature infants fed fortified human milk. *J Pediatr Gastroenterol Nutr* 2000;30:408-412.

118. Quan R, Yang C, Rubinstein S, Lewiston NJ, Stevenson DK, Kerner JA. The effect of nutritional additives on anti-infective factors in human milk. *Clin Pediatr* 1994;33:325-328.

119. Jocson MAL, Mason EO, Schanler RJ. The effects of nutrient fortification and varying storage conditions on host defense properties of human milk. *Pediatrics* 1997;100:240-243.

120. Simmer K. Choice of formula and human milk supplement for preterm infants in Australia. *J Paediatr Child Health* 2000;36:593-595.

121. Nutrition Committee, Canadian Paediatric Society. Nutrient needs and feeding of premature infants. *Can Med Assoc J* 1995;152:1765-1785.

122. Davidson M, Levine SZ, Bauer CH, Dann M. Feeding studies in low birth weight infants. I. Relationships of dietary protein, fat and electrolyte to rates of weight gain, clinical courses and serum chemical concentrations. *J Pediatr* 1967;70:695-713.

123. Babson SG, Bramhall JL. Diet and growth in the premature infant. The effect of different dietary intakes of ash electrolyte and protein on weight gain and linear growth. *J Pediatr* 1969;74:890-900.

124. Raiha NCR, Heinonen K, Rassin DK, Gaull GE. Milk protein quantity and quality in low birthweight infants: I. Metabolic responses and effects on growth. *Pediatrics* 1976;57:659-674.

125. Svenningsen NW, Lindroth M, Lindquist B. Growth in relation to protein intake of low birth weight infants. *Early Hum Dev* 1982;6:47-58.

126. Kashyap S, Forsyth M, Zucker C, Ramakrishnan R, Dell RB, Heird WC. Effects of varying protein and energy intakes on growth and metabolic response in low birth weight infants. *J Pediatr* 1986;108:955-963.

127. Goldman HI, Goldman JS, Kaufman I, Liebman OB. Late effects of early dietary protein intake on low birth weight infants. *J Pediatr* 1974;85:764-769.

128. Kashyap S, Okamoto E, Kanaya S, Zucker C, Abildskov K, Dell RB, Heird WC. Protein quality in feeding low birth weight infants: a comparison of whey-predominant versus casein-predominant formulas. *Pediatrics* 1987;79:748-755.

129. Brooke OG, Onubogu O, Heath R, Carter ND. Human milk and preterm formula compared for effects on growth and metabolism. *Arch Dis Child* 1987;62:917-923.

130. Ventura V, Brooke OG. Plasma amino acids in small preterm infants on human milk or formula. *Arch Dis Child* 1987;62:1257-1264.

131. Halken S, Host A, Hansen LG, Osterballo O. Effect of an allergy prevention programme on incidence of atopic symptoms in infancy. A prospective study of 159 'high-risk' infants. *Allergy* 1992;47:545-553.

132. Rigo J, Salle BL, Picaud JC, Putet G, Senterre J. Nutritional evaluation of protein hydrolysate formulas. *Eur J Clin Nutr* 1995;49(Suppl 1):S26-S38.

133. Weaver LT, Laker MF, Nelson R. Neonatal intestinal lactase activity. *Arch Dis Child* 1986;61:896-899.

134. Cicco R, Holzman I, Brown DR, Becker DJ. Glucose polymer tolerance in premature infants. *Pediatrics* 1981;67:498-501.

135. Mobassaleh M, Montgomery RK, Biller JA, Grand RJ. Development of carbohydrate absorption in the fetus and neonate. *Pediatrics* 1985;75:160-166.

136. Simmer K. Longchain polyunsaturated fatty acid supplementation in preterm infants (Cochrane Review). In: The Cochrane Library, 2, 2001. Oxford Update Software.

137. O'Connor DL, Hall R, Adamkin D, Auestad N, Castillo M, Connor WE, et al. Growth and development in preterm infants fed long-chain polyunsaturated fatty acids: a prospective, randomized controlled trial. *Pediatrics* 2001;108:359-371.

138. Huston RK, Reynolds JW, Jensen C, Buist NRM. Nutrient and mineral retention and Vitamin D absorption in low birth weight infants: effect of medium-chain triglycerides. *Pediatrics* 1983;72:44-48.

139. Whyte RK, Campbell D, Stanhope RN, Bayley HS, Sinclair JC. Energy balance in low birthweight infants fed formula of high or low medium-chain triglyceride content. *J Pediatr* 1986;106:964-971.

140. Bustamante SA, Fiello A, Pollack PF. Growth of premature infants fed formulas with 10%, 30% or 50% medium-chain triglycerides. *Am J Dis Child* 1987;141:516-519.

141. Hamosh M, Bitman J, Liao T, Mehta NR, Buczek RJ, Wood DL, Grylack LJ, Hamosh P. Gastric lipolysis and fat absorption in preterm infants: effect of medium-chain triglyceride or long-chain triglyceride containing formulas. *Pediatrics* 1989;83:86-92.

142. Wu PYK, Edmond J, Morrow JW, Auestad N, Ponder D, Benson J. Gastrointestinal tolerance, fat absorption, plasma ketone and urinary dicarboxylic acid levels in low birth weight infants fed different amounts of medium-chain triglycerides in formula. *J Pediatr Gastroenterol Nutr* 1993;17:145-152.

143. Carnielli VP, Rossi K, Badon T, Gregori B, Verlato G, Orzali A, Zacchello F. Medium-chain triacylglycerols in formulas for preterm infants: effect on plasma lipids, circulating concentrations of medium-chain fatty acids, and essential fatty acids. *Am J Clin Nutr* 1996;64:152-158.

144. Mercado M, Yu VYH, Gill A. Clinical experience with preterm formulas in very low birthweight infants. *J Sing Paediatr Soc* 1990;32:137-143.

145. Spencer SA, McKenna S, Stammers J, Hull D. Two different low birthweight formulae compared. *Early Hum Dev* 1992;30:21-31.

146. Rowe JC, Goetz CA, Carey DE, Horak E. Achievement of in utero retention of calcium and phosphorus accompanied by high calcium excretion in very low birth weight infants fed a fortified formula. *J Pediatr* 1987;110:581-585.

147. Brooke OG, Wood C, Barley J. Energy balance, nitrogen balance, and growth in preterm infants fed

expressed breast milk, a premature infant formula, and two low-solute adapted formulae. *Arch Dis Child* 1982;57:898-904.

148. Reichman B, Chessex P, Verellen G, Putet G, Smith JM, Heim T, Swyer PR. Dietary composition and macronutrient storage in preterm infants. *Pediatrics* 1983;72:322-328.

149. Calvert SA, Soltesz G, Jenkins PA, Harris D, Newman C, Adrian TE, Bloom SR, Aynsley-Green A. Feeding premature infants with human milk or preterm milk formula. *Biol Neonate* 1985;47:189-198.

150. Tudehope DI, Mitchell F, Cowley DM. A comparative study of a premature formula and preterm breast milk for low birthweight infants. *Aust Paediatr J* 1986;22:199-205.

151. Bell A, Halliday H, McClure G, Reid M. Controlled trial of new formulae for feeding low birthweight infants. *Early Hum Dev* 1986;13:97-105.

152. Lucas A, Morley R, Cole TJ, Gore SM, Lucas PJ, Crowle P, Pearse R, Boon AJ, Powell R. Early diet in preterm babies and developmental status at 18 months. *Lancet* 1990;335:1477-1481.

153. Lucas A, Morley R, Cole TJ, Gore SM, Davis JA, Bamford MF, Dossetor JF. Early diet in preterm babies and developmental status in infancy. *Arch Dis Child* 1989;64:1570-1578.

154. Lucas A, Morley R, Cole TJ, Gore SM. A randomised multicentre study of human milk versus formula and later development in preterm infants. *Arch Dis Child* 1994;70:F141-F146.

155. Stocks J. Effect of nasogastric tubes on nasal resistance during infancy. *Arch Dis Child* 1980;55:17-21.

156. Greenspan JS, Abbasi S, Bhutani VK. Sequential changes in pulmonary mechanics in the very low birthweight (less than or equal to 1000 grams) infant. *J Pediatr* 1988;113:732-737.

157. van Someren V, Linnett SJ, Stothers JK, Sullivan PG. An investigation into the benefits of resiting nasogastric feeding tubes. *Pediatrics* 1984;74: 379-383.

158. Wilkinson A, Yu VYH. Immediate effects of feeding on blood-gasses and some cardiorespiratory functions in ill newborn infants. *Lancet* 1974;1:1083-1085.

159. Yu VYH. Cardiorespiratory response to feeding in newborn infants. *Arch Dis Child* 1976;51:305-309.

160. Yu VYH, Rolfe P. Effect of feeding on ventilation and respiratory mechanics in newborn infants. *Arch Dis Child* 1976;51:310-313.

161. Patel BD, Dinwiddie R, Kumar SP, Fox WW. The effects of feeding on arterial blood gases and lung mechanics in newborn infants recovering from respiratory disease. *J Pediatr* 1977;90:435-438.

162. Krauss AN, Brown J, Waldman S, Gottlieb G, Auld PA. Pulmonary function following feeding in low-birthweight infants. *Am J Dis Child* 1978;132:139-142.

163. Pitcher-Wilmott R, Shutack JG, Fox WW. Decreased lung volume after nasogastric feeding of neonates recovering from respiratory disease. *J Pediatr* 1979;95:119-121.

164. Stothers JK, Warner RM. Effect of feeding on neonatal oxygen consumption. *Arch Dis Child* 1979;54:415-120.

165. Herrell N, Martin RJ, Fanaroff A. Arterial oxygen tension during nasogastric feeding in the preterm infant. *J Pediatr* 1980;96:914-916.

166. Heldt GP. The effect of gavage feeding on the mechanics of the lung, chest wall, and diaphragm of preterm infants. *Pediatr Res* 1988;24:55-58.

167. Blondheim O, Abbasi S, Fox WW, Bhutani VK. Effect of enteral gavage feeding rate on pulmonary functions of very low birth weight infants. *J Pediatr* 1993;122:751-755.

168. Nelle M, Hoecker C, Linderkamp O. Effects of bolus tube feeding on cerebral blood flow velocity in neonates. *Arch Dis Child* 1997;76:F54-F56.

169. Grant J, Denne SC. Effect of intermittent versus continuous enteral feeding on energy expenditure in premature infants. *J Pediatr* 1991;118:928-931.

170. Brooke OG, Barley J. Loss of energy during continuous infusions of breast milk. *Arch Dis Child* 1978;53:344-345.

171. Stocks RJ, Davies DP, Allen F, Sewell D. Loss of breast milk nutrients during tube feeding. *Arch Dis Child* 1985;60:164-166.

172. Narayanan I, Singh B, Harvey D. Fat loss during feeding of human milk. *Arch Dis Child* 1984;59: 475-477.

173. Bhatia J, Rassin DK. Human milk supplementation. Delivery of energy, calcium, phosphorus, magnesium, copper and zinc. *Am J Dis Child* 1988;142:445-447.

174. Voirin J, Le Coutour X, Bougle D, Mouhadjer M, Michel N, Oblin I. Development of maternal milk flora during continuous enteral feeding of premature infants. *Pediatrics* 1990;45:725-729.

175. Cooke RJ, Embleton ND. Feeding issues in preterm infants. *Arch Dis Child* 2000;83:F215-F218.

176. Premji S, Chessell L. Continuous nasogastric milk feeding versus intermittent bolus milk feeding for premature infants less than 1500 grams (Cochrane Review). In: The Cochrane Library, 2, 2001, Oxford: Update Software.

177. Wells DH, Zachman RD. Nasojejunal feedings in low birth weight infants. *J Pediatr* 1975;87:276-279.

178. Roy RN, Pollnitz RP, Hamilton JR, Chance GW. Impaired assimilation of nasojejunal feeds in healthy low birth weight newborn infants. *J Pediatr* 1977;90:431-434.

179. Drew JH, Johnston R, Finocchiaro C, Taylor PS, Goldberg HJA. A comparison of nasojejunal with nasogastric feedings in low birth weight infants. *Aust Paediatr J* 1979;15:98-100.

180. Pereira GR, Lemons JA. A controlled study of transpyloric and intermittent gavage feeding in the small preterm infant. *Pediatrics* 1981;67:68-72.

181. Whitefield MF. Poor weight gain of the low birthweight infant fed nasojejunally. *Arch Dis Child* 1982;57:597-601.

182. Van Caille M, Powell GK. Nasoduodenal versus nasogastric feeding in the very low birthweight infant. *Pediatrics* 1975;56:1065-1072.

183. Laing IA, Lang MA, Callaghan O, Hume R. compared with nasoduodenal feeding in low birthweight infants. *Arch Dis Child* 1986;61:138-141.

184. Steer PA, Lucas A, Sinclair JC. Feeding the low birthweight infant. In: Sinclair JC, Bracken MB (eds) Effective care of the newborn infant. Oxford University Press, Oxford 1992;94-140.

185. Vengusamy S, Pildes RS, Raffensperger JF, Levine HD, Cornblath M. A controlled study of feeding gastrostomy in low birth weight infants. *Pediatrics* 1969;43:815-820.

186. Pinelli J, Symington A. Non-nutritive sucking for promoting physiologic stability and nutrition in preterm infants (Cochrane Review). In: The Cochrane Review, 2, 2001. Oxford: Update Software.

187. Collins CT, Ryan P, Paterson S, Crowther CA, McPhee AJ. Transition to breast feeds for premature infants: does the use of artificial teats affect breast feeding success? A randomised controlled trial. Proc Perinatal Soc Aust NZ 5th Ann Congr. Canberra, 2001.

188. Gale CR, Martyn CN. Breastfeeding, dummy use and adult intelligence. *Lancet* 1996;347:1072-1075.

189. Olson M. The benign effects on rabbits' lungs of the aspiration of water compared with 5% glucose or milk. *Pediatrics* 1970;46:538-547.

190. Berseth CL. Gastrointestinal motility in the neonate. *Clin Perinatol* 1996;23:179-190.

191. Lucas A, Bloom SR, Aynsley-Green A. Gut hormones and "minimal enteral feedings". *Acta Paediatr Scand* 1986;75:19-23.

192. Tyson JE, Kennedy KA. Minimal enteral nutrition for promoting feeding tolerance and preventing morbidity in parenterally fed infants (Cochrane Review). In: The Cochrane Review, 2, 2001. Oxford: Update Software.

193. Kennedy KA, Tyson JE, Chamnanvanikij S. Early versus delayed initiation of progressive enteral feedings for parenterally fed low birth weight or preterm infants (Cochrane Review). In: The Cochrane Review, 2, 2001. Oxford: Update Software.

194. White KC. Harkavy KC. Hypertonic formula resulting from added oral medication. *Am J Dis Child* 1982;136:931-933.

195. Williams AF. Early enteral feeding of the preterm infant. *Arch Dis Child* 2000;83:F219-F220.

196. Dunn L, Hulman S, Weiner J, Kliegman R. Beneficial effects of early hypocaloric enteral feeding on neonatal gastrointestinal function: preliminary report of a randomized trial. *J Pediatr* 1988;112:622-629.

197. Slagle TA, Gross SJ. Effect of early low-volume enteral substrate on subsequent feeding tolerance in very low birth weight infants. *J Pediatr* 1988;13:526-531.

198. McClure RJ, Newell SJ. Randomised controlled trial of trophic feeding and gut motility. *Arch Dis Child*

1999;80:F54-F58..

199. McClure RJ, Newell SJ. Randomised controlled study of clinical outcome following trophic feeding. *Arch Dis Child* 2000;82:F29-F33.

200. Shulman RJ, Schanler RJ, Lau C, Heitkemper M, Ou C-N, Smith , EO. Early feeding, antenatal glucocorticoids, and human milk decrease intestinal permeability in preterm infants. *Pediatr Res* 1998;44:519-523.

201. Drew JH, Breheny JE, Gleeson M. Evaluation of non-graded 20 kilocalorie per 30 millilitre feedings to newborn infants. *Med J Aust* 1974;1:879-881.

202. Currao WJ, Cox C, Shapiro DL. Diluted formula for beginning the feeding of premature infants. *Am J Dis Child* 1988;142:730-731.

203. Baker JH, Berseth CL. Duodenal motor responses in preterm infants fed formula with varying concentrations and rates of infusion. *Pediatr Res* 1997;42:618-622.

204. Brown EG, Sweet AY. Preventing necrotizing enterocolitis in neonates. *JAMA* 1978;240:2452-2454.

205. Goldman HI. Feeding and necrotizing enterocolitis. *Am J Dis Child* 1980;134:553-555.

206. Spritzer R, Koolen AM, Baerts W, Fetter WP, Lafeber HN, Sauer PJ. A prolonged decline in the incidence of necrotizing enterocolitis after the introduction of a cautious feeding regimen. *Acta Paediatr Scand* 1988;77:909-911.

207. Zabielski PB, Groh-Wargo SL, Moore JJ. Necrotizing enterocolitis: feeding in endemic and epidemic periods. *JPEN* 1989;13:520-524.

208. Anderson DM, Kliegman RM. The relationship of neonatal alimentation practices to the occurrence of endemic necrotizing enterocolitis. *Am J Perinatol* 1991;8:62-67.

209. McKeown RE, Marsh TD, Amarnath U, Garrison CZ, Addy CL, Thompson SJ, Austin JL. Role of delayed feeding and of feeding increments in necrotizing enterocolitis. *J Pediatr* 1992;121:764-770.

210. Kennedy KA, Tyson JE, Chamnanvanakij S. Rapid versus slow rate of advancement of feedings for promoting growth and preventing necrotizing enterocolitis in parenterally fed low-birthweight

infants (Cochrane Review). In: The Cochrane Review, 2, 2001. Oxford: Update Software.

211. Collinge JM, Bradley K, Perks C, Rezny A, Topping P. Demand vs scheduled feedings for premature infants. *J Obstet Gynecol Nurs* 1982;11:362-367.

212. Raffles A, Schiller G, Exhardt P, Silverman M, Glucose polymer supplementation of feeds for very low birthweight infants. *BMJ* 1983;286:935-936.

213. Brooke OG. Energy balance and metabolic rate in preterm infants with standard and high energy formulas. *Br J Nutr* 1980;44:13-23.

214. Lucas A, Fewtrell Ms, Davies PS, Bishop NJ, Clough H, Cole TJ. Breastfeeding and catch-up growth in infants born small for gestational age. *Acta Paediatr* 1997;86:564-569.

215. Evans K, Evans R, Simmer K. Effect of method of breast feeding on breast engorgement, mastitis and infantile colic. *Acta Paediatr* 1995;84:849-852.

216. Coulie B, Tack J, Peeters T, Janssens J. Involvement of two different pathways in the motor effects of erythromycin on the gastric antrum in humans. *Gut* 1998;43:395-400.

217. Ng E, Shah V. Erythromycin for feeding intolerance in preterm infants (Cochrane Review). In: The Cochrane Review, 2, 2001. Oxford: Update Software.

218. Ng PC, So KW, Fung KSC, Lee CG, Fok TF, Wong E, Wong W, Cheung KL, Cheng AFB. Randomised controlled study of oral erythromycin for treatment of gastrointestinal dysmotility in preterm infants. *Arch Dis Child* 2001;84:F177-F182.

219. Ajuriaguwerra ME, Radvanyi-Boubet MF, Houn C, Moriette G. Gastro-esophageal reflux and apnoea in prematurely born infants during wakefulness and sleep. *Am J Dis Child* 1991;145:1132-1136.

220. Vandenplas Y, De Wolf D, Deneyer M, Sacre L. Incidence of gastro-esophageal reflux in sleep, awake, fasted and post-cibal periods in asymptomatic infants. *J Pediatr Gastroenterol Nutr* 1988;7:177-80.

221. Hampton FJ, MacFadyen UM, Simpson H. Reproducibility of 24 hour oesophageal pH studies in infants. *Arch Dis Child* 1990;65:1249-1254.

222. Bailey DJ, Andres JM, Danek GD, Pinneiro-Carrero VM. Lack of efficacy of thickened feeding as a treatment for gastro-oesophageal reflux. *J Pediatr*

1987;110:187-189.

223. Orenstien SR. Thickened feedings as a cause of increased coughing when used as therapy for gastro-oesophageal reflux in infants. *J Pediatr* 1992;121:913-915.

224. Cucchiara S, Staiano A, Boccieri A, De Stefano M, Capozzi C, Manzi G, Camerlingo F, Paone FM. Effects of cisapride on parameters of oesophageal motility and on the prolonged intraoesophageal pH test in infants with gastro-oesophageal reflux disease. *Gut* 1990;31:21-25.

225. Justo RN, Gray PH. Fundoplication in preterm infants with gastro-oesophageal reflux. *J Paediatr Child Health* 1991;27:250-254.

226. Enriquez A, Bolisetty S, Patole S, Garvey PA, Campbell PJ. Randomised controlled trial of cisapride in feed tolerance in preterm infants. *Arch Dis Child* 1998;79:F110-F113.

227. McClure RJ, Kristensen JH, Grauaug A. Randomised controlled trial of cisapride in preterm infants. *Arch Dis Child* 1999;80:F174-F177.

228. Lander A. The risk and benefits of cisapride in preterm neonates, infants, and children. *Arch Dis Child* 1998;79:469-471.

229. Clark DA, Miller MJS. Intraluminal pathogenesis of necrotizing enterocolitis. *J Pediatr* 1990;117:S64-S67.

230. Modler S, Kerner JA, Castillo RO, Breman HJ, Stevenson DK. Relationship between breath and total body hydrogen excretion rates in neonates. *J Pediatr Gastroenterol Nutr* 1988;7:554-558.

231. Kien CL. Colonic fermentation of carbohydrate in the premature infant: possible relevance to necrotizing enterocolitis. *J Pediatr* 1990;117:S52-S58.

232. Chew F, Villar J, Solomons NW, Figueroa R. In vitro hydrolysis with a beta-galactosidase for treatment of intolerance to human milk in very low-birthweight infants. *Acta Paediatr Scand* 1988;77:601-602.

233. Newell SJ. Enteral feeding of the micropremie. *Clin Perinatol* 2000;27:221-234.

234. Gill G, Yu VYH, Bajuk B, Astbury J. Postnatal growth in infants born before 30 weeks' gestation. *Arch Dis Child* 1986;61:549-553.

235. Pauls J, Bauer K, Versmold H. Postnatal body weight curves for infants below 1000 g birth weight receiving early enteral and parenteral nutrition. *Eur J Pediatr* 1998;17:416-421.

236. Lee JKF, Yu VYH. Calorie intake in sick versus respiratory stable very low birthweight babies. *Act Paediatr Jap* 1996;38:449-454.

Human Milk

Richard J. Schanler, M.D. and Stephanie A. Atkinson, Ph.D.

Reviewed by Hildegard Przyrembel, M.D., Ph.D., and Josef Neu, M.D.

Introduction

In its 1998 policy statement on the use of human milk, The American Academy of Pediatrics acknowledged that human milk is beneficial in the management of premature infants.[1] The beneficial effects generally relate to improvements in host defenses, digestion and absorption of nutrients, gastrointestinal function, neurodevelopmental outcomes, and maternal psychological well-being. However, the special needs of the premature infant that arise as a result of metabolic and gastrointestinal immaturity, immunologic compromise, and associated medical conditions, must be considered so that adequate nutrition can be provided to meet the needs for intrauterine rates of growth and nutrient accretion.[2] Human milk is capable of satisfying most of the needs of premature infants if careful attention is given to nutritional status. This review will focus on the benefits of feeding human milk and the practical approaches that enable the nutritional needs of the premature infant to be met.

Composition of Preterm Milk

Milk from mothers who give birth prematurely (preterm milk) has been studied extensively since 1978 when the first report was published of higher concentrations of nitrogen in preterm milk compared with milk of mothers giving birth at term (term milk).[3] Greater concentrations in preterm compared with term milk were subsequently reported for immune proteins, total lipid, medium chain fatty acids, energy, vitamins, some minerals (eg, calcium and sodium), and trace elements.[4,5,6,7] There are now compositional data for some 17 trace elements in preterm milk

compared with term milk.[6] While findings of higher concentrations of nutrients in preterm compared with term milk are not consistent among studies, no studies have found concentrations of nutrients in preterm milk to be less than term milk at similar stages of lactation.

The nutrient composition of preterm milk for early or transitional milk (approximately 6 to 10 days of lactation) and mature milk (approximately 22 to 30 days of lactation) in comparison with published values for mature term milk (approximately 30 days of lactation) are listed in Tables 1 and 2. Preterm milk is generally either higher in concentration for individual nutrients or within the normal range for term milk. There is a trend for nutrient concentrations in preterm milk to decline as lactation progresses, a pattern of change also observed in term milk. Thus, while the higher nutrient concentrations of "early" milk might meet the nutrient needs of the premature infant, exclusive feeding of mature preterm milk from two weeks postnatally and onward may lead to nutrient deficiencies in the rapidly growing premature infant (see further discussion below).

The physiological basis for reported differences in nutrient density between preterm and term milk is unlikely to be teleologic in origin. Early interruption of pregnancy might invoke incomplete maturation of the mammary gland to support normal lactation and thus permit paracellular leakage of serum proteins (eg, immune proteins) and ions (eg, sodium and chloride) through tight junctions that have not completely closed.[8] Although reported at weaning, it is unclear if paracellular leakage is a cause of the physiological differences in preterm milk.[9] Differences in milk composition also might be caused by a variable hormonal profile at parturition in women who deliver prematurely compared with those delivering at term.[10] In this regard, it is known that lactation may be repressed in some animal species by high placental luteal hormone concentrations.[11] It has been suggested that the greater nutrient density in preterm milk simply might be a function of the concentration of nutrients in a lower volume of milk secondary to the artificial expression of milk by pumping rather than suckling at the breast.[10,12] Maternal factors in the perinatal period also may influence the volume of milk produced and/or the synthesis and transport of nutrients into milk. Such events include: delay in initiation of pumping, maternal anxiety (interference with oxytocin secretion and milk production), medications (such as antenatal glucocorticoids), an early return of menses, and the use of contraceptive hormones.[4]

Benefits of Human Milk for Premature Infants
Host Defense Benefits

From clinical studies in nurseries throughout the world, there appears to be a decrease in the rate of a variety of infections in premature infants fed unsupplemented human milk compared with the feeding of formula. Narayanan[13] reported a lower incidence of a variety of infections in premature infants in India fed their mothers' milk during the daytime (and formula at night) compared with similar infants fed formula exclusively. A further reduction in the incidence of infection eventually was reported in that nursery following the implementation of exclusive feeding of human milk.[14] The lower rate of infections also is reported whether fresh or pasteurized human milk is fed.[15] In Mexico City, premature infants had fewer episodes of necrotizing enterocolitis, diarrhea, and urinary tract infection, and needed less antibiotic therapy when fed their own mothers' milk compared with similar infants fed term formula.[16]

Necrotizing enterocolitis occurs less frequently when the prior diet is human milk compared with formula.[17] A large, non-randomized study of hospitalized premature infants reported that the incidence of necrotizing enterocolitis was significantly lower in infants fed unsupplemented human milk, either exclusively or partially, compared with infants fed formula.[18] That study reported cases confirmed by surgery or autopsy and found that the incidence of necrotizing enterocolitis was significantly greater in premature infants solely fed formula.

Host defense factors in milk. Specific bioactive factors such as sIgA, lactoferrin, lysozyme, oligosaccharides, nucleotides, cytokines (such as Il-10), growth factors (such as epidermal growth factor), enzymes (such as platelet activating factor-acetylhydrolase), antioxidants, and cellular components all may affect the host defense of the premature infant. Nutrients, such as glutamine, taurine, and inositol also serve dual roles to protect the host. Perhaps no one factor will be identified, but interactions among these factors may provide the host with optimal immune defense.

Potential mechanisms of protection. One of the major protective effects of human milk on the recipient infant operates through the enteromammary immune system. It is reasonable to expect that exposure of the mother to the environment of the neonatal nursery through skin-to-skin contact with her premature infant may be advantageous to the infant. In this manner, mothers can be "induced" to make specific antibodies against the nosocomial pathogens in the nursery environment.

A lower incidence of necrotizing enterocolitis in formula-fed premature infants has been associated with receipt of an enteral supplement of serum-derived immunoglobulins A and G (IgA-IgG).[19] Infants fed the IgA-IgG preparation, in quantities approximating the intake from human milk, had a significantly higher fecal excretion of IgA than controls, consistent with a local protective effect throughout the gastrointestinal tract. Enteral supplementation with only human plasma-derived IgG, however, failed to provide protection against necrotizing enterocolitis or sepsis in low birth weight infants.[20] A greater content of IgA and lactoferrin also has been observed in feces and urine of premature infants fed human milk compared with similar infants fed formula.[21,22] From additional studies it appears that human milk-derived lactoferrin may be absorbed intact and excreted in the urine of premature infants.[23] Based on these results, human milk may potentiate the premature infant's host defenses through local and systemic actions.

In animal models, pretreatment with recombinant human acetylhydrolase protected against necrotizing enterocolitis.[24] In another series of studies, supplementation of the diet with polyunsaturated fatty acids reduced the incidence of NEC in the animal model.[25] The latter observation also has been noted in one human clinical trial of polyunsaturated fatty acid-supplementation of formula.[26] It may be argued that because of the significant concentrations of acetylhydrolase and polyunsaturated fatty acids in human milk, the susceptible infant fed human milk particularly may be protected from necrotizing enterocolitis. Diet also may affect fecal flora. The human milk-fed premature infant has a fecal flora that contains fewer pathogenic organisms than flora from an infant fed bovine-derived formula. Thus, the relationship between feeding of human milk and reduced incidence of infection and/or necrotizing enterocolitis reported in these descriptive studies supports the suitability of human milk for premature infants.

Neurodevelopment

Several studies have linked improved cognitive development later in childhood and adolescence to breastfeeding in term as well as premature infants.[27] In the multicenter British studies of premature infants weighing less than 1850 grams at birth, considerable advantages in growth, neurological development, and health outcomes were associated with the feeding of human milk compared with infant formula.[28,29,30] An advantage of human milk remained at 7.5 to 8 years of age with respect to a higher intelligence quotient for the group fed human milk even after controlling for mother's education and social class.[30] The investigators also reported a significant dose-response relationship; the more human milk fed, the greater the scores in follow-up. Even if those infants who were breastfed after hospital discharge were excluded from

the analysis, the differences between groups remained significant. Thus, it appears that these positive associations might be related more to the composition of the milk rather than the actual method (breastfeeding) in which it is fed. Moreover, despite slower rates of growth, premature infants fed pasteurized donor human milk in another study had advantages in psychomotor development at 18 months compared with infants fed preterm formula.[29] Significantly higher mental developmental index scores (mean differences of 7.4 points) were reported in very low birth weight infants < 1250 g at 18 months of age who received human milk compared to those who never received human milk in-hospital.[31]

In the one study in which infants were fed human milk with a multinutrient fortifier containing additional protein, minerals, and vitamins, no significant differences in neurodevelopmental outcome at 18 months were observed compared with infants fed human milk supplemented minimally with minerals and vitamins.[32] The authors attributed this observation to inadequate sample size since a 6.2-point advantage in mental development index was observed for males (but not females) who had received fortified human milk, and the total sample size had been estimated for a 6 point difference in this index.[32] To further complicate the interpretation, the outcomes also may have been affected by the large quantity of preterm formula received by infants in both groups.[33]

In summary, small but statistically significant neurodevelopmental advantages in children who were formerly fed human milk have been demonstrated at all points from 2 to 9 years of age. Long-term advantage was more consistently demonstrated for cognitive than for motor skills. Although results of the studies cannot be assumed to be representative of all preterm infants there is some evidence of a dose-response. Although the size effect is small, human milk offers at least the potential for enhancing the premature infant's development at no risk and little cost.

A note of caution in the interpretation of available studies on neurodevelopmental outcomes has been addressed.[34] There are inherent dangers of

Component (unit/L)	Ref	Preterm Transitional 6-10 days	Preterm Mature 22-30 days	Term Mature ≥30 days
Total Protein, g	A	19 ± 0.5	15 ± 1	12 ± 1.5
IgA, mg/g protein	A	92 ± 63	64 ± 70	83 ± 25
Non-protein nitrogen, % total nitrogen	A	18 ± 4	17 ± 7	24
Fat, g	B	34 ± 6	36 ± 7	34 ± 4
Carbohydrate, g	B	63 ± 5	67 ± 4	67 ± 5
Energy, kcal	B	660 ± 60	690 ± 50	640 ± 80
Ca, mmol	A	8.0 ± 1.8	7.2 ± 1.3	6.5 ± 1.5
P, mmol	A	4.9 ± 1.4	3.0 ± 0.8	4.8 ± 0.8
Mg, mmol	A	1.1 ± 0.2	1.0 ± 0.3	1.3 ± 0.3
Iron, mmol (mg)	B	23 (0.4)	22 (0.4)	22 (0.4)
Zn, µmol	B	58 ± 13	33 ± 14	15 - 46
Cu, µmol B	9.2 ± 2.1	8.0 ± 3.1	3.2 - 6.3	
Mn, µg (median)	B	6 ± 8.9	7.3 ± 6.6	3 - 6
Na, mmol	A	11.6 ± 6.0	8.8 ± 2.0	9.0 ± 4.1
K, mmol	A	13.5 ± 2.2	12.5 ± 3.2	13.9 ± 2.0
Cl, mmol	B	21.3 ± 3.5	14.8 ± 2.1	12.8 ± 1.5

[1]Values are mean ± SD.

A = Average ± SD of values summarized by Atkinson[4]

B = Average ± SD of values taken from the following reports in which milk samples were representative of a 24 hour milk collection and lactational stages analyzed were similar. Atkinson et al 1980[117], Anderson et al 1981, Anderson et al 1983[118], Gross et al 1981, Hibberd et al[119], Lemons et al 1982, Sann et al 1981[120], Friel et al 1999[6,121,122,123,124,125]

C[126]

D (Moran et al 1983)[127]

Table 1: Nutrient composition of transitional and mature preterm human milk compared with mature term milk.

over-interpreting the associations between higher developmental scores achieved by premature infants at 18 months and "intention" to breast feed by mothers compared with those who did not. Although similar strong relationships were found linking breastfeeding decisions to higher scores at 5 and 10 years of age, these associations have been linked to "positive" health behavior in mothers. Intention to breast feed a premature infant may not always result in substantial breast milk consumption.[35] Importantly, with the exception of one study that was under-powered for the outcome of interest,[32] the influence of fortification of human milk with single or multinutrient fortifiers on neurodevelopmental outcomes has not been investigated.

Visual function may be improved by feeding of human milk in premature infants, possibly due to the high quantity of very long-chain polyunsaturated fatty acids as well as high antioxidant activity.[36] Because of the antioxidant activity in human milk and

Component (units)	Premature Recommended Nutrient Intakes (P-RNI) (unit/kg/day)	Volume of Premature Human Milk to Meet P-RNI (mL/kg/day)
Energy, kcal	105-135	145-185
Protein, g	3.0-3.6	180-210
Potassium, mmol	2.5-3.5	155-220
Zinc, μmol	7.7-12.3	120-190
Copper, μmol	0.1-1.9	115-200
Vitamin E, mg	0.5-0.9	120-200

Table 2: Premature recommended nutrient intakes (P-RNI) for stable-growing premature infants >1 kg birth weight and the volume of human milk needed to meet the P-RNI for selected nutrients.[44]

predilection of polyunsaturated fatty acids for retinal membranes, the relationship between diet and retinopathy of prematurity was examined.[37] The diagnosis of retinopathy of prematurity and the severity of retinopathy were significantly greater in formula-fed infants than human milk-fed infants. Fewer infants fed human milk (exclusive or partial) progressed to advanced retinopathy, and none required retinal surgery.

It is not clear why the feeding of human milk affects neurodevelopmental outcome. Milk composition probably plays a significant role. Potential factors that might contribute to neurodevelopment include the very long-chain polyunsaturated fatty acids (eg, docosahexanoic acid, discussed elsewhere in this textbook), cholesterol, antioxidants (Vitamin E, cysteine), taurine, specialized growth factors, micronutrients, or the effect may be mediated through an improved health of the human milk-fed infant. Human milk serves as the model on which polyunsaturated fatty acid supplementation of formula for premature infants has been studied and reported to be beneficial. Studies in the premature infant reporting the beneficial effects of polyunsaturated fatty acid supplementation of formula use the human milk-fed premature infant as the control population. The same positive outcomes favoring polyunsaturated fatty acid supplementation of formula also are observed in the group of premature infants fed human milk.[38,39] These associations require further validation, but the marked effects of human milk on neurodevelopmental function in the premature infant receiving human milk should not be underestimated.

Gastrointestinal Effects

There is a consensus that human milk promotes more rapid gastric emptying than formula.[40] In studies of early "trophic feeding (day 4 to 14)" in premature infants, those infants fed human milk had significantly greater intestinal lactase activity than infants fed preterm formula.[41] Further studies indicate that feeding of human milk favors a decrease in intestinal permeability early in life compared with preterm formula.[42] Many of the bioactive factors in human milk function at the level of the gastrointestinal tract to protect the infant from foreign antigens.

Other Effects

The feeding of human milk in early neonatal life in premature infants was reported to be associated with lower blood pressure at 13-16 years of age compared to infants fed formula.[43]

Limitations in the Use of Human Milk for Premature Infants

Availability

Despite the desire to provide milk for their premature infants, mothers often do not sustain adequate milk production to meet their infants' needs. Several factors have been implicated: delayed initiation of lactation and/or feeding, infrequent milk expression, stress, fatigue, return to work, poor maternal health, sudden changes in the infant's condition, and, possibly, biological immaturity. Indeed, fatigue and pain result in stimulation of prolactin inhibitory factor, which serves to blunt milk synthesis induced by prolactin.

In addition, fluid administration to premature infants often is limited because infants do not feed ad libitum. Fluid restriction also is practiced for many infants because of their clinical condition. The volume of human milk required to meet the Canadian Premature Infant Recommended Nutrient Intakes (P-RNIs) for a selection of nutrients is shown in Table 2. Usually premature infants, especially those of extremely low birth weight, do not easily tolerate volumes of intake above 180 ml/kg body weight/day; many such infants are restricted to fluid intakes more in the range of 150 - 160 ml/kg/day. As observed in Table 2, to achieve the P-RNI for protein would require a minimum of 180 ml/kg/day of early lactation milk and the upper level of recommended intake for selected other nutrients could not be met unless 200 ml/kg/day or more were tolerated by the infant.[44] Even if human milk is available, many infants do not achieve full enteral feedings for several weeks after birth. Thus, adequacy of nutrient intake may be jeopardized by the unavailability of milk and limited fluid volume that can be tolerated by the infant.[45]

Variability in Milk Composition

The adequacy of nutrient intake is further compromised by the variability in nutrient composition, both inherent to milk and imposed by circumstances of collection and distribution of the milk. A large variation in the energy and protein contents of human milk brought to the neonatal nursery by the mother is observed.[46] This variation may arise because of differences in methods of milk collection and storage, the feeding of "spot" samples (individual samples of expressed milk from one or both breasts, or milk partially expressed from one breast), the use of feeding tubes, and the differences in length of lactation.[47]

The most variable nutrient in human milk is fat, the content of which differs during lactation, throughout the day, from mother to mother, and within a single milk expression.[48,49] As human milk is not homogenized, upon standing, the fat content separates from the body of milk. Much of the variation in energy content of milk as used in the nursery is a result of differences in and/or losses of fat in the unfortified milk.[47] In one report, the range in fat contents of milk brought to the nursery was 2.2 to 4.7 g/dL.[46] Therefore, when collecting, mixing, and/or storing milk, efforts must be directed to avoid allowing the fat to separate from the milk and be discarded inadvertently. When feeding, the use of continuous tube-feeding methods reduces fat delivery to the infant compared with intermittent-bolus feeding.[50] Should the clinical condition mandate continuous tube-feeding, the milk syringe should be oriented with tip upright, a short length of feeding tube should be used, and the syringe should be emptied completely into the infant at end of the infusion. This practice will ensure the least loss of fat because the fat will flow along with the remainder of the milk. The bolus tube-feeding method, however, is associated with the least loss of fat. The within-feed change in fat content, however, also can be used to benefit the infant if the mother's milk production is in excess of the infant's need. Hindmilk may have two- to three-fold greater fat content than foremilk and can be utilized to provide significantly more fat and, therefore, energy for growth.[48] As fat is the most variable nutrient and many mothers do not produce sufficient volumes to allow fractionation into foremilk and hindmilk, the use of vegetable oil supplements has been recommended. Because exogenous fat does not mix with human milk, the fat should be given in divided doses directly into the feeding tube before a tube-feeding.

There is a significant decline in the content of protein from transitional to mature milk which contributes to the problem of nutrient variability (Table 1). Although concentrations of protein and sodium decline through lactation, the nutrient needs of the premature infant remain higher than those of term infants until sometime after term postmenstrual age. Therefore, the decline in milk concentration precedes the reduction in nutrient needs and results in an inadequate nutrient supply from human milk for the premature infant. The content of other nutrients (eg, calcium, phosphorus) have less variability through lactation but remain too low with respect to the needs of the premature infant. Technical reasons associated with collection, storage, and delivery of milk to the infant also result in a decreased quantity of available nutrients (eg, Vitamin C, Vitamin A, riboflavin).

Consequences of Feeding Unfortified Human Milk

Growth

The exclusive feeding of unfortified human milk in premature infants, generally infants with birth weights less than 1500 g, has been associated with poorer rates of growth and nutritional deficits, during and beyond the period of hospital stay.[51-55] As growth rates in excess of 15 g/kg/day are desired, unfortified human milk would not meet this target.

Protein Status

Serum indices of protein nutritional status, urea nitrogen, albumin, total protein, and transthyretin, are lower and continue to decline over time when premature infants are fed unfortified human milk.[51,54,56]

Mineral Status

As a consequence of the low intakes of calcium and phosphorus, infants fed unfortified human milk have progressive decreases in serum phosphorus, increases in serum calcium, and increases in serum alkaline phosphatase activity compared with infants fed preterm formula.[52,57,58] Follow-up investigations of such infants at 18 months report that infants having the highest alkaline phosphatase in-hospital have as

much as a 2 cm reduction in linear growth.[59]

The low milk sodium intake, especially if diuretics are given to the infant, may be associated with late hyponatremia.[60]

Human Milk Fortification

The nutrient deficits that arise from feeding unfortified human milk can be corrected with nutrient supplementation.[45] Multinutrient supplementation of human milk is associated with improvements in growth (positive increments in body weight, length, and head circumference) and nutritional status.[61]

Protein and energy supplementation are associated with improved rates of weight gain, nitrogen balance, and indices of protein nutritional status: blood urea nitrogen, serum albumin, total protein, and transthyretin.[54,62] The efficacy of protein fortification of human milk on growth outcomes was recently reviewed.[63] An analysis of four randomized or quasi-randomized trials in premature infants (n=90) where the fortifier was derived from human milk protein or hydrolysate protein observed that protein supplementation (~ 1.5 g protein/kg/d added to human milk) was of short-term benefit resulting in increases in weight gain and increments in length and head circumference growth. Although the measured gains were small, the effects were cumulative. It was concluded that even a small advantage in growth (weight, length, or head circumference) could have a significant impact and even effect the duration of hospitalization.[63] The source of protein in the fortifier also has been studied. Similar responses to bovine compared with human milk protein sources have been reported.[64]

Single or combined mineral supplementation has been evaluated in hospitalized premature infants. Supplementation with both calcium and phosphorus results in normalization of biochemical indices of mineral status: serum calcium, phosphorus, and alkaline phosphatase activity, and urinary excretion of calcium and phosphorus.[57,65] Mineral supplementation of unfortified human milk has been associated with improved linear growth and increased bone mineralization during and beyond the neonatal period.[61] A normalization of serum sodium has been reported following the supplementation of unfortified human milk with sodium.[66]

A systematic review that addressed multinutrient fortification of human milk included a meta-analysis of ten controlled trials (n=596 infants in total with birth weight generally < 1850 grams) using either random or quasi-random allocation to human milk fortification compared with the feeding of unfortified human milk.[61] Based on this analysis, the addition of multinutrient fortifiers to human milk resulted in short-term improvements in weight gain and increments in both length and head circumference growth during hospital stay. For ethical reasons, it is now unlikely that further studies evaluating fortification of human milk in comparison with no fortification will be conducted.

More recent studies have compared randomized trials of newly formulated commercial human milk fortifiers. There are several issues relating to the desire to reformulate earlier human milk fortifiers. The desire to improve the intake of protein was a major factor in the design of recent human milk fortifiers. At the same time the concern about the lower fat absorption reported with fortified human milk was addressed by adding a fat source to the fortifier and by altering the mineral suspension.[67] In two such studies, comparisons of premature infants assigned randomly to one of two human milk fortifiers from different manufacturers, containing varying protein and mineral composition, there were benefits to growth in infants fed the formulations containing the greater quantities of protein and fat.[68,69] Beneficial effects on growth were observed in response to mean differences in protein intake of 0.3 - 0.4 g/kg/d fed over 20 to 29 days while in-hospital. Higher plasma alkaline phosphatase in the group receiving higher protein intake was considered a supportive indicator of enhanced linear growth.[69] In addition, since energy intakes were similar between treatment groups within each study, and since no apparent nutrient deficiencies were observed (normal plasma protein and mineral status), there is support for the hypothesis that the higher protein intakes, even of < 0.5 g/kg/d over only 3-5 weeks were responsible for

the benefits to growth.[62,68,69] Furthermore, the reported rates of growth were similar to those achieved in utero.[68-70] However, no catch-up growth has been observed, possibly since the average protein intake was limited to approximately 3 g/kg/d.

The use of multinutrient fortification of human milk for premature infants is recommended.[67,71-73] Further research is required to improve commercial fortifiers for human milk so that optimal growth and feeding tolerance can be achieved even in the extremely low birth weight infant.

Non-Nutritional Outcomes of Feeding Fortified Human Milk

Feeding Tolerance

Questions have been raised as to whether the addition of bovine-derived human milk fortifiers affect feeding tolerance in premature infants. Gastric residual volumes often are used to assess feeding tolerance. The residual volume may be affected by gastric emptying. The data on gastric emptying, however, are controversial. Novel ultrasound techniques to assess gastric cross-sectional areas have reported conflicting results.[74,75] In contrast, it clearly has been reported that use of fortified human milk is not associated with feeding intolerance, as manifest by abdominal distention, vomiting, changes in stool frequency, or volume of gastric aspirate.[32] An investigation of feeding tolerance indices 5 days before vs 5 days after addition of human milk fortifier revealed that of the ten indices assessed, only gastric residual volume > 2 ml/kg and emesis were statistically greater after the addition of HMF. However, infants manifesting these feeding intolerance indices were no more likely to have delays in achieving full tube-feeding or full oral feeding than infants not experiencing increases in feeding intolerance indices. Furthermore, no differences in feeding tolerance were reported in a meta-analysis comparing premature infants fed fortified human milk or unfortified human milk.[61] Moreover, premature infants fed human milk fortified with a variety of commercial multinutrient fortifiers have not manifested any differences in feeding tolerance.[68,69,76] Lastly, in comparison with infants fed preterm formula, those fed fortified human milk had similar tolerance to feeding.[67] Thus, concerns about feeding tolerance should not dissuade clinicians from using human milk fortifier.

Host Defense

A major concern with human milk fortification is that the added nutrients may affect the intrinsic host defense system of the milk. The relationship between diet and the incidence of infection in premature infants has been examined. Human milk-fed infants had a 26% incidence of documented infection compared with 49% in formula-fed infants.[37] Results of a randomized trial of fortified human milk indicated no increases in the incidence of either confirmed infection or necrotizing enterocolitis compared with controls.[32] When the latter two events were combined, however, the group fed fortified human milk had more events than infants in the control group. The data, however, are difficult to interpret because study infants in both groups received more than 50% of their diet as preterm formula.[33] Although it is difficult to conclude that use of fortifiers is harmful, these data support the need for continued surveillance of these events.

When compared with premature infants fed preterm formula, those infants fed exclusively fortified human milk had a significantly lower incidence of necrotizing enterocolitis and/or sepsis, fewer positive blood cultures, and less antibiotic usage.[67] In that study, infants receiving the most human milk had the fewest positive blood cultures. Infants fed exclusively fortified human milk also had more episodes of skin-to-skin contact with their mothers and shorter hospital stays. From these data, it appears that feeding premature infants fortified human milk might have a marked effect on reducing the cost of medical care.

The effect of nutrient fortification on some of the general host defense properties of milk have been evaluated.[77,78] Fortification did not affect the concentration of IgA in milk.[77,78] When fortified human milk was evaluated under simulated nursery conditions, bacterial colony counts were not significantly different after 20-hours storage at refrigerator temperature, but did increase from 20 to 24 hours when maintained at incubator temperature. The overall increase in bacterial colony counts at 24 hours, however, was back to the original values.[77] Based on these data, changes are unlikely to be necessary in regard to the current practice of how fortifiers are used in the nursery.

Other Outcomes

Unfortunately, there have been insufficient data to evaluate long-term outcomes of fortification of human milk on growth or neurodevelopment. One limited study found no differences in neurodevelopmental outcome at 18 months in premature infants fed fortified or minimally-supplemented human milk in-hospital.[32] Accordingly, several investigators have made a plea for further research that is designed to address both the short-term and long-term outcomes of protein and multinutrient fortification of human milk.[61]

Nutritional Issues with Human Milk Fortifiers
Powder vs Liquid Fortifiers

The fortification of human milk can be performed using a liquid commercial formula mixed with human milk or a powdered commercial product. The powdered product has the obvious advantage of not diluting the human milk and has been reported to be preferred by parents, and to have a positive impact on duration of breastfeeding.[79] Few randomized comparisons among fortifiers have been reported. A casual comparison between a liquid preterm formula mixed with human milk (1:1, vol:vol) and a powdered human milk fortifier can be derived from the literature.[67,80] Protein intake and net retention were lower with the liquid preparation than the powder. Calcium, phosphorus, and zinc intakes also were lower with the liquid compared with the powdered preparation used in the early 1990s. Not only are the nutrient intakes lower with the liquid preparation, but the achieved net nutrient retentions are well below expected rates of intrauterine nutrient accretion.[2] The use of a liquid fortifier should be reserved for situations when the mother is unable to provide sufficient milk to meet her infant's needs. However, when sufficient human milk is unavailable, an alternative approach is to feed fortified human milk (using powdered fortifier) for as many feedings as there is milk available, then alternating with preterm formula for the remaining feedings.

Growth

The growth of premature infants fed fortified human milk has been reported to be lower than that of similar infants receiving preterm formula in some but not all studies.[65,67,81] Several explanations have been advanced for this observation. The protein intake from fortified human milk is lower than preterm formula, especially if comparisons are made of fortified mature milk and formula. Studies of formulations of fortified human milk in the early 1990s reported lower fat absorption than infants fed preterm formula.[67] Thus, a slower rate of growth was observed as a consequence of lower energy absorption in the infants fed fortified human milk when compared with infants fed preterm formula.[32,38,82] The variability in the fat content of human milk, the lack of fat in the human milk fortifiers used in the 1990s, and the soluble mineral preparations interacting with the fat globule, together, could result in lower rates of fat absorption. The addition of a large quantity of minerals to human milk may have created an unfavorable milieu for the human milk lipid system. The fat globule may be disrupted by osmotic forces generated by the high mineral content of the fortifier, and result in the liberation of free fatty acids. The free fatty acids may bind minerals and form soaps. In the intestinal tract soap formation may hinder fat absorption.[83,84]

Paradoxically, it appears that slower rate of growth is not associated with poorer nutritional status. Biochemical indices for infants fed fortified human milk are within the normal range. Furthermore, premature infants fed fortified human milk have shorter hospital stays and less infection and necrotizing enterocolitis than infants fed preterm formula.[67] Thus, because of nutrient need and widespread use of human milk fortifiers, and because adequate safety features

have been demonstrated, efforts to improve human milk fortifier contents are needed.

To address issues of protein intake, growth, and fat absorption, two randomized trials of powdered human milk fortifier were conducted in the late 1990s.[68,69] The greater contents of protein, sodium, and fat were associated with improved growth. In one of the trials, increments in body weight, length, and head circumference were associated with the greater nutrient-containing human milk fortifier.[69] The group receiving the higher nutrient-containing human milk fortifier required a lower milk volume to achieve the greater rates of growth.[68] Although infants receiving the greater protein intake also had higher (more normal) blood urea nitrogen values,[68] indices of protein nutritional status tended to decline during the study.[69] From these data, it appears that optimal protein intakes were not achieved.

To address issues of highly soluble calcium-phosphorus salts and their association with hypercalcemia and hyperphosphatemia, as well as possible interaction with the human milk fat globule, the mineral suspension also was tested in one of the trials.[69] Serum calcium and phosphorus were lower in a group receiving a new fortifier containing less soluble mineral sources.[69] In addition, the human milk fortifier trials used formulations that differed markedly in their contents of zinc and copper. Despite no added copper to one of the fortifiers, no differences in serum copper or ceruloplasmin concentration were observed between infants fed a human milk fortifier not containing copper compared with infants fed a fortifier containing copper.[68] Neither randomized trial reported any safety issues or differences in morbidity between study groups.

Future Research Issues

To date, based on the randomized trials of fortified human milk, greater protein and fat (available energy) intakes appear to be needed to optimize growth and body composition of premature infants. Nevertheless, there exist a number of further research issues in the design of human milk fortifiers. The optimal protein quantity has not been established. As most milk is

Nutrient	Enfamil HMF	Similac HMF	SMA BMF	Milupa Eoprotin	Nutriprem Cow & Gate	Aptamil FMS Milupa	FM85 Nestle
How supplied	4 packets	4 packets	2 sachets	3 scoops	2 sachets	powder	powder
Quantity	4 g	4 g	4 g	3 g	3 g	3.4 g	5 g
Energy, kcal	14	14	15	11	10	12	18
Protein, g	1.1	1	1	0.6	0.7	0.8	0.8
Fat, g	0.65	0.36	0.16	0.02	0	0	0.015
Carbohydrate, g	1.1	1.8	2.4	2.1	2	2.2	3.6
Calcium, mg	90	117	90	38	60	69	51
Phosphorus. mg	45	67	45	26	40	46	34
Magnesium, mg	1	7	3	2.1	6	6.8	2
Iron, mg	1.44	0.35	0	0	0	0	0
Manganese, mcg	10	7.2	4.6	0	6	10	0
Zinc, mcg	720	1000	260	0	300	350	0
Copper, mcg	44	170	0	0	26	30	0
Sodium, mmol	0.5	0.7	0.8	0.9	0.3	0.3	1.2
Potassium, mmol	0.5	1.6	0.7	0.006	0.1	0.1	0.3
Chloride, mmol	0.3	1.1	0.5	0.4	0.2	0.2	0.5
Increment in Osmolality, mOsm	63	90	137	70	60	57	105
Vitamin A, mcg	285	186	270	30	130	150	0
Vitamin D, mcg	4	3	7.6	0	5	5.7	0
Vitamin E, mg	4.6	3.2	3	0.3	2.6	2.9	0
Vitamin K_1, mcg	4.4	8.3	11	0.2	6.3	7.1	0
Thiamin, mcg	150	233	220	0	130	150	0
Riboflavin, mcg	220	417	260	0	170	190	0
Vitamin B_6, mcg	115	211	260	0	110	120	0
Vitamin B_{12}, mcg	0.18	0.64	0.3	0	0.2	0.2	0
Niacin, mg	3	3.57	3.6	0	2.5	2.8	0
Folic acid, mcg	25	23	0	0	50	57	0
Pantothenic acid, mg	0.73	1.5	0	0	0.75	0.85	0
Biotin, mcg	2.7	26	0	0	2.5	2.8	0
Vitamin C, mg	12	25	40	15	12	14	0

Enfamil Human Milk Fortifier (Mead Johnson Nutritionals, Evansville, IN), Similac Human Milk Fortifier (Ross Laboratories, Columbus, OH), SMA Breast Milk Fortifier (Wyeth Nutritionals International, Philadelphia, PA), Eoprotin (Milupa, Friedrichsdorf, Germany), FM85 (Nestle, Vevey, Switzerland), Nutriprem (Cow & Gate), Aptamil FMS (Milupa)

Table 3: Nutrient composition of commercial human milk fortifiers.

"mature," efforts to augment the protein content of that milk are warranted. It also appears that the addition of fat to the fortifier may facilitate higher net fat absorption and lead to improved weight gain. As fat is the most variable nutrient in human milk, added fat supplement is appropriate, but the type of fat source has not been addressed. A variety of calcium-phosphorus sources have been used in human milk fortification, but no data exist to determine optimal bone mineralization (See full discussion in Chapter Nine, "Calcium, Magnesium, Phosphorus and Vitamin D"). The divergent views on zinc and copper supplementation also should be explored. Lastly, no studies have been conducted to determine whether iron should be included in the human milk fortifier.

In-Hospital Feeding Practices

A variety of protocols are used for feeding fortified human milk. In one such protocol, human milk is fortified when the infant achieves an enteral intake of 100 ml/kg/day.[67] The volume is maintained for approximately 2 days while the concentration is increased by the addition of fortifier. The intake of fortified human milk is then advanced daily to maintain a body weight gain of greater than 15 g/kg/day. No additional vitamin supplements are needed. To support the low iron stores of the premature infant, if the fortifier has insufficient iron content, an exogenous source of elemental iron is supplied after complete enteral feeding is achieved. By knowledge of the lactational stage of the milk being fed

1. Collection	3. Storage

A. Preparation
   a. Wash hands
   b. Clean nails
   c. Breast cleansing
      i. Daily shower adequate
      ii. Natural lubricants exist
      iii. No special cleansing
   d. Nipple lubricants are unnecessary
B. Breast pumps
   a. Hospital grade electric pump
   b. Hand pumps (e.g., bicycle horn variety) should not be used
   c. Cleaning of pumping kit
      i. Clean with hot soapy water
      ii. Dishwasher cleaning
      iii. Air drying
C. Parent instructions
   a. Clear and repeated
   b. Label milk
      i. Medications
      ii. Illnesses in the home
   c. Provide list of contact personnel
   d. Support groups
D. Containers
   a. Sterile, air tight caps
   b. Use rigid plastic or glass
   c. Discourage plastic bags
	A. Refrigerate immediately if to be used completely by 48 hours
	B. Freeze milk that will not be used completely by 48 h after expression
	C. Initially feed milk expressed in first 2 weeks
	D. Subsequently match feeding with newest milk collected
	E. Freezer storage adequate for 3 months

	4. Transport A. Thermally insulated cooler

	5. Delivery of milk to infant
	A. Thawing of frozen milk in storage container
	   a. Rapid, held under stream of lukewarm water
	   b. In water bath
	   c. Never use microwave oven
	   d. Avoid excessive heat
	B. Warming of thawed, refrigerated milk
	   a. Avoid excess heat
	   b. Hold under running lukewarm tap water
	   c. Short time in a dry heat incubator
	   d. Do not reuse after warming

2. Initiation of milk collection A. Begin milk expression soon after delivery B. Don't discard milk C. Each expression should be collected separately D. Package milk in feeding size portions	**6. Quality control issues** A. Bacteriological culture of milk not required B. Bacteriological screening of milk may identify improper collection techniques C. Hospital pumps should be cleaned and monitored daily D. Temperature of storage refrigerators/freezers monitored E. Milk storage in secure location F. Milk handling as other body fluids a. Dual staff signatures for each feeding to match mother and infant G. Document advice given to mother H. Document medications/illnesses recorded by mother

Adapted from Recommendations for Collection, Storage, and Handling of a Mother's Milk for Her Own Infant in the Hospital Setting. The Human Milk Banking Association of North America, 1993.[128]

Table 4: Human milk collection, storage, transport, and delivery to the hospitalized infant.

and then using the average milk composition of transitional or mature preterm milk in Table 1, one can estimate the intake achieved from human milk. Further addition of the fortifier contents (Table 3) then provides the actual intake of the infant.

Fortified human milk is prepared daily and stored at refrigerator temperature in individual feeding syringes until used within 24 hours. Milk should be handled and checked carefully to ensure that the donor and recipient identities match.

If maternal milk volume is inadequate to meet the infant's needs completely, either of two protocols have been practiced. A liquid preterm formula or liquid human milk fortifier has been used, mixed 1:1 (vol:vol) with human milk.[80] Another approach has been to alternate feedings of available fortified (powder) human milk with preterm formula.

Lactation Support

The importance of human milk for the premature infant is established. There are major concerns that mothers may be unable to produce sufficient milk to meet the needs of their premature infants. Milk production may not match milk demand. An aggressive approach toward lactation support, therefore, is critical for success.

Initiation

Clinicians should inquire as soon as possible following delivery of the premature infant as to the mother's plans regarding feeding. Many mothers who had no intention of breastfeeding their term infant, are willing, and even grateful, for the chance to contribute to their premature infant's care in a unique way. Mothers should hear an unequivocal message that their milk is preferable for feeding their infant. Parents who are concerned that they will be unable to provide milk for the entire hospital stay should be counseled that "any" of their milk is better than none of their milk. Mothers should begin milk expression as soon as possible after delivery.

Milk Production

Maternal milk volume is directly related to frequency of stimulation and degree of breast emptying.[85,86] Without a suckling infant, this is accomplished with the use of a mechanical breast pump. A hospital-grade electric breast pump, with a cycling pattern of 40 to 50 times per minute, is associated with the best compliance among mothers and is most often recommended for long-term milk volume maintenance.[87] Collection systems that allow for simultaneous pumping of both breasts (double pumping system) are available and preferred to shorten the time spent for this procedure and to enable the greatest milk production. Mothers should be instructed to pump at least every 3 hours during the day with no more than a 5 hour non-pumping interval at night. In the first week or so following delivery, mothers benefit from a pumping duration of 15 minutes when double pumping, or 20 minutes (10 minutes per breast) when single pumping. Alternating breasts, approximately 5 minutes on one, then 5 minutes on the other breast, followed by light massage of the breasts and then repeating the process, may be useful in synchronizing the milk ejection reflex with milk expression. Mothers should be encouraged to continue to express their milk until after the last droplets cease to flow. In that way, the breast will be emptied completely.

Milk Collection and Storage

Key guidelines for the collection and handling of expressed milk are outlined in Table 4. Milk should be collected in either glass or rigid plastic containers. Plastic bags should be discouraged because of the loss of immune components and the potential for contamination. One milk expression should be collected separately in each milk container. Milk to be

fed within 24 hours can be refrigerated after collection. Milk to be fed beyond that time should be frozen immediately at -15° to -20° C. All milk must be transported to the hospital in an enclosed thermally protected container. Maternal compliance with milk collection occasionally can be monitored by bacteriological screening of a milk sample.[88]

Maintaining Milk Volume

The maintenance of an adequate milk volume to meet her infant's needs is a concern of all breastfeeding mothers. The mother of a premature infant is in a unique position in that her milk volume, if adequate, will exceed her infant's volume needs in the early weeks following delivery. Maternal milk production with a suckling infant averages approximately 750 to 800 ml per day, or about 30 ml per hour.[89] For mothers who must express milk, this volume should be the target for the mother to reach by the end of the second week in order to allow for a safeguard in the event the volume diminishes during hospitalization. However, the inability to immediately produce such a volume does not represent lactation failure for the mother having to mechanically express her milk. Although a milk volume of 500 to 600 ml per day may be considered adequate for a small premature infant, as the duration of hospital stay is increased the volume may decline as a result of a static pumping schedule. In contrast to the term breastfeeding infant whose feeding schedule fluctuates to meet increased appetite and growth needs, the mother of a premature infant usually keeps the same milk expression frequency.

Milk production of less than 350 ml per day requires prompt attention. Strategies to deal with a low milk volume include relaxation techniques before pumping sessions, manual milk expression before mechanical pumping, increased frequency of milk expression, breast massage during pumping, prompt treatment of nipple and/or breast soreness or other abnormalities, and consideration of pharmacological therapy.[90] Pharmacological therapy with metoclopramide has been used with some success in women who have low, but measurable milk volume and are pumping frequently.[91]

Breastfeeding in the Premature Infant

Skin-to-skin contact

Kangaroo care or skin-to-skin holding of the infant has been shown to be of benefit to premature infants and their mothers in a variety of physiological and psychological ways.[82,92] Improved thermoregulation, heart rate, oxygen saturation, and weight gain are some of the benefits to the infant that have been reported.[93] A significant increase in maternal milk volume is observed in women who practice skin-to-skin holding of their premature infants.[94] Skin-to-skin holding also is an ideal prerequisite to early breastfeeding of the premature infant. Holding her infant close for prolonged periods each day allows the mother to observe early feeding cues, such as sucking on the feeding tube and the rooting reflex. This practice has facilitated maternal requests to initiate breastfeeding.

Initiation of Breastfeeding

Breastfeeding success requires not only adequate milk supply from the mother, but also adequate oral feeding skills from the infant. The timing of the initial breastfeeding episode is variable, depending on a variety of factors, not always related to the physiological ability of the infant. Traditional criteria to decide when to initiate oral feeding used the infant's ability to tolerate bolus tube-feedings, overall "clinical stability," and attainment of specific gestational age (~34 weeks) and body weight (~1.5 kg).[90] However, these criteria have not been proven to correlate with oral feeding success. Indeed, those criteria may delay the introduction of oral feeding. Behaviorally based criteria may be more meaningful. Observations of oral activity in the infant, sucking on the feeding tube, rooting reflex during skin-to-skin sessions, and brief periods of active or alert states, provide a better assessment of when to initiate breastfeeding.[90]

As compared with bottle-feeding, breastfeeding is a more active process. Because of the protractility and elasticity of the breast nipple, the infant must be able to grasp and hold the tissue while sucking is initiated. This contrasts with bottle feeding where the infant is not required to retain the rubber nipple in the mouth. Milk flow with bottle feeding, if necessary, can be regulated through external interventions.[95] In contrast, with breastfeeding, the sudden increase in flow during the let-down may lead to the incoordination of suck-swallow-breathe actions. As such, the infant's state and physiological stability become critical factors of breastfeeding success. Studies in premature infants have demonstrated improved oxygenation, heart and respiratory rate, and improved thermoregulation with breastfeeding as compared with bottle feeding.[96,97] However, due to the lack of early training or insufficient attention given to the feeding session, milk transfer during early breastfeeding may be less than that achieved using the bottle.[97] Recently, investigators have reported safety with an alternate method, the cup feeding method.[98]

Estimating Milk Intake at the Breast

Milk intake during breastfeeding can be estimated in several ways: by observing the infant's suck and swallow; from maternal perceptions of the milk ejection reflex; by the degree of change in breast fullness; by aspiration of the contents of indwelling orogastric tubes to measure gastric milk volume; and by test-weighing procedures. The first three methods generally have less accuracy because of their subjective nature. Measurement of gastric contents may be an underestimate of intake due to faster gastric motility rates that occur with human milk feedings.[40] Milk intake can be evaluated more accurately by test-weighing, a procedure in which the clothed infant is weighed on an electronic scale immediately before and after breastfeeding.[96,99] The test-weighing procedure also provides some assurance to mothers who want to know how much milk the infant is receiving, especially during the early breastfeeding sessions.

Strategies to Enhance the Success of Early Breastfeeding

The above methods to estimate milk intake provide the mother with the assurance that the baby is receiving a satisfactory intake. Sometimes it is helpful to encourage the mother to express milk before the breastfeeding session if she has a very active let-down, or to pump just before feeding to stimulate her let-down. Pumping on the opposite breast also may increase milk flow on the breast used for feeding. Nipple shields serve to increase milk transfer in premature infants.[100] The shield may compensate for the weak intraoral suction pressure exerted by the infant. Thin silicone shields are constructed so that the infant's nose is not blocked by the shield. Contrary to earlier reports, use of the newer nipple shields do not reduce the duration of breastfeeding.[100] Lastly, supplemental feeding devices may be used to augment milk intake during a breastfeeding session.[90] These devices generally utilize a soft feeding tube connected to a reservoir of milk. The tube is taped to the mother's breast, so that as the infant suckles, milk flows from the tube and the mother at the same time.

Progression of Breastfeedings

As breastfeeding progresses from the early practice session on the emptied breast to nutritive feeding, a primary concern for the mother and the clinician is the evaluation of milk intake during breastfeeding and management of complementary or supplementary feedings. As skin-to-skin holding sessions progress to "practice" feeding sessions at the emptied breast, the mother's availability should be assessed to determine a plan for advancing breastfeeding. Mothers may be available for only one feeding a day, as many mothers may have transportation problems or other family obligations. As the infant demonstrates success at more than one feeding per day, arrangements can be made with the mother to block a 6 to 8 hour interval to allow self-regulatory breastfeeding. In that interval, the mother may breastfeed as often as she receives cues from her infant. Throughout this transition to breastfeeding, the pattern of the infant's weight gain is monitored.

Discharge Planning

At the time when discharge planning begins, the status of the infant's milk intake during breastfeeding (use of the test-weighing procedure) and the maternal pumped milk volume (adequacy to meet the infant's daily needs at home) should be considered to develop a rational feeding plan. The discharge plan should be tailored to the needs of the particular infant. Premature infants unable to breastfeed all of their feedings, or those who cannot attain adequate growth while feeding unfortified human milk ad libitum need close scrutiny in the post-discharge period. In addition, those infants whose biochemical profile suggests ongoing inadequate nutrient intake (eg, unmeasurable blood urea nitrogen, low albumin, elevated alkaline phosphatase) also are at risk. The discharge plan should be prepared well in advance of the date of discharge. Infants receiving fortified human milk should be given at least a week to feed unfortified human milk so that appropriate assessments can be made.

It should be cautioned that in some circumstances counseling mothers to feed the infant "on-demand" may potentiate breastfeeding failure because of inadequate milk volume and/or inability of the infant to ingest adequate volume. Because of their concern about adequacy of their infants' intake at the breast, many mothers use additional feedings following breastfeeding sessions to ensure the adequacy of milk intake. The care plan should include these feedings if there are concerns that intake and/or weight gain will be suboptimal. Test-weighing procedures post-discharge, therefore, are useful to assist mothers in assessing milk transfer during breastfeeding and the management of additional feedings. Electronic infant scales are available for home use. This practice usually is useful for the first few days or week after discharge until the mother is confident that the infant's intake and growth are adequate.

Post-Discharge Use of Human Milk

Post-discharge, enriched formulas are now available for the formula-feeding premature infant. There is an array of milks from which to choose when the discharge of the premature infant is approaching. However, there are no data to support reference intakes to use for the premature infant who is breastfed post-discharge. It is neither practical, nor appropriate, routinely to use human milk fortifiers in the post-discharge period. The addition of supplemental nutrients to the milk prevents continued feeding at the breast. Furthermore, the concentration of the nutrients in human milk fortifiers may be too great when the infant surpasses near-term gestational age (~36 weeks). Feeding of human milk compared with standard infant formula after reaching term age may result in differences in growth and body composition. Thus, there remains a dilemma when making recommendations for the premature infant who is breastfed post-discharge.

The dilemma is heightened because of conflicting data in the few studies that have been reported. Premature infants fed unsupplemented human milk after hospital discharge appear to have a slower accretion in both radius[101,102] and whole body[81] bone mass when compared with infants fed standard formula. The lower bone mass is presumably due to a lower amount of calcium and phosphorus in human milk than in term formula. Mineral-deficient bone disease or osteopenia has been described in human milk-fed premature infants after hospital discharge,[103] and there is some suggestion that this is linked to fractures early in life[104] and reduced linear growth even at eighteen months of age.[59] Only a few studies have followed bone mineral accretion in premature infants after hospital discharge. One descriptive study comparing human milk vs standard term formula after discharge observed no differences in weight and length gains, although the sample size may have limited ability to detect differences.[70] An important observation in that study, however, was that both mean weight and length of these breastfed premature infants were within the 5th- to 50th-reference centiles for term breastfed infants over the first year of life.[70] The infants fed human milk did have a significantly higher percent body fat than those fed standard formula. One possible explanation was that protein intake was lower in the infants receiving human milk compared with formula. Since energy intakes were similar, the lower protein:energy ratio consumed by the human milk-fed group may have led to less deposition of lean mass with excess energy deposited as fat.

In contrast to the latter findings, one study showed that infants (birthweight 1.4 kg, gestational age 31 wk) predominantly fed their mother's milk for at least 6 weeks after discharge had lower weight and length gain and less lean mass (as computed from skinfold thickness measurements) compared with infants fed either enriched formula or term formula. The difference in growth parameters remained at 9-months-corrected age despite the termination of exclusive breastfeeding well before that time. Based on several studies in formula-fed premature infants, there appear to be short-term advantages in bone mineral accretion and linear growth after hospital discharge when an enriched vs standard formula is fed.[105-109] Persistence of benefits in growth and bone mineralization from an enriched formula were observed to twelve months, six months after the period of dietary intervention.[110] A small, but significantly greater body length was noted in another study at eighteen months, nine months after cessation of the enriched formula feeding compared with term formula. However, in studies where fortification of human milk supported greater bone mineral accretion of infants while in-hospital and through twelve months of age, the advantage to bone mass accretion was no longer apparent at twenty-four months of age.[111] In a retrospective study, no deficits in radius bone mineral after one year of age were noted in former premature infants fed human milk with moderate supplementation of calcium, phosphorus and protein in-hospital.[102]

To add to the conflict in the data, it appears that "catch-up" bone mineral accretion occurs once infants are weaned to formula, bovine milk, and solid foods.[81,102,111] In fact, there is evidence that human milk feeding, with relatively low intakes of calcium and phosphorus, is associated with a greater bone mineral content at five years of age.[112] Furthermore, in term breastfed infants, breastfeeding beyond three months has a positive advantage to bone mass in later life.[113] However, other data indicate that an elevated plasma alkaline phosphatase in the neonatal period has an inverse relationship to linear growth up to twelve years of age.[114]

The data on growth responses to the feeding of human milk remain conflicting. It appears that despite slower rates of growth in the neonatal period, attained growth parameters at eight years of former human milk-fed premature infants are similar to former premature infants fed formula in the neonatal period.[115] Although the data are conflicting, there may be implications of the effects of diet in early life on long-term bone growth and mineralization. Nevertheless, more studies are needed to substantiate such a hypothesis.

Thus, for the post-discharge management of the human milk-fed premature infant, close observation is warranted. Infants at risk should be breastfed, but their diet may need to be supplemented with enriched formula (once to twice per day). That formula may be prepared as a concentrated mixture (~30 kcal/oz or 100 kcal/100 ml) to provide added nutrients. The infant should have close follow-up of growth and serial measurement of selected biochemical indices of nutritional status.[116]

Conclusion

Consensus is emerging that human milk is beneficial in many aspects for premature infants. Research to date supports the clinical practice of using human milk for feeding premature infants. While velocity of growth and bone mineral accretion may be slower than in infants fed formula, there is no indication that slower growth in early life is an impediment to growth attained in childhood. Fortification of human milk with multiple nutrients during the time infants receive tube-feedings will serve to maintain normal protein and mineral status and promote growth. Mounting evidence underlines the positive influence of human milk over formula feeding of premature infants on health outcomes and neurodevelopment. Components of human milk may be important contributors to "programming" of metabolism that impacts on later growth and development. Clearly, this is an exciting area of research that needs to be expanded. The potential stimulation of an enteromammary pathway through skin-to-skin contact may be a means of providing species-specific antimicrobial protection for the premature infant. Human milk can only support the needs of the premature infant if adequate milk volumes are produced. Intensive efforts at lactation support are desirable. Neonatal centers should encourage the feeding of fortified human milk for premature infants along with skin-to-skin contact as a reasonable method to enhance milk production and initiate early breastfeeding, while potentially facilitating the development of an enteromammary response.

Acknowledgments

This review was supported by the National Institute of Child Health and Human Development, Grant No. RO-1-HD-28140 and the General Clinical Research Center, Baylor College of Medicine/Texas Children's Hospital Clinical Research Center, Grant No. MO-1-RR-00188, National Institutes of Health. Partial funding also has been provided from the USDA/ARS under Cooperative Agreement No. 58-6250-1-003. This work is a publication of the USDA/ARS Children's Nutrition Research Center, Department of Pediatrics, Baylor College of Medicine and Texas Children's Hospital, Houston, TX. The contents of this publication do not necessarily reflect the views or policies of the USDA, nor does mention of trade names, commercial products, or organizations imply endorsement by the US Government.

Case History

Baby boy JK, now 62 days of age, was an 810 g, 26-week-gestation infant who had moderate respiratory distress that resulted in chronic lung disease. He was extubated after 40 days hospitalization and now is receiving 1/2 liter of oxygen by nasal cannula. He had a grade 1 IVH bilaterally; subsequent cranial ultrasound exams were unremarkable. He has been fed his mother's milk beginning day 35 with 20 cc/kg/day (divided into feedings every 3 hours via orogastric tube). Currently he is receiving 200 cc/kg/day by OG tube and refuses to suck from a bottle. In the last 3 weeks he has gained approximately 12 g/day. He now weighs 1372 g. He has mild intercostal retractions and edema in his lower extremities. He has never received steroids. The following biochemical data were obtained on routine blood screening this week:

    Albumin: 1.9 g/dL
    Blood urea nitrogen: 2.0 mg/dL

Creatinine: 0.3 mg/dL

Na: 124 mEq/L (124 mmol/L)

K: 4.3 mEq/L (4.3 mmol/L)

Calcium: 11.3 mg/dL (2.8 mmol/L)

Phosphorus: 2.8 mg/dL (0.9 mmol/L)

Alkaline phosphatase: 998 IU/L

1. **Is the growth rate adequate?** *No. We still expect a rate of growth similar to or greater than the rate of intrauterine growth, > 15 g/kg/day. The use of human milk fortifier earlier in the hospital course would have benefited this infant.*

2. **Are the biochemical indices within normal limits?** *The use of unfortified human milk resulted in an abnormal protein and mineral nutritional status. The blood urea nitrogen and serum albumin are very low suggesting an inadequate intake of protein currently and previously for several weeks. The low serum phosphorus and high calcium and alkaline phosphatase indicate an inadequate intake of both calcium and phosphorus. The low serum sodium also reflects a low sodium intake.*

3. **Provide a nutrition plan for this infant.** *The infant requires greater intakes of protein, calcium, phosphorus, and sodium. He also would benefit from additional energy which should be provided as hindmilk, if the mother has sufficient volume to fractionate her milk collections into foremilk and hindmilk. If she is unable to do so, a simple vegetable oil supplement (approximately 2 ml/kg/day) given as a bolus in divided doses 4x per day would provide the needed calories. As fat is the most variable nutrient in human milk, it is the first choice for energy supplementation. We give the fat in divided doses, via the feeding tube just before every other milk feeding, because it doesn't mix easily with the milk.*

4. **Describe a plan for oral feeding.** *We would have initiated skin-to-skin contact between this infant and his mother in the first weeks after delivery. This is usually followed by "nonnutritive" feeding at the emptied breast and then a small "nutritive" feeding. Once appropriate latch-on is observed, one breastfeeding in place of a tube-feeding is given. Sometimes it is helpful for the mother to use a thin silicone nipple*

shield to aid the premature infant's suction. Test weighing procedures before and after a breastfeeding can provide useful information on milk intake. Breastfeeding is then practiced more than once per day. As mothers generally are unable to stay with their hospitalized premature infant for a whole day, it is helpful to define a given interval (eg, 6-8 hours) where breastfeeding is practiced frequently.

References

1. American Academy of Pediatrics, Work Group on Breastfeeding. Breastfeeding and the use of human milk. *Pediatrics* 1997;100:1035-1039.

2. Ziegler EE, O'Donnell AM, Nelson SE, Fomon SJ. Body composition of the reference fetus. *Growth* 1976;40:329-341.

3. Atkinson SA, Bryan MH, Anderson GH. Human milk: Difference in nitrogen concentration in milk from mothers of term and premature infants. *J Pediatr* 1978;93:67-69.

4. Atkinson SA. The effects of gestational stage at delivery on human milk components. In: Jensen RG. ed. *Handbook of Milk Composition.* San Diego: Academic Press; 1995:222-237.

5. Aquilio E, Spagnoli R, Seri S, Bottone G, Spennati G. Trace element content in human milk during lactation of preterm newborns. *Biol Trace Elem Res* 1996;51: 63-70.

6. Friel JK, Andrews WL, Jackson SE, et al. Elemental composition of human milk from mothers of premature and full-tern infants during the first 3 months of lactation. *Biol Trace Elem Res* 1999;67:225-247.

7. Perrone L, Di Palma L, Di Toro R, Gialanella G, Moro R. Interaction of trace elements in a longitudinal study of human milk from full-term and preterm mothers. *Biol Trace Elem Res* 1994;41:321-330.

8. Linzell JL, Peaker M. Changes in colostrum composition and in permeability of mammary epithelium at about the time of parturition in the goat. *J Physiol* (London) 1974;243:129-151.

9. Garza C, Johnson CA, Smith EO, Nichols BL. Changes in the nutrient composition of human milk during gradual weaning. *Am J Clin Nutr* 1983;37:61-65.

10. Anderson GH. The effect of prematurity on milk

composition and its physiological basis. *Fed Proc* 1984;43:2438-2442.

11. Djiane J, Durand P, Öhlin A. Prolactin-progesterone antagonism in self-regulation of prolactin receptors in the mammary gland during pregnancy and lactation. *Nature* 1977;266:641-643.

12. Lucas A, Hudson G. Preterm milk as a source of protein for low birthweight infants. *Arch Dis Child* 1984;59:831-836.

13. Narayanan I, Prakash K, Bala S, Verma RK, Gujral VV. Partial supplementation with expressed breast-milk for prevention of infection in low-birthweight infants. *Lancet* 1980;2:561-563.

14. Narayanan I, Prakash K, Gujral VV. The value of human milk in the prevention of infection in the high-risk low-birth-weight infant. *J Pediatr* 1981;99:496-498.

15. Schanler RJ. Suitability of human milk for the low birthweight infant. *Clin Perinatol* 1995;22:207-222.

16. Contreras-Lemus J, Flores-Huerta S, Cisneros-Silva I, et al. Disminucion de la morbilidad en neonatos pretermino alimentados con leche de su propia madre. *Biol Med Hosp Infant Mex* 1992;49:671-677.

17. Yu VYH, Jamieson J, Bajuk B. Breast milk feeding in very low birthweight infants. *Aust Paediatr J* 1981;17:186-190.

18. Lucas A, Cole TJ. Breast milk and neonatal necrotizing enterocolitis. *Lancet* 1990;336:1519-1523.

19. Eibl MM, Wolf HM, Fürnkranz H, Rosenkranz A. Prevention of necrotizing enterocolitis in low-birthweight infants by IgA-IgG feeding. *N Engl J Med* 1988;319:1-7.

20. Lawrence G, Tudehope D, Baumann K, et al. Enteral human IgG for prevention of necrotising enterocolitis: a placebo-controlled, randomised trial. *Lancet* 2001;357:2090-2094.

21. Goldblum RM, Schanler RJ, Garza C, Goldman AS. Human milk feeding enhances the urinary excretion of immunologic factors in low birth weight infants. *Pediatr Res* 1989;25:184-188.

22. Schanler RJ, Goldblum RM, Garza C, Goldman AS. Enhanced fecal excretion of selected immune factors in very low birth weight infants fed fortified human milk. *Pediatr Res* 1986;20:711-715.

23. Hutchens TW, Henry JF, Yip T-T, et al. Origin of intact lactoferrin and its DNA-binding fragments found in the urine of human milk-fed preterm infants. Evaluation by stable isotope enrichment. *Pediatr Res* 1991;29:243-250.

24. Caplan MS, Lickerman M, Adler L, Dietsch GN, Yu A. The role of recombinant platelet-activating factor acetylhydrolase in a neonatal rat model of necrotizing enterocolitis. *Pediatr Res* 1997;42:779-783.

25. Caplan MS, Russell T, Xiao Y, Amer M, Kaup S, Jilling T. Effect of polyunsaturated fatty acid (PUFA) supplementation on intestinal inflammation and necrotizing enterocolitis (NEC) in a neonatal rat model. *Pediatr Res* 2001;49:647-652.

26. Carlson SE, Montalto MB, Ponder DL, Werkman SH, Korones SB. Lower incidence of necrotizing enterocolitis in infants fed a preterm formula with egg phospholipids. *Pediatr Res* 1998;44:491-498.

27. Anderson JW, Johnstone BM, Remley DT. Breastfeeding and cognitive development: a meta-analysis. *Am J Clin Nutr* 1999;70:525-535.

28. Lucas A, Morley R, Cole TJ, et al. Early diet in preterm babies and developmental status in infancy. *Arch Dis Child* 1989;64:1570-1578.

29. Lucas A, Morley R, Cole TJ, Gore SM. A randomised multicentre study of human milk versus formula and later development in preterm infants. *Arch Dis Child* 1994;70:F141-F146.

30. Lucas A, Morley R, Cole TJ, Lister G, Leeson-Payne C. Breast milk and subsequent intelligence quotient in children born preterm. *Lancet* 1992;339:261-264.

31. McKinley LT, Thorp JW, Tucker R. Outcomes at 18 months corrected age of very low birth weight (VLBW) infants who received human milk during hospitalization. *Pediatr Res* 2000;47:1720A.

32. Lucas A, Fewtrell MS, Morley R, et al. Randomized outcome trial of human milk fortification and developmental outcome in preterm infants. *Am J Clin Nutr* 1996;64:142-151.

33. Schanler RJ. Human milk fortification for premature infants. *Am J Clin Nutr* 1996;64:249-250.

34. Morley R, Cole TJ, Powell R, Lucas A. Mother's choice to provide breast milk and developmental outcome. *Arch Dis Child* 1988;63:1382-1385.

35. Lucas A, Cole TJ, Morley R, et al. Factors associated with maternal choice to provide breastmilk for low birthweight infants. *Arch Dis Child* 1988;59:722-730.

36. Carlson SE, Werkman SH, Rhodes PG, Tolley EA. Visual-acuity development in healthy preterm infants: effect of marine-oil supplementation. *Am J Clin Nutr* 1993;58:35-42.

37. Hylander MA, Strobino DM, Pezzullo JC, Dhanireddy R. Association of human milk feedings with a reduction in retinopathy of prematurity among very low birthweight infants. *J Perinatol* 2001;21: 356-362.

38. Uauy R, Hoffman DR. Essential fatty acid requirements for normal eye and brain development. *Semin Perinatol* 1991;15:449-455.

39. O'Connor DL, Hall R, Adamkin D, et al. Growth and development in preterm infants fed long-chain polyunsaturated fatty acids: A prospective, randomized controlled trial. *Pediatrics* 2001;108:359-371.

40. Cavell B. Gastric emptying in infants fed human milk or infant formula. *Acta Paediatr Scand* 1981;70: 639-641.

41. Shulman RJ, Schanler RJ, Lau C, Heitkemper M, Ou CN, Smith EO. Early feeding, feeding tolerance, and lactase activity in preterm infants. *J Pediatr* 1998;133:645-649.

42. Shulman RJ, Schanler RJ, Ou C, Heitkemper M, Lau C. Intestinal permeability in the premature infant is related to urinary cortisol excretion. *Gastroenterology* 1996;110:A839.

43. Singhal A, Cole TJ, Lucas A. Early nutrition in preterm infants and later blood pressure: two cohorts after randomized trials. *Lancet* 2001;357:413-419.

44. Nutrition Committee, Canadian Paediatric Society. Nutrient needs and feeding of premature infants. *Can Med Assoc J* 1995;152:1765-1785.

45. Schanler RJ. The use of human milk for premature infants. *Pediatr Clin North Am* 2001;48:207-220.

46. Polberger S. Quality of growth in preterm neonates fed individually fortified human milk. In: Battaglia FC, Pedraz C, Sawatzki G, et al. eds. *Maternal and Extrauterine Nutritional Factors. Their Influence on Fetal and Infant Growth.* Madrid: Ediciones Ergon, S.A.; 1996:395-403.

47. Weber A, Loui A, Jochum F, Bührer C, Obladen M. Breast milk from mothers of very low birthweight infants: variability in fat and protein content. *Acta Pediatr* 2001;90:772-775.

48. Neville MC, Keller RP, Seacat J, Casey CE, Allen JC, Archer P. Studies on human lactation. I. Within-feed and between-breast variation in selected components of human milk. *Am J Clin Nutr* 1984;40:635-646.

49. Valentine CJ, Hurst NM, Schanler RJ. Hindmilk improves weight gain in low-birthweight infants fed human milk. *J Pediatr Gastroenterol Nutr* 1994;18: 474-477.

50. Greer FR, McCormick A, Loker J. Changes in fat concentration of human milk during delivery by intermittent bolus and continuous mechanical pump infusion. *J Pediatr* 1984;105:745-749.

51. Atkinson SA, Bryan MH, Anderson GH. Human milk feeding in premature infants: Protein, fat and carbohydrate balances in the first two weeks of life. *J Pediatr* 1981;99:617-624.

52. Atkinson SA, Radde IC, Anderson GH. Macromineral balances in premature infants fed their own mothers' milk or formula. *J Pediatr* 1983;102:99-106.

53. Cooper PA, Rothberg AD, Pettifor JM, Bolton KD, Devenhuis S. Growth and biochemical response of premature infants fed pooled preterm milk or special formula. *J Pediatr Gastroenterol Nutr* 1984;3:749-754.

54. Kashyap S, Schulze KF, Forsyth M, Dell RB, Ramakrishnan R, Heird WC. Growth, nutrient retention, and metabolic response of low-birthweight infants fed supplemented and unsupplemented preterm human milk. *Am J Clin Nutr* 1990;52:254-262.

55. Gross SJ. Growth and biochemical response of preterm infants fed human milk or modified infant formula. *N Engl J Med* 1983;308:237-241.

56. Polberger SKT, Axelsson IE, Räihä NCR. Urinary and serum urea as indicators of protein metabolism in very low birthweight infants fed varying human milk protein intakes. *Acta Paediatr Scand* 1990;79:737-742.

57. Rowe JC, Wood DH, Rowe DW, Raisz LG. Nutritional hypophosphatemic rickets in a premature infant fed breast milk. *N Engl J Med* 1979;300:293-296.

58. Pettifor JM, Rajah R, Venter A. Bone mineralization and mineral homeostasis in very low-birthweight

infants fed either human milk or fortified human milk. *J Pediatr Gastroenterol Nutr* 1989;8:217-224.

59. Lucas A, Brooke OG, Baker BA, Bishop N, Morley R. High alkaline phosphatase activity and growth in preterm neonates. *Arch Dis Child* 1989;64:902-909.

60. Roy RN, Chance GW, Radde IC, Hill DE, Willis DM, Sheepers J. Late hyponatremia in very low birthweight infants. *Pediatr Res* 1976;526-53l.

61. Kuschel CA, Harding JE. Multicomponent fortified human milk for promoting growth in preterm infants (Cochrane Review). The Cochrane Library 2001; Issue 3:http://www.cochranelibrary.com/enter

62. Polberger SKT, Axelsson IA, Raiha NCR. Growth of very low birth weight infants on varying amounts of human milk protein. *Pediatr Res* 1989;25:414-419.

63. Kuschel CA, Harding JE. Protein supplementation of human milk for promoting growth in preterm infants (Cochrane Review). The Cochrane Library 2001;http://www.cochranelibrary.com/enter

64. Polberger S, Räihä NC, Juvonen P, Moro GE, Minoli I, Warm A. Individualized protein fortification of human milk for preterm infants: comparison of ultrafiltrated human milk protein and a bovine whey fortifier. *J Pediatr Gastroenterol Nutr* 1999;29:332-338.

65. Schanler RJ, Garza C. Improved mineral balance in very low birthweight infants fed fortified human milk. *J Pediatr* 1987;112:452-456.

66. Kumar SP, Sacks LM. Hyponatremia in very low-birthweight infants and human milk feedings. *J Pediatr* 1978;93:1026-1027.

67. Schanler RJ, Shulman RJ, Lau C. Feeding strategies for premature infants: Beneficial outcomes of feeding fortified human milk vs preterm formula. *Pediatrics* 1999;103:1150-1157.

68. Porcelli P, Schanler R, Greer F, et al. Growth in human milk-fed very low birth weight infants receiving a new human milk fortifier. *Ann Nutr Metab* 2000;44:2-10.

69. Barrett-Reis B, Hall RT, Schanler RJ, et al. Enhanced growth of preterm infants fed a new powdered human milk fortifier: a randomized controlled trial. *Pediatrics* 2000;106:581-588.

70. Wauben IPM, Atkinson SA, Shah JK, Paes B. Growth and body composition of preterm infants: influence of nutrient fortification of mother's milk in hospital and

breast feeding post-hospital discharge. *Acta Paediatr* 1998;87:780-785.

71. Greer FR, McCormick A. Improved bone mineralization and growth in premature infants fed fortified own mother's milk. *J Pediatr* 1988;112:961-969.

72. Schanler RJ, Abrams SA. Postnatal attainment of intrauterine macromineral accretion rates in low birthweight infants fed fortified human milk. *J Pediatr* 1995;126:441-447.

73. Ziegler EE. Breast-milk fortification. *Acta Pædiatr* 2001;90:720-723.

74. Ewer AK, Yu VYH. Gastric emptying in pre-term infants: The effect of breast milk fortifier. *Acta Paediatr* 1996;85:1112-1115.

75. McClure RJ, Newell SJ. Effect of fortifying breast milk on gastric emptying. *Arch Dis Child* 1996;74:F60-F62.

76. Lau C. Effect of stress on lactation. *Pediatr Clin North Am* 2001;48:221-234.

77. Jocson MAL, Mason EO, Schanler RJ. The effects of nutrient fortification and varying storage conditions on host defense properties of human milk. *Pediatrics* 1997;100:240-243.

78. Quan R, Yang C, Rubinstein S, Lewiston NJ, Stevenson DK, Kerner JA. The effect of nutritional additives on anti-infective factors in human milk. *Clin Pediatr* 1994;33:325-328.

79. Fenton TR, Tough SC, Belik J. Breast milk supplementation for preterm infants: Parental preferences and postdischarge lactation duration. *Am J Perinatol* 2000;17:329-333.

80. Schanler RJ, Abrams SA, Garza C. Bioavailability of calcium and phosphorus in human milk fortifiers and formula for very low birthweight infants. *J Pediatr* 1988;113:95-100.

81. Wauben IP, Atkinson SA, Grad TL, Shah JK, Paes B. Moderate nutrient supplementation of mother's milk for preterm infants support adequate bone mass and short-term growth: a randomized, controlled trial. *Am J Clin Nutr* 1998;67:465-472.

82. Affonso D, Bosque E, Brady JP. Reconciliation and healing for mothers through skin-to-skin contact provided in an American tertiary level intensive care nursery. *Neonatal Network* 1994;12:25-32.

83. Schanler RJ, Henderson TR, Hamosh M. Fatty acid

soaps may be responsible for poor fat absorption in premature infants fed fortified human milk. *Pediatr Res* 1999;45:290A-290A.

84. Chappell JE, Clandinin MT, Kearney-Volpe C, Reichman B, Swyer PW. Fatty acid balance studies in premature infants fed human milk or formula: effect of calcium supplementation. *J Pediatr* 1986;108:439-447.

85. Daly SE, Kent JC, Owens RA, Hartmann PE. Frequency and degree of milk removal and the short-term control of human milk synthesis. *Exp Physiol Sep* 1996;81:861-875.

86. DeCarvalho M, Anderson DM, Giangreco A, Pittard WB. Frequency of milk expression and milk production by mothers of nonnursing premature neonates. *Am J Dis Child* 1985;13:483-485.

87. Hill PD, Aldag JC, Chatterton RT. The effect of sequential and simultaneous breast pumping on milk volume and prolactin levels: a pilot study. *J Hum Lact* 1996;12:193-199.

88. Hurst NM, Myatt A, Schanler RJ. Growth and development of a hospital-based lactation program and mother's own milk bank. *J Obstet Gynecol Neonatal Nurs* 1998;27:503-510.

89. Neville MC, Allen JC, Archer PC, et al. Studies in human lactation: milk volume and nutrient composition during weaning and lactogenesis. *Am J Clin Nutr* 1991;54:81-92 .

90. Schanler RJ, Hurst NM, Lau C. The use of human milk and breastfeeding in premature infants. *Clin Perinatol* 1999;26:379-398.

91. Ehrenkranz RA, Ackerman BA. Metoclopramide effect on faltering milk production by mothers of premature infants. *Pediatrics* 1986;78:614-620.

92. Charpak N, Ruiz-Peláez JG, Figueroa ZD, Charpak Y. Kangaroo mother versus traditional care for newborn infants less than or equal to 2000 grams: A randomized, controlled trial. *Pediatrics* 1997;100:682-688.

93. Anderson GC. Current knowledge about skin-to-skin (Kangaroo) care for preterm infants. *J Perinatol* 1991;11:216-226.

94. Hurst NM, Valentine C, Renfro L, Burns PA, Ferlic L. Skin-to-skin holding in the neonatal intensive care unit influences maternal milk volume. *J Perinatol* 1997;17:213-217.

95. Lau C, Sheena HR, Shulman RJ, Schanler RJ. Oral feeding in low birthweight infants. *J Pediatr* 1997;130:561-569.

96. Meier P, Lysakowski TY, Engstrom JL. The accuracy of test weighing for preterm infants. *J Pediatr Gastroenterol Nutr* 1990;10:62-65.

97. Bier JB, Ferguson AE, Morales Y, Liebling JA, Oh W, Vohr BR. Breastfeeding infants who were extremely low birthweight. *Pediatrics* 1997;http://pediatrics.org/cgi/content/full/100/6/e3.

98. Marinelli KA, Burke GS, Dodd VL. A comparison of the safety of cupfeedings and bottlefeedings in premature infants whose mothers intend to breastfeed. *J Perinatol* 2001;21:355.

99. Meier P, Engstrom JL, Crichton CL, Clark DR, Williams MM, Mangurten HH. A new scale for in-home test-weighing for mothers of preterm and high risk infants. *J Hum Lact* 1994;10:163-168.

100. Meier PP. Breastfeeding in the special care nursery: prematures and infants with medical problems. *Pediatr Clin North Am* 2001;48:425-442.

101. Chan GM. Growth and bone mineral status of discharged very low birth weight infants fed different formulas or human milk. *J Pediatr* 1993;123:439-443.

102. Rubinacci A, Sirtori P, Moro G, Galli L, Minoli I, Tessari L. Is there an impact of birth weight and early life nutrition on bone mineral content in preterm born infants and children? *Acta Paediatr* 1993;82:711-713.

103. Koo WWK, Sherman R, Succop P, et al. Sequential bone mineral content in small preterm infants with and without fractures and rickets. *J Bone Miner Res* 1988;3:193-197.

104. Tsang RC, Namgung R. Newborn bone development. In: Ross Products Division. ed. *Posthospital Nutrition in the Preterm Infant, Report of the 106th Ross Conference on Pediatric Research*. Columbus: Ross Products Division/Abbott Laboratories; 1996:21-26.

105. Bishop NJ, King FJ, Lucas A. Increased bone mineral content of preterm infants fed with a nutrient enriched formula after discharge from hospital. *Arch Dis Child* 1993;68:573-578.

106. Lucas A, Bishop NJ, King FJ, Cole TJ. Randomized

trial of nutrition for preterm infants after discharge. *Arch Dis Child* 1992;67:324-327.

107. Cooke RJ, Griffin IJ, McCormick K, et al. Feeding preterm infants after hospital discharge: effect of dietary manipulation on nutrient intake and growth. *Pediatr Res* 1998;43:355-360.

108. Cooke RJ, McCormick K, Griffin IJ, et al. Feeding preterm infants after hospital discharge: effect of diet on body composition. *Pediatr Res* 1999;46:461-464.

109. Brunton JA, Saigal S, Atkinson SA. Growth and body composition in infants with bronchopulmonary dysplasia up to 3-months-corrected age: A randomized trial of a high-energy, nutrient-enriched formula fed after hospital discharge. *J Pediatr* 1998;133:340-345.

110. Cooke RJ, Embleton ND, Griffin IJ, Wells JC, McCormick KP. Feeding preterm infants after hospital discharge: growth and development at 18 months of age. *Pediatr Res* 2001;49:719-722.

111. Schanler RJ, Burns PA, Abrams SA, Garza C. Bone mineralization outcomes in human milk-fed preterm infants. *Pediatr Res* 1992;31:583-586.

112. Bishop NJ, Dahlenburg SL, Fewtrell MS, Morley R, Lucas A. Early diet of preterm infants and bone mineralization at age five years. *Acta Paediatr* 1996;85:230-236.

113. Jones G, Riley M, Dwyer T. Breastfeeding in early life and bone mass in prepubertal children: a longitudinal study. *Osteoporosis International* 2000;11:146-152.

114. Fewtrell MS, Cole TJ, Bishop NJ, Lucas A. Neonatal factors predicting childhood height in preterm infants: Evidence for a persisting effect of early metabolic bone disease? *J Pediatr* 2000;137:668-673.

115. Morley R, Lucas A. Randomized diet in the neonatal period and growth performance until 7.5-8 years of age in preterm children. *Am J Clin Nutr* 2000;71:822-828.

116. Hall RT. Nutritional follow-up of the breastfeeding premature infant after hospital discharge. *Pediatr Clin North Am* 2001;48:453-460.

117. Atkinson SA, Radde IC, Chance GW, Bryan MH, Anderson GH. Macro-mineral content of milk obtained during early lactation from mothers of premature infants. *Early Hum Dev* 1980;4:5-14.

118. Anderson DM, Williams FH, Merkatz RB, Schulman PK, Kerr DS, Pittard WB. Length of gestation and nutritional composition of human milk. *Am J Clin Nutr* 1983;37:810-814.

119. Hibberd CM, Brooke OG, Carter ND, Haug M, Harzer G. Variation in the composition of breast milk during the first 5 weeks of lactation: implications for the feeding of preterm infants. *Arch Dis Child* 1982;57:658-662.

120. Sann L, Bienvenu F, Lahet C, Bienvenu J, Bethenod M. Comparison of the composition of breast milk from mothers of term and preterm infants. *Acta Paediatr Scand* 1981;70:115-116.

121. Jensen RG, Bitman J, Carlson SE, Couch SC, Hamosh M, Newburg DS. Milk lipids. In: Jensen RG. ed. *Handbook of Milk Composition.* San Diego: Academic Press; 1995:495-575.

122. Neville MC. Volume and caloric density of human milk. In: Jensen RG. ed. *Handbook of Milk Composition.* San Diego: Academic Press; 1995: 99-113.

123. Newburg DS, Neubauer SH. Carbohydrates in milks: analysis, quantities, and significance. In: Jensen RG. ed. *Handbook of Milk Composition.* San Diego: Academic Press; 1995:273-349 .

124. Atkinson SA, Alston-Mills B, Lonnerdal B, Neville MC. Major minerals and ionic constituents of human and bovine milks. In: Jensen RG. ed. *Handbook of Milk Composition.* San Diego: Academic Press; 1995:593-622.

125. Casey C, Smith A, Zhang S. Microminerals in human and animal milks. In: Jensen RG. ed. *Handbook of Milk Composition.* San Diego: Academic Press; 1995:622-674.

126. Chappell JE, Francis T, Clandinin MT. Vitamin A and E content of human milk at early stages of lactation. *Early Hum Dev* 1985;11:157-167.

127. Moran JR, Vaughan R, Stroop S, Coy S, Johnston H, Greene HL. Concentrations and total daily output of micronutrients in breast milk of mothers delivering preterm: a longitudinal study. *J Pediatr Gastroenterol Nutr* 1983;2:629-634.

128. Human Milk Banking Association of North America. Recommendations for collection, storage, and

handling of a mother's milk for her own infant in the hospital setting. West Hartford, CT: Human Milk Banking Association of North America, 1993.

Feeding After Discharge: Growth, Development and Long-Term Effects

Susan E. Carlson, Ph.D.

Reviewed by Reg Sauve, M.D., and Jane Carver, Ph.D.

Growth, Development and Long-Term Effects

During the past 20 years, much research has been devoted to describing and improving the nutritional status of VLBW infants in the hospital. By comparison, there is relatively little work on post-discharge nutritional status of very-low-birth-weight infants, the subject of this chapter. An attempt has been made to address individual nutrients that influence growth and development. Most research has centered on variations in protein concentration and the effects on short- and long-term growth. Because of the number of nutrients essential for growth and development of preterm infants and the effort and cost required to study each, research for individual nutrients is not uniform.

The chapter acknowledges that improvements in nutrition in hospital are a major uncontrolled variable for post-discharge nutritional status of preterm infants. The change that has had the most impact is the use of special preterm formulas or human milk fortifiers in hospital compared with formulas designed for term infants or unfortified human milk, respectively. The best evidence for the need to provide additional amounts of any given nutrient after discharge comes from studies that show low status of that nutrient among infants who have received either preterm formula or fortified human milk, the current standard of care for nutritional management in hospital.

The chapter is included in the Practical Applications section of the book, and so it concludes with general guidelines for nutritional management. The reader will realize that "practical" sometimes means that the guidelines are based on a combination of theory and evidence that is quite limited. There is much that is not known about nutritional status of these infants post-discharge, and, therefore, best practice should continue to evolve. By acknowledging that, work that is needed may be encouraged.

As noted above, preterm formulas designed for the higher nutrient needs of VLBW infants as well as human milk fortifiers for infants receiving human milk are now employed routinely to provide nutrition in hospital. In these formulations many nutrients were increased simultaneously, which is a practical rather than a scientific approach. In general, studies have shown such formulas and supplements safely promoted faster weight gain and more "optimal" biochemical profiles in the hospital.[1-5] Despite the availability of higher-nutrient formulas and awareness of the importance of rapidly reinstating nutrition following VLBW delivery in hospital, percentiles for growth are below birth at discharge,[6-10] providing evidence that nutritional management of VLBW infants in the hospital could be improved.

The physiologic immaturity and disease processes of VLBW preterm infants impose limitations for nutrition. However, overly conservative introduction of nutrition in some NICUs results in infants with slower nutritional recovery than necessary, which could be avoided. Fear of NEC may be one of the major reasons for conservative feeding of preterm infants in hospital.[6] However, the risk of NEC diminishes long before many infants are discharged. Preterm infants in most nurseries are not allowed to ad libitum feed until very late in their hospital course, if ever.

Considering the large number of infants who have

been discharged from NICUs in the past 20 years, it is somewhat surprising that the subject of post-discharge nutrition has received so little study. In the early 1990s, a few reports suggested low post-discharge status of Vitamin A[11] and zinc.[12-14] Others reports indicated inadequate phosphorus status for normal bone mineralization, especially in the infant fed human milk.[15,16] Lucas and coworkers[17] reported that nutrient-enriched formula enhanced growth in LBW and VLBW infants discharged at 2400g body weight. Results of these early studies suggested a plausible mechanism for the poor growth and development and more frequent infections of growing preterm infants compared to term infants, ie, low status of one or more essential nutrients after discharge.

Despite this, formulas designed for the nutrient needs of much larger, well-nourished infants, and unfortified human milk remained the standard for post-discharge nutrition even as infants began to be discharged at increasingly lower weights. The 1995 Ross Conference "Posthospital Nutrition in the Preterm Infant"[18] called attention to the poor nutritional status of preterm infants after discharge and the need for research in this area. Since that time, infant formulas have been designed for nutritional management of infants fed formula after discharge, so called "post-discharge" formulas. The formulas have a nutrient and energy content that is generally intermediate between term and preterm formulas. Use of these formulas after discharge currently represents common practice for post-discharge nutritional management of infants who are formula fed.

Despite this, there are no published data about the status of individual nutrients of infants fed these intermediate nutrient formulas designed for post-discharge feeding. There are limited data for the status of several individual nutrients in VLBW infants maintained on preterm formula for several months after discharge. Infants discharged on preterm formula rapidly attain plasma concentrations of several nutrients comparable to those of term infants of the same corrected age.[11,19,20,21] No such evidence exists for infants fed the new post-discharge formulas. It is

reasonable to suggest that the rate at which nutritional recovery occurs decreases when infants are changed from a preterm to a post-discharge formula at hospital discharge. Unnecessary delays in recovery of normal nutrient status during the period that tissues and organs are developing rapidly, raise theoretical concerns for development.

This chapter contains advice on nutritional management of VLBW infants for pediatricians and family practice physicians who manage these infants after discharge. An extensive treatment of this subject and protocols for management are provided in the chapter entitled "Nutritional Concerns at Transfer or Discharge"[22] of the 3rd Edition of *Nutritional Care for High-Risk Newborns*. The chapter is an excellent, comprehensive and practical guide for nutritional care of infants born before 37-weeks gestation. Recommendations for management are based on characteristics that influence nutrient needs of these infants such as birth weight, discharge weight, growth achievement and disease burden. That chapter and a companion chapter, "Routine Nutrition Care During Follow-Up"[23] contain much practical information that physicians and other health professionals caring for these infants need to know for their nutritional management. Other resources are also available and may be useful to the reader.[24,25]

Growth

How Do VLBW Infants Grow After Discharge?
After birth, VLBW infants are typically smaller in weight and length than would be expected for their in utero growth percentiles.[6-10] Because most nurseries now provide TPN followed by preterm formula or fortified human milk, a decline in growth percentiles following VLBW delivery is likely the result of too little total energy, albeit from a proper balance of nutrients, rather than too low intake of any individual nutrient. Other factors such as corticosteroids can also reduce linear growth even when energy intake is not low.[26]

The literature on long-term growth performance of VLBW infants post-discharge is quite extensive. For purposes of discussion, it is convenient to divide the studies into two groups. The first group includes studies done when infants were routinely discharged on formulas designed for the nutrient needs of larger, term infants, hereafter referred to as term formulas, at approximately 1800 grams body weight. The second group includes studies of infants discharged on a nutrient-enriched formula or fortified human milk. The second group of studies is quite small.

VLBW Infants Fed Lower Nutrient Feeds at Discharge. Growth studies of infants discharged beginning in the middle 1980s do not necessarily describe the discharge diet, but it may be inferred that term formulas were provided at discharge to those on formula and unsupplemented human milk to those who were human milk fed. These were the standards of care at that time. Given the improvements in in-hospital nutrition management that have occurred since that time, it is safe to assume that many of these infants had a relatively poor nutritional status at discharge compared to now. Georgieff et al[27] compared post-discharge growth in infants who had similar post-discharge nutritional management but different in-hospital nutritional management. Infants born in 1982 were compared with those born in the same hospital in 1986. The second group had more aggressive use of parenteral and enteral nutrition than the first. At 12-months-corrected age (CA), those cared for in 1986 had less than half the incidence of weights less than the 5th percentile on the NCHS growth charts[28,29] compared to infants cared for in 1982 (24% vs 49%).

A large retrospective study examined growth of LBW infants among 374,554 children less than 2 years of age from the Centers for Disease Control Pediatric Nutrition Surveillance System.[30] The researchers determined the prevalence of LBW as 9.2%, 13.4% and 9.2% for white, black and Hispanic children, respectively. The authors determined that the proportion of low length-for-age (<5th percentile) under 2 years of age due to LBW was 29%, 28% and 21% for these respective groups. Thus LBW results in a disproportionate amount of infants with failure to thrive before 2 years of age.

In a large prospective study, Casey and coworkers[31] reported growth to 3-years-corrected age in 985 infants

in three birth weight groups, <1250 g (Group 1), n=149, 1250 to 1999 g (Group 2), n=474, and 2000 to 2500 g (Group 3), n=362. All three groups in the study of Casey et al[31] had growth lower than NCHS reference standards[29] for growth of term infants of the same corrected age and sex. Although some catch-up in length occurred in the first year of life in both boys and girls, there was no further "catch-up" between 1 and 3 years of age.

Several smaller studies of VLBW infants followed for varying numbers of years after discharge also demonstrate a high incidence of poor growth in the years following discharge. Most importantly, none reported normal growth in childhood compared to term infants. Hack[32] reported that 22% and 33% of <750 g infants born between 1982 and 1986 had weights and heights, respectively, below the 3rd percentile at 6-7 years of age. Kitchen et al[33] determined height and weight of three birth weight groups: 1) 500-999 g, 2) 1000-1499 g, and 3) >2500 g. At 8 years of age, infants of the smallest size at birth were shorter than those 1000-1499 g at birth, but they had similar weights at 8 years of age. Both VLBW groups were shorter and lighter than normal birth weight infants at 8 years of age. However, the proportion of VLBW infants below the NCHS reference 10th percentiles for weight and height at 2 years of age decreased by about half by 8 years of age.

Bowman and Yu[34] followed 800-1000 g infants born during the same era until 2 years of age and found 44% and 45% to be below the 10th percentile for weight and length of the pre-2000 NCHS reference. Ernst et al[35] reported that 30%, 21% and 14% of infants, respectively, were below the 5th percentiles for weight, length and head circumference at 12-months-corrected age.

Several studies have shown that preterm girls grow better long term than boys, with major factors being similar. Casey et al[31] found that boys in all three birth weight groups differed in weight, length and head circumference growth during the first 36 months, whereas girls differed significantly at all study ages only with regard to head circumference. By 30 and 36 months, weights of girls still differed by birth weight

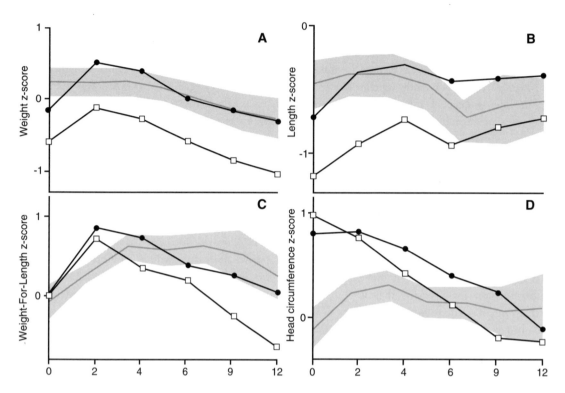

Figure 1: Figures 1A, B, C, and D show mean weight, length, weight-for-length and head circumference Z-scores in reference to the NCHS growth charts for term infants that existed prior to 2000. Infants had a mean birth weight of approximately 1100g, were fed a preterm infant formula until discharge and a term formula after discharge.[8] The shaded area shows the mean ± SEM for first year growth of 61 term infants enrolled in the same center. Both term and preterm infants were mostly of African-American descent and receiving Medicare support, a government assistance program.[8,53] Regular preterm and term formula during hospital and post-discharge, respectively (●). Fish oil-supplemented preterm and term formula providing DHA and EPA (1:15) (□).

group (p<0.02) although the actual size of the difference was small. Lengths did not differ by birth weight group. Ernst et al[35] reported that AGA females had higher percentiles on NCHS reference data for term infants than did AGA males.

Because of these differences in growth related to gender, studies that do not balance groups for gender or that do not include equal numbers of boys and girls in each group are not strictly comparable to those in which groups are weighted toward one gender. Commonly there are more girl than boy infants in NICUs who fit the inclusion criteria for nutrient studies of VLBW infants, and, frequently, gender does not distribute equally for groups in small studies with 30 or fewer infants per group.

Intrauterine growth retardation is an independent risk factor for poor first year growth in VLBW infants. Ernst et al[35] reported that male infants, whether AGA or SGA, and female SGA infants all grew similarly and had lower percentiles than female AGA infants. Strauss and Dietz[36] found that symmetrically and asymmetrically growth retarded infants continued to have growth deficits at 3-years-corrected age (CA) compared with AGA preterm infants and the NCHS reference group. Karniski et al[37] found that AGA infants had approximately normal growth at 29 months of age while SGA infants still had subnormal growth.

As with gender, there are differences in the proportion of AGA to SGA infants among studies.

Moreover, even when infants in some lower SES populations are above the 5th percentile at birth, they may have some degree of growth restriction relative to other populations, which could result in relatively lower growth performance. This has been observed in studies of predominantly African-American infants whose length in particular is below the NCHS reference group at term.

The first year growth of lower SES preterm infants from Memphis was compared with that of term infants from the same hospital population[38] (Figure 1). The comparison illustrates the value in having a reference group of term infants for growth from the same population as the VLBW infants studied. Compared to the NCHS reference group during the first 12-months CA, weight Z-scores of VLBW infants were lower at 0-months CA, higher at 2- and 4-months CA, similar at 6 months and lower at 9- and 12-months CA.[38] At the same time, growth of VLBW infants was lower for length and higher for head circumference compared to the NCHS reference group during the first 12-months CA.[38] However, weight and length growth of the VLBW infants was excellent compared to formula- and breast-fed term infants enrolled in the same center and whose mothers had similar characteristics to those of the VLBW group[38] (Figure 1). It is important to note that the VLBW infants in this study had more females than males and only 10% had bronchopulmonary dysplasia (BPD), which typically affects 40% of VLBW infants.[9] These characteristics of the study group could have resulted in better growth than otherwise.

LBW infants fed high nutrient formulas but discharged on lower nutrient formulas designed for term infants in the mid-1980s have now reached adolescence. Peralta-Carcelen et al[39] found that infants less than 1000 g birth weight continued to be shorter by 4.8 cm and lighter by 9.1 kg compared to controls at adolescence, although they had similar relative body composition and normal sexual maturation.

There is evidence that a member of the health team who acts specifically as an advocate for nutrition can influence growth. Bryson et al[40] found that post-discharge growth of VLBW infants was greater if a registered dietitian (RD) was a member of the multidisciplinary team that cared for the infant after discharge. At 8-months CA, 72% of infants cared for without an RD had lengths less than the 5th percentile compared with 36% of infants cared for by a team with an RD. By 12-months CA, the number of infants with length <5th percentile had declined to 43% and 13%, respectively, for groups without and with care from an RD. The absolute difference between groups was more pronounced than at the earlier age.

Lucas has emphasized the high voluntary energy intakes of VLBW infants after discharge.[41] Others have emphasized the psychosocial factors that lead to failure to thrive among LBW infants.[42] An advocate for nutrition can ensure that parents know how to encourage ad libitum feeding and have the training to identify feeding problems before growth delays occur; and advocates can help families with their specific barriers to optimal nutritional care. VLBW infants should be discharged to the care of health professionals prepared to give individualized nutritional care. This may not always be the case.

Growth of VLBW Infants fed a Nutrient-Enriched Feeding at Discharge.

Post-discharge formulas have been available for a relatively short period. Few studies have been published, and these have not determined growth beyond 12-months CA. Several studies have shown higher growth with higher nutrient compared to lower nutrient formula. The higher nutrient formulas contain more protein than those with lower nutrients, and, in most cases, increases in vitamins and minerals compared to term formulas. However, there is a great deal of variability in nutrient content among the higher-nutrient formulas fed, and other nutrients could result in different growth effects among studies.

Using a prototype "post-discharge formula", Lucas et al[17] compared growth of groups of preterm infants discharged at approximately 2400 g and 37-weeks-postmenstrual age on either a post-discharge, nutrient-enriched formula or a term formula available in the UK. Infants in their study weighed <1800 g at birth and had a mean birth weight of approximately 1500 g.

Weight and length were higher in the group fed the post-discharge formula until 40-weeks CA when compared with the term formula group. Infants fed the post-discharge formula came close to achieving the 50th percentile for term norms used in the UK (Gairdner-Pearson charts),[43] whereas the group discharged on term formula had a linear growth between the 10th and 25th percentiles on these charts.

A strength of the study was that the number of male and female infants in the diet groups were balanced. The major limitations were the absence of information about the nutritional content of the comparison diet (term formula), absence of information about the nutritional content of the formula fed prior to discharge (all infants were formula fed), and the small sizes of the groups (n~16). The post-discharge formula contained 2.6 g protein /100 kcal, which is typical of post-discharge formulas now available commercially in the US. If the infants did not receive a preterm formula in hospital (~3 g of protein/100 kcal), which is common in the US, and the term formula at discharge was lower than the 2.1 g of protein/100 kcal that is standard in the US, the effect of the post-discharge formula on growth could have been overestimated relative to what would be expected with the standard of care in the US.

The post-discharge formula was the prototype for formulas that were subsequently developed for discharge formulas in the United States. Carver et al[44] compared growth to 12-months CA of infants fed a commercial post-discharge formula or a commercially available term formula. One hundred twenty-five infants were randomized, and 53 completed study to 12-months CA. The study involved a number of centers and infants studied were discharged between 1800 and 2300 g. As in the study by Lucas et al[17] study, infants weighed less than 1800 g at birth, but the mean weight in this study was approximately 1300 g, 200 g lower than in the Lucas study. Therefore, the study likely included more VLBW infants than the study by Lucas et al.[17] The post-discharge formula contained 2.6 g protein per 100 kcal and was formulated at 22 kcal per ounce. The term formula contained 20 kcal per ounce.

The main effects of nutrient-enriched formula on growth were observed only at the earliest time points, and only for weight at 1- and 2-months CA and length at 3-months CA.[44] However, there were interactions between birth weight and feeding, the net effect of which was that among infants of <1250 g birth weight, the nutrient-enriched formulas resulted in higher weight at 0-, 6- and 12-months CA. Infants who weighed <1250 g at birth, and who were fed nutrient-enriched compared to term formula at 6 months, had greater length at 6-months CA and greater head circumference at 0-,1-,3-,6- and 12-months CA.[44]

The study is limited by the fact that the groups were not balanced for gender and had dissimilar proportions of male and female infants assigned to the two diet groups. In addition, 58% of the consented group exited the study before 12 months. At 12-months CA, data were available from only 53 infants. It is not known how early exit from the study influenced the balance of male and female infants studied at each age. The nutritional management of the infants prior to discharge was not controlled and was not reported. Given the apparent differences in gender, there is the potential that the effects of the post-discharge formula on growth could be underestimated, because a larger proportion of girls were fed the lower nutrient formula than the post-discharge formula. As noted before, girls grow better than boys in relation to growth standards of term infants during the first year following preterm delivery.

Cooke et al[45,46] published serial reports on growth and development of preterm infants after hospital discharge in the UK. Infants were fed a preterm formula before discharge. The preterm infants that were studied weighed <1751 g at birth and were without evidence of systemic disease and growing at >25 g/day immediately prior to discharge. At discharge, infants (n=86) were assigned randomly to one of three groups: 1) a commercial formula designed for term infants, 2) a preterm formula designed for preterm infants or 3) a preterm formula fed until expected term followed by a term formula until 6-months CA. Randomization was stratified for birth weight less than or greater than 1250 g. The term and preterm formulas contained 2.1 g and 2.75 g protein per 100 kcal, respectively, and the preterm formula was enriched in most vitamins and minerals compared to the term formula. The enrichment included iron, although the iron content of the preterm formula was still below that of US formulas for term and preterm infants. Vitamin and mineral content of the formulas were in some cases similar and in others quite dissimilar to formulas provided in the US, reflecting differences in formulas in the UK compared to the US.

For girls, growth velocity was similar in the three diet groups. However, boys fed preterm formula until 6-months CA had higher weight, length and head circumference at 6-months CA compared to the other two groups, ie, boys fed preterm formula from discharge until expected term followed by term formula to 6-months CA or boys fed term formula after discharge. When infants were fed a preterm formula from discharge until 6 months, boys grew faster than girls. Absolute differences in growth by gender were not found for the groups of infants fed term formula from discharge to 6-months CA or fed term formula from expected term to 6-months CA.[45] However, male infants had lower Z-scores for length, head circumference and weight than females with these two latter diet assignments.

When the infants were 18 months of age, Cooke et al[46] measured growth of the infants again. More infants were studied[46] than reported initially[45] suggesting that the original group had increased by new enrollment. Boys fed a preterm formula until 6-months CA continued to weigh more at 12- and 18-months CA than the other diet groups,[46] continuing the pattern established before 6-months CA.[45] Girls continued to have similar growth among diet groups at 12- and 18-months CA just as in the initial report at 6-months CA.[45]

A major strength of the study is that the growth data were shown as Z-scores compared to growth reference data for term infants in the UK,[46] permitting the reader to make a number of observations not possible from absolute measurements of size. For example, the group of males fed preterm formula for 6 months after discharge had linear growth that closely approached

that of term infants. The preterm formula group was the only group of males that did not have significantly lower head circumference scores than females at 6-, 12- and 18-months CA whereas the other two groups did. In general, it is clear from the normalized data of term and preterm infants that preterm infants have growth patterns quite different form term infants in the first 18 months of life. The studies suggest that this is true even when attention is given to continuing the period of nutrient-enrichment begun in hospital by providing nutrient-enriched feedings after discharge.

A limitation of the study was that the groups were not balanced for male and female infants and did not include a similar proportion of male and female infants. Males accounted for 55% of the infants fed preterm formula at discharge until 6 months and only 35% of the group fed term formula from discharge until 6 months. Because males in the study grew better than females when fed preterm compared to term formula, the fact that the group discharged on preterm formula contained more male infants could have biased results toward the conclusion of higher growth with the preterm compared to the term formula.[45] It is not clear how the additional infants added to the study affected the balance of gender in each diet group.[46] Z-scores take into account differences in growth for gender that occur in healthy term infants; however, male and female VLBW infants appear to have different relationships to term norms for growth.

Wheeler and Hall[47] studied a group of 43 infants with a mean birth weight of ~1375 g for 8 weeks after discharge using a prototype post-discharge formula fed at 20 kcal per ounce like the term formula used for comparison. The protein content of the post-discharge formula was higher than that of the term formula (1.83 g/dL vs 1.5 g/dL). Head circumference and length were greater at the end of the study in the group provided the post-discharge formula compared to the term formula.

While most of the studies of growth have compared groups of infants fed formulas with different levels of protein and other essential nutrients, two consecutive studies from Memphis compared growth of infants fed formulas with identical concentrations of essential

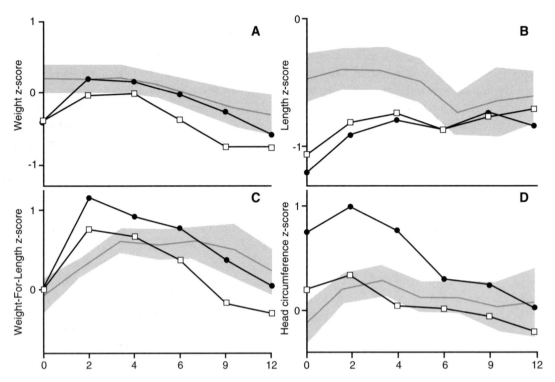

Figure 2: Figures 2A, B, C, and D show mean weight, length, weight-for-length and head circumference Z-scores in reference to the NCHS growth charts for term infants that existed prior to 2000. Infants had a mean birth weight of approximately 1050g, were fed a preterm infant formula until 2 months CA and a term formula from 2 until 12 months CA.[9] The shaded area shows the mean ± SEM for first year growth of 61 term infants enrolled in the same center. Both term and preterm infants were mostly of African-American descent and receiving Medicare support, a government assistance program.[9,53] Regular preterm and term formula during hospital and post-discharge, respectively (●). Fish oil-supplemented preterm and term formula providing DHA and EPA (1/0.25) until 2 months CA and regular term formula from 2 to 12 months CA (□).

nutrients, but different amounts of docosahexaenoic acid (DHA) and eicosapentaenoic acid (EPA) from fish oil. Longitudinal growth was studied to 12-months CA.[8,9] These studies, and a study by Ryan et al[48] suggest that DHA and EPA can reduce the growth performance of at least some VLBW infants.

The arachidonic acid (AA) status of VLBW infants in this population was found to be lower when formula containing fish oil was fed.[49] Most importantly, higher AA status was associated with higher growth performance in the first year of life even among infants in the group fed formula without long chain polyunsaturated fatty acids (LCPUFA). In other words, some VLBW infants have low amounts of AA

that are related to lower growth performance. Both AA and EPA (the precursor of DHA) share a common biosynthetic pathway. There is already good evidence that preformed DHA enhances function in preterm infants, but because of a common biosynthetic pathway, infants who benefit from DHA for neural development may also benefit from AA for growth.[50] Two large randomized clinical trials have provided both AA and DHA (n-6 and n-3 LCPUFA, respectively) in formula to preterm[51] and term[52] infants until 12-months CA. In both studies, growth of the LCPUFA supplemented group did not differ from growth of the group that did not receive the supplement. A number of smaller trials with sufficient power to detect a meaningful effect on growth (reviewed in reference 38) have fed both DHA and AA. Unlike several studies that found lower growth in preterm infants fed only DHA (or DHA with EPA), none has found lower growth in infants fed LCPUFA compared to infants fed formulas without LCPUFA. These recent studies suggest that a diet that includes both DHA and AA can prevent lower growth caused by feeding n-3 LCPUFA alone. The US government has now cleared the way for DHA to be added to infant formula in the US, and it appears this will happen in 2002, most likely paired with AA.

Table 1 includes absolute growth infants from the Lucas et al[17], Cooke et al[45,46] and Carver et al[44] studies in which infants discharged on term formula were compared to a group fed a nutrient enriched formula after discharge. Data from two consecutive studies in Memphis are also included in the table. In the first of these latter studies, infants were fed a preterm formula until discharge at approximately 1.8 kg and a term formula from discharge to 12-months CA.[8] In the second of these studies, infants were fed a preterm formula until 2-months CA. After 2-months CA, they were fed the same term formula as the control group from 2- to 12-months CA.[9] Although infants in the Memphis studies were cared for in the same unit with similar practices, their studies are not directly comparable just as none of the other individual studies shown in the table is directly comparable. Nevertheless, one is struck by the similarity of growth among these studies especially given the dissimilarity of the nutrient mixtures fed post-discharge.

Growth of infants in the two Memphis studies is expressed as Z-scores for the NCHS reference group prior to 2000 (Figures 1 and 2, A, B, C, and D for weight, length, weight-for-length and head circumference respectively). The shaded area in each figure illustrates growth of 61 term infants (mean ± SEM) enrolled in the same hospital and who were fed either human milk or term formula throughout the first year of life.[53]

Several points about first year growth are illustrated by these figures. First, term infants from the same low SES population grow very differently from the NCHS reference group, as was noted earlier. Second, compared to the term reference group, weight and length performances in the first year of the groups fed regular formulas were at least as good, although VLBW infants tended to be on the lower end of normal for weight-for-length. Third, as noted above, growth in the groups fed DHA and EPA was less than the group of infants fed formula without DHA and EPA and the term reference group, although this was restricted to lower weight-for-length in the group in Figure 2. Fourth, weight-for-length diverged progressively from the term reference group between 2- and 12-months CA for both preterm groups but more so for the groups supplemented with DHA and EPA. Fifth, head circumference Z-scores are difficult to use for evaluating normal brain growth as brain growth measurement is confounded by decreases in head circumference that occur as head shape returns to normal, from an elliptical to a more spherical shape.[54]

A major limitation of the study illustrated in Figure 1 was that the groups were not balanced for gender. In addition, male infants were a higher proportion of those assigned to receive n-3 LCPUFA. Because female VLBW infants generally have superior growth to male VLBW infants, the lower growth with n-3 LCPUFA might have been more pronounced had the groups been balanced for gender.

From data on the comparison of growth with a reference group from the same population, we suggest that growth recovery, especially linear growth, is excellent whereas using the NCHS reference data for reference depicts a failure to catch up. Thus, among lower SES infants of mainly African-American descent, comparison with the NCHS reference group may underestimate the degree of growth recovery that occurs in the first year. There was no reason to suspect that growth of these term infants reflected less than optimal nutrition. Their parents were given advice about how to give ad libitum feeding, and they were not restricted in the amount of formula provided. Both should have promoted optimal growth.

How Do Measures of Size in Studies Compare?

Comparisons of growth between studies should be done with the awareness that there are multiple differences in design, formula composition, etc. that could influence individual outcomes. Table 1 includes a summary of linear growth in centimeters for a few studies that fed nutrient-enriched formulas after discharge and a couple of studies that did not. Absolute measures of growth may be more useful for comparing growth among studies, because not all use the NCHS reference data. There are new NCHS reference data since 2000, further complicating use when comparing results of different studies.

Only minor differences in mean length can be observed among the studies, and these seem especially insignificant given the variations in birth weight, gestational age and gender among the subjects studied. In the two Memphis studies, growth of infants appeared to be virtually identical (Table 1), a somewhat surprising observation given that there were a number of differences between the groups studied including the nutrient content of the formulas fed at discharge.

Body Composition. At discharge, VLBW infants have a higher proportion of body fat than infants who remain in utero until the same gestational ages.[7, 55,56] Kashyap et al[57] found that the ratio of protein to fat accretion reflected the protein to energy ratio of the feeding when they varied the protein:energy concentration of infant formula. However, they concluded that catch-up by discharge is impossible without fat accretion in excess of intrauterine rates. Atkinson and coworkers[55] reported that preterm infants had a higher proportion of body fat and more absolute body fat when fed their own mothers' milks than did infants fed formula until 3-months CA.

Body composition of VLBW infants does eventually normalize between 1 and 2 years of age.[58] Increases in weight gain in VLBW infants are highly related to increases in both lean body mass and fat mass.[46, 59] Many VLBW infants experience a disproportionate increase in weight for length in the early months after

discharge, and this should not be used as evidence for restriction of intake. As noted previously, weight of ad libitum-fed infants studied in Memphis initially increased above the 50th percentile for the NCHS charts, but declined below the 50th percentile by 12 months CA. Until 6-months CA, mean weight-for-length exceeded the NCHS norms (Figure 1C and 2C). From 6 months to 12-months CA, weight-for-length was normal to low. One possible interpretation of these data is that the early increase in weight-for-length is permissive for growth achievement by 12-months CA. It would be interesting to know if endocrine differences between growing term and VLBW infants could explain differences in growth and body composition during the first year of life. Plasma insulin-like growth factor (IGF)-I and IGF binding protein (BP)-3 concentrations have been determined in preterm infants given corticosteroids[60], which are known to compromise physical growth.[26,60] Poor growth during steroid treatment was associated with lower IGF-I and IGFBP-3 concentrations.[60] Plasma IGF-I and IGFBP-3 concentrations were determined in preterm infants from one Memphis study, in which infants were fed a preterm formula until 2-months CA.[61] The comparison group was the group of term infants used as a reference for growth in Figures 1 and 2. In preterm infants, plasma IGF-I concentration increased linearly from 3 months before expected term delivery until 2-months CA (an 11-fold increase) then declined until 9-months CA and rose again between 9 and 12-months CA. IGFBP-3 increased 4-fold from 3 months before term until 2-months CA; then the concentration stayed constant through 9-months CA before increasing again at 12-months CA.

Compared to term infants, the plasma IGF-I concentration in the preterm infants was significantly higher at 2-, 4-, 6- and 12-months CA.[59] Plasma IGFBP-3 was significantly higher in VLBW infants at 2- and 4-months CA, similar at 6-months CA and lower at 12-months CA when compared with the group of term infants. Apparently first year concentrations of plasma IGF-I and IGFBP-3 are influenced by postnatal age and gestational age at birth even after adjusting for early birth. Plasma growth factors continued to be different in the two groups even at 12-months CA.

The ratio of IGF-I to IGFBP-3 at 12-months CA was higher in VLBW compared to term infants. It has been suggested that the pubertal surge in IGF-I accompanied by a less prominent increase in IGFBP-3 could favor growth.[62,63] It remains to be determined if these changes relate to growth in term and VLBW preterm infants. The availability of normal data obtained longitudinally could be useful to compare with other populations of growing VLBW infants. It would be interesting to know if VLBW infants continue to have a different pattern of growth factors compared to term infants beyond 12-months CA and if these patterns differ in infants of African-American descent compared to other groups of infants.

Growth Assessment

Growth assessment is an integral part of follow-up and can be critical in identifying, elucidating and addressing problems with feeding. The need for standardized growth curves for growth assessment of preterm infants is no less important than for term infants. These growth curves might be more important given the problems with growth of VLBW infants noted earlier. There are two kinds of growth curves available. Those that include normalized growth of a population of term infants such as the new 2000 NCHS growth charts and those that include normalized growth of a population of preterm infants to 3-years CA such as the 1999 Infant Health and Development Program Growth Percentiles for LBW and VLBW infants (Ross Products Division, Abbott Laboratories, Inc., Columbus, OH). The 1999 National Institute of Child Health and Human Development Neonatal Research Network Postnatal Growth Charts[64] represent the experience of this network for in-hospital growth of VLBW infants by 100 g increments of birth weight from birth until discharge.

The NCHS growth charts and those for in-hospital nutrition reflect normalized growth achievement expected with current standards of nutritional management of term and preterm infants. The Ross charts, while only recently developed, are based on growth of infants in the era before post-discharge feedings were nutrient-enriched and so may represent slightly less than currently achievable growth rates.

The problem with normalized growth for VLBW infants is that growth of preterm infants is not normal, and they have the potential to lead to acceptance of abnormal growth instead of efforts to find solutions for improvement. If the limitations of the charts are kept in mind, they have some utility for health professionals who would like to compare how an infant is growing in relation to growth obtained by other centers. Also, growth of infants who are outside of the 3rd and 97th percentiles on the term growth chart can be plotted and followed more easily with preterm charts. It is probably useful to plot growth of VLBW infants on both types of charts routinely. The term growth charts reinforce the need for continued growth promotion.

In summary of this section, growth continues to be sub-optimal in VLBW infants after discharge and it is not clear if as a group they ever achieve growth similar to their term peers. Infants fed a nutrient-enriched formula post-discharge appear to grow somewhat better than those fed formulas for term infants after discharge. In the two most recent studies of post-discharge nutrition, however, infants did not achieve growth similar to term infants of the same CA by the end of the studies. Whether or not long-term growth will be improved as the result of these formulas remains to be seen. Data from VLBW infants fed a nutrient-enriched preterm formula from the first week of life until 2-months CA showed that compared to term infants from the same hospital, they had similar mean concentrations of plasma IGF-I and IGFBP-3 at corrected age of term, but different concentrations and patterns through 12-months CA.[61] Despite this, or perhaps because of this, by 12-months CA, the preterm infants had achieved similar size to the term infants. Studies in other populations and in older infants could help determine if there continue to be underlying endocrine differences between term and preterm infants long-term.

Status of Specific Nutrients and Post-Discharge Feeding

While growth is the most commonly measured outcome related to nutrition after discharge, some attention has been given to the biochemical status of individual nutrients after discharge. Data are not available for these nutrients with post-discharge formula, which contain a "stepped down" nutrient content for most vitamins and minerals compared to preterm formula but which are "stepped up" from the nutrient concentration of term formula. Discharge on term formulas can delay the attainment of normal concentrations of plasma nutrients in comparison to term infants fed term formula or accepted standards of normal status. In theory, post-discharge preterm formula should result in more rapid attainment of normal nutrient status than discharge on a term formula, but this has not been tested for any nutrient. Similarly, the use of human milk fortifier should enhance nutritional status of breast fed infants. The human milk fortifiers are quite variable in nutrient content. Most provide protein, another source of energy, and calcium and phosphorus. The main outcomes that have been studied, in post discharge infants provided human milk with fortifiers, relate to bone health and growth.

Calcium and Phosphorus. Beginning during parenteral nutrition, VLBW infants require high calcium and phosphorus intake and Vitamin D. Better attention to these nutrients during parenteral nutrition and a change from term to higher nutrient preterm formulas in the past 15 years led to the apparent disappearance of neonatal rickets in rapidly growing VLBW infants. After discharge, it is VLBW infants fed human milk who are most vulnerable to develop osteopenia due to inadequate intake of phosphorus, because of the increased demands for phosphorus with rapid growth.

After discharge, Schanler et al[65] followed VLBW infants (mean birth weight 1.1 kg) who had been fed fortified human milk in the hospital. At discharge they were fed by parental choice either term formula or human milk without fortification. Six, 15 and 42 weeks later, infants who were breast-fed after discharge had significantly lower mineral content in the distal third of the radius compared to infants fed term formula. Infants who were breast-fed also had lower serum phosphorus and higher alkaline phosphatase activity. Bone mineralization of infants fed term formula after discharge caught up to term infants by 6-months CA, but did not catch up in breast-fed infants who continued to receive human milk for >6 months after discharge, until sometime between 1 and 2 years of age.

Hall et al[66] studied two groups of <1800 g birth weight, breast-fed infants after discharge. One group received a supplement with 100 and 50 mg/kg per day of calcium and phosphorus, respectively. Another group was fed a term formula after discharge. Both groups received 400 IU of Vitamin D. Infants were evaluated for plasma calcium, phosphorus and alkaline phosphatase levels at study entry, discharge and 8 weeks later. By 8 weeks after discharge, both groups of human milk-fed infants had lower serum phosphorus than infants fed term formula. Hypophosphatemia (phosphorus <4.5 mg/dL) occurred in 0 of 6 supplemented and 4 of 9 unsupplemented breast-fed infants. When infants were included who had illnesses but who continued to receive exclusive human milk feeding, 1 of 12 supplemented and 7 of 15 unsupplemented infants had hypophosphatemia. The authors concluded that breast-fed infants who do not receive calcium and phosphorus supplementation after hospital discharge are at significant risk for developing hypophosphatemia despite receiving supplementation in hospital. They recommended that plasma phosphorus and alkaline phosphatase activity of breast fed infants be measured in VLBW infants 4 to 8 weeks after discharge.

Bishop et al[67] reported that a prototype post-discharge formula with 70 mg calcium and 35 mg phosphorus/dL compared with a term formula containing 35 mg calcium and 29 mg phosphorus/dL resulted in higher bone mineral content. They noted, however, that infants who received even the nutrient-enriched formula did not reach a level of 2 standard deviations below the mean for bone mineral content of term infants until 9-months CA.

All of the above studies measured the radius at the one-third distal site using single photon absorptiometry. Dual energy X-ray absorptiometry was used by Fewtrell et al[68] to evaluate children at 9 and 12 years of age formerly fed donor human milk or preterm formula in hospital. They were the subjects of another study as infants.[69] At 9 to 12 years of age, the researchers could not find any relationship between early diet in hospital and bone mineral content.[68] It would have been quite surprising if a diet effect had been found, because the interval between the diet and assessment of bone mineral content was so long and the period the original diet differed so short (approximately 4 weeks). Cooke et al[59] reported higher bone mineral mass and bone area in preterm infants fed a preterm formula after discharge compared to a term formula. The differences were significant in males through at least 12-months CA but females were different only until sometime between 3- and 6-months CA.

Vitamin A (Retinol). Plasma retinol concentrations in hospitalized VLBW infants declined after they were changed from parenteral administration of retinol to administration in preterm formula fed at 120 kcal/kg per day.[11] When infants reached full enteral feeding with a preterm formula, 9% of VLBW infants had plasma retinol concentrations considered indicative of Vitamin A deficiency (<0.35 mmol/L). At discharge, all received a term formula. When they returned for their followup visit, approximately 3 weeks later, 48% (32 of 67) VLBW infants had this indicator of Vitamin A deficiency and another 45% (30 of 67) had hyperetinolemia (plasma retinol of 0.35 to 0.67 mmol/L) Plasma concentrations of retinol did not reach normal for all infants until 6-months CA, or approximately 7 months after discharge on term formula. A possible reason for the high incidence of this indicator of vitamin A deficiency and the long interval required for it to normalize was the practice of discharging infants <2 kg on formulas designed for term infants.[11]

Based on this response, we chose to continue preterm formula until 2-months CA in a subsequent study of VLBW infants[19] and to measure the same indicators of vitamin A status. After 2-months CA, infants were fed a term formula from 2- to 12-months CA.[19] Although the studies were sequential rather than concomitant, the infants received similar in-hospital nutrition management compared to those in the study that discharged infants on term formula, received term formula with the same nutrient composition, and had similar mean birth weights and ranges (mean 1110 g, range 750-1398 g or 1042 g, range 747-1275 g, respectively). By expected term gestation, most infants in the second study already had normal plasma retinol concentrations (>0.67 mmol/L), and all infants had normal plasma retinol concentrations by 2-months CA.

Infants continued to be monitored for the remaining 10 months of infancy for plasma retinol, retinol-binding protein (RBP) concentration and the molar ratio of retinol to RBP. Even though they received a lower nutrient (term) formula after 2-months CA, all continued to have a normal plasma retinol concentration at 4-, 6-, 9- and 12-months CA. Mean retinol intake (RE/kg per day) was 379 at 0-months CA and 282 at 2-months CA. Between 2-months and 12-months CA, retinol intake declined to < 100 RE/kg per day based on estimates from reported formula intake. From this study[19], we suggested that postdischarge use of a nutrient-enriched formula designed for in-hospital care of preterm infants can rapidly produce normal vitamin A status by 2 months postdischarge, after which a term formula contains sufficient Vitamin A to meet needs. In comparison with infants from the historical study, normal plasma retinal concentrations occurred at least 4 months sooner and there was no evidence that Vitamin A intake exceeded desirable levels, since the retinol to RBP ratio remained between 0.8 and 0.9 throughout infancy.

Zinc and Copper. Friel et al[70] randomly allocated VLBW infants to term formula with or without zinc supplements (4.4 mg/L) post-discharge. While in the hospital these infants were fed a preterm formula in hospital that provided 12.2 mg of zinc/L. The study formula used post-discharge contained a basal level of

6.7 mg of zinc/L. Infants consumed the formulas for 6 months and were evaluated at 3-, 6-, 9- and 12-months CA. The group that received additional zinc had higher plasma zinc concentrations at 1 and 3 months and higher linear growth velocity over the study period for the group as a whole and for girls alone.

In another study, preterm VLBW and ELBW infants were fed a preterm formula with 12.2 mg zinc/L in hospital and until 2-months CA, followed by a term formula with 5.1 mg zinc/L from 2- until 12-months CA.[20] A reference group of term infants fed term formula was the comparison group. Mean plasma zinc concentrations in the preterm infants increased from 80 to 101 µg/dl between expected term and 2-months CA and remained between 101-107 µg/dl from 4- to 12-months CA. These values were similar to values found in term infants of the same adjusted ages fed term formula. Because RBP concentrations are dependent upon zinc status, these values were measured and found to be normal at all ages from 2- to 12-months CA.[19] Such was not the case in a previous study of VLBW and ELBW infants who were fed a term formula after discharge. These infants had low plasma RBP concentrations and a high molar ratio of plasma retinol to RBP, especially at 9- and 12-months CA.[11] A high molar ratio of plasma retinol to RBP and a low RBP concentration are changes that would be expected with suboptimal zinc status, and may have been evidence of relatively poor zinc status.

Plasma copper was also studied in the same group of infants discharged on preterm formula. All infants received a formula with 2 mg of copper/L until 2-months CA and 0.6 mg of copper/L from 2- to 12-months CA. Plasma copper rose progressively from 0- to 12-months CA. The values observed were virtually identical at all ages to those of term infants fed term formula. L'Abbe and Friel[21] reported a progressive rise in plasma copper concentrations in VLBW infants post-discharge on term formula that were virtually identical to VLBW infants discharged on preterm formula.[20] This may be taken as evidence that preterm infants do not need more copper than is in term formula.

Long chain fatty acids. All term and preterm formulas available in the US contain the essential fatty acids of the n-6 and n-3 families, linoleic acid and α-linolenic acid, respectively. While the long chain polyunsaturated products of these fatty acids, arachidonic acid (AA) and docosahexaenoic acid (DHA) are found in human milk, they have been added only to experimental formulas fed in the US. Sanders et al[71] first noted that infants fed human milk had higher circulating levels of DHA than infants fed formula, which we confirmed in US infants.[72] There are now dozens of reports demonstrating higher levels of DHA in plasma or red blood cells of infants fed human milk or DHA-enriched formulas compared to infants fed formulas without DHA. While suggestive of lower status, differences in blood levels of DHA could not be interpreted as such without functional data that infants performed better and had higher body DHA status when they were fed DHA. A large number of studies in the past 10 years have focused on the neural development of infants randomized to formulas with or without DHA.[73,74] As will be discussed in the section on development, these reports are evidence that DHA is a conditionally essential nutrient for preterm infants. Studies have shown that DHA accumulation is greater in brains of breast-fed infants compared to brains of infants fed formulas without DHA,[75,76] further evidence of a link between brain DHA and neural function. Only a few brains of preterm infants have been studied at autopsy, but the results confirm the early hypothesis that formula-fed preterm infants have lower DHA accumulation in brain than formula-fed term infants.[75]

In summary, there is relatively little data on the status of individual nutrients during the first year of life after VLBW infants are discharged. Even those data are not definitive in that they mainly raise concerns due to low plasma nutrient concentrations while offering almost no data on functional outcomes. The data that are available are mainly for nutrients such as zinc, Vitamin A, calcium and phosphorus. Zinc and Vitamin A have important roles in immunity, growth and neurodevelopment. Infants discharged on preterm formula appear to develop normal plasma concentrations of these nutrients as much as 4 months before infants discharged on term formula. There are no published data on the amount of time needed for full recovery of Vitamin A and zinc in infants receiving any of the post-discharge formulas that are currently available for infant feeding.

Now that early enteral nutrition with preterm formulas and human milk fortifier are the standard for in-hospital care of formula and human milk-fed infants, rickets in the hospital is thought to be rare. The greatest risk for osteopenia occurs after discharge when rapid growth combines with discontinuation of human milk fortifiers. VLBW infants discharged on breast-milk should be monitored for plasma phosphorus concentrations and activity of alkaline phosphatase at 4 and 8 weeks after discharge, especially if they are not provided human milk fortifier after discharge. About half of the infants discharged without human milk fortifier developed osteopenia in one study.[66] Higher calcium and phosphorus in a prototype post-discharge formula led to higher bone mineral content that a term formula, but even the nutrient-enriched formula resulted in bone mineralization that was two standard deviations below the mean for term infants by 9-months CA.[67] There is a high correlation between bone mineralization and body weight, further emphasizing the importance of promoting early catch-up growth.[77,78]

The use of glucocorticoids in hospital continues to be a major risk factor for poor bone mineralization and reduced linear growth in the first year of life. The goal for bone development should focus on normal bone accretion rather than avoiding osteopenia. More research is needed to determine if there is a causal relationship between bone mineralization and linear growth using post-discharge diets with different amounts and ratios of calcium and phosphorus.

Nutrition and Developmental Outcomes

Growth is the most commonly measured outcome of nutritional studies, but much of the interest in growth as an outcome relates to the fact that it is linked to development, which in turn is linked to physiologic function. The problem for this chapter is that there are

many developmental systems, all of which have the potential to be influenced by nutritional status of VLBW infants, and few of which have been studied in relation to nutrition, much less post-discharge nutrition. Development of physiological systems is under the influence of programming that is age-related to at least some degree. Researchers interested specifically in the effect of postdischarge nutrition on development are limited by the lack of control over nutrition during hospitalization in the same way that researchers interested in studying nutrition in hospital are limited by a lack of control over prenatal nutrition. Programming might be important during any of these periods, and is likely to depend upon the physiologic system of interest.

In the real world, the ideal experiment cannot be done. Poor maternal nutritional status is known to be an etiological factor for preterm birth, and infant nutrient status is well-known to reflect maternal nutrient status (even though biochemical indices of most nutrients demonstrate higher fetal than maternal status). For all of these reasons, the status of individual nutrients is often less than perfect at the time of VLBW delivery, and nutrient status generally declines in hospital. In addition, many of the medical problems and interventions are confounders for development. For example, glucocorticoids given to enhance gut and lung maturation prematurely have known adverse effects on other developing systems including skeletal, endocrine and immunesystems.[26,79] Singer[80] has written an excellent chapter on some of the methodological considerations involved in studying aspects of neural development in high-risk infants.

In the area of neurodevelopment, there are still questions about the best outcomes to use after discharge to assess the risk of adverse neurological outcomes long term. Global measures of behavior such as the Bayley Mental Developmental Index (MDI) and Psychomotor Developmental Index (PDI) are often used because there are standardized methods available from studies of normal term infants. While these permit the researcher to compare preterm infant development to that of normal term infants, global measures are not able to detect effects on specific behavioral domains. Depending upon the effect of a given nutrient, some but not all domains of behavior may be affected.

More exploratory outcomes for which standardized tests do not exist may have a better potential for elucidating the underlying problem so an intervention can be designed. However, in the absence of a standardized method, other investigators may have difficulty replicating results. The same methodological issues are bound to apply for other developmental systems. For example, what outcome can be studied in infancy to detect long-term risk for hypertension? Without a reliable marker, risks cannot be identified and theoretical interventions undertaken before developmental "programming" occurs. These are the kinds of problems that affect the ability to study long-term development, even when an investigator might be willing to devote the time required to do such studies.

Studies of nutrition during development of VLBW infants would be worthwhile if development of a system is shown to differ from that of normal term infants. While differences in development could be the result of many factors, marginal nutrient status needs to be considered among the factors possible and may be one of the most easily correctable, once the data are available. This is the underlying theoretical basis for our attempts to provide optimal nutritional management both in the hospital and after discharge. It seems reasonable to correct marginal status of nutrients when this can be done without risk. Moreover, it is not practical to insist that development of every system be studied and improvements demonstrated before setting a goal to achieve nutrient status that is at least at the level accepted for term infants.

It may be worth noting here that low plasma concentrations of a nutrient are not always evidence of too little of that nutrient in the body. Sometimes carrier proteins are too low because of immaturity or less than optimal amounts of another nutrient. VLBW infants frequently have low circulating proteins during the period before they reach full enteral feeding, and this fact can complicate interpretation of nutrient status.

There are more studies of nutrient intervention post-discharge and its relationship to behavior than there are equivalent studies for other systems. There is little doubt that the focus of research on the developing brain development reflects its societal premium. However, all aspects of development are important. In the long-term, the individual quality of life for VLBW infants may have more to do with proper functioning of immunity, respiratory or other function.

Neural Development. Preterm infants are at increased risk for poor developmental outcomes compared to term infants.[81] Among the problems that occur in preterm infants with greater frequency than in term infants are impaired vision, visual-motor integration, neuromotor function, cognitive function, and problems with behavior and temperament. Factors that influence development include maternal health and nutrition during pregnancy, maternal interaction and stimulation of the infant, chronic illnesses, and the nutritional status of the infant him- or herself.

The first evidence that nutrition in hospital could affect developmental outcome came from Lucas et al.[82] In one cohort of infants, those fed a nutrient-enriched formula for approximately 4 weeks in hospital compared to a term formula had significantly higher Bayley PDI scores at 18-months CA. The advantages of receiving the nutrient-enriched compared to the term formula were greater for SGA infants and male infants, who had higher Bayley MDI scores as well as higher scores on the PDI.

In a parallel study from these authors, infants of mothers who were not offered their own milk were randomly assigned to donor human milk or preterm formula in hospital.[69] Even though the nutrient intakes of infants fed human milk were presumed to be much lower than those of infants fed preterm formula, the two diet groups showed little difference in MDI or PDI at 18-months CA.

In another analysis of data from this group, children whose mothers chose to provide human milk performed better than those whose mothers chose not to when studied at 18-months CA and also at 7.5 to

8 years of age.[83] These results led to speculation about some component in human milk that could plausibly provide such an advantage. Speculation centered on the fact that donor milk contains long chain fatty acids such as DHA, which were not in formulas in Europe at that time. This fit with the data reported just prior, which showed higher retinal function in hospitalized preterm infants[84] and visual development of preterm infants after discharge[85,86] when formula contained n-3 LCPUFA from fish oil.

LCPUFA are not the only factors in human milk that could affect development, and it will probably never be known if these are the factors that conferred benefit in the Lucas, Morley studies. However, a number of randomized studies have provided formulas with and without added DHA from a variety of sources and the effects on normal first year development have been assessed. These studies have just been reviewed.[74,75] Development of visual acuity has been the most commonly measured outcome in both term and preterm infants, but a few studies have measured global development, problem-solving, and attention duration and concluded that these were positively influenced by DHA supplementation of formula. Two independent systematic reviews published this year concluded that there were short-term benefits on visual development of feeding long chain polyunsaturated fatty acids to preterm infants,[87,88] and one reached the same conclusion for term infants.[89]

Long-term visual development has not been studied in randomized trials, but Williams et al[90] report that 3.5 year-old term infants were more likely to have achieved high-grade stereoacuity if their mothers ate oily fish that contain considerable amounts of n-3 LCPUFA during pregnancy. Term infants breast fed for at least 4 months were also more likely to achieve high-grade stereoscopic vision at 3.5 years of age than infants fed formula. Both maternal intake of oily fish during pregnancy and breast-feeding would be expected to increase the amount of DHA available to the infant relative to no fish or formula feeding. The evidence that DHA is a conditionally essential nutrient is stronger for preterm than for term infants, who have

the opportunity to accumulate brain DHA in utero.

DHA may provide a cautionary tale for the poor status of other nutrients such as iron, zinc and Vitamin A. Like DHA, these nutrients when marginal do not result in obvious health problems, but they are critical to normal brain development. There is evidence from some though not all studies that iron deficiency with[91] or without[92] anemia has adverse effects on brain development in term infants and that these effects might not be reversible.[92-94] One could imagine preterm infants would be more vulnerable to iron-deficiency than term infants, but there has been only one study of development in LBW infants assigned to one of two levels of iron fortification. In that study, Friel et al[95] compared the development (Griffith's Developmental Assessment) of LBW infants fed formula with 13.4 mg/L of iron compared to infants fed high iron formula (21 mg/L) until one year after hospital discharge. The researchers concluded that the higher iron did not enhance development. Moreover, higher iron intake was associated with lower concentrations of plasma copper and zinc at 12 months and more respiratory infections, both of which could be regarded as undesirable effects. Iron-fortified term and post-discharge formulas available in the US contain 1.8 mg of iron/100 kcal, equivalent to the "normal" iron fed by Friel and coworkers.

It should be emphasized that infants in the Friel et al study[95] were enrolled and were fed the amount of iron available in a commercially available post-discharge formula well before discharge from the hospital. The best practice is to provide for adequate iron while preterm infants are hospitalized and a meta-analysis has confirmed a marked reduction in iron-deficient anemia among hospitalized preterm infants given iron supplements.[96]

In an earlier study, Friel et al[70] found that VLBW infants who received a commercially available term formula with zinc supplements (4.4 mg/L for a total of 11 mg/L) and who were assessed at 3-, 6-, 9- and 12-months CA with the Griffith's Developmental Assessment had significantly higher motor development scores.

In summary, the neurodevelopment of VLBW infants is not normal compared to term infants. Insults to the developing nervous system prenatally and during intensive care are components of this picture, and may not be avoided easily. Low/declining nutrient status during the postnatal and post-discharge period and extended periods of nutritional recovery may be layered on top of these other problems. Improvements in nutritional management can still be made and these could be functionally important. The goal should be to achieve fully normal indices for nutrient status rather than to prevent obvious nutritional deficiencies. It is reasonable to speculate that some of the damage to developing systems that occurs during clinical care is made more severe by low nutrient states or could be ameliorated by better nutrition. Georgieff and Rao[97] have provided an excellent review of the relationships between nutrition and infant cognitive development including a review of the underlying mechanisms that nutrients play in development.

Post-discharge formulas represent an advance over term formula for preterm infants who routinely have suboptimal nutrient status at hospital discharge. However, these formulas should continue to be studied and improved. With regard to development, it seems more ideal to "catch up" in nutritional status sooner rather than later. From studies of a few selected nutrients, preterm infants fed a nutrient-enriched formula to 2-months CA had normal indices of nutrient status and they remained normal on a term formula until 12-months CA. Neurodevelopment occurs through age-related "programming" and this may be true for other aspects of development as well. Delays in returning nutritional status indices to normal theoretically could compromise both early and long-term development.

Nutritional Management and Monitoring for Preterm Infants After Discharge

A number of groups and individuals have provided guidelines for nutritional management after discharge.[22,24,25,98] For the most part, these recommendations are quite consistent given the paucity of data available about the nutritional status

of preterm infants fed the various milk alternatives after discharge.

A necessary prerequisite for discharge from the hospital is physiologic maturity that includes cardiopulmonary stability and the ability to maintain body temperature in an open bed. In addition, with rare exceptions, infants are not discharged until they demonstrate the ability to gain weight adequately when fed by mouth. Infants within a wide range of ages and sizes meet these criteria. Often, discharge is initiated based upon the infant achieving a criterion for weight defined within a given hospital even though the AAP Committee on the Fetus and Newborn[99] has proposed that early discharge be based on a sustained pattern of weight gain rather than a specific achieved weight. The variability in discharge weights among hospitals is relevant here, because relatively smaller infants are less likely than larger ones to have caught up from nutritional deficits suffered during the typical hospitalization.

Although there are not comprehensive studies of all nutrients at the time of hospital discharge, the nutrients that have been studied show a fairly consistent pattern of lower than normal status for what would be expected in term infants fed human milk or formula. Consequently, there have been attempts to improve nutritional status of infants post-discharge through a couple of different means. For the preterm infants who is formula fed, preterm formula or one of the post-discharge formulas that are intermediate in nutrient content between term and preterm formulas could be fed for some period after discharge. For the infant fed human milk, the options for providing additional nutrients include a human milk fortifier or limited supplementation with preterm formula.

Two studies that were done consecutively could be used to support continued feeding of preterm formula after discharge as a means to return Vitamin A and zinc status to normal between 0- and 2-months CA.[11,19] After 2-months CA, the status indicators for these nutrients remained normal on a term formula, and no evidence of negative effects on plasma electrolytes or evidence of toxicity was found.[19,20] Vitamin A and zinc are important nutrients for cognitive and motor development, and it could be argued that they should be normalized as soon as possible. Theoretically, because they contain lower amounts of these nutrients, post-discharge formulas would return Vitamin A and zinc status to normal more slowly than preterm formula. Four studies have been reported comparing a post-discharge formula or prototype post-discharge formula with a term formula. Each found some evidence of improved post-discharge growth compared to a term formula.[17,44-47]

It has been said that preterm formulas are inappropriate for infants who weigh more than 2.5 kg due to the increased nutrient content and concerns about nutrient toxicity.[98] It is difficult to accept this premise in light of a report that infants discharged on preterm formula did not have normal Vitamin A content until 2-months CA.[19] At that time, the infants weighed on average just over 10 pounds (4.84 kg).[9] The chances of toxicity of a nutrient developing are small in any given period when nutrient status is below normal and growth is very rapid. These conditions characterize the period immediately after discharge for healthy VLBW infants. Infants in that study[9] gained ~6.6 pounds in the first 12 weeks after discharge.

At the same time that there is an absence of negative findings, there are positive findings that preterm formula after discharge helped preterm infants catch up in status for important nutrients such as zinc and Vitamin A by 2-months CA. Unfortunately, similar evaluations of many other vitamins were not made.

Recommendations for Formula-Fed Infants

Although data to inform the choice of type of formula post-discharge are limited, there is considerable evidence that nutrient status has not caught up to normal at discharge even when in-hospital nutrition is managed optimally. Moreover, it is plausible to suggest that low status of any number of nutrients prevents optimal infant development. For this reason, either a preterm formula until 2-months CA or a post-discharge formula during the first year of life are recommended (Table 2). With either option,

supplemental vitamins and iron would not be needed above those in the preterm or post-discharge formulas, and available evidence would not suggest a need for additional vitamins and iron at any time during infancy, even after infants were changed to a term formula. These two strategies have been used experimentally without apparent problems.

Caregivers should be encouraged to ad libitum feed preterm infants by putting more formula in the bottle than the infant is expected to consume, and by permitting the infant to stop the feeding when he/she desires. It is important not to restrict feeding of these infants simply because their weight-for-length becomes disproportionately high compared to NCHS reference values for term infants, as it frequently does. Lucas et al[41] reported that 50% of the infants they studied consumed >165 kcal/kg per day for many months after hospital discharge. In general, weight and length become proportional around the end of the first year. Length percentiles by 12-months CA may exceed weight percentiles. From our data, we suggest that as a group, increases in weight percentiles in the first half of infancy may help determine linear growth achievement in the second half of infancy (Figures 1, 2).

Preterm infants fed human milk after discharge should receive a supplemental multivitamin and iron until 5 kg.[22] If breast milk is insufficient, a post-discharge formula or standard term formula with iron could be used for occasional supplemental feedings.[24] If formula becomes the major source of milk, supplemental vitamins and iron may be unnecessary. VLBW infants who are breast fed after discharge should be monitored for plasma phosphorus concentrations and activity of alkaline phosphatase at 4 and 8 weeks after discharge, especially if they are not provided human milk fortifier after discharge. There is not a consensus among professionals that these infants should receive a human milk fortifier; however, evidence in favor of such a course of action can be found.[66,67] Although not all infants fed human milk develop osteopenia without fortification, a good percentage can be expected to develop this problem. Given that there are no known adverse effects of continuing the fortifiers, it seems prudent to continue their use for some time after discharge to avoid osteopenia in infants who would develop the problem. If osteopenia develops, either a high-protein, high-mineral supplement or human milk fortifier are recommended until the nutrient deficiency is corrected.[22]

In the final analysis, the goal of post-discharge nutrition should be to ensure that nutrient status of infants is within normal indicators as soon as possible whenever possible. There is accumulating evidence that this does not occur with term formula or unfortified human milk. Until some data are available on the nutrient status of infants fed post-discharge formulas, one could argue the merits of preterm vs post-discharge formulas. However, post-discharge formulas at least provide more nutrients than term formulas and they have been fed without obvious adverse effects to 12-months CA.

Case History

AGA male of African descent born at 29-weeks postmenstrual age weighing 1.077 kg, 38.5 cm long and 26.5 cm head circumference. He was born to a 20-year-old G2P1 by C-section due to breech and preterm labor. He was resuscitated in the operating room by endotracheal tube, continued to require ventilator support for 248.5 hours, and was weaned to an oxyhood. He continued to receive supplemental oxygen for an additional 18 days or for a total of 28 days.

Parenteral nutrition was started at 11 hours of age and given by umbilical artery catheter until 284 hours of age. Intralipid and parenteral nutrition with 10% glucose were tapered gradually and discontinued at 22 days of life. Enteral feeding with Similac Special Care® and Iron, a preterm formula, was initiated at 91 hours of life and advanced gradually to 101 kcal/kg per day on preterm formula on the 24th day of life. He progressed on enteral feeding from continuous nasogastric to intermittent nipple feeding without any interruption in enteral feeding until discharge on day 47 of life. Between full enteral feeding and discharge, his daily energy intake on preterm formula ranged from 108 to 122 kcal/kg per day. He was discharged at 1.83 kg on preterm formula (24 kcal/oz).

Prior to discharge, he received 56 ml of packed red blood cells, 4 doses of Survanta® for HMD, had mild

BPD and required furosamide. He was given theophyline for apnea of prematurity, and phototherapy for increased bilirubin. On his 14th day of life, he had increased blood pressure and received an abdominal ultrasound. An aortic clot was observed below the kidneys extending to the iliac crest with good perfusion of the extremities. The infant had some difficulty weaning from the ventilator and oxygen (he was reintubated twice). On day of life 29, he had decreased oxygen saturation and tachypnea and was given ampicillin/gentamycin and vancomycin for 3 days prophylactically.

He returned for his term visit at 39.5-weeks-postmentstrual age. At that time, his mother reported he was consuming 3.5 oz of formula every 3 hours around the clock, or a total of 28 oz/day. He weighed 2.89 kg so his intake was estimated at 232 kcal/kg per day. He had a 35.1 cm head circumference and was 48.4 cm long. At 48-weeks-postmenstrual age (2-months CA), his mother reported feeding 32 oz of formula/day in 5 total feedings between 7 AM and 10 PM. He weighed 5.33 kg and was consuming 144 kcal/kg/day. He was 56.5 cm long and had a head circumference of 39.4 cm. Weight and head circumference at 2-months CA were at the 50th percentile for the pre-2000 NICHD growth charts.

After 2-months CA, the infant was fed Similac with Iron®, a term formula, until one-year-corrected age. His reported energy intake from formula was 98, 79, 79 and 84 kcal/kg per day at 4-, 6-, 9- and 12-months corrected age. Throughout that time, his length was at the 25th percentile and his weight gradually declined from the 50th to the 25th percentile. His head circumference decreased from the 55th percentile at 2-months-corrected age to the 45th, 25th, 25th and 15th at 4-, 6-, 9- and 12-months-corrected age, respectively.

This infant demonstrates the high energy intakes that can be consumed when preterm infants are encouraged to consume formula ad libitum. At the same time, his growth during the first year was excellent in-so-far as weight and length were concerned. The case illustrates how well infants can grow in weight and length when they remain well in hospital, are started early on enteral feeding with a nutrient-enriched formula, and energy intake can be maintained at approximately 120 kcal/kg throughout most of the hospital stay. The decrease in head circumference percentiles with time is frequently observed. The head circumference percentiles early on may mask lower brain growth. Head circumference was low at 1 year of age (15th percentile) compared to the excellent weight and length growth of this infant. Although his visual development and hearing were within normal limits, the infant was reported to be slow to test and to show little interest in pictures used for a standardized test for infant development at 6, 9 and 12 months. Moreover, he did not show a preference for pictures of novel faces when tested at 6- and 9-months CA, suggesting he processed information more slowly than normal. Coupled with his slower than normal head growth, it appears some degree of subtle neurological impairment is possible. Based on his relatively uneventful history, his early problems with oxygenation would be the most likely cause.

References

1. Brooke OG, Onubogu O, Heath R, Carter ND. Human milk and preterm formula compared for effects on growth and metabolism. *Arch Dis Child* 1987;62:917-923.

2. Reis BB, Hall RT, Schanler RJ, Berseth CL, Chan G, Ernst JA, Lemons J, Adamkin D, Baggs G, O'Connor D. Enhanced growth of preterm infants fed a new powdered human milk fortifier: A randomized, controlled trial. *Pediatr* 2000;106:581-588.

3. Koo WWK, Sherman R, Succop P, Oestreich E, Tsang RC, Krug-Wispe SK, Steichen JJ. Sequential bone mineral content in small preterm infants with and without fractures and rickets. *J Bone Miner Res* 1988; 3:193-197.

4. Putet G, Senterre J, Rigo J, Salle B. Nutrient balance, energy utilization and composition of weight gain in very low birth weight infants fed pooled human milk or a preterm formula. *J Pediatr* 1984;105:79-85.

5. Schanler RJ, Garza C, Nichols BL. Fortified mothers' milk for very low birthweight infants: Results of growth and nutrient balance studies. *J Pediatr* 1985;107:437-445.

6. Hay WW. IV. Posthospital nutrition of the preterm infant requires improved predischarge nutrition, in Posthospital Nutrition in the Preterm Infant (Report of the 106th Ross Conference on Pediatric Research, Col-

orado Springs, August 18-20, 1995), eds, Silverman E, Redfern DE, Columbus, OH: Ross Products Division Abbott Laboratories, 1996; 76-81.

7. Heird WC, Wu C. Nutrition, growth and body composition, Ibid; 7-16.

8. Carlson SE, Cooke RJ, Werkman SH, Tolley EA. First year growth of preterm infants fed standard compared to marine oil n-3 supplemented formula. *Lipids* 1992; 27:901-907.

9. Carlson SE, Werkman SH, Tolley EA. The effect of long chain n-3 fatty acid supplementation on visual acuity and growth of preterm infants with and without bronchopulmonary dysplasia. *Am J Clin Nutr* 1996; 63: 687-697.

10. Ehrenkrantz RA. Growth outcomes of very low-birthweight infants in the newborn intensive care unit. *Clin Perinatol* 2000;27:325-345.

11. Peeples JM, Carlson SE, Werkman SH, Cooke RJ. Vitamin A status of preterm infants during infancy. *Am J Clin Nutr* 1991; 53:1455-1459.

12. Tyrala EE, Manser JI, Brodsky NL, Tran N. Serum zinc concentrations in growing premature infants. *Acta Paediatr Scand* 1983;72:695-698.

13. Koo WW, Succop P, Hambidge KM. Serum alkaline phosphatase and serum zinc concentrations in preterm infants with rickets and fractures. *Am J Dis Child* 1989;143:1342-1345.

14. Tyrala EE. Zinc and copper balances in preterm infants. *Pediatr* 1986;77:513-517.

15. Mimouni F, Tsang RC. Vitamin D metabolism and requirements in pregnancy, lactation,the term and the preterm infants. In: *Annales Nestle* 53/2, 1995, Vitamins in Infancy and Pregnancy, Vevey, Switzerland: Nestec Ltd: 1995; 52-60.

16. Tsang R, Namgung R. Newborn bone development. In Posthospital Nutrition in the Preterm Infant. Report of the 106th Ross Conference on Pediatric Research; August 18-20, 1995: Colorado Springs. eds. Silverman E, Redfern DE, Columbus, OH: Ross Products Division Abbott Laboratories, 1996; 21-26.

17. Lucas A, Bishop NJ, King FJ, Cole TJ. Randomized trial of nutrition for preterm infants after discharge. *Arch Dis Chil* 1992; 67:324-327.

18. Posthospital Nutrition in the Preterm Infant. Report of

the 106th Ross Conference on Pediatric Research; August 18-20, 1995: Colorado Springs. eds. Silverman E, Redfern DE, Columbus, OH: Ross Products Division Abbott Laboratories, 1996;

19. Carlson SE, Peeples JM, Werkman SH, Koo WWK. Plasma retinol and retinol binding protein concentrations in premature infants fed preterm formula past hospital discharge. *European J Clin Nutr* 1995; 49: 134-136.

20. Rajaram S, Carlson SE, Koo WWK, Braselton EW. Plasma mineral concentrations in preterm infants fed a nutrient-enriched formula after hospital discharge. *J Pediatr* 1995; 126:791-796.

21. L'Abbe MR, Friel JK. Copper status of very low birthweight infants during the first 12 months of infancy. *Pediatr Res* 1992; 32:183-188.

22. Hovasi Cox J, Doorlag D. Nutritional concerns at discharge. In: *Nutritional Care for High-Risk Newborns* (3rd. Ed), eds. Groh-Wargo S, Thompson M, Cox J, Chicago, Precept Press, Inc.: 2000:549-565.

23. Theriot L. Routine nutrition care during follow-up. In Ibid:567-583.

24. De Curtis M, Pieltain C, Rigo J. Nutrition of preterm infants on discharge from the hospital. In: *Infant Formula: Closer to the Reference*. eds. Raiha NCR, Rubaltelli FF, Nestle Nutrition Workshop Series Pediatric Program, Vol. 47. Philadelphia: Williams and Wilkins; 2002:149-161.

25. Greer FR. Feeding the preterm infant after hospital discharge. *Pediatr Ann* 2001; 30: 658-665.

26. Weiler H, Paes B, Shah JK, Atkinson SA. Longitudinal assessment of growth and bone mineral accretion in prematurely born infants treated for chronic lung disease with dexamethasone. *Early Hum Dev* 1997;47:271-286.

27. Georgieff MK, Mills MM, Lindeke L, Iverson S, Johnson DE, Thompson TR. Changes in nutritional management and outcome of very low birthweight infants. *Am J Dis Child* 1989; 143:82-85.

28. Dibley MJ, Goldsby JB, Staehling NW, Trowbridge FL. Development of normalized curves for the international growth reference: historical and technical considerations. *Am J Clin Nutr* 1987; 46: 736-748.

29. Hamill PV, Drizd TA, Johnson CL, Reed RB, Roche AS, Moore WM. Physical growth: National Center for Health Statistics percentiles. *Am J Clin Nutr* 1979; 32:607-629.

30. Gayle HD, Dibley MJ, Marks JS, Trowbridge FL. Malnutrition in the first two years of life. The contribution of low birth weight to population estimates in the United States. *Am J Dis Child* 1987;141:531-534.

31. Casey PH, Kraemer HC, Bernbaum J, Yogman MW, Sells JC. Growth status and growth rates of a varied sample of low birth weight, preterm infants: A longitudinal cohort from birth to three years of age. *J Pediatr* 1991;119:599-605.

32. Hack M, Borawski-Clark E. Postdischarge growth of very-low-birth-weight children. In: Posthospital Nutrition in the Preterm Infant. Report of the 106th Ross Conference on Pediatric Research, August 18-20, 1995: Colorado Springs. eds. Silverman E, Redfern DE, Columbus, OH: Ross Products Division Abbott Laboratories, 1996; 58-63.

33. Kitchen WH, Doyle LW, Ford GW, Callanan C. Very low birth weight and growth to age 8 years. *Am J Dis Child* 1992; 146:40-45.

34. Bowman E, Yu VY. Continuing morbidity in extremely low birthweight infants. *Early Hum Dev* 1988;18: 165-174.

35. Ernst JA, Bull MJ, Rickard KA, Brady MS, Lemons JA. Growth outcome and feeding practices of the very low birthweight infant less than 1500 grams) within the first year of life. *J Pediatr* 1990;117:S156-166.

36. Strauss RS, Dietz WH. Effects of intrauterine growth retardation in premature infants on early childhood growth. *J Pediatr* 1997; 130: 95-102.

37. Karniski W, Blair C, Vitucci JS. The illusion of catch-up growth in premature infants. Use of the growth index and age correction. *Am J Dis Chld* 1987;141:520-526.

38. Lapillone A, Carlson SE. Polyunsaturated fatty acids and infant growth. *Lipids* 2001; 36: 901-912.

39. Peralta-Carcelen M, Jackson DS, Goran MI, Royal SA, Mayo MS, Nelson KG. Growth of adolescents who were born at extremely low birth weight without major disability. *J Pediatr* 2000; 136:633-640.

40. Bryson SR, Theriot L, Ryan NJ, Pope J, Tolman N, Rhoades P. Primary follow-up care in a multidiscipli-

nary setting enhances catch-up growth of very low birthweight infants. *J Am Diet Assoc* 1997;97:386-390.

41. Lucas A. Nutrition, growth and development of postdischarge, preterm infants in Posthospital Nutrition in the Preterm Infant. Report of the 106th Ross Conference on Pediatric Research, August 18-20, 1995: Colorado Springs. eds. Silverman E, Redfern DE, Columbus, OH: Ross Products Division Abbott Laboratories, 1996; 81-89

42. Kelleher KJ, Casey PH, Bradley RH, Pope SK, Whiteside L, Barrett KW, Swanson ME, Kirby RS. Risk factors and outcomes for failure to thrive in low birthweight preterm infants. *Pediatr* 1993;91: 941-948.

43. Gardner-Pearson charts, UK:Castlemead.

44. Carver JD, Wu PY, Hall RT, Zeigler EE, Sosa R, Jabocbs J, Baggs G, Auestad N, Lloyd B. Growth of preterm infants fed nutrient-enriched or term formula after hospital discharge. *Pediatr* 2001;107:683-689.

45. Cooke RJ, Griffin IJ, McCormick K, Wells JCK, Smith JS, Robinson SJ, Leighton M. Feeding preterm infants after hospital discharge: effect of dietary manipulation on nutrient intake and growth. *Pediatr Res* 1998; 43:355-360.

46. Cooke RJ, Embleton ND, Griffin IJ, Wells JC, McCormick KP. Feeding preterm infants after hospital discharge: growth and development at 18 months of age. *Pediatr Res* 2001; 49:719-722.

47. Wheeler RE, Hall RT. Feeding of premature infant formula after hospital discharge of infants weighing less than 1800 grams at birth. *J Perinatol* 1996; 16: 111-116.

48. Ryan AS, Montalto MB, Groh-Wargo S, Mimouni F, Sentipal-Walerius J, Doyle J, Siegman JS, Thomas AJ. Effect of DHA-containing formula on growth of preterm infants to 59 weeks postmenstrual age. *Am J Hum Biol* 1999; 11:457-467.

49. Carlson SE, Cooke RJ, Rhodes PG, Peeples JM, Werkman SH, Tolley EA. Long-term feeding of formulas high in linolenic acid and marine oil to very low birthweight infants: Phospholipid fatty acids. *Pediatr Res* 1991; 30:404-412.

50. Carlson SE, Werkman SH, Peeples JM, Cooker RJ, Tolley EA. Arachidonic acid status correlates with first year growth in preterm infants. *PNAS* 1993;90:1073-1077.

51. O'Connor D, Hall R, Adamkin D, Auestad N, Castillo M., Connor WE. Connor SL, Fitzgerald K, Groh-Wargo S, Hartmann EE, Jacobs J, Janowksi J, Lucas A, Margeson D, Mena P, Neuringer M, Nesin M, Singer L, Stephenson T, Szabo J, Zemon V on behalf of the Ross Preterm Lipid Study. Growth and development in preterm infants fed long-chain polyunsaturated fatty acids: A prospective randomized controlled trial. *Pediatr* 2001; 359-371.

52. Auestad N, Halter R, Hall RT, Blatter M, Bogle ML, Burks W, Erickson JR, Fitzgerald KM, Dobson V, Innis SM, Singer LT, Montalto MB, Jacobs JR, Qiu W, Bornstein MH. Growth and development in term infants fed long-chain polyunsaturated fatty acids: A double-masked, randomized, parallel, prospective, multivariate study. *Pediatr* 2001; 108: 372-381.

53. Carlson SE, Ford AJ, Werkman SH, Peeples JM, Koo WWK. Visual acuity and fatty acid status of term infants fed human milk and formula with and without docosahexaenoate and arachidonate from egg yolk lecithin. *Pediatr Res* 1996; 39:1-7.

54. Atkinson SA. Body composition of premature infants to the 1st-year corrected age, in Posthospital Nutrition in the Preterm Infant (Report of the 106th Ross Conference on Pediatric Research, Colorado Springs, August 18-20, 1995), eds, Silverman E, Redfern DE, Columbus, OH: Ross Products Division Abbott Laboratories, 1996, p. 127-131.

55. Elliman AM, Bryan EM, Elliman AD, Starte D. Narrow heads of preterm infants – do they matter? *Dev Med Child Neurol* 1986;28:745-748.

56. Putet G, Senterre J, Rigo J, Salle B. Energy balance and composition of body weight. *Biol Neonate* 1987;52:S117-124.

57. Kashyap S, Schulze KF, Ramakrishnan R, Dell RB, Heird WC. Evaluation of a mathematical model for predicting the relationship between protein and energy intakes of low-birth-weight infants and the rate and composition of weight gain. *Pediatr Res* 1994;35: 704-712.

58. de Gamarra ME, Schutz Y, Catzeflis C, Freymond D, Cauderay M, Calame A, Micheli JL, Jequier E. of weight gain during the neonatal period and

longitudinal growth follow-up in premature babies. *Biol Neonate* 1987;52:181-187.

59. Cooke RJ, McCormick K, Griffin IJ, Embleton N, Faulkner K, Wells JC, Rawlings DC. Feeding preterm infants after hospital discharge: Effect of diet on body composition. *Pediatr Res* 1999;46:461-464.

60. Skinner AM, Battin M, Solimano A, Daaboul J, Kitson HF. Growth and growth factrs in premature infants receiving dexamethasone for bronchopulmonary dysplasia. *Am J Perinatol* 1997;14:539-546.

61. Rajaram S. Carlson SE, Koo WWK, Kelly DP, Rangachari A. Insulin-like growth factor (IGF-I) and IGF-binding protein 3 during the first year in term and preterm infants. *Pediatr Res* 1995; 37:581-585.

62. Blum WF, Albertsson-Wikland K, Rosberg S, Ranke MB. Serum levels of insulin-like growth factor I (IGF-I) and IGF binding protein 3 reflect spontaneous growth hormone secretion. *J Clin Endocrinol Metab* 1993; 76:1610-1616.

63. Argente J, Barrios V, Pozo J, Munoz MT, Hervas S, Stene M, Hernandez M. Normative data for insulin-like growth factors (IGFs), IGF-binding proteins, and growth hormone-binding protein in a healthy Spanish pediatric population: age- and sex-related changes. *J Clin Endocrinol Metab* 1993; 77:1522-1528.

64. Ehrenkrantz RA, Youndes N, Lemons J, Fanaroff AA, Donovan EF, Wright LL, Katsikiotis V, Tyson JE, Oh W, Shankaran S, Bauer CR, Korones SB, Stoll BJ, Stevenson DK, Papile LA. Longitudinal growth of hospitalized very low birth weight infants [National Institute of Child Health and Human Development Neonatal Research Network Postnatal Growth Charts]. *Pediatr* 1999; 104: 280-289.

65. Schanler RJ, Abrams SA. Postnatal attainment of intrauterine macromineral accretion rates in low birthweight infants fed fortified human milk. *J Pediatr* 1995;126:441-447.

66. Hall RT, Wheeler RE, Rippetoe LE. Calcium and phosphorus supplementation after initial hospital discharge in breast-fed infants of less than 1800 grams birthweight. *J Perinatol* 1993:XIII:272-278.

67. Bishop NJ, King FJ, Lucas A. Increased bone mineral content of preterm infants fed with a nutrient enriched formula after discharge from hospital. *Arch Dis Child*

1993; 68: 573-578.

68. Fewtrell MS, Cole TJ, Bishop NJ, Lucas A. Neonatal factors predicting childhood height in preterm infants: evidence for a persisting effect of early metabolic bone disease. *J Pediatr* 2000;137:668-673.

69. Lucas A, Morley R, Cole TJ, Gore SM. A randomized multicentre study of human milk versus formula and later development in preterm infants. *Arch Dis Child* 1994;70:F141-146.

70. Friel JK, Andrews WL, Matthew JD, Long DR. Cornel AM, Cox M, McKim E, Zerbe GO. Zinc supplementation in very-low-birth-weight infants. *J Pediatr Gastroenterol Nutr* 1993; 17:97-104.

71. Sanders TAB, Naismith DJ. A comparison of the influence of breast-feeding and bottle-feeding on the fatty acid composition of the erythrocytes. *Br J Nutr* 1979; 41: 619-623.

72. Putnam JC, Carlson SE, DeVoe PW, Barness LA. The effect of variations in dietary fatty acids on the fatty acid composition of erythrocyte phosphatidylcholine and phosphatidylethanolamine in human infants. *Am J Clin Nutr* 1982;36:106-114.

73. Gibson RA, Chen W, Makrides M. Randomized trials with polyunsaturated fatty acid interventions in preterm and term infants: functional and clinical outcomes. *Lipids* 2001; 36: 873-883

74. Uauy R, Hoffman DR, Peraino P, Birch DG, Birch EE. Essential fatty acids in visual and brain development. *Lipids* 2001; 36: 885-895.

75. Farquharson J, Cockburn F, Patrick WA, Jamieson EC, Logan RW. Infant cerebral cortex phospholipid fatty-acid composition and diet. *Lancet* 1992; 340: 810-813.

76. Makrides M, Neumann MA, Byard RW, Simmer K, Gibson RA. Fatty acid composition of brain, retina, and erythrocytes in breast- and formula-fed infants. *Am J Clin Nutr* 1994;60: 189-194.

77. Koo WWK, Walters J, Bush AJ, Chesney RW, Carlson SE. Dual-energy-x-ray absorptiometry studies of bone mineral status in newborn infants. *J Bone Miner Res* 1996;11:997-1002.

78. Rigo J, Nyamugabo K, Picaud JC, Gerard P, Peiltain C, DeCurtis M. Reference values of body composition obtained by dual energy X-ray absorptiometry in preterm and term neonates. *J Pediatr Gastroenterol Nutr*

1998; 27:184-190.

79. Pelkonen AS, Suomalainen H, Hallman M, Turpeinen M. Peripheral blood lymphocyte subpopulations in schoolchildren born very preterm. *Arch Dis Child Fetal Neonatal Ed* 1999;81:F188-193.

80. Singer LT. Methodological considerations in longitudinal studies of infant risk. In: *Developing Brain and Behavior*. ed. Dobbing J, London: Academic Press Limited; 1997: 209-231.

81. Bregman J. Developmental outcome in very low birthweight infants: Current status and future trends. *Pediatr Clin N Am* 1998;45:673-690.

82. Morley R, Cole TJ, Powell R, Lucas A. Mother's choice to provide breast milk and developmental outcome. *Arch Dis Child* 1988;63:1382-1385.

83. Lucas A, Morley R. Breast milk and subsequent intelligence quotient in children born preterm. *Lancet* 1991;339:261-264.

84. Uauy R, Birch DG, Birch EE, Tyson JE, Hoffman DR. Effect of dietary omega-3 fatty acids on retinal function of very low birthweight neonates. *Pediatr Res* 1990; 28:485-492.

85. Birch EE, Birch DG, Hoffman DR, Uauy RD. Dietary essential fatty acid supply and visual acuity development. *Invest Ophthalmol Vis Sci* 1992; 33: 3242-3253.

86. Carlson SE, Werkman SH, Rhodes PG, Tolley EA. Visual acuity development in healthy preterm infants: Effect of marine oil supplementation. *Am J Clin Nutr* 1993; 58:35-42.

87. San Giovanni JP, Parra-Cabrera S, Colditz GA, Berkey CS, Dwyer JT. Meta-analysis of dietary essential fatty acids and long chain polyunsaturated fatty acids as they relate to visual resolution in healthy preterm infants. *Pediatr* 2000;105: 1292-1298.

88. Simmer K. Long chain polyunsaturated fatty acid supplementation in preterm infants. *Cochrane Database Syst Rev.* 2000.

89. San Giovanni JP, Berkey CS, Dwyer JT, Colditz GA. Dietary essential fatty acids, long chain polyunsaturated fatty acids and visual resolution acuity in healthy, full-term infants. A Systematic Review. *Early Hum Dev* 2000;57:165-188.

90. Williams C, Birch EE, Emmet P, North K and ALPAC Team. Stereoacuity at 3.5 years of age in children born full-term is associated with prenatal and postnatal dietary factors, a report from a population based cohort study. *Am J Clin Nutr* 2001; 73: 316-322.

91. Lozoff B, Brittenham GM, Viteri FE, Wolf AW, Urrutia JJ. Developmental deficits in iron deficient infants: effects of age and severity of iron lack. *J Pediatr* 1982;101:351-357.

92. Oski FA, Honig AS, Helu B, Howanitz P. Effect of iron therapy on behavior performances in nonanemic iron deficient infants. *Pediatr* 1983; 71:877-880.

93. Moffat ME, Oongstaff S, Besant J, Dureski C. Prevention of iron deficiency and psychomotor decline in high risk infants through the use of iron fortified formula: a randomized trial. *J Pediatr* 1994;125: 527-534.

94. Williams J, Wolff A, Daily A, MacDonald A, Aukett A, Booth IW. Iron supplemented formula milk related to reduction in psychomotor decline in infants from inner city areas: a randomized study. *Br Med J* 1999;318: 693-697.

95. Friel JK, Andrews WL, Aziz K, Kwa PG, Lepage G, L'Abbe, MR. A randomized trial of two levels of iron supplementation and developmental outcome in low birthweight infants. *J Pediatr* 2001;139:254-260.

96. Doyle JJ, Zypurksy A. Neonatal blood disorders. In: *Effective Care of the Newborn Infant*. Sinclair JC, Bracken MR, eds. Oxford: Oxford University Press; 1992:425-451.

97. Georgieff MK, Rao R. The role of nutrition in cognitive development. In: *Handbook of Cognitive Neuroscience*. Cambridge, MA, MIT Press;2000.

98. Nutrition Practice Care Guidelines for Preterm Infants, Developed by Pediatric Nutrition Work Group, Child Development and Rehabilitation Center, 2001, http://cdrc.ohsu.edu/nutrition-services/a…les/files/5/premie_guidelines_for_WIC.htm

99. Hospital discharge of the high-risk neonate- Proposed guidelines. American Academy of Pediatrics Committee on Fetus and Newborn. *Pediatr* 1998;102: 411-417.

Conditions Requiring Special Nutritional Management
Patti J. Thureen, M.D. and William W. Hay, Jr., M.D.

Reviewed by David Clark, M.D., and Edward Bell, M.D.

There are a number of clinical conditions in preterm infants that may require changes in the nutritional strategies previously outlined in this book. Such conditions include hypoxic-ischemic encephalopathy, drug administration that alters feeding tolerance or metabolism (eg, indomethacin, dexamethasone, dopamine), drug withdrawal, and presumed catabolic states such as sepsis. Unfortunately, there have been few prospective trials in human infants of different nutritional strategies in these situations. Therefore, we have selected several common clinical conditions and disease states for which there is sufficient information to indicate that nutritional management should be altered. These include:

1. Gastrointestinal disorders such as necrotizing enterocolitis and short bowel syndrome.
2. Post-operative management of the infant who has undergone surgery.
3. Infants at risk for or with symptomatic patent ductus arteriosus.
4. Infants with suboptimal fetal growth (small for gestational age and intrauterine growth restricted infants).
5. Acute and chronic lung disease (hyaline membrane disease, pulmonary hypertension, bronchopulmonary dysplasia).
6. Sepsis.

Much of the data regarding the need for dietary alterations in these conditions is based on animal studies or investigations in small numbers of human infants rather than large, prospective investigations of specific feeding strategies. Thus, most of the following feeding strategies are tentative, as they are extrapolated from limited data and require further investigation before definitive recommendations can be made.

Interest also is shifting to the effect of ingredients of the diet on modifying development as well as aspects of clinical disorders. Vitamins A, C, and E, as well as the amino acids arginine and glutamine have been shown to boost immune function, as have ribonucleotides and a change from omega 6 to omega 3 free fatty acids. The latter are associated with a reduction in the production of proinflammatory mediators. Furthermore, these fatty acids function as important regulators of numerous cellular functions and affect many cell signaling pathways. Membrane fluidity, ion channel flow, and cell surface receptor function (as well as the generation of prostaglandins, leukotrienes, cytokines, and expression of inflammatory gene products) are some of the processes involved. There also is growing concern about and evidence for the role of inflammatory mediators and oxidants in the pathology of certain neonatal disorders, and that addition of immune-enhancing and antioxidant nutrients should be part of nutritional management of these infants, both to prevent as well as to treat the disorders. For example, Vitamin A, which is discussed below in the section on nutrition and respiratory disorders, has shown promise in its ability to ameliorate bronchopulmonary dysplasia. Glutamine also is being studied for its role in promoting gut development and immune function. And there may be a role for using larger amounts of eicosapentaenoic acid (an omega 3 polyunsaturated fatty acid) and γ-linolenic acid (an omega 6 polyunsaturated fatty acid) plus antioxidants in patients with systemic inflammatory response syndrome and more localized inflammatory processes in infants with respiratory distress syndrome, sepsis, pneumonia, and necrotizing enterocolitis. Despite such exciting potential advances, there is very little information in the literature for these issues to support specific recommendations. There should be considerable new information in future editions of this book to address this emerging area of using ingredients in the diet to promote development and inhibit clinical disorders and diseases.

Nutrition in Gastrointestinal Disorders (Necrotizing Enterocolitis, Short Bowel Syndrome)

Necrotizing Enterocolitis (NEC)

There are two principal questions regarding feeding and NEC: 1) Are there feeding strategies that might prevent NEC? and 2) How should the infant with established medical NEC (ie, NEC that does not require surgical intervention) be fed? Data regarding feeding and prevention of NEC are discussed in detail below. There are no definitive strategies for feeding in medical NEC, and guidelines tend to be institution specific. Our approach to feeding in medical NEC is presented under Recommendations for Feeding with NEC. NEC can affect all areas of the gastrointestinal tract, but most commonly involves the ileum, colon and jejunum. Nutrition in surgical NEC depends on the site and extent of intestinal resection and will be discussed below under Short Bowel Syndrome (SBS).

Etiology of NEC

The etiology of NEC has not been clearly established, but it is associated with prematurity and appears to represent a common pathologic response that is triggered by a variety of risk factors acting singly or in combination. Such factors include hypoxia, ischemia, infection, exotoxin (eg, from intestinal stasis and bacterial overgrowth) rapid advancement of feedings, polycythemia, and exchange transfusions.[1,2] Until recently, the most common approach to feeding infants at risk of NEC (primarily preterm infants) has been to withhold enteral feeding, often for many days. This practice has been fortified by the successful development of neonatal intravenous feeding in the

1970s and early 1980s.

Does exclusive parenteral nutrition prevent NEC? Nearly all infants with NEC have received enteral feedings.[1] However, NEC does not develop in the vast majority of infants who have been enterally fed, and there is no evidence that delaying enteral feedings and providing exclusive parenteral nutrition prevent the development of NEC.

What is the rationale for and against enteral feedings? Acute NEC is rare in the first days of life, but there often is significant concern for the ability of the GI tract of the preterm infant to handle enteral stimulation. Based on neonatal animal studies it is suggested that hypotension and asphyxia may predispose to gut injury when enteral feedings are given.[3-5] Physiological studies of enteral nutrition have not been conducted in very preterm neonates in the first days of life who have the risk factors for NEC noted above, but it is reasonable to assume some have compromised GI tract function and mucosal integrity. Unfortunately there are no good tests to identify these infants, so enteral nutrition is commonly withheld for several to many days. At the same time, there is evidence that delaying feedings has a negative impact on GI structure and function in the neonate. Enteral starvation quickly induces GI atrophy.[6] Furthermore, enteral feeding in both neonatal animals and humans produces significant beneficial effects on growth, structure, and physiological function of the GI tract.[7-15] Based on some of these observations, several investigators have studied the effects of small enteral feeding volumes on the subsequent capacity to feed these infants enterally and the associated risk of NEC.

Do early enteral feedings either cause or prevent NEC in very preterm neonates? It is difficult to summarize the outcome of studies of early enteral nutrition in very preterm and ill neonates because of large differences in a number of variables among the studies.[14,16-23] Nevertheless, none of these studies demonstrated an increased incidence of NEC in infants who received small enteral feeding volumes (called variably minimal enteral feeding or MEF, minimal enteral nutrition or MEN, as well as other terms such as trophic or priming feeds). However, it is likely that none of these studies had sufficient numbers of subjects to be able to conclude that MEF did not increase or even decrease the incidence of NEC compared with neonates who received exclusive parenteral nutrition. On balance, MEF appears to demonstrate some significant benefits in preterm neonates, but definitive conclusions about its safety and its effects on the incidence of NEC await larger randomized trials, particularly in very immature and critically ill preterm infants.

A number of issues regarding early MEF still need to be addressed regarding their relationship to cause or prevention of NEC, including: whether to use milk or formulas and which formulas to use; the composition of the formulas or supplemented ("fortified") milk; when the feedings are started; and how fast to advance the volume and concentration of the feedings. Compared to formula, human milk appears to confer an advantage for protection against infection, the development of allergies, and the incidence of NEC in preterm infants.[24-26] Potential mediators of a protective effect of human milk against development of NEC include the presence of a number of anti-infective agents such as lysozyme, immuoglobulins, complement, macrophages, lymphocytes and lactoferrin. Unfortified human milk may not be sufficient to sustain growth in very small, preterm neonates when it is the sole source of nutrition. It is, however, a sound choice for MEF, based on better tolerance and a lower incidence of associated NEC. In addition, human milk has better immunological properties than formulas.[27,28] Others have used dilute formulas, although from recent data they appear to demonstrate a disadvantage because they fail to induce normal gastrointestinal motor activity or peristalsis.[15,21] Few studies have investigated fortified human milk or preterm formula as the initial feed in very preterm infants.[29] No definite conclusions can be drawn about the relative tolerance of fortified versus regular strength formula or human milk. Fortification of human milk, however, does not delay gastric emptying.[30]

There have been no studies that specifically address the optimal time to start MEF in order to decrease the incidence of NEC. The rate of advancement of MEF varies greatly among studies and practices, ranging from increases started on day one of life[17] to continued small volume feedings until 14 days of age before volume is advanced.[26] Several studies have suggested that volume advances of <20 cc/kg/d do not increase the incidence of NEC compared with delayed feeding advancement.[16-19] A recent report demonstrated good tolerance of an advance of 35 cc/kg/d, even in very preterm neonates.[31] However, no studies to date have sufficient power to determine the optimal duration of MEF prior to nutritive advance or the effect of different rates of volume advance on the development of NEC.

A recent series of reviews of existing studies regarding various issues concerning the safety of MEF conclude that there are insufficient data to determine the benefits and risks of small enteral feedings on the development of NEC.[32-34] Clearly larger studies involving much larger numbers of infants are required to answer these questions.

Other strategies for possible prevention of NEC
Several studies suggest that antenatal steroids decrease the incidence of postnatal NEC,[35,36] though this has not been confirmed in other investigations.[37] Oral antibiotics decrease the incidence of NEC in preterm infants, but may not be indicated because of the development of bacterial resistance.[38] Other promising therapies not yet confirmed in large trials include oral immunoglobulin,[39,40] use of preterm formula with egg phospholipid,[41] and glutamine supplementation.[42]

Recommendations for Feeding with NEC
Preventing NEC

1. There is no evidence that brief or prolonged exclusive parenteral nutrition (PN) will prevent NEC.

2. Studies to date have not included sufficient numbers of patients to conclusively demonstrate that minimal enteral feedings or a specific rate of nutritive advance of enteral feedings either increase or decrease the incidence of NEC. Therefore, no specific enteral feeding strategy can

be recommended to prevent NEC.

3. Avoid hyperosmolar feedings and medications.

4. Human milk may be preventive for the development of NEC.

Feeding with Medical (ie, does not require surgical intervention) NEC

1. In non-surgical NEC, the period of "bowel rest" should be proportional to the severity of clinical disease. In the absence of significant systemic symptoms or marked abnormalities in laboratory tests, severity of medical NEC is commonly based on the degree of abnormality of abdominal X-ray findings. Portal venous gas or a persistently dilated and fixed bowel loop generally indicates advanced disease. Unfortunately, pneumatosis is not a reliable indicator of the severity of intestinal compromise, nor does its resolution necessarily indicate improvement.[43] Therefore, there are no clear guidelines for when to restart feeds after an episode of medical NEC, and strategies clearly vary among centers. One strategy with mild clinical disease is to provide 3-5 days of bowel rest after the last abnormal abdominal film or clinical abnormality, such as bloody stool. With severe disease, 7-10 days of bowel rest is recommended.

2. Since the degree of functional gastrointestinal tract compromise after medical NEC is difficult to predict, there is no clearly defined optimal feeding strategy for volume and type of initial feed or rate of nutritive advance, and enteral feeding must be individualized on a "trial and response" basis. Unless functional short bowel syndrome is suspected or is likely to exist, our approach is to start with undiluted human milk if available; if not, 20-calorie formula appropriate for age is used (ie, preterm formula for preterm infants). A number of centers, however, routinely start with dilute human milk or formula. Initial several feedings are small volume (5 ml/kg) to assess tolerance. If several feedings are tolerated, then feeds are advanced at 10-20 ml/kg/d (or more rapidly in very mild disease) depending on tolerance.

3. There is no proven advantage of bolus vs continuous feeds.

4. Advance to full volume feedings first, then increase caloric density.

5. With evidence of functional short bowel syndrome or significant feeding intolerance, use of elemental formulas, dilute formulas, and continuous feedings may be necessary.

Short Bowel Syndrome (SBS)

Short bowel syndrome is defined as malabsorption combined with fluid and electrolyte loss secondary to a significant shortening of functional bowel resulting in inadequate enteral nutrition. Generally it follows massive resection of the small intestine, but may include large bowel loss. Most cases occur after surgical removal of compromised or dead bowel, but some cases do occur where bowel is healthy but dysfunctional, such as in certain cases of gastroschisis and long-segment Hirschsprung's disease. The primary cause of SBS in neonates is necrotizing enterocolitis, accounting for 1/4 to 1/2 of all cases.[44,45] Other etiologies include intestinal atresias, gastroschisis, omphalocoele, midgut volvulus, and vascular abnormalities of the arterial blood supply to the gut.

Pathophysiology of SBS. The degree of malabsorption in cases of SBS is dependent on both the amount and site of intestinal loss. Figure 1 demonstrates the site-specific functions of the gastrointestinal tract and the changes in absorption that might be anticipated with resection of different portions of the GI tract. Additionally, severity and duration of nutrient intolerance is related to the degree of adaptation of the intestine after the primary insult.

The functions of the proximal and distal small intestine are quite different, and prognosis is highly dependent on which of these areas is resected as well as whether or not the ileocecal valve is preserved. The proximal intestine has a large surface area for nutrient absorption, is rich in digestive enzymes, and has a relatively high density of transport carrier proteins. The distal small intestine and the colon are major sites of water resorption back into the plasma; thus, their

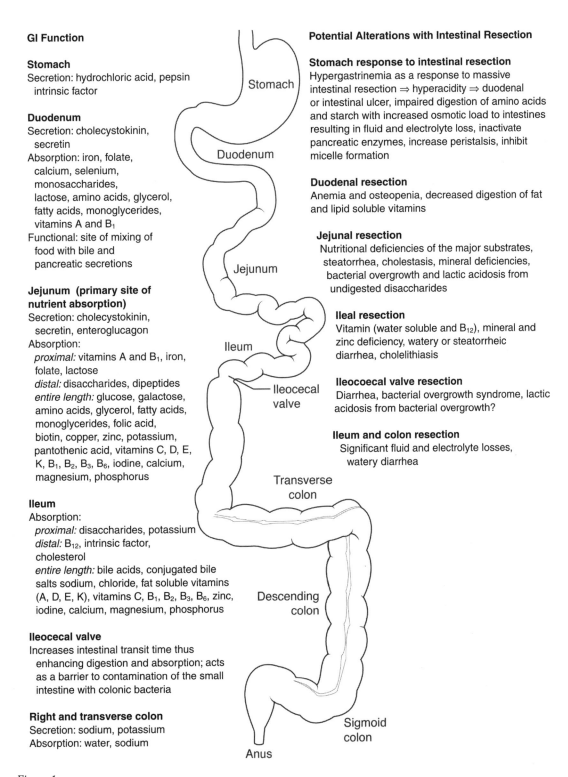

GI Function

Stomach
Secretion: hydrochloric acid, pepsin
   intrinsic factor

Duodenum
Secretion: cholecystokinin,
   secretin
Absorption: iron, folate,
   calcium, selenium,
   monosaccharides,
   lactose, amino acids, glycerol,
   fatty acids, monoglycerides,
   vitamins A and B_1
Functional: site of mixing of
   food with bile and
   pancreatic secretions

Jejunum (primary site of nutrient absorption)
Secretion: cholecystokinin,
   secretin, enteroglucagon
Absorption:
   proximal: vitamins A and B_1, iron,
   folate, lactose
   distal: disaccharides, dipeptides
   entire length: glucose, galactose,
   amino acids, glycerol, fatty acids,
   monoglycerides, folic acid,
   biotin, copper, zinc, potassium,
   pantothenic acid, vitamins C, D, E,
   K, B_1, B_2, B_3, B_6, iodine, calcium,
   magnesium, phosphorus

Ileum
Absorption:
   proximal: disaccharides, potassium
   distal: B_{12}, intrinsic factor,
   cholesterol
   entire length: bile acids, conjugated bile
   salts sodium, chloride, fat soluble vitamins
   (A, D, E, K), vitamins C, B_1, B_2, B_3, B_6, zinc,
   iodine, calcium, magnesium, phosphorus

Ileocecal valve
Increases intestinal transit time thus
   enhancing digestion and absorption; acts
   as a barrier to contamination of the small
   intestine with colonic bacteria

Right and transverse colon
Secretion: sodium, potassium
Absorption: water, sodium

Potential Alterations with Intestinal Resection

Stomach response to intestinal resection
Hypergastrinemia as a response to massive
intestinal resection $\Rightarrow$ hyperacidity $\Rightarrow$ duodenal
or intestinal ulcer, impaired digestion of amino acids
and starch with increased osmotic load to intestines
resulting in fluid and electrolyte loss, inactivate
pancreatic enzymes, increase peristalsis, inhibit
micelle formation

Duodenal resection
Anemia and osteopenia, decreased digestion of fat
and lipid soluble vitamins

Jejunal resection
Nutritional deficiencies of the major substrates,
steatorrhea, cholestasis, mineral deficiencies,
bacterial overgrowth and lactic acidosis from
undigested disaccharides

Ileal resection
Vitamin (water soluble and B_{12}), mineral and
zinc deficiency, watery or steatorrheic
diarrhea, cholelithiasis

Ileocoecal valve resection
Diarrhea, bacterial overgrowth syndrome, lactic
acidosis from bacterial overgrowth?

Ileum and colon resection
Significant fluid and electrolyte losses,
watery diarrhea

Stomach
Duodenum
Jejunum
Ileum
Ileocecal valve
Transverse colon
Descending colon
Sigmoid colon
Anus

Figure 1:

loss results in significant fluid and electrolyte losses. In general, the ileum can adapt and compensate for some of the absorptive function that is lost with resection of the jejunum, but the reverse is not true for the jejunum when the distal small intestine is lost.[46] "Maximal adaptation" already exists in the proximal small intestine in most neonates, and there is little increase in absorptive capacity after resection of other portions of the GI tract.[47] Because of the ability of the ileum but not the jejunum to undergo this process of adaptation, infants with jejunal resection tend to do better than those who undergo removal of the ileum.

Resection of the stomach or duodenum alone is rare. The absence of the stomach is reasonably well tolerated as long as Vitamin B_{12} (cobalamin) is supplemented to prevent pernicious anemia. However, there is significant alteration in stomach physiology with increased gastrin release in response to loss of a significant amount of other portions of the intestinal tract. This gastrin release is probably secondary to loss of an intestinal-mediated inhibition of gastrin secretion in response to the entry of acid from the stomach into the intestine. In approximately half of infants with significant intestinal loss, hyperacidity occurs which can impair protein and starch digestion, inactivate pancreatic digestive enzymes, stimulate peristalsis, inhibit micelle formation, and induce esophagitis and ulcer formation in the duodenum and small intestine. Additionally, impaired digestion presents an increased osmotic load to the colon, where it is augmented by bacterial action, predisposing to diarrhea.[48]

The duodenum and jejunum are the primary sites of amino acid, carbohydrate, and fat absorption and digestion, as well as absorption of fat- and water-soluble vitamins (with the exception of B_{12}) and most minerals. The jejunum has a significantly larger surface area for absorption compared to the distal small intestine, and serves as the site for major nutrient digestion and absorption.[48] Loss of the jejunum results in significant vitamin and mineral deficiencies (especially zinc). Additionally, the "porous" nature of the jejunal mucosa allows for back diffusion of fluid and electrolytes into the intestinal lumen, with loss of

these nutrients. However, if the ileum and colon are intact, water and electrolytes can usually be reabsorbed at these sites.

The ileum is a primary site for disaccharide and fat digestion and absorption of bile salts, bile acids, fat-soluble vitamins, and Vitamin B_{12}. Loss of the ileum thus can result in fat, carbohydrate, and vitamin malabsorption. Watery diarrhea may occur due to loss of sodium and chloride with associated water loss[49] or to bile acid induced colonic irritation. Loss of bile results in steatorrhea and calcium,[48,50] and depletion of bile acids can produce cholelithiasis.

Loss of the ileocecal valve produces unique difficulties in feeding. Its absence leads to reflux of colonic contents into the small intestine with subsequent diarrhea as well as bacterial contamination and subsequent overgrowth in the ileum. The ileocecal valve also slows intestinal transit time; its absence, therefore, limits digestion and absorption of nutrients. Absence of this valve significantly delays the process of "intestinal adaptation" (see below).[51,52]

The colon, particularly the right and transverse colon, reabsorbs water and electrolytes. Absence of these bowel segments predisposes to watery diarrhea and electrolyte loss with potential hypovolemia and dehydration.

Intestinal adaptation. In response to loss of significant intestinal mass, the remaining intestine adjusts to this loss by undergoing a series of anatomical and physiological alterations. This process is referred to as "intestinal adaptation."[44,53,54] There is a gradual increase in absorptive surface area in the remaining gut that is accomplished by a variety of mechanisms including mucosal hyperplasia, increases in length and crypt depth of the intestinal villi, changes in intestinal motility and hormonal response, and increases in both intestinal length and diameter. As noted above, the ileum has significant adaptive capabilities after jejunal resection with an estimated 70-100% structural and functional increase, while jejunal adaptation after ileal loss is only 20-30%.[46] Stimuli for intestinal adaptation include intraluminal nutrients, pancreatic and biliary digestive enzymes, and hormones such as enteroglucagon. Hormones found in milk but not in formulas, such as EGF and IGFs, also may enhance gut growth and development.[55-57]

Parenteral nutritional therapy of SBS. Parenteral nutrition (PN) is a key component of successful outcome in infants with SBS since it is the only means by which adequate nutrition can be provided to sustain growth in the infant until full enteral nutrition has been achieved. Unfortunately, hepatic disease associated with PN is a major cause of both morbidity and mortality that can occur in SBS. Cholestasis is the most common type of liver abnormality in infants with SBS who require prolonged PN therapy. Other liver disorders can include "biliary sludging," cholelithiasis, cholecystitis, cirrhosis, liver carcinoma, and hepatic failure. Cholestatic liver disease occurs in 30-60% of infants with SBS, with eventual hepatic failure reported in up to 19% of children with SBS in the neonatal period.[58-62] Specific mechanisms of liver disease in neonatal SBS are not known.

Several risk factors for cholestatic liver disease (with or without SBS) have been identified, including preterm birth with low birth weight,[63,64] episodes of sepsis,[60] early initiation of PN, duration of PN,[65] lack of enteral feeding, excessive administration of specific nutrients (particularly energy, and especially carbohydrate, overfeeding), imbalances of macro- or micro-nutrients in the PN solution, suboptimal gastrointestinal hormonal secretion, existence of mechanical or functional bowel disorders, bacterial overgrowth syndrome, and pre-existing malnutrition or liver disease.[62,66-69] In most centers, cholestatic liver disease associated with parenteral feeding either has been eliminated or reduced markedly in severity and duration in those clinical situations when early gastric and/or transpyloric feeding has been tolerated.

Guidelines for parenteral therapy in SBS are therefore directed at: 1) optimizing growth (see other chapters in this book and appendices for gestational-age specific growth recommendations); 2) monitoring for and treating specific deficiencies that develop during prolonged PN therapy; and 3) avoiding PN-associated toxicity.

The best method to avoid cholestasis in infants with SBS is to establish enteral nutrition. However, full enteral feedings are often not possible for extended periods. Once it is clear that an infant will require prolonged PN, weekly routine PN laboratory assessments should be made. Of particular interest are "liver function tests," abnormalities of which are often the first indication of development of PN-related hepatocellular damage and hepatic dysfunction. Asymptomatic increases in serum bile acids are often the first biochemical abnormality in PN associated cholestasis,[68] but they are not routinely monitored in many centers. The usual first evidence of PN associated hepatocellular damage is an elevated direct bilirubin concentration (>1.5 - 2.0 mg/dL or >40% of the total bilirubin concentration.[63,70] Alkaline phosphatase and gammaglutamyl transferase levels will also increase, but may not be as specific as the direct bilirubin concentration.[71] With progressive disease, markers of hepatic synthetic function will also be impaired.

There is considerable overlap among nutritional strategies designed to prevent and treat PN-related related hepatic dysfunction, and most strategies are primarily based on ameliorating the risk factors noted above. The most effective strategy for both prevention and treatment is to discontinue PN and provide exclusive enteral nutrition;[72] however, this is usually not possible. Providing enteral nutrition is key to both prevention and treatment, and even small-volume feeds are likely to decrease disease progression.[69] Meehan and Georgeson have advocated a protocol that has been successful in preventing liver failure in PN-dependent children with SBS. This includes meticulous catheter care, aggressive prevention and treatment of sepsis, enteral feeding when tolerated, use of taurine, early PN cycling, and use of strategies to inhibit bacterial translocation from the GI tract.[73]

Parenteral energy intake above that required to cover energy expenditure and growth requirements should be avoided.[63,64] This value will vary among infants, but one study demonstrated increased cholestasis in infants receiving more than 110 kcal/kg/d of energy.[74] It has been shown that infants with parenteral glucose intakes greater than approximately 18 g/kg/d change from primarily oxidative glucose metabolism to conversion of glucose to fat,[75-76] a situation which may predispose to fatty infiltration of the liver. Studies in adults receiving high energy intravenous nutrition ("energy overfeeding"), especially when hyperglycemia is present, have demonstrated increased rates of infection.[17,78] A possible mechanism for this may be an increase in the expression of tumor necrosis factor receptors induced by increased energy intake.[79]

Either an excess or an imbalance of amino acids has been implicated in liver dysfunction associated with PN. In the late 1980s a parenteral crystalline amino acid solution (TrophamineTM) for preterm infants was developed that was designed to produce plasma amino acid concentrations that were comparable to those seen in postprandial human milk fed infants of the same gestational age.[80] This solution improved nitrogen balance and resulted in normal blood urea nitrogen concentrations. Subsequently, several more "pediatric" PN amino acid preparations have been developed that are in common use today, though none was designed for the unique amino acid requirements of very preterm infants. There are no definitive data from studies using these current PN solutions that suggest either the maximal amino acid intake or the specific preparation that prevents or treats PN-associated hepatic dysfunction.[65,81,82] Therefore, until further data are available, PN intake in preterm infants with SBS should follow guidelines recommended in previous chapters for gestational age-specific growth. In established PN-associated liver disease, some centers "cycle" amino acid intake with alternating days of low and high amino acid administration in an attempt to minimize potential amino acid-associated toxicity. However, this technique has not been prospectively evaluated.

Because of the immaturity of metabolic pathways involved in its production, taurine is considered a conditionally essential amino acid in neonates. One of its functions is to conjugate bile acids to a less toxic form than that of glycine-conjugated bile acids. However, neither human nor animal studies of taurine-supplemented PN have demonstrated a benefit of preventing cholestasis.[83-85] There also are reports in the literature indicating that several components of PN

	Sodium	Potassium	Chloride	Bicarbonate
Gastric fluid	140	15	155	0
Ieostomy fluid	80-140	15	115	40
Colonic fluid	50-80	10-30	40	20-25
Diarrhea	10-90	10-80	10-110	30-40

Table 1: Electrolyte content (mEq/L) of intestinal fluid losses for replacement calculation.

may break down to potentially hepatotoxic products when exposed to UV light, phototherapy, and elevated ambient temperatures.[86,87] Whether or not these toxic products produce significantly adverse clinical effects is unclear. Until this risk is clearly defined, some investigators have advocated covering PN and lipid solutions and their delivery tubing with opaque material. Intravenous cholecystokinin and oral ursodeoxycholic acid have shown some promise in stimulating gall bladder secretion and bile flow to prevent or treat the formation of "biliary sludge" and cholelithiasis, although data in neonates to support this practice are limited.[88,89]

There is no consensus on beneficial effects of "cycling" of PN in preterm or term neonates even though it has been advocated to both prevent[71] and treat[91] cholestasis. PN "cycling" is a technique in which PN is infused over a period of less than 24 hours per day. There is evidence in adults that liver dysfunction is decreased with this technique.[90] Reports of its efficacy in infants are limited.[73,91] There are various cycling regimens used in infants with significant cholestatic disease.

Parenteral replacement of electrolyte deficiencies is critical in infants with significant intestinal fluid and electrolyte losses. A separate cc per cc of infusion of replacement solution based on anticipated site-specific GI tract losses should be used in the treatment of SBS, particularly during the early phase of therapy when nasogastric, ostomy, and/or diarrheal losses may be significant.[47] Composition of electrolyte losses from various sites is shown in Table 1[92-94] and these values can be used to guide replacement therapy. However, in individual patients with highly variable serum electrolyte concentrations, it may be beneficial to measure electrolyte concentrations of the specific intestinal fluids. In addition to the usual trace mineral supplementation for prolonged PN, infants with ileostomies generally need additional parenteral zinc supplementation.

In patients with established cholestatic disease, various alterations may be made in the PN solution. Manganese and copper are both essential trace elements routinely added to PN solutions that are primarily excreted by the biliary tract. Both may accumulate in cholestatic disorders leading to possible neurotoxicity (manganese) and hepatotoxicity (copper).[62,95] One approach is to halve copper intake and delete manganese with cholestatic liver disease.

Enteral therapy of SBS.[48,96,97] Several studies have demonstrated the efficacy of elemental diets consisting of medium chain triglycerides, glucose polymers, and protein hydrolysates or amino acids in short bowel syndrome.[98,99] However, the ideal fat:carbohydrate mix in these patients has not been well studied.

In general, protein and amino acid digestion are preserved to a greater extent than that of carbohydrate or fat. Protein in the diet is best tolerated in a predigested form. Protein hydrolysates are more rapidly absorbed than intact proteins. Rarely, elemental amino acid formulas are required. There is a theoretical consideration that an injured, immature gut may be less prone to developing intestinal protein allergy with protein hydrolysate or elemental amino acid formulas. Carbohydrates, particularly lactose and sucrose, are poorly tolerated because of the loss of carbohydrate digestive enzymes, and often are associated with significant osmotic diarrhea.

Glucose (a monosaccharide) is easily absorbed, but it significantly increases osmolality, which may promote water and electrolyte loss. In significant malabsorption states, low osmolality glucose polymers or starch, both of which can be digested by the relatively preserved enzyme maltase, may be the most effective source of carbohydrate.[97,100] Fructose (a monosaccharide) and sucrose (a disaccharide composed of fructose and glucose) are also used.

Ileal resection leads to fat malabsorption. This problem is augmented by the associated bile acid loss since fat solubilization and absorption depend on bile acids. In order to meet dietary requirements, fat may need to be administered as medium chain triglycerides, which are water soluble and do not require bile acids for digestion. A combination of both medium- and long-chain fats may be desirable because long chain fats appear to stimulate the process of intestinal adaptation.[101]

Early enteral feeding appears to be a primary stimulus for intestinal adaptation.[48,50,102] Continuous drip feedings are preferred to maximize absorption while minimizing stimulation of peristalsis.[103] Generally, a predigested or semi-elemental formula is used.[96] Dilute formulas should not be used because of the associated poor caloric intake unless extreme malabsorption occurs. Feedings should be decreased if ostomy output exceeds 20 mL/kg/d or stool losses are greater than 40-50 mL/kg/d.[47] When significant diarrhea occurs, carbohydrate malabsorption (noted by decreased stool pH or presence of reducing substances) and/or bacterial overgrowth should be suspected.

Fat soluble vitamins generally need to be replaced. Serum electrolytes, calcium, phosphorus, and magnesium concentrations need to be monitored. Supplementation with iron, Vitamin B_{12}, and zinc are commonly required. Trace elements need to be administered and their intake monitored, particularly to avoid zinc and copper deficiencies seen with high ostomy output.

Other therapy in SBS. Gastric acid hypersecretion can be treated with H_2-antagonists, though therapy is indicated only for a limited time (several months) because this post-operative complication resolves with time and long-term H_2-antagonist therapy may decrease B_{12} absorption as well as predispose to bacterial overgrowth.[104] Cholestyramine resin can decrease intestinal bile salt loss and intestinal motility, but this therapy also has the potential to increase fat malabsorption and constipation, as well as exacerbate metabolic bone disease.[105] Antiperistaltic drugs such as loperamide can decrease transit time. In cases of bacterial overgrowth, antibiotic therapy can improve digestion and absorption.[105] It is unclear if other therapies such as enzyme, hormone, or specific nutrient supplementation can be used to improve absorption or enhance intestinal adaptation.

Animal studies have demonstrated conflicting results on whether intravenous or enteral glutamine supplementation enhances GI adaptation.[106-108] There are no conclusive data advocating their clinical use. Animal studies involving administration of enteroglucagon, pancreatic secretions, prostaglandins, epidermal growth factor, growth hormone, and short-chain fatty acids (supplied directly or as a product of fiber fermentation by bacteria) have shown some promise for inducing intestinal adaptation.[109]

Nutritional Management of the Surgical Neonate

The endocrine response to surgery in adults results in endogenous protein breakdown, lipolysis, glycogenolysis, and gluconeogenesis. These result in a combination of beneficial (production of protective cytokines) and undesirable (nutrient intolerance and catabolism) effects. It was not until the mid 1980s that the neonatal metabolic response to pain and surgery were studied.[110-111] Studies showed that anesthesia without post-operative analgesia in neonates undergoing surgery resulted in increased concentrations of blood glucose, lactate, pyruvate, ketone bodies, and glycerol. Adrenaline and noradrenaline concentrations also were increased, likely contributing to sustained increases in the concentrations of blood glucose and lactate for several hours postoperatively.[112]

Studies in adults[113] and neonates[114] have shown that the use of perioperative fentanyl analgesia can limit the stress response, contributing to improved homeostasis. When compared to those infants who did not receive narcotic analgesia, infants treated with fentanyl post-operatively have been shown to have lower plasma levels of adrenaline, glucagon, adrenocorticoids, lactate, and pyruvate.[114] In adults the suppression of the stress response and associated protein catabolism appeared to correlate with the dose of narcotic analgesia.[113] Although there were no control infants, a study of six parenterally fed preterm infants undergoing PDA ligation with fentanyl and pancuronium anesthesia showed no change in

nitrogen balance before and after surgery, suggesting a significant attenuation of the stress response to pain and surgery.[115]

A more recent study was designed to determine if post-surgical neonates could achieve a positive protein balance without protein toxicity in the immediate newborn period.[116] Ten 36-37 week gestational age newborns undergoing major surgery (gastroschisis or diaphragmatic hernia repair) in the first 24 hours of life were prospectively randomized to immediate post-operative administration of 1.5 vs 2.5 g/kg/day amino acids. All infants were maintained on fentanyl continuous infusion for 48 hours post-operatively. Protein balance was positive and significantly higher in the 2.5 g/kg/d amino acid intake group. Serum ammonia concentrations (as an indicator of protein toxicity) were normal in both groups.

Several studies of substrate and energy metabolism in surgical neonates who were at least 3 days post-operative and receiving exclusive parenteral nutrition[76,117-119] have shown that the addition of intravenous fat to the parenteral nutrition regimen not only enhanced nitrogen retention[117] but decreased carbon dioxide production, presumably by decreasing glucose oxidation.[118] In these patients, net fat synthesis from glucose occurred at glucose intake rates greater than ~12 mg/kg/min, resulting in increased carbon dioxide production.[76] The findings noted above, plus those regarding the partitioning of energy expenditure,[119] do not appear to be different from those reported in the non-surgical neonate. This may be because these infants were out of the immediate post-operative period when studied and thus past the acute neonatal stress response to surgery. Whether these findings also exist in the immediate post-surgical period will require further study.

In summary, a combination of anesthesia with fentanyl analgesia in term and preterm neonates undergoing surgery appears to sufficiently blunt the operative stress response to allow for improved tolerance of administered substrates. Though some degree of both lipid and glucose intolerance may prevent high energy intakes, both substrates can be given with monitoring in the immediate post-operative period. Additionally, it appears that both term and preterm infants can tolerate sufficiently high intravenous intake rates of amino acids to be "anabolic" following surgery when administered general anesthesia with continuous post-operative narcotic infusion.

Feeding with Patent Ductus Arteriosus and/or Indomethacin Therapy

The ductus arteriosus of many extremely low birthweight infants remains open for days or weeks.[120] Its persistent patency is associated with significant neonatal morbidity which can be significantly reduced with its closure.[121] Studies in preterm infants with patent ductus arteriosus (PDA) have demonstrated decreased flow in the descending aorta, superior mesenteric artery, and celiac artery.[122,123] This occurs as a result of the "diastolic ductal steal" phenomenon,[124,125] as well as increased vascular resistance in the superior mesenteric and celiac arteries.[122,123] This hypoperfusion of the gut has been implicated as an etiology in the increased incidence of NEC seen with PDA.[126,127]

Indomethacin is the primary non-surgical therapy for symptomatic PDA in preterm infants. Indomethacin use in preterm infants for closure of a symptomatic PDA is associated with lowered gastrointestinal blood supply by Doppler ultrasound measurements,[128,129] and its administration in treatment of symptomatic PDA has also been implicated in neonatal NEC.[126,130]

Feeding practices in infants with symptomatic PDA, with or without indomethacin therapy, have not been studied. Fluid administration is usually restricted because of the association of high parenteral fluid volume intake with an increased incidence of clinically significant PDA.[131] Most centers withhold feedings because of the already increased risk of NEC and the abnormal mesenteric blood flow patterns seen with both the PDA and treatment doses of indomethacin. However, in one study comparing bolus versus continuous infusion of indomethacin, the slower indomethacin infusion seemed to mitigate the negative effects of indomethacin on blood flow velocities.[132]

Whether minimal enteral feedings, particularly with slow indomethacin infusion, might have a beneficial effect even with symptomatic PDA, has not been studied.

Low-dose indomethacin has been used in preterm infants without PDA for prophylaxis against development of severe grades of intraventricular hemorrhage.[133-135] However, prophylactic indomethacin without the confounding effect of a symptomatic PDA, and at both lower doses and less frequent intervals than are commonly used therapeutically for treatment of a PDA, was still associated with a significant decrease in both mean- and end-diastolic mesenteric blood flow velocities.[136] Two recent publications, one a meta-analysis of existing studies[137] and the other an NICHD sponsored multicenter study,[138] have looked at the effect of prophylactic indomethacin use on outcome. Both reports noted a significantly decreased incidence of both symptomatic PDA and severe intraventricular hemorrhage. The former report also suggested a trend towards an increased incidence of NEC; however, feeding strategies were not discussed, and dosages as well as timing of indomethacin administration varied significantly from one study to another. The NICHD trial used a consistent low dose of indomethacin (0.1 mg/kg/d) for three days, and did not demonstrate any increased incidence of NEC, though concomitant feeding was not described. Anecdotally, many centers provide at least minimal enteral feedings with low-dose prophylactic indomethacin because of reluctance to withhold feeds for several days. Further studies are needed to clarify this issue.

Nutrition in Infants with Suboptimal Fetal Growth

Intrauterine Growth Restricted (IUGR) and Small for Gestational Age (SGA) Neonates

SGA infants are those whose birth weight is more than 2 standard deviations below the mean birth weight for gestational age or below the 10th percentile of the birthweight-gestational age relationship. Small for gestational age infants can be normally small (because their parents were, for example) or abnormally small because they did not grow at their growth capacity in utero (ie, they experienced intrauturine growth restriction). Thus, infants with intrauterine growth restriction are SGA from growing at a slower than normal rate due to pathophysiological processes that either limit fetal nutrition or limit the capacity of the fetus to grow when provided with nutrients. Intrauterine growth restriction and its consequences remain a major health problem in this country.[139] IUGR contributes significantly to perinatal morbidity and mortality[140] and has been implicated by epidemiological studies to lead to a higher incidence of adult disorders of hypertension, insulin resistance, obesity, and adult onset, or Type 2, diabetes mellitus.[141]

SGA and IUGR infants comprise a disproportionately large fraction of the usual population of infants in neonatal intensive care units,[142] yet there have been no systematic studies on feeding these infants. Studies regarding feeding strategies and growth outcomes in infants born small for their gestational age (SGA) have resulted in very conflicting results, particularly when the goal has been to achieve catch-up growth. SGA infants comprise a very heterogeneous group and differ in terms of their absolute size and the degree of pathophysiologic alteration they have undergone. At one extreme are those SGA infants who simply have a birth weight less than 2 standard deviations below the mean for infants of the same gestational age, but who have the capacity to grow normally. These infants are generally healthy and grow along growth curves at a similar percentile as their birth size. The next category of infants is those with mildly decreased rates of fetal growth. These infants commonly demonstrate "catch-up" growth, but may have a slightly increased risk of adverse adult health outcomes. At the other end of the spectrum of SGA and IUGR infants is a subpopulation with more severe intrauterine growth restriction resulting from a more marked failure of normal fetal growth due to inadequate fetal nutrient delivery. There is growing evidence that these infants with severe IUGR undergo in utero physiological adaptations that can produce fetal, neonatal, and potentially adult adverse consequences, and that trying to "overfeed" this group of IUGR infants to

produce catch-up growth may lead to acute metabolic disturbances and actually promote adult disease.[141]

Markers that can accurately differentiate the more severe IUGR subpopulation of SGA infants at birth are limited. Pardi and colleagues suggest that these IUGR neonates can be suspected based on evidence of placental insufficiency with associated progressive growth failure in utero, and on abnormal in utero umbilical blood flow and fetal heart rate patterns.[143] Subsequent studies have validated that the severity of fetal growth failure and blood flow and heart rate patterns correlates with severity of a variety of fetal metabolic abnormalities including increased lactate concentrations and hypoxia,[143-145] decreased placental system A amino acid transporter activity,[144] and evidence of increased fetal protein breakdown (based on decreased fetal/maternal plasma enrichment ratios after maternal infusion of stable isotopic leucine).[146] These alterations in fetal metabolism may persist postnatally. These infants who have severe in utero growth restriction (IUGR) caused by fetal nutrient deprivation represent an extreme subpopulation of the larger groups of SGA infants; it is likely that they should receive unique nutrition and feeding strategies. The majority of nutrition and feeding studies to date that have included SGA infants make little or no distinction regarding the causes of small size at birth. Thus, only general recommendations can be made based on the literature regarding nutrition and feeding strategies of SGA and IUGR infants.

Metabolic and Body Composition Differences Between SGA and AGA Infants

Information about protein metabolism in SGA infants immediately after birth is scarce and has generally been extrapolated either from studies done in the fetus or from studies done in older infants. Studies using stable isotopes have produced conflicting results regarding the difference in protein metabolism in SGA compared to AGA infants. Pencharz et al concluded that SGA infants have a 20-30% increase in rates of protein turnover, catabolism, and synthesis compared with AGA infants.[147] In contrast, a study by Cauderay et al demonstrated that SGA infants had a 20%

decrease in rates of protein turnover, catabolism, and synthesis compared to AGA infants.[148] In the latter study, AGA and SGA infants had equal weight gain and composition of weight gain, and it was concluded that the lower protein synthesis rate in SGA infants resulted in a more efficient protein gain:protein synthesis ratio. Two other studies concluded that AGA and SGA infants had equal protein turnover rates, but in one of these investigations nitrogen balance was increased in SGA infants[149] while in the other it was not.[150] In the only study specifically measuring rates of protein oxidation, leucine oxidation was decreased in SGA infants.[150]

One of the major limitations to making conclusions about the metabolism of SGA infants from existing studies is that these studies have included very heterogeneous groups of infants. Some studies compare AGA and SGA groups of infants who are of comparable gestational age and therefore, presumably of comparable metabolic maturity, while others compare groups of similar weight but at different gestational ages who are therefore of different "maturity." Also, feeding schedules and food composition have not always been comparable. The definition of SGA infants has varied, with some studies including infants who might be considered "mildly" SGA along with infants who very likely had more severe growth restriction. It also has been suggested that protein turnover, synthesis, catabolism, and oxidation should be normalized to fat free mass, the metabolically active component of the body, and not to total body mass as is generally reported, given the significantly lower fat mass in the SGA compared to the AGA infant.

Glycogen content is markedly reduced in both liver and skeletal muscle of SGA infants. Hypoglycemia is a very common event early in the life of SGA infants, increasing with the severity of the growth restriction. This increased incidence of hypoglycemia appears secondary to reduced glycogen and fat stores, as well as decreased rates of gluconeogenesis in some SGA infants.

A number of studies have indicated increased resting energy expenditure per kg body weight in SGA infants,[151] indicating a need for postnatal increased energy delivery in addition to that required for catch-up growth. Again, because these infants represent a very heterogeneous group, quantitative protein and energy intake recommendations have not been established. Although few comprehensive studies have been performed of energy expenditure in the SGA infant, numerous investigators have examined resting metabolic rate (RMR). These studies have shown that RMR is elevated in the growth restricted infant relative to the AGA LBW infant, although the magnitude of the reported increase in expenditure is quite variable, ranging from 6.3% to 44%.[148,151,152] A number of authors also have found an increased total energy expenditure (TEE) in SGA infants.[148,151] The hypermetabolism observed in the SGA infant in part is the product of a large brain:body weight ratio.[153] However, the energy cost of protein metabolism is estimated to be 20% of TEE, and increases in protein metabolic rate also could be responsible for a significant portion of the increases in energy expenditure seen in SGA infants.

A few investigators have documented digestibility of nutrients in SGA infants, but with inconsistent results. Chessex et al[151] found SGA preterm infants to have an 11-14% lower fat and protein digestibility than AGA preterm infants, despite the greater maturity of the SGA infants studied. Cauderay et al[148] however, found digestibility to be similar for SGA and AGA LBW infants fed a formula diet.

Knowing that SGA infants are born with a body composition that is decreased in protein and fat content relative to appropriately grown (AGA) infants,[154] most clinicians currently recommend increased protein and energy intakes per kg body weight compared to normally grown infants in order to achieve catch-up growth. The data of Lucas also support this approach in the SGA preterm infant (particularly males), where higher protein intakes resulted in improved developmental outcome at 7-8 years of age.[155]

Catch-up Growth and Outcome in SGA Infants

Population studies of catch-up growth in SGA infants

indicate highly variable growth outcomes.[156] It appears that the slower the rate of intrauterine growth, the less the likelihood the infant will "catch up" and eventually grow normally.[141] Thus it seems reasonable that less-affected and healthier SGA infants are more likely to respond to nutritional intervention. From several studies it is suggested that SGA infants are prone to persistent deficits in muscle mass, but normal or excessive gain in fat.[154,157]

There is increasing evidence that early diet can have long-term effects on developmental outcome.[158,159] There have been few prospective trials of nutrient interventions in SGA infants and effects on growth outcome.[160,161] Population studies have shown that the majority of SGA infants achieve catch-up growth over the first 2 years of life, but there is evidence that a failure to demonstrate early compensatory growth may be associated with permanently decreased growth.[162,163] Whether this is due to inadequate early nutrition or to permanent programming for decreased growth is unknown.

Nutrition in Infants with Respiratory Disorders

Acute Respiratory Distress

Nutritional requirements for increased work of breathing. The literature contains little information that specifically addresses nutritional requirements for newborn infants with acute respiratory disorders, such as respiratory distress syndrome or clinical hyaline membrane disease due to surfactant deficiency, pneumonia, meconium aspiration syndrome, and congenital diaphragmatic hernia. A primary concern of the few studies conducted and reported is an assumed need for more non-protein calories in infants with respiratory distress.[164] Such infants appear to have increased work of breathing and presumably increased energy expenditure. Wahlig et al[167] showed a positive correlation between oxygen consumption and the ventilatory index (mean airway pressure x intermittent mandatory ventilation rate) in a small number (n=12) of infants. Fetal lambs stimulated to breathe (by electrical stimulation of the diaphragm and intercostal muscles) can have increased rates of oxygen

consumption of up to 30% above basal, accounting for an additional caloric expenditure of about 25 kcal/kg/day.[168] Such high rates of oxygen consumption and energy expenditure have not been measured consistently in newborn infants with respiratory distress, even when not receiving mechanical ventilation, largely due to technical deficiencies in the measurement of oxygen consumption rates.[164] There have been no studies to show that increased non-protein calorie intake beneficially affects the respiratory disorder. Wahlig et al showed no significant correlation between nitrogen balance and ventilatory index in infants with acute respiratory distress syndrome.[167] In general, such infants have not been fed as much, IV or enterally, as infants without respiratory distress. This practice has limited their growth, but whether or not it has adversely affected their respiratory function has not been determined. Many of these infants suffer additional stresses, leading to increased rates of protein breakdown from associated factors such as increased circulating concentrations of catecholamines, cortisol, and cytokines such as TNF-α, interleukin 6, and interleukin 1b. Increased supply of amino acids intravenously may be helpful to reduce the associated protein breakdown, enhance protein synthesis, and maintain protein balance and earlier muscle growth under such circumstances. There has been little study of this, however.

Maximal glucose oxidative capacity. Additional studies have addressed which non-protein calorie source, carbohydrate or lipid, is optimal for infants. High carbohydrate intakes, above 40 kcal/kg/day in a term infant, lead to lipogenesis from glucose and thus high rates of CO_2 production, which has been documented in infants[169-171] as well as older children and surgical patients.[172] High carbohydrate intakes also have been thought to stimulate adrenergic activity leading to increased energy expenditure from brown fat turnover.[169,173,174] While these theoretical concerns appear valid, practical evidence from controlled trials do not document quantitatively important contributions of glucose-induced increases in energy expenditure to overall nutritional requirements.[171] In such infants who are ventilated, increased respiratory rate by infants above that of the respirator may be part of the compensation that limits the adverse effects of glucose-generated increased CO_2 production and hypercapnia.[175] Whether such increased respiratory rates affect energy balance significantly or contribute to clinical problems such as fatigue of breathing or growth failure are not known.

At least two studies[176,177] have shown improved nitrogen balance in infants fed a high ratio of lipid to glucose; it is not known whether this beneficially affects lung disorders. Furthermore, despite potentially positive benefits of a higher lipid to glucose ratio, high intravenous lipid infusion rates have been associated with a variety of adverse effects on pulmonary structure and function. Not all of these adverse effects have been confirmed, though, leaving some confusion about the appropriate lipid:glucose ratio for nutrition of infants with acute pulmonary disorders. For example, early reports of lipid droplet accumulation in the lungs (and other organs)[178-180] subsequently have been attributed to postmortem lipid deposition from de-emulsification of serum lipids due to hydrolysis of triglycerides in the lipoprotein coat, followed by postmortem agglomeration of triglyceride particles to larger fat particles and not to intravenous lipid infusion.[17,81-183] In contrast, other possibly adverse effects have been seen and reported more consistently and should temper excessive use of high lipid infusion rates.[184] For example, adverse effects of lipid infusion on pulmonary diffusing capacity, hemorrhagic pulmonary edema, and vascular tone have been observed,[185-192] probably through higher production rates of free fatty acids, particularly free oleic acid, and eicosanoids (prostaglandins, thromboxanes, and leukotrienes) derived from fatty acid in the lipid emulsions.[178,193-197] The literature is quite mixed on these effects, not surprisingly, given that individual eicosanoids have relaxant, constrictive, or mixed effects on vasculature.[198-200] In different infants with different rates of lipid infusion; associated conditions (acidosis, hypoxia, hypovolemia, sepsis); other drug infusions; use of heparin; different types of lipid infused; and different gestational ages; a large variety of effects from marked vasodilation to marked vasoconstriction can be seen.[201-206] Still other studies have noted conflicting effects of polyunsaturated fatty acids (PUFAs) on pulmonary vascular function, including a protective effect of PUFAs on hyperoxic injury versus increased lung injury from lipid peroxides derived from PUFAs[87,217-212] Fortunately, with IV lipid nutritional regimens that advance lipid infusions slowly and to final rates not exceeding 2-3 grams/kg/day, given over 24 hours of the day rather than shorter duration, such adverse effects have not proved clinically significant. Both Brans et al and Adamkin et al found no difference in oxygenation between infants randomly assigned to various lipid doses (including controls without lipid) when using lower rates and longer infusion times.[213,214] Adamkin also found no difference in the lecithin/sphingomyelin ratio of tracheal phospholipids between the two study groups and failed to support the hypothesis that essential fatty acid deficiency, which was assumed to have developed in the control group without lipid, adversely affects pulmonary maturation (at least over the study period). Future studies in this area are indicated.

Bronchopulmonary Dysplasia
Relationship of Nutritional Factors and Their Possible Role in Bronchopulmonary Dysplasia

The premature infant is at risk for development for hyaline membrane disease and subsequent bronchopulmonary dysplasia (BPD). Both disease processes increase energy expenditure requirements by as much as 25% above basal needs in infants who, by virtue of their immaturity, are severely compromised in their ability to have appropriate nutrition established.[165,215] Infants with BPD recover more quickly if they have adequate caloric intake, yet the metabolism of this energy results in increased CO_2 production and O_2 consumption in infants whose respiratory function is already stressed. There are a number of animal studies and a few clinical studies that indicate which nutrient deficiencies may play a role in the development and exacerbation of BPD. From these reports, some rationale for feeding the infant with BPD can be developed.

Decreased energy reserves	Decreased replacement of damaged cells[4,8,24,25]
Early onset of catabolic state[1,2] Effects on Respiratory Distress Syndrome	Decreased replacement of damaged extracellular components (elastin, collagen)[4,26] Lung growth and replication
Altered surfactant production[3-7]	Decreased lung biosynthesis[4,8,24,25]
Decreased respiratory muscle function[4,8-10] Protection from hyperoxia and barotrauma	Decreased lung structural maturation[4,8,24,25] Susceptibility to infection
Decreased epithelial integrity (insufficient Vitamin A)[4,11-18] Decreased antioxidant defense systems (antioxidant enzymes, glutathione, Vitamin E, Vitamin C, polyunsaturated fatty acids (PUFAs)[3,4,19-23]	Decreased cellular/humoral defenses[27-29]
	Decreased epithelial cell integrity[4,8,11,13,24,25]
Decreased lung biosynthesis/cell replication for lung repair[4,8,24,25] Lung repair and development of BPD	Decreased clearance mechanisms[4,8]

1. Kashyap S. Nutritional management of the extremely-low-birth-weight infant. In: Cowett RM, Hay WW, Jr., eds. *The micropremie: the next frontier. Report of the 99th Ross Conference on Pediatric Research:* Ross Laboratories, Columbus, OH; 1990:115-122.
2. American Academy of Pediatrics CoN. Nutritional needs of low-birth-weight infants. *Pediatrics* 1985;75:976-986.
3. Farrell P. Nutrition and infant lung functions. *Pediatr Pulmonol* 1986;2:44-59.
4. Edelman NH, Rucker RB, Peavy HH. NIH Workshop Summary. Nutrition and the respiratory system. *Am Rev Respir Dis* 1986;134:347-352.
5. Gail DB, Massaro GD. Influence of fasting on the lung. *J Appl Physiol* 1977;42:88-92.
6. Gross I, Ilie I, Wilson CM, Rooney SA. The influence of postnatal nutritional deprivation on the phospholipid content of developing rat lung. *Biochem Biophys Acta* 1976;441:412-422.
7. Gross I, Rooney SA, Warshaw JB. The inhibition of enzymes related to pulmonary fatty acid and phospholipid synthesis by dietary deprivation in the rat. *Biochem Biophys Res Commun* 1975;64:59-63.
8. O'Brodovich HM, Mellins RB. Bronchopulmonary dysplasia: unresolved neonatal acute lung injury. *Am Rev Respir Dis* 1985;132:694-709.
9. Arora N, Rochester D. Respiratory muscle strength and maximal voluntary ventilation in undernourished patients. *Am Rev Respir Dis* 1982;126:6-8.
10. Kelsen S, Ference M, Kapoor S. Effects of prolonged undernutrition on structure and function of the diaphragm. *J Appl Physiol* 1985;58:1354-1359.
11. Zachman RD. Vitamin A. In: Farrell PM, Taussig LM, eds. *Bronchopulmonary dysplasia and related chronic respiratory disorders. Report of the 90th Ross Conference on Pediatric Research.* Columbus, OH: Ross Laboratories; 1986:86-96.
12. Hustead V, Gutcher G, Anderson S. Relationship of vitamin A status to lung disease in the preterm infant. *J Pediatr* 1984;105:610-615.
13. Anzano MA, Olson JA, Lamb AJ. Morphologic alterations in the trachea and the salivary gland following the induction of rapid synchronous vitamin A deficiency in rats. *Am J Pathol* 1980;98:7171-7180.
14. Blomhoff R, Green MH, Norum KR. Vitamin A: physiological and biochemical processing. *Annu Rev Nutr* 1992;12:37-57.
15. Shenai J, Kennedy K, Chytil F, Stahlman M. Clinical trial of vitamin A supplementation in infants susceptible to bronchopulmonary dysplasia. *Journal of Pediatrics* 1987;111:269-277.
16. Pearson E, Bose C, Snidow T, et al. Trial of vitamin A supplementation in very low birth weight infants at risk for bronchopulmonary dysplasia. *Journal of Pediatrics* 1992;121.
17. Massaro GD, Massaro D. Formation of pulmonary alveoli and gas-exchanging surface area: Quantitation and regulaton. *Annu Rev Physiol* 1996;58:73-92.
18. Tyson J, LL W, Oh W, et al. Vitamin A supplementation for extremely-low-birth-weight infants. *New England Journal of Medicine* 1999;340:1962-1968.
19. Sullivan J. Iron, plasma antioxidants, and the oxygen radical disease of prematurity. *Am J Dis Child* 1988;132:1341-1344.
20. Deneke S, Gershoff S, Fanburg B. Potentiation of oxygen toxicity in rats by dietary protein or amino acid deficiency. *J Appl Physiol* 1983;54:147-151.
21. Cross C, Haegawa G, Reddy K, Omaye ST. Enhanced lung toxicity of oxygen in selenium-deficient rats. *Res Commun Chem Pathol Pharmacol* 1977;16:695-706.
22. Ehrenkranz RA, Ablow RC. Effect of vitamin E on the development of oxygen-induced lung injury in neonates. *Ann NY Acad Sci* 1982;93:452-466.
23. Sosenko IRS, Innis SM, Frank L. Polyunsaturated fatty acids and protection of newborn rats from oxygen toxicity. *J Pediatr* 1988;112:630-637.
24. Roberts RJ. Implications of nutrition in oxygen-related pulmonary diseases in the human premature infant. *Adv Pharmacol Ther* 1978;8:53-64.
25. Frank L, Groseclose EE. Oxygen toxicity in newborns: the adverse effect of undernutrition. *J Appl Physiol* 1982;53:1248-1255.
26. Sahebjami H, Vassalo C. Effects of starvation and refeeding on lung mechanics and morphometry. *Am Rev Respir Dis* 1979;119:443-451.
27. Martin T, Altman Z, Alvares L. The effects of severe protein-calorie malnutrition on antibacterial defense mechanisms in the rat lung. *Am Rev Respir Dis* 1983;128:1013-1019.
28. Chandra RK. Nutrition, immunity and infection. Present knowledge and future directions. *Lancet* 1983;1:688-691.
29. Mata L. The malnutrition-infection complex and its environmental factors. *Proc Nutr Soc* 1979;38:29-40.

Table 2: Potential pulmonary effects of undernutrition in the VLBW infant susceptible to BPD.

There are many mechanisms that contribute to development and persistence of BPD. Nutritional deficiencies in the premature infant that may exacerbate these mechanisms are summarized in Table 2 and have been reviewed by Van Aerde.[216] Of particular note, a recent trial has been completed of Vitamin A administration to preterm infants at risk of BPD conducted by the NICHD Neonatal Research Network[217] in over 800 infants less than 1000g birth weight. This study showed that a dose of 5000 IU of Vitamin A administered intramuscularly for the first 4 weeks of life reduced the incidence of BPD at 36 weeks post-conceptional age from 62% to 55% (P<0.03, 95% confidence interval 0.8 to 0.99), without any evidence for Vitamin A toxicity. Importantly, despite this much higher than conventional dose of 1000 IU/d, 24-40% of retinol-supplemented infants failed to achieve a "normal" Vitamin A status, versus 50-70% of the placebo-treated group.

Specific energy and nutrient requirements in BPD

Failure to thrive is a major complication of BPD. Theoretical possibilities for growth impairment include increased energy expenditure, suboptimal energy intake (often secondary to fluid restriction), chronic hypoxia, chronic respiratory acidosis, metabolic disturbances related to drug therapy, decreased gastrointestinal absorption of nutrients, and congestive heart failure.

Hypotheses for increased energy expenditure in infants with BPD include increased work of breathing, higher basal metabolic rate (perhaps secondary to medications such as theophylline), and increased energy expenditure and CO_2 production accompanying the metabolism of high caloric density (particularly high carbohydrate) formula.[218] Although most clinicians have concluded that energy expenditure is increased in infants with BPD, actual measurements of such energy expenditures have not revealed large or even consistent values.[164-166,218] In adults, respiratory muscles make only a small contribution to overall energy expenditure.[220] Additionally, as pointed out in a review by Kalhan and Denne,[164] there have been a number of difficulties with interpreting studies of infants, particularly those who require supplemental oxygen.[165,174,219,221] Such studies are prone to error because current calorimetry systems are inaccurate under conditions of increased inspired oxygen concentration.

Energy requirements in the infant with BPD, therefore, include not only increased total energy because of the disease process itself, but also additional energy to try to prevent the slower rate of growth observed in these infants. The magnitude of growth delay in these infants is directly related to severity and duration of disease.[216] The portion of intake that is distributed to each of these demands is not clear, and undoubtedly varies depending on such factors as severity of disease and infant maturity.

Despite the focus to date on the need for more energy in infants with BPD, it is a common clinical observation that many of these infants develop excessive body fat, indicating that their intakes of lipids and carbohydrates exceed their non-protein caloric expenditures. Most infants in these studies were receiving less than 3 grams/kg/day of protein, which is less than the protein requirements for preterm infants to meet normal rates of in utero growth. Thus it is reasonable to conclude that growth rates in these infants are limited more by protein deficiency than non-protein caloric intake. Higher protein intakes also may prove more valuable in supporting protein synthesis and growth of respiratory muscles, although there is no specific evidence for this.

In general, infants with BPD are treated with relative fluid restriction, because pulmonary edema appears to complicate the pathology of BPD.[222] The presence of a PDA also is associated with large fluid intakes and with increased risk of developing BPD.[222] Van Marter et al suggested that excessive fluid therapy, even in the first days of life, might increase the risk of BPD in low-birthweight infants.[223] Based on this information, it is advisable to refrain from excessive water administration during all stages of BPD.

It has been demonstrated that infants with BPD have improved growth if oxygenation is maintained in a higher range according to pulse oximetry.[224] This fits with general clinical experience and is consistent with the observation of reduced growth in infants with cyanotic congenital heart disease and infants purposefully kept hypoxic to maintain patency of cardiac mixing shunts. The mechanisms responsible for the effect of oxygen on growth are not known. However, animal studies have documented decreased protein synthesis rates[225] and DNA synthesis rates[226] under experimental conditions of hypoxia.

As noted earlier in this chapter, the dietary distribution of energy clearly influences metabolic rate, CO_2 production, and O_2 consumption in studies of intravenous feedings in infants[169,216,227-229] and enteral alimentation in adults.[230,231] Glucose:lipid calorie ratios of 3:1 or 2:1 minimize CO_2 production.[216] Further research also is needed to determine optimal feeding methods and routes, as well as formula supplements.

Recommendations for Feeding with Respiratory Disease

As discussed elsewhere in this chapter and this book, preterm infants need improved (increased) protein nutrition whether they have respiratory problems or not. Although it seems reasonable to conclude that a higher protein intake that produces increased nitrogen:protein balance and lean body mass would include growth of respiratory muscles and thus the capacity to breathe better, there are no studies to support such a conclusion. Non-protein calorie intakes above 80 (for IV feeding)-120 (for enteral feeding) kcal/kg/day add more to adiposity than to improved growth of lean body mass.[232] The optimal non-protein calorie:protein ratio and nutritional regimen varies considerably by type of feeding (IV vs enteral) and the size and condition of the infant. There are no studies or experimental evidence to show that higher non-protein calorie intakes promote respiratory muscle growth or improve physiological function in infants with either acute or chronic respiratory disorders and increased respiratory work. Practical problems (increased incidence and degree of hyperglycemia and fatty infiltration of organs such as the liver and heart) and theoretical concerns (increased adrenergic activity,

high CO_2 production rates) should temper the use of high carbohydrate intakes (especially high intravenous glucose infusion rates). Intravenous feeding regimens should have a greater proportion of amino acids (at least 3 grams/kg/day in preterm infants) than has been customary in the past. Glucose infusion rates should not exceed 10-12 mg/min/kg and lipid infusion rates should not exceed 3 grams/kg/day. As for enteral feedings, Ziegler (personal comment) has suggested that premature infant formulas may still not contain sufficient protein for optimal protein nutrition, particularly for the infant who cannot tolerate large volume feeds, and there is a need for higher protein concentrations in formulas designed for earlier feedings when increased volumes and rates of feedings have been associated with increased risks of NEC. There is no evidence to support supplementing milk or formulas with carbohydrates or lipids to achieve improved growth or respiratory function in preterm or term infants with acute or chronic respiratory problems.

Sepsis

In adults, sepsis induces profound changes in both energy and protein metabolism. There have been several neonatal studies demonstrating glucose and lipid intolerance in neonates with sepsis.[233-235] There is little information on protein metabolism in neonatal sepsis. In adults, the marked catabolic response to systemic infection releases amino acids from skeletal muscle that are then taken up by the liver for gluconeogenesis and for use in the synthesis of acute phase proteins. In a recent study on the effect of sepsis on metabolism in neonates, oxygen consumption was increased and there was a significant negative effect on nitrogen balance that was proportional to the severity of illness.[236]

In terms of feeding strategies to prevent sepsis, there have been few studies on immunonutrition in neonates. From recent data it is suggested that enteral glutamine supplementation decreases both the incidence of sepsis and feeding intolerance in the preterm infant.[42] This finding needs to be confirmed.

Case Study

Baby GH was a 29-day-old female infant, 789 g and 26-weeks gestation at birth, born to a mother with chorioamnionitis. She was born vaginally and required immediate intubation for poor respiratory effort. Her Apgar scores were 1 at one minute and 4 at five minutes. She received surfactant in the delivery room. Initial chest radiograph showed bilateral opacification of the lungs. Her early course suggested probable sepsis with left-shifted white blood cell count and low absolute neutrophil count, and need for pressor support for the first 5 days of life. By one week of age she was still requiring significant ventilator support with FiO$_2$ of 0.8 and radiographic changes consistent with early chronic lung disease (CLD). She was supported with PN from day 2 of life. Enteral feedings were started on day of life 8, and she was advanced to full volume feedings by day of life 19. On day of life 23 she developed NEC and enteral feedings were withheld for a 10-day period. She received intermittent diuretic therapy for her CLD. She was on conventional ventilation with a rate of 25 breaths per minute, peak inspiratory pressure of 17 cm H$_2$O, positive end expiratory pressure of 4 cm H$_2$O, and FiO$_2$ of 0.45. Arterial blood gases demonstrated pH values of 7.41-7.43 and PaCO$_2$ of 54-59 mm Hg. CXR showed moderate CLD, and attempts to wean the ventilator rate resulted in further CO$_2$ retention. Her weight was 824 grams at 20 days of life, and she had demonstrated poor weight gain (approximately 5-6 g/kg/d) despite non-protein parenteral energy intake of 125 kcal/kg/d. Consultation with the nutrition team was obtained. It was determined that the patient was receiving 25 g/kg/d of glucose and 4 g/kg/d of intravenous lipid. Indirect calorimetry was performed. Resting energy expenditure was 78 kcal/kg/d with a VCO$_2$ of 10.1 mL/kg/min. Resting heart rate was 162 beats per minute. The patient's glucose intake was gradually decreased over the next 2 days to 16 g/kg/d. Two days later indirect calorimetry was repeated. Resting energy expenditure was now 64 kcal/kg/d with VCO$_2$ of 8.2 mL/kg/min. The infant was noted by the nursing staff to be significantly less "jittery" and require less sedation. Resting heart rate was now 140 beats per minute. Over the next week the PaCO$_2$ decreased allowing for weaning of the ventilator rate. Despite being on a lower caloric intake (95 non-protein cals/kg/d) she started growing at a consistent rate of 10-13 g/kg/d.

This case demonstrates the hypermetabolism and carbon dioxide retention that can result from excessive carbohydrate intake. In this case, decreasing glucose intake below the presumed maximal glucose oxidative capacity decreased both energy expenditure and carbon dioxide retention, resulting in an improved rate of growth.

References

1. Kliegman RM, Fanaroff AA. Necrotizing enterocolitis. *New England Journal of Medicine* 1984;310:1093-1103.

2. Neu J, Weiss MD. Necrotizing enterocolitis: pathophysiology and prevention. *Journal of Parenteral and Enteral Nutrition* 1999;23:S13-S17.

3. Crissinger KD, Burney DL, Velasquez OR, Gonzalez E. An animal model of necrotizing enterocolitis induced by infant formula and ischemia in developing piglets. *Gastroenterology* 1994;106:1215-1222.

4. Szabo JS, Mayfield SR, Oh W, Stonestreet BS. Postprandial gastrointesinal blood flow and oxygen consumption: effects of hypoxia in neonatal piglets. *Pediatric Research* 1987;21:93-98.

5. Crissinger KD, Granger DN. Mucosal injury induced by ischemia and reperfusion in the piglet intestine: influences of age and feeding. *Gastroenterology* 1989;97:920-926.

6. Hughes C, Dowling R. Speed of onset of adaptive mucosal hypoplasia and hypofunction in the intestine of parenterally fed rats. *Clinical Science* 1980;59:317-327.

7. Widdowson E, Colombo V, Artavanis C. Changes in the organs of pigs in response to feeding for the first 24 hours after birth. II. The digestive Tract. *Biology of the Neonate* 1976;28:272-281.

8. Heird WC, Schwarz SM, Hansen TH. Colostrum-induced enteric mucosal growth in beagle puppies. *Pediatric Research* 1984;18:512-515.

9. Lucas A, Adrian T, Christofides N, Bloom S, Aynsley-Green A. Plasma motilin, gastrin and enteroglucagon and feeding in the human newborn. *Arch Dis Child* 1980;55:673-677.

10. Klagsbrun M. Human milk stimulates DNA synthesis and cellular proliferation in cultured fibroblasts. *Proc Natl Acad Sci USA* 1978;7511:5057-5061.

11. Lucas A, Bloom S, Aynsley-Green A. The development of gut hormone response to feeding in neonates. *Arch Dis Child* 1980;55:678-682.

12. Lucas A, Bloom S, Aynsley-Green A. Postnatal surges in plasma gut hormones in term and preterm infants. *Biol Neonate* 1982;41:63-67.

13. Aynsley-Green A, Adtrian T, Bloom S. Feeding and the development of enteroinsular hormone secretion in the preterm infant: Effects of continuous gastric infusions of human milk compared with intermittent boluses. *Acta Paediatr Scand* 1982;71:379-383.

14. Berseth CL. Effect of early feeding on maturation of the preterm infant's small intestine. *Journal of Pediatrics* 1992;120:947-953.

15. Koenig WJ, Amarnath RP, Hench V, Berseth CL. Manometrics for preterm and term infants: A new tool for old questions. *Pediatrics* 1995;95:203-206.

16. LaGamma EF, Ostertag SG, Birenbaum H. Failure of delayed oral feedings to prevent necrotizing enterocolitis. *American Journal of Diseases of Childhood* 1985;139:385-389.

17. Ostertag SG, LaGamma EF, Reisen CE, Ferrentino FL. Early enteral feeding does not affect the incidence of necrotizing enterocolitis. *Pediatrics* 1986;77:275-280.

18. Slagle TA, Gross SJ. Effect of early low-volume enteral substrate on subsequent feeding tolerance in very-low-birth-weight infants. *Journal of Pediatrics* 1988;113: 526-531.

19. Dunn L, Hulman S, Weiner J, Kliegman R. Beneficial effects of early hypocaloric enteral feeding on neonatal gastrointestinal function: Preliminary report of a randomized trial. *Journal of Pediatrics* 1988;112:622-629.

20. Meetze WH, Valentine C, McGuigan JE, Conlon M, Sacks N, Neu J. Gastrointestinal priming prior to full enteral nutrition in very low birth weight infants. *Journal of Pediatric Gastroenterology and Nutrition* 1992;15:163-170.

21. Berseth CL, Nordyke C. Enteral nutrients promote postnatal maturation of intestinal motor activity in preterm infants. *American Journal of Physiology* 1993; 264:G1046-G1051.

22. Troche B, Harvey-Wilkes K, Engle WD, et al. Early minimal feedings promote growth in critically ill premature infants. *Biology of the Neonate* 1995;67: 172-181.

23. McClure RJ, Newell SJ. Randomised controlled study of clinical outcome following trophic feeding. *Arch Dis Child* 2000;82:F29-F33.

24. Atkinson SA. Human milk feeding of the micropremie. *Clinics in Perinatology* 2000;27:235-247.

25. Lucas A, Cole TJ. Breast milk and necrotising enterocolitis. *Lancet* 1990;366:1519-1523.

26. Schanler R, Shulman R, Lau C, Smith E, Heitkemper M. Feeding strategies for premature infants: randomized trial of gastrointestinal priming and tube-feeding method. *Pediatrics* 1999;103:434-439.

27. Slusser W, Powers NG. Breastfeeding update 1: Immunology, nutrition, and advocacy. *Pediatric Reviews* 1997;18:111-119.

28. Pittard WB, 3rd. Breast milk immunology. A frontier of infant nutrition. *American Journal of Diseases in Children* 1979;133:83-87.

29. Jadcherla SR, Berseth CL. Acute and chronic intestinal motor activity responses to two infant formulas. *Pediatrics* 1995;96:331-335.

30. McClure RJ, Newell SJ. Effect of fortifying breast milk on gastric emptying. *Archives of Disease in Childhood* 1996;74:F60-F62.

31. Rayyis S, Ambalavanan N, Wright L, Carlo W. Randomized trial of "slow" versus "fast" advancements on the incidence of necrotizing enterocolitis in very-low-birth-weight infants. *Journal of Pediatrics* 1999;134:293-297.

32. Kennedy KA, Tyson JE, Chamnanvanakij S. Early versus delayed initiation of progressive enteral feedings for parenterally fed low birth weight or preterm infants. The Cochrane Database of Systematic Reviews. 2000:CD001970.

33. Tyson JE, Kennedy KA. Minimal enteral nutrition for promoting feeding tolerance and preventing morbidity in parenterally fed infants. The Cochrane Database of Systematic Reviews. 2000:CD000504.

34. Kennedy KA, Tyson JD, Chamnanvanakij S. Rapid versus slow rate of advancement of feedings for promoting growth and preventing necrotizing enterocolotis in parenterally fed low-birth-weight infants. The Cochrane Database of Systematic Reviews. 2000:CD001241.

35. Van Marter LJ, Allred EN, Leviton A, Pagano M, Parad R, Moore M. Antenatal glucocorticoid treatment does not reduce chronic lung disease among surviving preterm infants. *Journal of Pediatrics* 2001;138:198-204.

36. Halac J, Begue EF, Casanas JM, et al. Prenatal and postnatal corticosteroid therapy to prevent neonatal necrotizing enterocolitis: a controlled trial. *Journal of Pediatrics* 1990;117:132-188.

37. Wright LL, Verter J, Younes N, et al. Antenatal corticosteroid administration and neonatal outcome in very low birth weight infants: the NICHD Neonatal Research Network. *American Journal of Obstetrics and Gynecology* 1995;173:269-274.

38. Bury RG, Tudehope D. Enteral antibiotics for preventing necrotizing enterocolitis in low-birth-weight or preterm infants. The Cochrane Database of Systematic Reviews. 2001:CD000405.

39. Eibl MM, Wolf HM, Furnkranz H, Rosenkranz A. Prevention of necrotizing enterocolitis in low-birth-weight infants by IgA-IgG feeding. *New England Journal of Medicine* 1988;319:1-7.

40. Foster J, Cole M. Oral immunoglobulin for preventing necrotizing enterocolitis in preterm and low-birth-weight neonates (Cochrane Review). The Cochrane Library. 2001.

41. Carlson SE, Montalto MB, Ponder DL, Werkman SH, Korones SB. Lower incidence of necrotizing enterocolitis "in infants fed a preterm formula with egg phospholipids. *Pediatric Research* 1998;44:491-498.

42. Neu J, Roig JC, Meetze WH et al. Enteral glutamine supplementation for very low birthwieght infants decreases morbidity. *Journal of Pediatrics* 1997;131:691-699.

43. Bates MD, Balistreri WF. The neonatal gastrointestinal tract. In: Fanaroff AA, Martin RJ, eds. *Neonatal-Perinatal Medicine: Diseases of the Fetus and Infant*. 2 vol. 7th ed. St. Louis: Mosby; 2002:1255-1307.

44. Ricketts RR. Surgical treatment of necrotizing enterocolitis and the short bowel syndrome. *Clinics in Perinatology* 1994;21:365-387.

45. Warner BW, Ziegler MM. Management of the short bowel syndrome in the pediatric population. *Pediatric Clinics of North America* 1993;40:1335-1350.

46. Dowling RH. Small bowel adaptation and its regulation. *Scandanavian Journal of Gastroenterology Suppl* 1982;74:53-74.

47. Vanderhoof JA. Short bowel syndrome. *Clinics in Perinatology* 1996;23:377-386.

48. Clark J. Management of short bowel syndrome in the high-risk infant. *Clinics in Perinatology* 1984;11:189-197.

49. Fordtran JS, Rector FC, Carter NW. The mechanisms of sodium absorption in the human intestine. *Journal of Clinical Investigation* 1968;47:884-900.

50. Purdum PP, III, Kirby DF. Short-bowel syndrome: A review of the role of nutrition support. *Journal of Parenteral and Enteral Nutrition* 1991;15:93-101.

51. Georgeson KE, Breux CW, Jr. Outcome and intestinal adaptation in neonatal short-bowel syndrome. *Journal of Pediatric Surgery* 1992;27:344-348.

52. Goulet OJ, Revillon Y, Jan D et al. Neonatal short bowel syndrome. *Journal of Pediatrics* 1991;119:18-23.

53. Weber TR, Tracy T, Jr., Connors RH. Short-bowel syndrome in children--quality of life in an era of improved survival. *Archives of Surgery* 1991;126:841-846.

54. Vanderhoof JA. Short bowel syndrome and intestinal adaptation. In: Walker WA, Durie PR, Hamilton JR, Walker-Smith JA, Watkins JB, eds. *Pediatric Gastrointestinal Disease: Pathophysiology, Diagnosis, Management*. 3rd ed. St. Louis: Mosby-Year Book, Inc.; 2000.

55. Koldovsky O. Hormones in milk. In: Litwack G, ed. *Vitamins and Hormones*. New York: Academic Press, Inc.; 1995:77-149.

56. Philipps AF, Anderson GG, Dvorak B et al. Growth of artificially fed infant rats: effect of supplementation with insulin-like growth factor 1. *American Journal of Physiology* 1997;272:R1532-R1539.

57. Dvorak B, Philipps AF, Koldovsky O. Milk-borne growth factors and gut development. In: Ziegler E, Lucas A, Moro G, eds. *Nutrition of the Very Low Birthweight Infant*. New York: Lippincott-Raven Press; 1999.

58. Teitelbaum DH, Drongowski R, Spivak D. Rapid development of hyperbilirubinemia in infants with short bowel syndrome as a correlate to mortality: Possible indications for early small bowel transplant. *Transplant Proceedings* 1996;28:2699-2700.

59. Caniano DA, Starr J, Ginn-Pease ME. Extensive short bowel syndrome in neonates: Outcome in the 1980's. *Surgery* 1989;105:119-124.

60. Sondheimer J, Asturias E, Cadnapaphornchai M. Infection and cholestasis in neonates with intestinal resection and long-term parenteral nutrition. *Journal of Pediatric Gastroenterology and Nutrition* 1998;27:131-137.

61. Simmons MG, Georgeson KE, Figueroa R, Mock DL.

Liver failure in parenteral nutrition dependent children with short bowel syndrome. *Transplant Proceedings* 1996;28:2701.

62. Suita S, Masumoto K, Yamanouchi T, Nagano M, Nakamura M. Complications in neonates with short bowel syndrome and long-term parenteral nutrition. *Journal of Parenteral and Enteral Nutrition* 1999;23:S106-S109.

63. Beale EF, Nelson RM, Bucciarelli RL, Donnelly WH, Eitzman DV. Intrahepatic cholestasis associated with parenteral nutrition in premature infants. *Pediatrics* 1979;64:342-347.

64. Merritt RJ. Cholestasis associated with total parenteral nutrition. *Journal of Pediatric Gastoenterology and Nutrition* 1986;5:9-22.

65. Forchielli ML, Gura KM, Sandler R, Lo C. Aminosyn PF or trophamine: which provides more protection from cholestasis associated with total parenteral nutrition? *Journal of Pediatric Gastroenterology and Nutrition* 1995;21:374-382.

66. Andorsky DJ, Lund DP, Lillehei CW et al. Nutritional and other postoperative management of neonates with short bowel syndrome correlates with clinical outcomes. *Journal of Pediatrics* 2001;139:27-33.

67. Bines JE. Cholestatsis associated with parenteral nutrition therapy. In: Walker WA, Durie PR, Hamilton JR, Walker-Smith JA, Watkins JB, eds. *Pediatric Gastrointestinal Disease: Pathophysiology, Diagnosis, Management.* 3rd ed. St. Louis: Mosby-Year Book, Inc.; 2000:1219-1228.

68. Sokol RJ. Total parenteral nutrition-related liver disease. *Zhonghua Min Guo Xiao Er Ke Yi Xue Hui Za Zhi (Acta Paed Sin)* 1997;38:418-428.

69. Kleinman RE, Sandler RH. Cholestasis associated with parenteral nutrition. In: Walker WA, Durie PR, Hamilton JR, Walker-Smith JA, Watkins JB, eds. *Pediatric Gastrointestinal Disease: Pathophysiology, Diagnosis, Management.* 2 vol. 2nd ed. St. Louis: Mosby-Year Book, Inc.; 1996:1271-1281.

70. Whitington PF. Cholestasis associated with total parenteral nutrition in infants. *Hepatology* 1985;5:693-696.

71. Naji AA, Anderson FH. Sensitivity and specificity of liver function tests in the detection of parenteral nutrition associated cholestasis. *Journal of Parenteral and Enteral Nutrition* 1985;9:307-307.

72. Moss RL, Amii LA. New approaches to understanding the etiology and treatment of total nutrition associated cholestasis. *Seminars in Pediatric Surgery* 1999;8:140-147.

73. Meehan JJ, Georgeson KE. Prevention of liver failure in parenteral nutrition-dependent children with short bowel syndrome. *Journal of Pediatric Surgery* 1997;32:473-475.

74. Kubota A, Okada A, Nezu R, Kamata S, Imura K, Takagi Y. Hyperbilirubinemia in neonates associated with total parenteral nutrition. *Journal of Parenteral and Enteral Nutrition* 1988;12:602-606.

75. Bresson JL, Narcy P, Putet G, Ricour C, Sachs C, Rey J. Energy substrate utilization in infants receiving total parenteral nutrition with different glucose to fat ratios. *Pediatric Research* 1989;25:645-648.

76. Jones MO, Pierro A, Hammond P, Nunn A, Lloyd DA. Glucose utilization in the surgical newborn infant receiving total parenteral nutrition. *Journal of Pediatric Surgery* 1993;28:1121-1125.

77. Golden SH, Peart-Vigilance C, Brancatai FL, Kao WH. Perioperative glycemic control and the risk of infectious complications in a cohort of adults with diabetes. *Diabetes Care* 1999;22:1408-1414.

78. Kudsk KA, Croce MA, Fabian TC, et al. Enteral versus parenteral feeding. *Annals of Surgery* 1992;215:503-513.

79. Jeejeebhoy KN. Total parenteral nutrition: potion or poison? *American Journal of Clinical Nutrition* 2001;74:160-163.

80. Heird WC, Hay WW, Jr., Helms RA, Storm MC, Kashyap S, Dell RB. Pediatric parenteral amino acid mixture in low birthweight infants. *Pediatrics* 1988;81:41-50.

81. Helms RA, Christensen ML, C. ME, Storm MC. Comparison of a pediatric versus standard amino acid formulation in preterm neonates requiring parenteral nutrition. *Journal of Pediatrics* 1987;110:466-470.

82. Coran AG, Drongowski RA. Studies on the toxicity and efficacy of a new amino acid solution in pediatric parenteral nutrition. *Journal of Parenteral and Enteral Nutrition* 1987;11:368-377.

83. Howard D, Thompson DF. Taurine: an essential amino acid to prevent cholestasis in neonates? *Annals of Pharmacotherapy* 1992;26:1390-1392.

84. Guertin F, Roy CC, Lepage G, Perea A GR, Youse fl, B. T. Effect of taurine on total parenteral nutrition-associated

cholestasis. *Journal of Parenteral and Enteral Nutrition* 1991;15:247-251.

85. Cooke RJ, Whitington PF, Kelts D. Effect of taurine supplementation on hepatic function during short-term parenteral nutrition in the premature infant. *Journal of Pediatric Gastroenterology and Nutrition* 1984;3:234-238.

86. Shattuck KE, Bhatia J, Grinnell C, Rassin DK. The effects of light exposure on the in vitro hepatic response to an amino acid-vitamin solution. *Journal of Parenteral and Enteral Nutrition* 1995;19:398-402.

87. Neuzil J, Darlow BA, Inder TE, Sluis KB, Winterbourn CC, Stocker R. Oxidation of parenteral lipid emulsion by ambient and phototherapy lights: potential toxicity of routine parenteral feeding. *Journal of Pediatrics* 1995;126:785-790.

88. Collier S, Lo C. Advances in parenteral nutrition. *Current Opinion in Pediatrics* 1996;8:476-482.

89. Schwartz JB, Merritt RJ, Rosenthal P, Diament M, Sinatra FR, Ramos A. Ceruletide to treat neonatal cholestasis. *Lancet* 1988:1219-1220.

90. Collier S, Crough J, Hendricks K, Caballero B. Use of cyclic parenteral nutrition in infants less than 6 months of age. *Nutrition in Clinical Practice* 1994;9:65-68.

91. Georgeson K, Halpin D, Figueroa R, Vincente Y, Hardin WJ. Sequential intestinal lengthening procedures for refractory short bowel syndrome. *Journal of Pediatric Surgery* 1994;29:316-320.

92. Ein SH. The pediatric ostomy. In: Walker WA, Durie PR, Hamilton JR, Walker-Smith JA, Watkins JB, eds. *Pediatric Gastrointestinal Disease: Pathophysiology, Diagnosis, Management.* 2 vol. 2nd ed. St. Louis: Mosby-Year Book, Inc.; 1996:2095-2113.

93. Heird WD, Winters RW. Fluid therapy for the pediatric surgical patient. In: Winters RW, ed. *Principles of Pediatric Fluid Therapy.* 2nd ed. Boston: Little, Brown;1982:595.

94. Winters RW, Heird WD. Special problems of the pediatric surgical patient. In: Winters RW, ed. *Principles of Pediatric Fluid Therapy.* 2nd ed. Boston: Little, Brown;1982.

95. Hambidge KM, Sokol RJ, Fidanza SJ, Goodall MA. Plasma manganese concentrations in infants and children receiving parenteral nutrition. *Journal of Parenteral and Enteral Nutrition* 1989;13:168-171.

96. Warner BW, Vanderhoof JA, Reyes JD. What's new in the management of short gut syndrome in children. *Journal of*

the American College of Surgeons 2000;190:725-736.

97. Ziegler MM. Short bowel syndrome in infants: Etiology and management. *Clinics in Perinatology* 1986;13:163-173.

98. Christie DS, Ament ME. Dilute elemental diet and continuous-infusion technique for management of short bowel syndrome. *Journal of Pediatrics* 1975;87:705-708.

99. Voitk AJ, Echave V, Brown RA, Gurd FN. Use of elemental diet during the adaptive stage of short gut syndrome. *Gastroenterology* 1973;65:419-426.

100. Weser E. Short gut adaptation. *American Journal of Medicine* 1979;67:1014-1020.

101. Vanderhoof JA, Grandjean CJ, Kaufman SS, Burkley KT, Antonson DL. Effect of high percentage medium-chain triglyceride diet on mucosal adaptation following massive bowel resection in rats. *Journal of Parenteral and Enteral Nutrition* 1984;8:685-689.

102. Feldman EJ, Dowling RH, McNaughton J, Peters TJ. Effects of oral versus intravenous nutrition on intestinal adaptation after small bowel resection in the dog. *Gastroenterology* 1976;70:712-719.

103. Parker P, Stroop S, Greene H. A controlled comparison of continuous versus intermittent feeding in the treatment of infants with intestinal disease. *Journal of Pediatrics* 1981;99:360-364.

104. Taylor SF, Sokol RJ. Infants with short bowel syndrome. In: Hay WW, Jr., ed. *Neonatal Nutrition and Metabolism.* 1 vol. St. Louis, MO: Mosby Year Book; 1991:432-450.

105. Wilschanski M, Shamir R. Short bowel syndrome. In: Altschuler SM, Liacouras CA, eds. *Clinical Pediatric Gastroenterology.* Philadelphia: Churcill Livingstone; 1998.

106. Michail S, Mohammadpour J, Park JHY, Vanderhoof JA. Effect of glutamine supplemented diet on mucosal adaptation following bowel resection. *Journal of Pediatric Gastroenterology and Nutrition* 1995;21:394-398.

107. Booth IW. Enteral nutrition of primary therapy in short bowel syndrome. *Gut* 1994;1:S69-S72.

108. Vanderhoof JA, Blackwood DJ, Mohammadpour H, Park JHY. Effects of oral supplementation of glutamine on small intestinal mucosal mass following resection. *American College of Nutrition* 1992;11:223-227.

109. Treem WR. Short bowel syndrome. In: Wyllie R, Hyams JS, eds. *Pediatric Gastrointestinal Disease.*

Philadelphia: W.B. Saunders Co.; 1999:315-333.

110. Schmeling DJ, Coran AG. Hormonal and metabolic response to operative stress in the neonate. *Journal of Parenteral and Enteral Nutrition* 1991;15:215-238.

111. Anand KJS, Brown MJ, Causon RC, et al. Can the human neonate mount an endocrine and metabolic response to surgery? *Journal of Pediatric Surgery* 1985;20:41-48.

112. Anand KJS, Brown MJ, Bloom SR, et al. Studies on the hormonal regulation of fuel metabolism in the human newborn infant undergoing anesthesia and surgery. *Hormone Research* 1985;22:115-128.

113. Giesecke K, Klingstedt C, Ljungqvist O, Hagenfeldt L. The modifying influence of anaesthesia on postoperative protein catabolism. *British Journal of Anaesthesia* 1994;72:697-699.

114. Anand KJS, Sippell WG, Aynsley-Green A. Randomized trial of fentanyl anesthesia in preterm babies undergoing surgery: Effects on the stress response. *Lancet* 1987;8527:243-248.

115. Keshen TH, Jaksic T, Jahoor F. Measurement of the protein metabolic response to surgical stress in extremely-low-birthweight (ELBW) neonates (Abst). *Pediatric Research* 1997;41:234A.

116. Anderson M, Thureen P, Baron K, Bass K, Melara D, Hay W, Jr. Achieving positive protein balance in the immediate post-operative period in neonates with amino acid administration and narcotic analgesia. *Pediatric Research* 1999:Abst.

117. Pierro A, Carnielli V, Filler RM, Smith J, Heim T. Characteristics of protein sparing effect of total parenteral nutrition in the surgical infant. *Journal of Pediatric Surgery* 1988;23:538-542.

118. Pierro A, Carnielli V, Filler RM, Smith J, Heim T. Metabolism of intravenous fat emulsion in the surgical newborn. *Journal of Pediatric Surgery* 1989;24:95-102.

119. Pierro A, Carnielli V, Filler RM, Kicak L, Smith J, Heim TF. Partition of energy metabolism in the surgical newborn. *Journal of Pediatric Surgery* 1991;26:581-586.

120. Dudell GG, Gersony WM. Patent ductus arteriosus in neonates with severe respiratory disease. *Journal of Pediatrics* 1984;104:915.

121. Cotton RB, Stahlman MR, Bender HW, Graham TP, Catterton WZ, Kovar I. Randomized trial of early closure of symptomatic patent ductus arteriosus in small preterm infants. *Journal of Pediatrics* 1978;93:647-651.

122. Wong SN, Lo RNS, Hui PW. Abnormal renal and splanchnic arterial doppler pattern in premature babies with symptomatic patent ductus arteriosus. *Journal of Ultrasound Medicine* 1990;9:125-130.

123. Shimada S, T. K, Konishi M, Fujiwara T. Effects of patent ductus arteriosus on left ventricular output and organ blood flows in preterm infants with respiratory distress syndrome treated with surfactant. *Journal of Pediatrics* 1994;125:270-277.

124. Spach MS, Serwer GA, Anderson PA, Canent RVJ, Levin AR. Pulsatile aortopulmonary pressure-flow dynamics of patent ductus arteriosus in patients with varying hemodynamic states. *Circulation* 1980; 61:110-122.

125. Perlman JM, Hill A, Volpe JJ. The effect of patent ductus arteriosus on flow velocity in the anterior cerebral arteries: ductal steal in the premature newborn infant. *Journal of Pediatrics* 1981;99:767-771.

126. Kitterman JA. Effects of intestinal ischemia in necrotizing enterocolitis in the newborn infant. In: Moore TD, ed. Report of the 68th Ross Conference of Pediatric Research. 38 vol. Columbus: Ross Laboratories; 1975.

127. Walsh MC, Kliegman RM. Nectrotizing enterocolitis: Treatment based on staging criteria. *Pediatric Clinics of North America* 1986;33:179.

128. Van Bel F, Van Zoeren D, Schipper J, Guit GL, Baan J. Effect of indomethacin on superior mesenteric artery blood flow velocity in preterm infants. *Journal of Pediatrics* 1990;116:965-970.

129. Vangi PM, Bertini BR, Cianciulli D, Rubaltelli FF. Effects of indomethacin and ibuprofen on mesenteric and renal blood flow in preterm infants with patent ductus arteriosus. *Journal of Pediatrics* 1999;135:733-738.

130. Walters M. Tolerance in intravenous indomethacin treatment for premature infants with patent ductus arteriosus. *British Medical Journal* 1988;297:773-773.

131. Bell EF, Warburton D, Stonestreet BS, Oh W. Effect of fluid administration on the development of symptomatic patent ductus arteriosus and congestive heart failure in premature infants. *New England Journal of Medicine* 1980;302:598-604.

132. Hammerman C, Glaser J, Schimmel JS, Ferber B, Kaplan M, Eidelman AL. Continuous versus multiple rapid infusions of indomethacin: effects on cerebral blood flow velocity. *Pediatrics* 1995;95:244-248.

133. Bandstra ES, Montalvo BM, Goldberg RN et al. Prophylactic indomethacin for prevention of intraventricular hemorrhage in premature infants. *Pediatrics* 1988;82:533-542.

134. Bada HS, Green RS, Pourcyrous M et al. Indomethacin reduces the risks of severe intraventricular hemorrhage. *Journal of Pediatrics* 1989;115:631-637.

135. Ment LR, Oh W, Ehrenkranz RA et al. Low-dose indomethacin and prevention of intraventricular hemorrhage: a multicenter randomized trial. *Pediatrics* 1994;93:543-550.

136. Yanowitz TD, Yao AC, Werner JC, Pettigrew KD, Oh W, Stonestreet BS. Effects of prophylactic low-dose indomethacin on hemodynamics in very-low-birth-weight infants. *Journal of Pediatrics* 1998;132:28-34.

137. Fowlie PW. Intravenous indomethacin for preventing mortality and morbidity in very low birthweight infants. The Cochrane Database of Systematic Reviews. 2001:CD000174.

138. Schmidt B, Davis P, Moddemann D et al. Long-term effects of indomethacin prophylaxis in extremely-low-birth-weight infants. *New England Journal of Medicine* 2001;344:1966-1972.

139. Hay WW, Jr., Catz CS, Grave GD, Yaffe SJ. Workshop summary: fetal growth: its regulation and disorders. *Pediatrics* 1997;99:585-591.

140. Fanaroff AA, Wright LL, Stevenson DK. Very-low-birth-weight outcomes of the National Institute of Child Health and Human Development Neonatal Research Network, May 1991 through December 1992. *American Journal of Obstetrics and Gynecology* 1995;167:1499-1505.

141. Hales CN. Metabolic consequences of intrauterine growth retardation. *Acta Paediatrica Scandinavica Supplement* 1997;423:184-187.

142. Lucas A. Nutrition, growth and development of postdischarge, preterm infants. In: Hay WW, Jr., Lucas A, eds. Posthospital Nutrition in the Preterm Infant. Report of the 106th Ross Conference vol: Ross Laboratories, Columbus, OH; 1995:81-89.

143. Pardi G, Cetin I, Marconi AM et al. Diagnostic value of blood sampling in fetuses with growth retardation. *New England Journal of Medicine* 1993;328:692-696.

144. Glazier JD, Cetin I, Perugino G et al. Association between the activity of the system A amino acid transporter in the microvillous plasma membrane of the human placenta and severity of fetal compromise in intrauerine growth restriction. *Pediatric Research* 1997;42:514-519.

145. Marconi AM, Cetin I, Ferrazzi E, Ferrari MM, Pardi G, Battaglia FC. Lactate metabolism in normal and growth retarded human fetuses. *Pediatric Research* 1990;28:652-656.

146. Marconi A, Paolini C, Stramare L et al. Steady state maternal-fetal leucine enrichments in normal and intrauterine growth-restricted pregnancies. *Pediatric Research* 1999;46:114-119.

147. Pencharz PB, Masson M, Desgranges F, Papageorgiou A. Total-body protein turnover in human premature neonates: effects of birthweight, intra-uterine nutritional status and diet. *Clinical Science* 1981;61:207-215.

148. Cauderay M, Schutz Y, Micheli JL, Calame A, Jequier E. Energy-nitrogen balances and protein turnover in small and appropriate for gestational age low birthweight infants. *European Journal of Clinical Nutrition* 1988;42:125-136.

149. van Goudoever JB, Sulkers EJ, Halliday D et al. Whole body protein turnover in preterm appropriate for gestational age and small for gestational age infants: comparison of [15N]glycine and [1-13C]leucine administered simultaneously. *Pediatric Research* 1995;37:381-388.

150. Kandil H, Darwish O, Hammad S, Zagloul N, Halliday D, Millward J. Nitrogen balance and protein turnover during the growth failure in newly born low-birth-weight infants. *American Journal of Clinical Nutrition* 1991;53:1411-1417.

151. Chessex P, Reichman B, Verellen G et al. Metabolic consequences of intrauterine growth retardation in very-low-birth-weight infants. *Pediatric Research* 1984;18:709-713.

152. Sinclair JC, Silverman WA. Relative hypermetabolism in undergrown human neonates. *Lancet* 1964;2:49.

153. Holliday M, Potter D, Jarrah A, et al. Relation of metabolic rate to body weight and organ size. A review. *Journal of Physiology* 1967;199:685-703.

154. Yau K, Chang M. Growth and body composition of preterm, small-for-gestational-age infants at a postmenstrual age of 37-40 weeks. *Early Human Development* 1993;33:117-131.

155. Lucas A, Morley R, Cole TJ. Randomised trial of early diet in preterm babies and later intelligence quotient. *British Medical Journal* 1998;317:1481-1487.

156. Hediger M, Overpeck M, Maurer K, Kuczmarski R, McGlynn A, Davis W. Growth of infants and young children born small or large for gestational age: findings from the Third National Health and Nutrition Examination Survey. *Archives of Pediatrics & Adolescent Medicine* 1998;152:1225-1231.

157. Hediger M, Overpeck M, Kuczmarski R, McGlynn A, Maurer K, Davis W. Muscularity and fatness of infants and young children born small- or large-for-gestational-age. *Pediatrics* 1998;1025:e60.

158. Lucas A, Morely RM, Cole TJ, Gore SM. A randomised multicentre study of human milk versus formula and later development in preterm infants. *Archives of Disease in Childhood* 1994;70:F141-F146.

159. Lucas A, Morley R, Cole TJ, Lister G, Leeson-Payne C. Breast milk and subsequent intelligence quotient in children born preterm. *Lancet* 1992;339:261-264.

160. Brooke OG, Kinsey JM. High energy feeding in small for gestation infants. *Archives of Disease in Childhood* 1985;60:42-46.

161. Lucas A, Fewtrell MS, Davies PS, Bishop NJ, Clough H, Cole TJ. Breastfeeding and catch-up growth in infants born small for gestational age. *Acta Paediatrica Scandinavica* 1997;86:564-569.

162. Karlberg J, Albertsson-Wikland K, Baber FM, Low LC, Yeung CY. Born small for gestational age: consequences for growth. *Acta Paediatrica Scandinavica Supplement* 1996;417:8-13.

163. Albertsson-Wikland K, Karlberg J. Postnatal growth of children born small for gestational age. *Acta Paediatrica Scandinavica Supplement* 1997;423:193-195.

164. Kalhan SC, Denne SC. Energy consumption in infants with bronchopulmonary dysplasia. *J Pediatr* 1990;116:662-664.

165. Kurzner SI, Garg M, Bautitsa DB, Sargent CW, Bowman CM, Keens TG. Growth failure in bronchopulmonary dysplasia: elevated metabolic rates and pulmonary mechanics. *J Pediatr* 1988;112:73-80.

166. Kurzner SI, Garg M, Bautista DB, et al. Growth failure in infants with bronchopulmonary dysplasia: nutrition and elevated resting metabolic expenditure. *Pediatrics* 1988;81:379-384.

167. Wahlig TM, Gatto CW, Boros SJ, Mammel MC, Mills MM, Georgieff MK. Metabolic response of preterm infants to variable degrees of respiratory illness. *Journal of Pediatrics* 1994;124:283-288.

168. Rurak DW, Gruber NC. Increased oxygen consumption associated with breathing activity in fetal lambs. *Journal of Applied Physiology* 1983;54:701-707.

169. Van Aerde JEE, Sauer PJJ, Pencharz PB, Smith JM, Swyer PR. Effect of replacing glucose with lipid on the energy metabolism of newborn infants. *Clinical Science* 1989;76:581-588.

170. Pereira GR, Baumgart S, Bennet MJ, et al. High fat formula for premature infants with bronchopulmonary dysplasia; metabolic, pulmonary, and nutritional studies. *Journal of Pediatrics* 1994;124:605-611.

171. Piedboeuf B, Chessex P, Hazan J, Pineault M, Lavoie JC. Total parenteral nutrition in the newborn infant: energy substrates and respiratory gas exchange. *Journal of Pediatrics* 1991;118:97-102.

172. Rodriguez JL, Askanazi J, Weissman C, Hensle TW, Rosenbaum SH, Kinney JM. Ventilatory and metabolic effects of glucose infusions. *Chest* 1985;88:512-518.

173. Chessex P, Gagne G, Pineault M, Vaucher J, Bisaillon S, G.B. Metabolic and clinical consequences of changing from high-glucose to high-fat regimens in parenterally fed newborn infants. *Journal of Pediatrics* 1989;115:992-997.

174. Yunis KA, Oh W. Effects of intravenous glucose loading on oxygen consumption, carbon dioxide production, and resting energy expenditure in infants with bronchopulmonary dysplasia. *J Pediatr* 1989;115: 127-132.

175. Chessex P, Belanger S, Piedboeuf B, Pineault M. Influence of energy substrates on respiratory gas exchange during conventional mechanical ventilation of preterm infants. *Journal of Pediatrics* 1995;126:619-624.

176. Pineault M, Chessex P, Bisaillon S, Brisson G. Total parenteral nutrition in the newborn: impact of the quality of infused energy on nitrogen metabolism. *Am J Clin Nutr* 1988;47:298-304.

177. Van Aerde JE, Sauer PJ, Pencharz PB, Smith JM, Heim T, Swyer PR. Metabolic consequences of increasing energy intake by adding lipid to parenteral nutrition in full-term infants. *Am J Clin Nutr* 1994;59:659-62.

178. Friedman Z, Frolich JC. Essential fatty acids and the major urinary metabolites of the E prostaglandins in thriving neonates and in infants receiving parenteral fat emulsion. *Pediatr Res* 1979;13:932-936.

179. Levene MI, Wigglesworth JS, Desai R. Pulmonary fat accumulation after Intralipid infusion in the preterm infant. *Lancet* 1980;2:815-818.

180. Dahms BB, Halpin TC. Pulmonary arterial lipid desposit in newborn infants receiving infusion in the very-low-birth-weight infant. *Journal of Pediatrics* 1980;97:800.

181. Hertel J, Tygstrup I, Anderson EE. Intravascular fat accumulation after Intralipid infusion in the very-low-birth-weight infant. *Journal of Pediatrics* 1982;100:975-976.

182. Schroder H, Paust H, Schmidt R. Pulmonary fat embolism after Intralipid therapy–a post-mortem artifact? Light and electron microscopic investigations in low-birth-weight infants. *Acta Paediatrica Scandinavica* 1984;73:461-464.

183. Allardyce DB. The postmortem interval as a factor in fat embolism. *Arch Pathol* 1971;92:248.

184. Stahl GE, Spear ML, Hamosh M. Physiologic effects of lipid infusions. In: Polin RA, Fox WW, eds. *Fetal and Neonatal Physiology.* 1 vol. 2nd ed. Philadelphia: W.B. Saunders Co.; 1998:514-527.

185. Kimura T, Toung JK, Margolis S, Permutt S, Cameron JL. Respiratory failure in acute pancreatitis: a possible role for triglycerides. *Ann Surg* 1979; 189:509-514.

186. Kimura T, Toung JK, Margolis S, Bell W, Cameron JL. Respiratory failure in acute pancreatitis: the role of free fatty acids. *Surgery* 1980;87:509-513.

187. Ali J, Wood LD. Does increased pulmonary blood flow redistribute towards edematous lung units? *J Surg Res* 1983;35:188-194.

188. Ali J, Wood LD. Pulmonary vascular effects of furosemide on gas exchange in pulmonary edema. *J Appl Physiol* 1984;57:160-167.

189. Breen PH, Schumacker PT, Hedenstierna G, Ali J, Wagner PD, Wood LD. How does increased cardiac output increase shunt in pulmonary edema? *J Appl Physiol* 1982;53:1273-1280.

190. Derks CM, Jacobvitz-Derks D. Embolic pneumopathy induced by oleic acid: a systematic morphologic study. *Am J Pathol* 1977;87:143-158.

191. Grossman RF, Jones JG, Murray JF. Effects of oleic acid-induced pulmonary edema on lung mechanics. *J Appl Physiol* 1980;48:1045-1051.

192. Ali J, Wood LD. The acute effects of Intralipid on lung function. *J Surg Res* 1985;38:599-605.

193. Hyman AL, Spannhake EW, Kadowitz PJ. Prostaglandins and the lung. *Am Rev Respir Dis* 1978;117:111-136.

194. Wooley PVI, Hunter MJ. Binding and circular dichroism data on bilirubin-albumin in the presence of oleate and salicylate. *Arch Biochem Biophys* 1970;140:197.

195. Hwang DH, Carroll AE. Decreased formation of prostaglandins derived from arachidonic acid by dietary linolenate in rats. *Am J Clin Nutr* 1980;33:590-597.

196. Seyberth HW, Oelz O, Kennedy T, et al. Increased arachidonate in lipids after administration to man: effects on prostaglandin biosynthesis. *Clin Pharmacol* 1975;18:521-529.

197. Wicks TC, Rose JC, Johnson M, Ramwell PW, Kot PA. Vascular responses to arachidonic acid in the perfused canine lung. *Circ Res* 1976;38:167-171.

198. Wiberg T, Vaage J, Bjertnaes L, Hauge A, Gautvik KM. Prostaglandin content in blood and lung tissue during alveolar hypoxia. *Acta Physiol Scand* 1978;102:181-190.

199. Hyman AL, Spannhake EW, Kadowitz PJ. Divergent responses to arachidonic acid in the feline pulmonary vascular bed. *Am J Physiol* 1980;239:H40-H46.

200. Spannhake EW, Hyman AL, Kadowitz PJ. Dependence of the airway and pulmonary vascular effects of arachidonic acid upon route and rate of administration. *J Pharmacol Exp Ther* 1980;212:584-590.

201. McKeen CR, Brigham KL, Bowers RE, Harris TR. Pulmonary vascular effects of fat emulsion infusion in unanesthetized sheep. Prevention by indomethacin. *J Clin Invest* 1978;61:1291-1297.

202. Inwood RJ, Gora P, Hunt CE. Indomethacin inhibition of Intralipid-induced lung dysfunction. *Prostaglandins Med* 1981;6:503-514.

203. Hunt CE, Gora P, Inwood RJ. Pulmonary effects of Intralipid: the role of Intralipid as a prostaglandin

precursor. *Prog Lipid Res* 1981;20:199-204.

204. Hageman JR, McCulloch K, Gora P, Olsen EK, Pachman L, Hunt CE. Intralipid alterations in pulmonary prostaglandin metabolism and gas exchange. *Critical Care Medicine* 1983;10:794-798.

205. Gurtner GH, Knoblauch A, Smith PL, Sies H, Adkinson NF. Oxidant- and lipid-induced pulmonary vasoconstriction mediated by arachidonic acid metabolites. *American Journal of Physiology* 1983;55: 949-954.

206. Teague WGJ, Raj JU, Braun D, Berner ME, Clyman RI, Bland RD. Lung vascular effects of lipid infusion in awake lambs. *Pediatr Res* 1987;22:714-719.

207. Sosenko IRS, Innis SM, Frank L. Polyunsaturated fatty acids and protection of newborn rats from oxygen toxicity. *J Pediatr* 1988;112:630-637.

208. Sosenko IR, Innis SM, Frank L. Intralipid increases lung polyunsaturated fatty acids and protects newborn rats from oxygen toxicity. *Pediatr Res* 1991;30:413-417.

209. Dennery PA, Kramer CM, Alpert SE. Effect of fatty acid profiles on the susceptibility of cultures of rabbit tracheal epithelial cells to hyperoxic injury. *Am J Respir Cell Mol Biol* 1990;3:137-144.

210. Spitz DR, Kinter MT, Kehrer JP, Roberts RJ. The effect of monosaturated and polyunsaturated fatty acids on oxygen toxicity in cultured cells. *Pediatr Res* 1992;32: 366-372.

211. Helbock HJ, Motchnik PA, Ames BN. Toxic hydroperoxides in intravenous lipid emulsions used in preterm infants. *Pediatrics* 1993;91:83-87.

212. Pitkanen O, Hallman M, Anderson S. Generation of free radicals in lipid emulsion used in parenteral nutrition. *Pediatric Research* 1991;29:56-59.

213. Brans YW, Dutton EB, Andrew DS, Menchaca EM, West DL. Fat emulsion tolerance in very-low-birth-weight neonates: Effect on diffusion of oxygen in the lungs and on blood pH. *Pediatrics* 1986;78:79-84.

214. Adamkin DH, Gelke KN, Wilkerson SA. Clinical and laboratory observations; influence of intravenous fat therapy on tracheal effluent phospholipids and oxygenation in severe respiratory distress syndrome. *Journal of Pediatrics* 1985;106:122-124.

215. Weinstein MR, Oh W. Oxygen consumption in infants with bronchopulmonary dysplasia.

Journal of Pediatrics 1981;99:958-961.

216. Van Aerde JEE. Acute respiratory failure and bronchopulmonary dysplasia. In: Hay WW, Jr., ed. *Neonatal Nutrition and Metabolism.* St. Louis: Mosby-Year Book, Inc.; 1991:476-506.

217. Tyson J, LL W, Oh W et al. Vitamin A supplementation for extremely-low-birth-weight infants. *New England Journal of Medicine* 1999;340:1962-1968.

218. Van Aerde JE, Sauer R, Heim T, Smith J, Swyer P. Is bountiful nutrient intake beneficial for the orally fed very-low-birth-weight infant? *Pediatr Res* 1988;23:427A.

219. Kao LC, Durand DJ, Nickerson BG. Improving pulmonary function does not decrease oxygen consumption in infants with bronchopulmonary dysplasia. *J Pediatr* 1988;112:616-621.

220. Roussos C, Macklem PT. The respiratory muscles. *New England Journal of Medicine* 1982;307:786-797.

221. Yeh TF, McClenan DA, Ayahi OA, Pildes RS. Metabolic rate and energy balance in infants with bronchopulmonary dysplasia. *J Pediatr* 1989;114:448-451.

222. Brown E, Stark A, Sosenko I, Lawson EE, Avery ME. Bronchopulmonary dysplasia: possible relationship to pulmonary edema. *J Pediatr* 1978;92:982-984.

223. Van Marter LJ, Leviton A, Allred EN, Pagano M, Kuban KCK. Hydration during the first days of life and the risk of bronchopulmonary dysplasia in low-birth-weight infants. *J Pediatr* 1990;116:942-949.

224. Groothuis J, Rosenberg A. Home oxygen promotes weight gain in infants with bronchopulmonary dysplasia. *Am J Dis Child* 1987;141:992-995.

225. Milley JR. Ovine fetal leucine kinetics and protein metabolism during decreased oxygen availability. *American Journal of Physiology* 1998;274:E618-E626.

226. Green LR, Kawagoe Y, Hill. D J, Richardson BS, Han VK. The effect of intermittent umbilical cord occlusion on insulin-like growth factors and their binding proteins in preterm and near-term ovine fetuses. *Journal of Endocrinology* 2000;166:565-577.

227. Van Aerde JE, Sauer PJ, Heim T et al. Effect of increasing glucose loads on respiratory exchange in the newborn infant. *Pediatr Res* 1986;20:420A.

228. Nose O, Tipton JR, Ament ME, Yabuuchi J. Effect of the energy source on changes in energy expenditure,

respiratory quotient and nitrogen balance during total parenteral nutrition in children. *Pediatric Research* 1987;21:538-541.

229. Heim T, Putet G, Verellen G, et al. Energy cost of intravenous alimentation in the newborn infant. In: Stern L, Salle B, Friis-Hansen B, eds. *Intensive Care in the Newborn III.* New York: Masson Publishing; 1981:219-238.

230. Heymsfield SB, Erbland M, Casper K et al. Enteral nutritional support: metabolic, cardiovascular, and pulmonary interrelations. *Clin Chest Med* 1986;7: 41-67.

231. Heymsfield SB, Head CA, McManus CB, Seitz S, Staton GW, Grossman GD. Respiratory, cardiovascular and metabolic effects of enteral hyperalimentation: influence of formula dose and composition. *American Journal of Clinical Nutrition* 1984;40:116-130.

232. Kashyap S, Forsyth M, Zucker C, Ramakrishnan R, Dell RB, Heird WC. Effects of varying protein and every intakes on growth and metabolic response in low-birth-weight infants. *Journal of Pediatrics* 1986;108:955-963.

233. Fitzgerald MJ, Goto M, Myers TF, Zeller WP. Early metabolic effects of sepsis in the preterm infant: Lactic acidosis and increased glucose requirement. *Journal of Pediatrics* 1992;121:951-955.

234. Leake RD, Fiser RH, Oh W. Rapid glucose disappearance in infants with infection. *Clinical Pediatrics* 1981;20:397-401.

235. Park W, Paust H, Brosicke H, Knoblach G, Helge H. Impaired fat utilization in parenterally fed low-birth-weight infants suffering from sepsis. *Journal of Parenteral and Enteral Nutrition* 1986;10:627-630.

236. Mrozek JD, Georgieff MK, Blazar BR, Mammel MC, Schwarzenberg SJ. Effect of sepsis syndrome on neonatal protein and energy metabolism. *Journal of Perinatology* 2000;20:96-100.

Appendix 1 - Nutrient Composition of Infant Formulas

Preterm Infant Formulas

Manufacturer:		Bristol-Myers Squibb Mead Johnson						Ross Laboratories			Wyeth	Nestle		Milupa		Humana		
		Enfamil Premature LIPIL	Enfalac Premature/Enfamil A+ Premature/Enfamil Premature Premium	Enfamil/Enfalac Premature LCPUFA Formula (Powder)	Enfamil/Enfalac Premature Formula (Powder)	Enfalac Premature Formula	EnfaCARE LIPIL (RTU) (Powder)	Similac Special Care	Similac NeoSure	Similac Natural Care	S-26 LBW RTF	Aletemil Premature Formula (Powder)	Bebe Premature Formula	Aptamil Prematil (Powder)	Aptamil Prematil HA (Powder)	Humana 0	Humana 0-HA (Powder)	Humana 0-VLB
Mass of powder prod	g	.*	-	20.4	20.4	-	19.1	-	-	-	-	19.96	-	19.25	19.25	-	20	-
Volume, 20 kcal/fl.oz.	mL	148	148	148	148	148	-	148	-	-	-	-	-	-	-	-	-	-
Volume, 22 kcal/fl.oz.	mL	-	-	-	-	-	135	-	134	-	-	-	-	-	-	133	133	133
Volume, 24 kcal/fl.oz.	mL	124	124	124	124	124	-	124	-	124	125	125	125	125	125	-	-	-
Water, 20 kcal/fl.oz.	mL	134	134	135	135	133	-	133	-	-	-	-	-	-	-	-	-	-
Water, 22 kcal/fl.oz.	mL	-	-	-	-	-	120	-	120	-	-	-	-	-	-	-	115	-
Water, 24 kcal/fl.oz.	mL	108	108	109	108	108	-	109	-	109	109	112	112	113	113	-	-	-
Energy	kcal	100	100	100	100	100	100	100	100	100	100	100	100	100	100	100	100	100
Protein	g	3	3	3	3	3	2.8	2.71	2.6	2.71	2.4	2.9	2.89	3	3	2.67	2.67	3.07
Carbohydrate	g	11	11	11	11.1	11.1	10.4	10.6	10.3	10.6	10.5	10.7	10.7	9.75	9.63	10.4	10.4	10
Lactose	g	4.4	4.5	5.3	4.7	4.5	4.1	5.3	5.15	5.3	5.25	6.95	6.95	7.5	6	7.33	7.33	3.33
Glucose Oligomer	g	6.5	6.4	5.7	6.4	6.5	6.2	5.3	5.15	5.3	5.25	3.75	3.75	2.05	3.67	3.07	3.07	6.67
Fat	g	5.1	5.1	5.1	5.1	5.1	5.3	5.43	5.5	5.43	5.4	5.19	5.19	5.5	5.5	5.33	5.33	5.33
MCT oil	%	40	38	38	40	40	20	50	25	50	11.5	30	30			25	25	25
Linoleic	mg	810	810	810	1170	1000	950	700	750	700	670	740	740	1	2.5	750	750	1000
alpha-Linolenic	mg	90	110	110	90	130	95				82	80	79.8			80	76	85
Arachidonic	mg	34	34	34			34				31					10.7		
Docosahexaenoic	mg	17	17	17			17				21					10.7	10.7	10.7
Vitamin A	IU	1250	1250	500	390	1250	450	1250	460	1250	366	367	352	467	625	311	312	311
Vitamin D	IU	240	240	100	63	270	80	150	70	150	73	104	104	120	120	88	88	88
Vitamin E	IU	6.3	6.3	6.3	2.5	6.3	4	4	3.6	4	2.2	1.8	1.8	3.75	3.75	1.33	1.34	1.33
Vitamin K	ug	8	14	8	9	8	8	12	11	12	9.8	8	8	7.5	9.63	8	8	8
Ascorbate	mg	20	20	20	19	20	16	37	15	37	13	16	16	20	20	15	15	15.1
Thiamin	ug	200	200	200	79	200	200	250	220	250	146	70	70	175	175	93	93	93
Riboflavin	ug	300	300	300	160	300	200	620	150	620	245	150	150	250	250	173	174	173
Pyridoxine	ug	150	150	150	75	150	100	250	100	250	88	76	76	150	150	107	107	107
Niacin	ug	4000	4000	4000	1200	4000	2000	5000	1950	5000	1610	1000	1000	3000	3750	2267	2270	1800
Pantothenate	ug	1200	1200	1200	460	1200	850	1900	800	1900	549	460	460	1250	1250	800	800	800
Biotin	ug	4	4	4	3	4	6	37	9	37	2.9	2.2	2.2	3.75	5.6	6.67	6.67	6.67
Folate	ug	40	40	40	36	40	26	37	25	37	59	70	70	60	43	40	40	40
Vitamin B12	ug	0.25	0.25	0.25	0.5	0.25	0.3	0.55	0.4	0.55	0.37	0.3	0.3	0.25	0.25	0.23	0.23	0.23
Sodium	mg	58	58	58	40	58	35	43	33	43	43	42	42	50	60	40	40	40
Potassium	mg	98	100	100	130	100	105	129	142	129	104	120	120	100	100	125	125	133
Chloride	mg	90	85	85	85	85	78	81	75	81	73	64	64	60	59	85	85	85
Calcium	mg	165	165	120	120	165	120	180	105	210	98	124	124	125	112.5	133	133	133
Phosphorus	mg	83	83	66	66	83	66	100	62	116	52	68	68	62.5	59	75	75	75
Magnesium	mg	9	9	9	12	9	8	12	9	12	9.8	10.4	10.4	12.5	12.5	10.7	10.7	10.7
Iron, low iron form	mg	0.5	0.5	0.5	0.2	0.25		0.4		0.37				1.13	1.13	1.47	1.5	1.47
Iron, with iron form	mg	1.8	1.8			1.8	1.8	1.8	1.8		1	1.5	1.5	0.88	0.88	1.11	1.11	1.11
Zinc	mg	1.5	1.5	1	1	1.5	1.25	1.5	1.2	1.5	1	0.8	0.8	0.88	0.88			
Copper	ug	120	120	120	120	121	120	250	120	250	90	100	100	100	100	93	93	147
Selenium	ug	2.8	2	2	2	2	2.8	1.8	2.3	1.8						4	4	13.3
Chromium	ug	0.2	0.2	0.2	0.2	0.2	0.2											
Manganese	ug	6.3	8	6.3	37	6.3	15	12	10	12	7.5	10	8	12.5	13	53	53	67
Molybdenum	ug	0.4	0.25	0.25	0.25	2	0.25									6	6	11.3
Iodine	ug	25	25	25	15	25	21	6	15	6	10	26	26	17.5	25	14	14	14.7
Taurine	mg	6	6	6	6	6	6				5.7				7.5			
Carnitine	mg	2.4	2	2	-	2	2					2.2	2.2	2.5	2.5	1.6	1.6	1.87
Inositol	mg	44	45	45	6	45	30	5.5	6	5.5	5.5	6.6	6.6	37.5		4.3	4.3	4
Choline	mg	20	18	18	12	18	24	10	16	10	16	15	15	12.5	26	7.5	7.5	7.33
AMP**	mg	0.5					0.5											
CMP	mg	2.5					2.5											
GMP	mg	0.3					0.3											
UMP	mg	0.9					0.9											

All values are in units per 100 kcal.

All product forms are liquid, ready-to-use (RTU) formulations except where "powder" is indicated

Missing values were either not specified, not available, or not applicable

* A dash (-) indicates this value is not relevant

** AMP = adenosine monophosphate; CMP = cytidine monophosphate; GMP = guanosine monophosphate; UMP = uridine monophosphate

Appendix 2 - Human Milk Fortifiers

		Amounts per 100 kcal						Amounts Added to 100 mL Milk						Amounts per 100 mL Mixed as Directed						
		Mead Johnson Enfamil Human Milk Fortifier (Powder)	Ross Similac Natural Care (Liquid)	Ross Similac Human Milk Fortifier (Powder)	Wyeth S-26 SMA HMF (Powder)	Nestle FM 85 Human Milk Fortifier (Powder)	Milupa Aptamil FMS Human Milk Fortifier (Powder)	Mead Johnson Enfamil Human Milk Fortifier (Powder)	Ross Similac Natural Care (Liquid)	Ross Similac Human Milk Fortifier (Powder)	Wyeth S-26 SMA HMF (Powder)	Nestle FM 85 Human Milk Fortifier (Powder)	Milupa Aptamil FMS Human Milk Fortifier (Powder)	Preterm Human Milk	Mead Johnson Enfamil Human Milk Fortifier (Powder)	Ross Similac Natural Care (Liquid)	Ross Similac Human Milk Fortifier (Powder)	Wyeth S-26 SMA HMF (Powder)	Nestle FM 85 Human Milk Fortifier (Powder)	Milupa Aptamil FMS Human Milk Fortifier (Powder)
Mass of powder produce	g	20.6	-	25.7	27.4	28	28.9	2.9	-	3.6	4	5	3	-	2.9	-	3.6	4	5	3
Volume, 20 kcal/fl.oz.	mL	-*	-	-	-	-	-	-	-	-	-	-	-	100	-	-	-	-	-	-
Volume, 22 kcal/fl.oz.	mL	-	-	-	-	-	-	-	-	-	-	-	-	-	-	-	-	-	-	-
Volume, 24 kcal/fl.oz.	mL	-	124	-	-	-	-	-	100	-	-	-	-	-	-	100	-	-	-	-
Water, 20 kcal/fl.oz.	mL	-	-	-	-	-	-	-	-	-	-	-	-	-	-	-	-	-	-	-
Water, 22 kcal/fl.oz.	mL	-	-	-	-	-	-	-	-	-	-	-	-	-	-	-	-	-	-	-
Water, 24 kcal/fl.oz.	mL	-	109	-	-	-	-	-	88	-	-	-	-	-	-	-	-	-	-	-
Energy	kcal	100	100	100	100	100	100	14	81	14.0	14.6	17.9	10.4	68	80.8	74.5	80.6	81.0	83.8	77.2
Protein	g	8.1	2.71	7.14	6.8	4.68	6.88	1.13	2.2	1.0	1	0.84	0.71	1.62	2.7	1.9	2.6	2.6	2.4	2.3
Carbohydrate	g	1.6	10.6	12.86	15.8	20.2	18.87	0.23	8.6	1.8	2.3	3.6	1.96	7.3	7.4	8.0	8.9	9.4	10.6	9.1
Lactose	g	0.1	5.3		7.9		0.32		4.3		1.15		0.03	7.3	7.2	5.8	7.2	8.3	7.1	7.2
Glucose Oligomer	g	0.3	5.3		7.9		16.53		4.3		1.15		1.72		0.0	2.2	0.0	1.1	0.0	1.7
Fat	g	7.4	5.43	2.57	1.0	0.08	0	1.03	4.4	0.36	0.15	0.01	0	3.5	4.5	4.0	3.8	3.6	3.4	3.4
MCT oil	%	70	50					70	40.5					-0	16	23	0	0	0	0
Linoleic	mg	1000	700					140	567					480	611	524	472	471	468	473
alpha-Linolenic	mg	121						17						30	46	15	29	29	29	30
Arachidonic	mg													20	20	10	20	20	20	20
Docosahexaenoic	mg													10	10	5	10	10	10	10
Vitamin A	IU	6800	1250	4429	6164		4133	950	1013	620	900		429	48	984	531	656	929	47	470
Vitamin D	IU	1070	150	857	2055		1931	150	122	120	300		200	8	156	65	126	302	8	205
Vitamin E	IU	33	4	23	31		25	4.6	3.2	3.2	4.5		2.6	0.39	4.9	1.8	3.5	4.8	0.4	2.9
Vitamin K	ug	31	12	59	75		61	4.4	9.7	8.3	11		6.3	2	6.3	5.9	10.1	12.7	2.0	8.2
Ascorbate	mg	86	37	179	274		116	12	30	25	40		12	4.4	16	17	29	44	4	16
Thiamin	ug	1070	250	1664	1541		1240	150	200	233	225		129	8.9	157	104	238	229	9	136
Riboflavin	ug	1570	620	2979	1712		1650	220	500	417	250		171	27	243	264	436	272	26	195
Pyridoxine	ug	820	250	1507	1712		1070	115	200	211	250		111	6.2	119	103	213	251	6	115
Niacin	ug	21400	5000	25500	23973		24080	3000	4000	3576	3500		2500	210	3164	2105	3719	3637	205	2670
Pantothenate	ug	5200	1900	10714	6164		7230	730	1540	1502	900		750	230	946	885	1701	1108	224	966
Biotin	ug	19.3	7	186	10.3		24	2.7	30	26.00	1.5		2.5	0.54	3.2	15.3	26.1	2.0	0.5	3.0
Folate	ug	179	37	164	205		483	25	30	23	30		50	3.1	27.7	16.6	25.6	32.5	3.0	52.3
Vitamin B12	ug	1.29	0.55	5	2.1		1.9	0.18	0.45	1	0.3		0.2	0.02	0.20	0.24	0.65	0.31	0.02	0.22
Sodium	mg	79	43	107	123	150	60	16	35	15	18	26.8	6.2	28	43	32	42	45	53	34
Potassium	mg	143	129	450	185	64.4	38	29	105	63	27	11.5	3.98	50	78	78	111	75	60	53
Chloride	mg	64	81	271	116	104	68	13	66	38	17	18.6	7.1	58	70	62	94	74	75	64
Calcium	mg	640	210	836	616	286	590	90	170	117	90	51.1	61	25	113	98	139	113	74	85
Phosphorus	mg	360	116	479	308	190	393	50	94	67	45	33.9	41	14.5	64	54	80	58	47	55
Magnesium	mg	7.1	12	50	21	11.2	58	1	9.7	7	3	2	60	3.3	4.5	6.5	10.1	6.2	5.2	62.4
Iron, low iron formula	mg		0.37	3					0.3				0	0.09	0.1	0.2	0.1	0.1	0.1	0.1
Iron, with iron formula	mg	10.3						1.44					-	0.09	1.5	0.0	0.1	0.1	0.1	0.1
Zinc	mg	5.1	1.5	7	1.7		2.95	0.72	1.22	1.0	0.25		0.31	0.37	1.07	0.80	1.35	0.61	0.36	0.67
Copper	ug	310	250	1214			246	44	200	170			26	38	81	119	204	37	37	63
Selenium	ug		1.8	4					1.46					2.4	2.4	1.9	2.4	2.4	2.3	2.4
Chromium	ug													-	-	-	-	-	-	-
Manganese	ug	71	12	51	31		58	10	9.7	7	4.5		6	0.36	10.2	5.0	7.2	4.8	0.4	6.3
Molybdenum	ug													-	-	-	-	-	-	-
Iodine	ug	-	6				106		4.9				11	17.8	17.5	11.4	17.5	17.5	17.4	28.4
Taurine	mg													4	3.9	2.0	3.9	3.9	3.9	3.9
Carnitine	mg													0.7	0.7	0.4	0.7	0.7	0.7	0.7
Inositol	mg		5.5	28					4.5	3.9										
Choline	mg		10	13					8.1	1.8										

* A dash (-) indicates this value is not relevant

Missing values were not specified, not available, or not applicable

Appendix 3 - Summary of Reasonable Nutrient Intakes (mass units) for Preterm Infants

		ELBW				VLBW			
		Day 0*	Transition**	Growing		Day 0*	Transition**	Growing	
		per kg/day	per kg/day	per kg/day	per 100 Cal***	per kg/day	per kg/day	per kg/day	per 100 Cal***
Energy	Parenteral	40-50	75-85	105-115	100	40-50	60-70	90-100	100
Cal	Enteral	50-60	90-100	130-150	100	50-60	75-90	110-130	100
FluidsΔ	Parenteral	90-120	90-140	140-180	122-171	70-90	90-140	120-160	120-178
mL	Enteral	90-120	90-140	160-220	107-169	70-90	90-140	135-190	104-173
Protein	Parenteral	2	3.5	3.5-4	3.0-3.8	2	3.5	3.2-3.8	3.2-4.2
g	Enteral	2	3.5	3.8-4.4	2.5-3.4	2	3.5	3.4-4.2	2.6-3.8
Carbohydrate	Parenteral	7	8-15	13-17	11.3-16.2	7	5-12	9.7-15	9.7-16.7
g	Enteral	7	8-15	9-20	6.0-15.4	7	5-12	7-17	5.4-15.5
Fat	Parenteral	1	1-3	3-4	2.6-3.8	1	1-3	3-4	3.0-4.4
g	Enteral	1	1-3	6.2-8.4	4.1-6.5	1	1-3	5.3-7.2	4.1-6.5
Linoleic acid	Parenteral	110	110-340	340-800	296-762	110	110-340	340-800	340-889
mg	Enteral	110	110-340	700-1680	467-1,292	110	110-340	600-1440	462-1,309
Linoleate:Linolenate		5-15	5-15	5-15	5-15	5-15	5-15	5-15	5-15
Docosahexaenoic acid	Parenteral	>=4	>=4	>=11	>=10	>=4	>=4	>=11	>=12
mg	Enteral	>=4	>=4	>=21	>=16	>=4	>=4	>=18	>=16
Arachidonic acid	Parenteral	>=5	>=5	>=14	>=13	>=5	>=5	>=14	>=16
mg	Enteral	>=5	>=5	>=28	>=22	>=5	>=5	>=24	>=22
Sodium	Parenteral	0-23	46-115	69-115 (161†)	60-110	0-23	46-115	69-115 (161†)	69-128
mg	Enteral	0-23	46-115	69-115 (161†)	46-88	0-23	46-115	69-115 (161†)	53-105
Potassium	Parenteral	0	0-78	78-117	68-111	0	0-78	78-117	78-130
mg	Enteral	0	0-78	78-117	52-90	0	0-78	78-117	60-106
Chloride	Parenteral	0-35.5	71-178	107-249	93-237	0-35.5	71-178	107-249	107-277
mg	Enteral	0-35.5	71-178	107-249	71-192	0-35.5	71-178	107-249	82-226
Calcium	Parenteral⊕	20-60	60	60-80	52-76	20-60	60	60-80	60-89
mg	Enteral	33-100	100	100-220	67-169	33-100	100	100-220	77-200
Phosphorus	Parenteral⊕	0♦	45-60	45-60	39-57	0♦	45-60	45-60	45-67
mg	Enteral	20-60	60-140	60-140	40-108	20-60	60-140	60-140	46-127
Magnesium	Parenteral	0	4.3-7.2	4.3-7.2	3.7-6.9	0	4.3-7.2	4.3-7.2	4.3-8.0
mg	Enteral	2.5-8	7.9-15	7.9-15	5.3-11.5	2.5-8	7.9-15	7.9-15	6.1-13.6
Iron	Parenteral	0	0	100-200	87-190	0	0	100-200	100-222
µg	Enteral	0	0	2000-4000	1,333-3,077	0	0	2000-4000	1,538-3,636
Zinc	Parenteral	0-150	150	400	348-381	0-150	150	400	400-444
µg	Enteral	0-1000	400-1200	1000-3000	667-2,308	0-1000	400-1200	1000-3000	769-2,727
Copper	Parenteral	0	≤20	20	17-19	0	≤20	20	20-22
µg	Enteral	0	≤150	120-150	80-115	0	≤150	120-150	92-136
Selenium	Parenteral	0	≤1.3	1.5-4.5	1.3-4.3	0	≤1.3	1.5-4.5	1.5-5.0
µg	Enteral	0	≤1.3	1.3-4.5	0.9-3.5	0	≤1.3	1.3-4.5	1.0-4.1
Chromium	Parenteral	0	≤0.05	0.05-0.3	0.04-0.29	0	≤0.05	0.05-0.3	0.05-0.33
µg	Enteral	0	≤0.1	0.1-2.25	0.07-1.73	0	≤0.1	0.1-2.25	0.08-2.05
Molybdenum	Parenteral	0	0	0.25	0.22-0.24	0	0	0.25	0.25-0.28
µg	Enteral	0	0	0.3	0.20-0.23	0	0	0.3	0.23-0.27
Manganese	Parenteral	0	≤0.75	1	0.87-0.95	0	≤0.75	1	1.00-1.11
µg	Enteral	0	≤7.5	0.7-7.5	0.5-5.8	0	≤7.5	0.7-7.5	0.5-6.8
Iodine	Parenteral	0	≤1	1	0.87-0.95	0	≤1	1	1.00-1.11
µg	Enteral	0	≤60	10-60	6.7-46.2	0	≤60	10-60	7.7-54.5
Vitamin A	Parenteral	700-1500	700-1500	700-1500	609-1,429	700-1500	700-1500	700-1500	700-1,667
IU	Enteral	700-1500	700-1500	700-1500	467-1,154	700-1500	700-1500	700-1500	538-1,364
Vitamin D	Parenteral◊	40-160	40-160	40-160	35-152	40-160	40-160	40-160	40-178
IU	Enteral◊◊	150-400	150-400	150-400	100-308	150-400	150-400	150-400	115-364
Vitamin E	Parenteral▲	2.8-3.5	2.8-3.5	2.8-3.5	2.4-3.3	2.8-3.5	2.8-3.5	2.8-3.5	2.8-3.9
IU	Enteral	6-12	6-12	6-12	4.0-9.2	6-12	6-12	6-12	4.6-10.9
Vitamin K	Parenteral	500 im/child	10	10	8.7-9.5	1000 im/child	10	10	10.0-11.1
µg	Enteral	500 im/child	8-10	8-10	5.3-7.7	1000 im/child	8-10	8-10	6.2-9.1
Thiamin	Parenteral	200-350	200-350	200-350	174-333	200-350	200-350	200-350	200-389
µg	Enteral	180-240	180-240	180-240	120-185	180-240	180-240	180-240	138-218
Riboflavin	Parenteral	150-200	150-200	150-200	130-190	150-200	150-200	150-200	150-222
µg	Enteral	250-360	250-360	250-360	167-277	250-360	250-360	250-360	192-327
Niacin	Parenteral	4-6.8	4-6.8	4-6.8	3.5-6.5	4-6.8	4-6.8	4-6.8	4.0-7.6
mg	Enteral	3.6-4.8	3.6-4.8	3.6-4.8	2.4-3.7	3.6-4.8	3.6-4.8	3.6-4.8	2.8-4.4
Vitamin B6	Parenteral	150-200	150-200	150-200	130-190	150-200	150-200	150-200	150-222
µγ	Enteral	150-210	150-210	150-210	100-162	150-210	150-210	150-210	115-191

Appendix 3 - Summary of Reasonable Nutrient Intakes (mass units) for Preterm Infants *(cont.)*

		ELBW				VLBW			
		Day 0* per kg/day	Transition** per kg/day	Growing per kg/day	Growing per 100 Cal***	Day 0* per kg/day	Transition** per kg/day	Growing per kg/day	Growing per 100 Cal***
Folate	Parenteral	56	56	56	49-53	56	56	56	56-62
µg	Enteral	25-50	25-50	25-50	17-38	25-50	25-50	25-50	19-45
Vitamin B12	Parenteral	0.3	0.3	0.3	0.26-0.29	0.3	0.3	0.3	0.30-0.33
µg	Enteral	0.3	0.3	0.3	0.20-0.23	0.3	0.3	0.3	0.23-0.27
Pantothenic acid	Parenteral	1-2	1-2	1-2	0.9-1.9	1-2	1-2	1-2	1.0-2.2
mg	Enteral	1.2-1.7	1.2-1.7	1.2-1.7	0.8-1.3	1.2-1.7	1.2-1.7	1.2-1.7	0.9-1.5
Biotin	Parenteral	5-8	5-8	5-8	4.3-7.6	5-8	5-8	5-8	5.0-8.9
µg	Enteral	3.6-6	3.6-6	3.6-6	2.4-4.6	3.6-6	3.6-6	3.6-6	2.8-5.5
Vitamin C	Parenteral	15-25	15-25	15-25	13.0-23.8	15-25	15-25	15-25	15.0-27.8
mg	Enteral	18-24	18-24	18-24	12.0-18.5	18-24	18-24	18-24	13.8-21.8
Taurine	Parenteral	0-3.75	1.88-3.75	1.88-3.75	1.6-3.6	0-3.75	1.88-3.75	1.88-3.75	1.9-4.2
mg	Enteral	0-9	4.5-9.0	4.5-9.0	3.0-6.9	0-9	4.5-9.0	4.5-9.0	3.5-8.2
Carnitine	Parenteral	0-2.9	~2.9	~2.9	~2.5-2.8	0-2.9	~2.9	~2.9	~2.9-3.2
mg	Enteral	0-2.9	~2.9	~2.9	~1.9-2.2	0-2.9	~2.9	~2.9	~2.2-2.6
Inositol	Parenteral	0-54	54	54	47-51	0-54	54	54	54-60
mg	Enteral	0-54	32-81	32-81	21-62	0-54	32-81	32-81	25-74
Choline	Parenteral	0-28	14.4-28	14.4-28	12.5-26.7	0-28	14.4-28	14.4-28	14.4-31.1
mg	Enteral	0-28	14.4-28	14.4-28	9.6-21.5	0-28	14.4-28	14.4-28	11.1-25.5
AMP‡	Parenteral	0	0.35-0.8	0.35-0.8	0.30-0.76	0	0.35-0.8	0.35-0.8	0.35-0.89
mg	Enteral	0.35-0.8	0.35-0.8	0.35-0.8	0.23-0.62	0.35-0.8	0.35-0.8	0.35-0.8	0.27-0.73
CMP	Parenteral	0	2.1-4.1	2.1-4.1	1.8-3.9	0	2.1-4.1	2.1-4.1	2.1-4.6
mg	Enteral	2.1-4.1	2.1-4.1	2.1-4.1	1.4-3.2	2.1-4.1	2.1-4.1	2.1-4.1	1.6-3.7
GMP	Parenteral	0	0.05-0.7	0.05-0.7	0.04-0.67	0	0.05-0.7	0.05-0.7	0.05-0.78
mg	Enteral	0.05-0.7	0.05-0.7	0.05-0.7	0.03-0.54	0.05-0.7	0.05-0.7	0.05-0.7	0.04-0.64
UMP	Parenteral	0	0.9-1.2	0.9-1.2	0.8-1.1	0	0.9-1.2	0.9-1.2	0.9-1.3
mg	Enteral	0.9-1.2	0.9-1.2	0.9-1.2	0.6-0.9	0.9-1.2	0.9-1.2	0.9-1.2	0.7-1.1

* Day 0: Appropriate starting points for the parenteral administration of each nutrient on the first day of life. If enteral feedings are appropriate on the first day, then the amount is determined by human milk or formula content and quantity administered.

** Transition: The period of physiologic and metabolic instability following birth which may last as long as 7 days. This period may differ in length and in appropriate progression for each nutrient.

*** Amounts per 100 Cal (kilocalories) are calculated from minimum nutrient level divided by maximum calories and from maximum nutrient level divided by minimum calories.

Δ Fluids/Water: Amounts shown are those likely required to deliver recommended nutrients. Actual water requirements are dictated by highly variable environmental and physiological factors for which the chapter on water should be consulted.

⊛ Calcium and Phosphorous, parenteral: higher amounts listed may require use of organic forms of these to avoid precipitation.

♦ Phosphorous: May give up to 30 mg/kg on first day if organic forms are available.

▲ Vitamin E need may be increased when using DHA and ARA parenterally: see chapter.

◊ Max Vitamin D: 400 IU/d

⦹ Aim Vitamin D: 400 IU/d

† May need up to 160 mg/kg/d for late hyponatremia

‡ AMP = adenosine monophosphate; CMP = cytidine monophosphate; GMP = guanosine monophosphate; UMP = uridine monophosphate

Appendix 4 - Summary of Reasonable Nutrient Intakes (SI units) for Preterm Infants

		ELBW				VLBW			
		Day 0* per kg/day	Transition** per kg/day	Growing per kg/day	Growing per 419 kJ***	Day 0* per kg/day	Transition** per kg/day	Growing per kg/day	Growing per 419 kJ***
Energy	Parenteral	168-210	314-356	440-482	419	168-210	251-293	377-419	419
kJ	Enteral	210-251	377-419	545-629	419	210-251	314-377	461-545	419
FluidsΔ	Parenteral	90-120	90-140	140-180	122-171	70-90	90-140	120-160	120-178
mL	Enteral	90-120	90-140	160-220	107-169	70-90	90-140	135-190	104-173
Protein	Parenteral	2	3.5	3.5-4	3.0-3.8	2	3.5	3.2-3.8	3.2-4.2
g	Enteral	2	3.5	3.8-4.4	2.5-3.4	2	3.5	3.4-4.2	2.6-3.8
Carbohydrate	Parenteral	7	8-15	13-17	11.3-16.2	7	5-12	9.7-15	9.7-16.7
g	Enteral	7	8-15	9-20	6.0-15.4	7	5-12	7-17	5.4-15.5
Fat	Parenteral	1	1-3	3-4	2.6-3.8	1	1-3	3-4	3.0-4.4
g	Enteral	1	1-3	6.2-8.4	4.1-6.5	1	1-3	5.3-7.2	4.1-6.5
Linoleic acid	Parenteral	0.4	0.4-1.2	1.2-2.9	1.1-2.7	0.4	0.4-1.2	1.2-2.9	1.2-3.2
mmol	Enteral	0.4	0.4-1.2	2.5-6.0	1.7-4.6	0.4	0.4-1.2	2.1-5.1	1.7-4.7
Linoleate:Linolenate		5-15	5-15	5-15		5-15	5-15	5-15	5-15
Docosahexaenoic acid	Parenteral	>=12	>=12	>=33	>=30	>=12	>=12	>=33	>=36
μmol	Enteral	>=12	>=12	>=64	>=49	>=12	>=12	>=55	>=49
Arachidonic acid	Parenteral	>=16	>=16	>=46	>=43	>=16	>=16	>=46	>=53
μmol	Enteral	>=16	>=16	>=92	>=72	>=16	>=16	>=79	>=72
Sodium	Parenteral	0.0-1.0	2.0-5.0	3-5(7†)	2.6-4.8	0.0-1.0	2.0-5.0	3-5(7†)	3.0-5.6
mEq	Enteral	0.0-1.0	2.0-5.0	3-5(7†)	2.0-3.8	0.0-1.0	2.0-5.0	3-5(7†)	2.3-4.6
Potassium	Parenteral	0	0.0-2.0	2.0-3.0	1.7-2.8	0	0.0-2.0	2.0-3.0	2.0-3.3
mEq	Enteral	0	0.0-2.0	2.0-3.0	1.3-2.3	0	0.0-2.0	2.0-3.0	1.5-2.7
Chloride	Parenteral	0.0-1.0	2.0-5.0	3.0-7.0	2.6-6.7	0.0-1.0	2.0-5.0	3.0-7.0	3.0-7.8
mEq	Enteral	0.0-1.0	2.0-5.0	3.0-7.0	2.0-5.4	0.0-1.0	2.0-5.0	3.0-7.0	2.3-6.4
Calcium	Parenteral⊞	0.5-1.5	1.5	1.5-2.0	1.3-1.9	0.5-1.5	1.5	1.5-2.0	1.5-2.2
mmol	Enteral	0.8-2.5	2.5	2.5-5.5	1.7-4.2	0.8-2.5	2.5	2.5-5.5	1.9-5.0
Phosphorus	Parenteral⊞	0♦	1.5-1.9	1.5-1.9	1.3-1.8	0♦	1.5-1.9	1.5-1.9	1.5-2.2
mmol	Enteral	0.6-1.9	1.9-4.5	1.9-4.5	1.3-3.5	0.6-1.9	1.9-4.5	1.9-4.5	1.5-4.1
Magnesium	Parenteral	0	0.2-0.3	0.2-0.3	0.2-0.3	0	0.2-0.3	0.2-0.3	0.2-0.3
mmol	Enteral	0.1-0.3	0.3-0.6	0.3-0.6	0.2-0.5	0.1-0.3	0.3-0.6	0.3-0.6	0.3-0.6
Iron	Parenteral	0	0	1.8-3.6	1.6-3.4	0	0	1.8-3.6	1.8-4.0
μmol	Enteral	0	0	35.8-71.6	23.8-55.0	0	0	35.8-71.6	27.5-65.0
Zinc	Parenteral	0.0-2.3	2.3	6.1	5.3-5.8	0.0-2.3	2.3	6.1	6.1-6.8
μmol	Enteral	0.0-15.3	6.1-18.3	15.3-45.9	10.2-35.3	0.0-15.3	6.1-18.3	15.3-45.9	11.8-41.7
Copper	Parenteral	0	<=0.3	0.3	0.3-0.3	0	<=0.3	0.3	0.3-0.3
μmol	Enteral	0	<=2.4	1.9-2.4	1.3-1.8	0	<=2.4	1.9-2.4	1.4-2.1
Selenium	Parenteral	0	<=16.5	19.0-57.0	16.5-54.4	0	<=16.5	19.0-57.0	19.0-63.3
nmol	Enteral	0	<=16.5	16.5-57.0	11.4-44.3	0	<=16.5	16.5-57.0	12.7-51.9
Chromium	Parenteral	0	<=1.0	1.0-5.8	0.8-5.6	0	<=1.0	1.0-5.8	1.0-6.3
nmol	Enteral	0	<=1.9	1.9-43.3	1.3-33.3	0	<=1.9	1.9-43.3	1.5-39.4
Molybdenum	Parenteral	0	0	2.6	2.3-2.5	0	0	2.6	2.6-2.9
nmol	Enteral	0	0	3.1	2.1-2.4	0	0	3.1	2.4-2.8
Manganese	Parenteral	0	<=13.7	18.2	16-17	0	<=13.7	18.2	18-20
nmol	Enteral	0	<=137	13-137	9-106	0	<=137	13-137	9-124
Iodine	Parenteral	0	<=8	7.9	7-7	0	<=8	7.9	8-9
nmol	Enteral	0	<=473	79-473	53-364	0	<=473	79-473	61-429
Vitamin A	Parenteral	700-1500	700-1500	700-1500	609-1,429	700-1500	700-1500	700-1500	700-1,667
IU	Enteral	700-1500	700-1500	700-1500	467-1,154	700-1500	700-1500	700-1500	538-1,364
Vitamin D	Parenteral◊	40-160	40-160	40-160	35-152	40-160	40-160	40-160	40-178
IU	Enteral◊◊	150-400	150-400	150-400	100-308	150-400	150-400	150-400	115-364
Vitamin E	Parenteral▲	2.8-3.5	2.8-3.5	2.8-3.5	2.4-3.3	2.8-3.5	2.8-3.5	2.8-3.5	2.8-3.9
IU	Enteral	6-12	6-12	6-12	4.0-9.2	6-12	6-12	6-12	4.6-10.9
Vitamin K	Parenteral	1100 im/child	22.0	22.0	19-21	1100 im/child	22.0	22.0	22-24
nmol	Enteral	1100 im/child	18-22	18-22	12-17	1100 im/child	18-22	18-22	14-20
Thiamin	Parenteral	0.6-1.0	0.6-1.0	0.6-1.0	0.5-1.0	0.6-1.0	0.6-1.0	0.6-1.0	0.6-1.2
μmol	Enteral	0.5-0.7	0.5-0.7	0.5-0.7	0.4-0.5	0.5-0.7	0.5-0.7	0.5-0.7	0.4-0.6
Riboflavin	Parenteral	0.4-0.5	0.4-0.5	0.4-0.5	0.3-0.5	0.4-0.5	0.4-0.5	0.4-0.5	0.4-0.6
μmol	Enteral	0.7-1.0	0.7-1.0	0.7-1.0	0.4-0.7	0.7-1.0	0.7-1.0	0.7-1.0	0.5-0.9
Niacin	Parenteral	33-56	33-56	33-56	29-54	33-56	33-56	33-56	33-63
μmol	Enteral	30-40	30-40	30-40	20-30	30-40	30-40	30-40	23-36
Vitamin B6	Parenteral	0.7-1.0	0.7-1.0	0.7-1.0	0.6-0.9	0.7-1.0	0.7-1.0	0.7-1.0	0.7-1.1
μmol	Enteral	0.7-1.0	0.7-1.0	0.7-1.0	0.5-0.8	0.7-1.0	0.7-1.0	0.7-1.0	0.6-0.9

Appendix 4 - Summary of Reasonable Nutrient Intakes (SI units) for Preterm Infants *(cont.)*

		ELBW				VLBW			
		Day 0* per kg/day	Transition** per kg/day	Growing per kg/day	Growing per 419 kJ***	Day 0* per kg/day	Transition** per kg/day	Growing per kg/day	Growing per 419 kJ***
Folate	Parenteral	126	126	126	111-120	126	126	126	126-140
nmol	Enteral	56-113	56-113	56-113	38-86	56-113	56-113	56-113	43-102
Vitamin B12	Parenteral	0.22	0.22	0.22	0.19-0.21	0.22	0.22	0.22	0.22-0.24
nmol	Enteral	0.22	0.22	0.22	0.15-0.17	0.22	0.22	0.22	0.17-0.20
Pantothenic acid	Parenteral	5-9	5-9	5-9	4-9	5-9	5-9	5-9	5-10
µmol	Enteral	5-8	5-8	5-8	4-6	5-8	5-8	5-8	4-7
Biotin	Parenteral	21-33	21-33	21-33	18-31	21-33	21-33	21-33	21-37
nmol	Enteral	15-25	15-25	15-25	10-19	15-25	15-25	15-25	12-23
Vitamin C	Parenteral	85-142	85-142	85-142	74-135	85-142	85-142	85-142	85-158
µmol	Enteral	102-136	102-136	102-136	68-105	102-136	102-136	102-136	78-124
Taurine	Parenteral	0-30	15-30	15-30	13-29	0-30	15-30	15-30	15-34
µmol	Enteral	0-72	36-72	36-72	24-55	0-72	36-72	36-72	28-66
Carnitine	Parenteral	0-18	~18	~18	~16-17	0-18	~18	~18	~18-20
µmol	Enteral	0-18	~18	~18	~12-14	0-18	~18	~18	~14-16
Inositol	Parenteral	0-300	300	300	261-283	0-300	300	300	300-333
µmol	Enteral	0-300	178-450	178-450	117-344	0-300	178-450	178-450	139-411
Choline	Parenteral	0-270	139-270	139-270	121-257	0-270	139-270	139-270	139-300
µmol	Enteral	0-270	139-270	139-270	93-207	0-270	139-270	139-270	107-246
AMP‡	Parenteral	0	1.0-2.3	1.0-2.3	0.9-2.2	0	1.0-2.3	1.0-2.3	1.0-2.6
µmol	Enteral	1.0-2.3	1.0-2.3	1.0-2.3	0.7-1.8	1.0-2.3	1.0-2.3	1.0-2.3	0.8-2.1
CMP	Parenteral	0	6.5-12.7	6.5-12.7	5.6-12.1	0	6.5-12.7	6.5-12.7	6.5-14.2
µmol	Enteral	6.5-12.7	6.5-12.7	6.5-12.7	4.3-9.9	6.5-12.7	6.5-12.7	6.5-12.7	5.0-11.5
GMP	Parenteral	0	0.1-1.9	0.1-1.9	0.1-1.8	0	0.1-1.9	0.1-1.9	0.1-2.1
µmol	Enteral	0.1-1.9	0.1-1.9	0.1-1.9	0.1-1.5	0.1-1.9	0.1-1.9	0.1-1.9	0.1-1.8
UMP	Parenteral	0	2.8-3.7	2.8-3.7	2.5-3.4	0	2.8-3.7	2.8-3.7	2.8-4.0
µmol	Enteral	2.8-3.7	2.8-3.7	2.8-3.7	1.9-2.8	2.8-3.7	2.8-3.7	2.8-3.7	2.2-3.4

* Day 0: Appropriate starting points for the parenteral administration of each nutrient on the first day of life. If enteral feedings are appropriate on the first day, then the amount is determined by human milk or formula content and quantity administered.

** Transition: The period of physiologic and metabolic instability following birth which may last as long as 7 days. This period may differ in length and in appropriate progression for each nutrient.

*** Amounts per 419 kJ (kiloJoules) are calculated from minimum nutrient level divided by maximum calories and from maximum nutrient level divided by minimum calories.

Δ Fluids/Water: Amounts shown are those likely required to deliver recommended nutrients. Actual water requirements are dictated by highly variable environmental and physiological factors for which the chapter on water should be consulted.

⊕ Calcium and Phosphorous, parenteral: higher amounts listed may require use of organic forms of these to avoid precipitation.

♦ Phosphorous: May give up to 30 mg/kg on first day if organic forms are available.

▲ Vitamin E need may be increased when using DHA and ARA parenterally: see chapter.

◊ Max Vitamin D: 400 IU/d

⊗ Aim Vitamin D: 400 IU/d

† May need up to 7 mEq/kg/d for late hyponatremia

‡ AMP = adenosine monophosphate; CMP = cytidine monophosphate; GMP = guanosine monophosphate; UMP = uridine monophosphate

Index